Gynecology: Advanced Surgical Procedures

Gynecology: Advanced Surgical Procedures

Edited by Juliette Brookes

hayle medical

New York

Hayle Medical,
750 Third Avenue, 9th Floor,
New York, NY 10017, USA

Visit us on the World Wide Web at:
www.haylemedical.com

ISBN: 978-1-63241-765-7

Cataloging-in-Publication Data

Gynecology : advanced surgical procedures / edited by Juliette Brookes.
  p. cm.
Includes bibliographical references and index.
ISBN 978-1-63241-765-7
1. Generative organs, Female--Surgery. 2. Gynecology. 3. Generative organs, Female--Diseases.
I. Brookes, Juliette.
RG104 .G85 2019
618.105 9--dc23

Table of Contents

Preface

This book has been an outcome of determined endeavour from a group of educationists in the field. The primary objective was to involve a broad spectrum of professionals from diverse cultural background involved in the field for developing new researches. The book not only targets students but also scholars pursuing higher research for further enhancement of the theoretical and practical applications of the subject.

The branch of science and medicine concerned with the health of the breasts and the female reproductive organs-the vagina, uterus and ovaries, is known as gynecology. The main tools of diagnosis in gynecology are physical examination and clinical history. A medical tool, called speculum, is often used to examine the female reproductive organs. Rectovaginal examination, abdominal ultrasound and vaginal ultrasound are some of the common ways to diagnose gynecological problems. Some of the common gynecological problems are incontinence of urine, infertility, amenorrhoea, dysmenorrhoea, menorrhagia, etc. This book is a compilation of chapters that discuss the most vital concepts and emerging trends in the field of gynecology. It aims to present researches that have transformed this discipline and aided its advancement. As this field is emerging at a rapid pace, the contents of this book will help the readers understand the modern concepts and applications of the subject.

It was an honour to edit such a profound book and also a challenging task to compile and examine all the relevant data for accuracy and originality. I wish to acknowledge the efforts of the contributors for submitting such brilliant and diverse chapters in the field and for endlessly working for the completion of the book. Last, but not the least; I thank my family for being a constant source of support in all my research endeavours.

Editor

Complete plastic lining of the abdominal cavity during laparoscopic electromechanical morcellation—a promising technique

Henrik Halvor Springborg · Olav Istre

Abstract The risk of intraperitoneal fragment dissemination of uterine tissue, especially the dissemination of unexpected leiomyosarcoma during electromechanical morcellation, has been increasingly debated during the last year. An improved technique for contained morcellation of uterine tissue inside an insufflated plastic bag during laparoscopy is presented. Twenty-one consecutive contained morcellations were carried out during the summer of 2014, at one institution. Five laparoscopic myomectomies and 16 hysterectomies were performed. Standard laparoscopic equipment was used and a transparent plastic bag was introduced into the abdominal cavity through the umbilical incision mounted on two curved blunt metal probes, which facilitated the placement of the uterine tissue into the bag. Morcellation was carried out inside the plastic bag through the opening in the umbilicus. All 21 morcellations during the study period were successfully performed. The median operative time was 105 min (range 45–180 min) and applying plastic bag and trocar median 10 min (range 4–30 min). Median specimen weight was 560 g (range 80–1265 g). No complications occurred, and no unintended bag perforation was identified. The presented improved contained morcellation technique is feasible in laparoscopic hysterectomy and myomectomy. Larger studies will however be required before the general introduction of the method.

Level of evidence: II-3

Tweetable abstract Twenty-one successful contained morcellations of uterine tissue during laparoscopic surgery are reported.

H. H. Springborg (✉) · O. Istre
Department of Minimal Invasive Gynaecology, Aleris Hamlet Hospital, Gyngemose Parkvej 66, 2860 Soeborg, Copenhagen, Denmark
e-mail: henrik.springborg@aleris-hamlet.dk

O. Istre
Center of Gynaecology, University of Southern Denmark, Odense, Denmark

Keywords Minimal invasive gynaecology · Morcellation · Leiomyosarcoma · Laparoscopic hysterectomy · Laparoscopic · Myomectomy · Uterine Fibroids

Introduction

Dissemination of benign myoma after electromechanical morcellation is a known complication and is estimated to occur after 0.1 to 1 % of procedures. The fragments of uterine tissue left in the abdomen can cause the implantation of fibroma, infection, pain and the need for reoperation [1–3]. The unintended morcellation of uterine leiomyosarcoma is of even greater concern and is suspected to worsen prognosis [4–6]. It is estimated that between 1:400 and 1:1000 hysterectomy specimens for presumed benign myoma will ultimately be confirmed as leiomyosarcoma [7]. These rare but serious problems not only occur in relation to electromechanical morcellation but probably also during manual morcellation through the vagina or mini-laparotomy. The cleaning and irrigation of the abdominal cavity after traditional electromechanical morcellation are often difficult and time consuming. Morcellation in an inflated transparent plastic bag may reduce these problems. The method may even reduce the risk of the unintended morcellation of the bowel since the bowel is kept away by the plastic bag, which lies flush against all aspects of the abdominal cavity during morcellation.

Morcellation is of great importance in benign gynaecological laparoscopic surgery. In laparoscopic myomectomy and supracervical hysterectomy, it is imperative. In total laparoscopic hysterectomy, morcellation is also required when the uterus, due to size, cannot be removed by the vaginal route. The US Food and Drug Administration (FDA) approved the first electromechanical morcellator in 1995.

During the latest years, the risk of intraperitoneal fragment dissemination, especially the dissemination of unexpected leiomyosarcoma, has been debated [1, 4, 6], and the US Food and Drug Administration in April 2014 issued a statement discouraging the use of electromechanical morcellation in most cases [7]. AAGL emphasizes in the report "Morcellation During Uterine Tissue Extraction" from May 2014 the great demand for a contained morcellation system and instrumentation to facilitate the safe removal of specimens [8]. It will be a great setback for minimal invasive gynaecology if laparotomy has to be reintroduced as a standard treatment for many benign gynaecological diseases.

In this report, we describe an innovative feasible technique to place and morcellate uterine and myoma tissue in a specimen retrieval pouch during laparoscopic procedures. Cohen et al. have recently described a technique for contained power morcellation [10]. Our study confirms the feasibility of the technique, presented by Cohen et al., and introduces additional improvement of the minimally invasive specimen retrieval technique.

Materials and methods

Twenty-one consecutive patients underwent uterine tissue morcellation from June to September 2014 for the removal of uterine tissue during laparoscopic myomectomy or laparoscopic hysterectomy at Aleris Hamlet Hospital in Copenhagen, Denmark. All morcellations were performed in a plastic bag, and no laparotomy was performed. The described technique is now a standard procedure at our institution, when removal of uterine tissue requires morcellation during laparoscopy. Informed consent was obtained from all patients for being included in the study.

The preoperative workup to evaluate risk of genital tract cancer included a recent Pap test, endometrial sampling in cases of irregular bleeding and imaging with abdominal and pelvic ultrasonography. Demographic information included patient age, obstetric history, body mass index, physical status, surgical history and indication for surgery. Perioperative information collected prospectively included type of procedure performed, operative time (time from incision to closure), time for placing bag in the abdomen including placement of uterine tissue in the bag and time for placing lateral port in bag (representing extra time used for performing this technique), estimated blood loss (anaesthetic nurse estimate recorded in the operative record), specimen weight, intact status of specimen retrieval pouch (obtained by visual inspection of the bag by the surgeon), length of hospital stay, intraoperative complications, readmission to hospital and reoperation.

A 12-mm port is placed in the umbilicus and additional three 5-mm ports. Two are placed on the level of the umbilicus, laterally on both sides, and one port approximately 6 cm above the umbilicus in the midline, in order to give a good overview when placing the bag (Fig. 1). To avoid slippage of the right lateral trocar from its location within the isolation bag and avoid spillage during morcellation, a balloon-tipped 5-mm trocar (Kii Fios, Applied Medical, Rancho Santa Margarita, CA, USA) is used (Fig. 2). Morcellation is performed with a reusable electromechanical 15 or 20 mm morcellator (Wolf, Hamburg, Germany) (Fig. 1). A standard 30° 5-mm optic (Olympus, Hamburg, Germany) is used enabling us to port jump. The plastic bag used is a standard (8 Euro) plastic isolation/transport bag 47 cm × 46 cm, with a strap in the rim, normally used for bowel placement during laparotomy (Microtec Medical, Zutphen Netherlands).

The plastic isolation bag, mounted on two curved blunt metal probes, is inserted through a 2-cm incision in the umbilicus after the laparoscopic hysterectomy or myomectomy (Fig. 3a, b). Inside the abdomen, the upper metal probe is turned 180°, and the two probes in the rim of the bag forms a ring like a traditional "endobag" which facilitates the placement of the uterine tissue into the bag (Fig. 3c, d). After the placement of the tissue in the bag, the strap in the rim of the bag is pulled back, the probes are retracted at the same time and the opening of the bag is brought extra-abdominally. A blunt 12-mm trocar is introduced through the opening of the bag in the umbilicus, and the bag is insufflated under laparoscopic guidance. The space outside the bag is desufflated through the vents of the other ports. When fully inflated, visual inspection through the 12-mm trocar is carried out to confirm that the uterine tissue is located inside the plastic bag and to check that the bag fully lines the abdominal cavity.

To facilitate insufflation and continuous laparoscopic visualization during the insertion of the morcellator through the umbilical incision, the inflated bag is pierced by the 5-mm balloon-tipped trocar in the right lateral port and the balloon tip is insufflated (Fig. 2). In order to facilitate the penetration of the plastic bag and to avoid lesions in the bowel, which may be relocated during the insufflation of the bag, a special technique is recommended: The tip of the balloon-tipped right

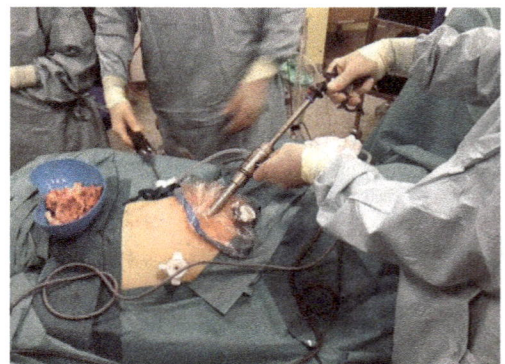

Fig. 1 Feasible placement of trocars during morcellation

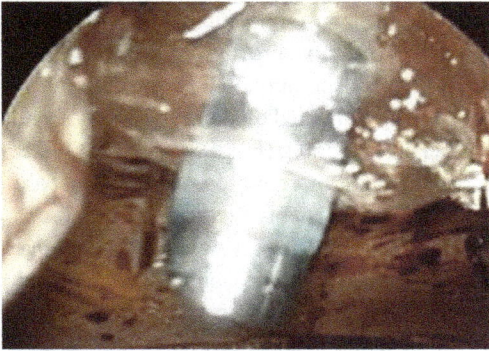

Fig. 2 A 5-mm balloon-tipped trocar (right lateral port)

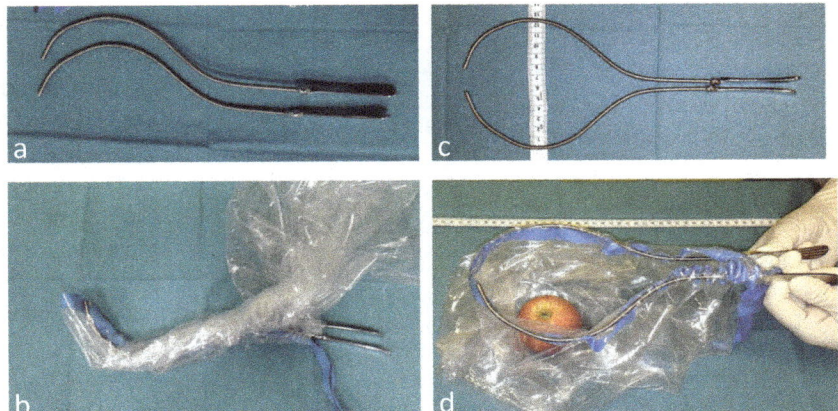

Fig. 4 Electromechanical morcellation in plastic bag

lateral 5-mm trocar is inserted into the tube of the 12-mm trocar, visually guided by the 5-mm optic located in the 12-mm trocar. When the two trocars are aligned, the optic is withdrawn, the 5-mm trocar is inserted into the tube of the 12-mm trocar and the plastic bag is easily penetrated. The balloon tip is then inflated again while retracting the 5-mm port from the tube of the 12-mm port. The defect in the bag is now "sealed" by the balloon (Fig. 2). The 5-mm optic and CO_2 insufflation are shifted to the right lateral 5-mm port. The 12-mm trocar is removed from the bag, and the morcellator device is introduced into the inflated bag through the umbilical incision. The morcellation is now performed under continuous laparoscopic visualization, and all remnants and blood are captured in the bag (Fig. 4). After morcellation, the lateral 5-mm trocar is removed after deflation of the tip, and the plastic bag is removed and tested for perforations. After the specimen is removed, a laparoscopic survey of the abdomen and pelvis is performed in order to watch haemostasis and secure that no morcellated tissue has escaped the bag.

Statistics

Descriptive statistics were performed using Microsoft Office Excel 2013. Median and range are presented for continuous variables. Categorical variables are presented as a number and percentage.

Results

Twenty-one consecutive cases of uterine morcellation were performed during the study period. Table 1 summarizes the baseline characteristics. The median patient age was 45 years (range 38–53 years), median body mass index (BMI) was 23 (range 20–30), median physical status (ASA) 1 (range 1–2) and median parity 1 (range 0–3). Prior abdominal surgery was noticed in 43 % of the patients. Table 2 summarizes the operative characteristics and outcome. Leiomyoma was the indication for the procedure in all cases, in combination with pain in 16 cases and bleeding disorders in 10 cases.

Total laparoscopic hysterectomy was performed in 2 patients, in 12 patients supracervical laparoscopic hysterectomy and in 5 patients a myomectomy. Nearly half of the cases included salpingectomy and 19 % oophorectomy or cystectomy. Major adhesiolysis were performed in 24 % of the cases.

Operative outcomes included mean operation time of 105 min (range 45–180 min). Mean time used for introducing the plastic bag into the abdomen, manipulating the uterine specimen into the bag, insufflating the bag and placement of

Fig. 3 Instrumentation for introduction of bag in the abdomen and placement of tissue in the bag. a Two parallel curved blunt uterine probes enabling insertion of the plastic bag through a 2-cm incision. b Probes placed in the rim of the plastic bag ready to be inserted in the abdomen. c Turning one probe 180° demonstrated without bag. d The bag is opened and the tissue can easily be brought into the bag

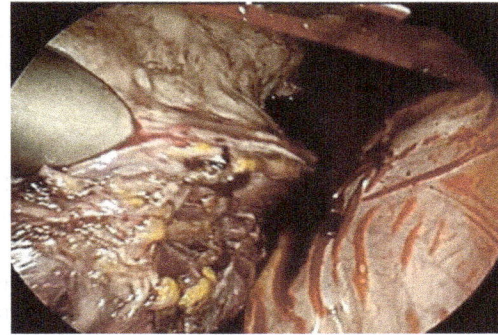

Table 1 Baseline characteristics of study population (N=21)

Characteristic	Value
Age (years)	45 (38–53)
Body mass index (BMI) (kg/m^2)	23 (20–30)
ASA	1 (1–2)
Parity	1 (0-3)
Prior abdominal surgery	
None	12 (57)
Laparoscopy	3 (14)
Laparotomy	6 (29)

Data are median (range) or n (%)

ASA American Society of Anaesthesiologists physical status classification system

the 5 mm trocar for gas and optic was 10 min (range 4–30 min). During the first 11 operations, the mean time used

Table 2 Operative characteristics and outcomes of study population (N=21)

Characteristic or outcome	Value
Surgical indications[a]	
Leiomyoma	21 (100)
Abnormal bleeding	10 (48)
Pelvic pain	16 (76)
Other	2 (14)
Procedure	
Supracervical laparoscopic hysterectomy	14 (67)
Total laparoscopic hysterectomy	2 (10)
Myomectomy	5 (24)
Additional procedures	
Adnexal removal or cystectomy	4 (19)
Salpingectomy	9 (43)
Adhesiolysis	5 (24)
Operative time (min)	105 (45–180)
Time for applying bag and trocar[b]	
All 21 patients (min)	10 (4–30)
First 11 patients (min)	16 (7–30)[c]
Last 10 patients (min)	7 (4–13)[c]
Estimated blood loss (ml)	80 (10–500)
Specimen weight (g)	560 (80–1265)
Bag intact at end of procedure	21 (100)
Length of hospital stay	
<24 h	20 (95)
24–48 h	1 (5)

Data are median (range) or n (%)

[a] Categories not mutually exclusive

[b] Total time used for introducing the bag into the abdomen, manipulating the uterine specimen into the bag, insufflating the bag and placement of the 5-mm balloon-tipped trocar for gas and optic

[c] Statistical analysis not performed since the patients were not comparable

was 16 min and the last 10 operations was 7 min. The patients and procedures were not directly comparable; however, the reduction in time consumption indicates a considerable learning curve. Median estimated blood loss was 80 ml and median specimen weight was 560 g (range 80–1265 g). No complications occurred; furthermore, no conversion to laparotomy or repeat surgery and all patients except one were discharged the following morning. One patient stayed 2 days in the hospital for a headache. All retrieval pouches were removed without macroscopic spillage, and the technique was successful with complete morcellation in all 21 cases. No bag perforation was identified, except the 5-mm intended puncture site for inspection and gas insufflation.

Discussion

In this study, we have demonstrated a feasible method, enabling the gynaecologist to continue minimal invasive surgery without risk of dissemination, even when treating larger uterine myomas. The operating time was not increased, because although insertion of the bag was time consuming (mean 10 min), time at the end was saved because of less need of cleaning and irrigating of the abdominal cavity for remnants of tissue fragments and blood.

The strengths of this study are that all morcellations of uterine tissue performed in the study period were contained in a plastic bag and no laparotomy was needed in the study period. The use of the balloon-tipped trocar prevented leakage from the perforation in the bag, and the visually controlled method of introducing the trocar in the plastic bag prevents bowel perforation during insertion. The procedure was furthermore based on standard laparoscopic equipment and with very low cost. Weaknesses include the small study size and that only two surgeons performed all operations. The deliberate perforation of the plastic bag by the trocar may cause unintended leakage of fluid and tissue despite the "sealing effect" of the balloon trocar. A small in vitro study of contained morcellation in a plastic bag similar to the one used in this study, however, suggests that the technique can effectively decrease or potentially eradicate tissue spillage [9]. A prospective cohort multicentre study, including 200 patients, is planned in Denmark to evaluate the safety and feasibility of the method.

The results in the multicentre cohort study of Cohen et al. [10], combined with the results of this study, confirm that morcellation of uterine tissue within a specimen retrieval pouch is feasible. Both techniques are based on the use of an inflated large bag made of clear plastic drape film. This results in a large intraabdominal space where bowel is kept away and morcellation is easily performed. The technique will probably be the basis of further development of contained morcellation.

Acknowledgments We thank Senior Consultant, MD, PhD, Lars Franch Andersen, for proofreading the manuscript.

Funding None.

Details of the contributions of individual authors Both authors contributed pertinent aspects of the planning, conducting and reporting of the work described in the article.

References

1. Heller DS, Cracchiole B (2014) Peritoneal nodules after laparoscopic surgery with uterine morcellation: review of a rare complication. J Minim Invasive Gynecol 21:384–388
2. Leren V, Langebrekke A, Qvigstad E (2012) Parasitic leiomyomas after laparoscopic surgery with morcellation. Acta Obstet Gynecol Scand 91:1233–1236
3. Cucinella G, Granese R, Calagna G, Somigliana E, Perino A (2011) Parasitic myomas after laparoscopic surgery: an emerging complication in the use of morcellator? Description of four cases. Fertil Steril 96:e90–e96
4. Park JY, Park SK, Kim DY, Kim JH, Kim YM, Kim YT et al (2011) The impact of tumor morcellation during surgery on the prognosis of patients with apparently early uterine leiomyosarcoma. Gynecol Oncol 122:255–259
5. Einstein MH, Barakat RR, Chi DS, Sonoda Y, Alektiar KM, Hensley ML et al (2008) Management of uterine malignancy found incidentally after supracervical hysterectomy or uterine morcellation for presumed benign disease. Int J Gynecol Cancer 18:1065–1070
6. Della Badia C, Karini H (2010) Endometrial stromal sarcoma diagnosed after uterine morcellation in laparoscopic supracervical hysterectomy. J Minim Invasive Gynecol 17:791–793
7. Laparoscopic uterine power morcellation in hysterectomy and myomectomy: FDA Safety Communication, April 17, 2014. (http://www.fda.gov/MedicalDevices/Safety/AlertsandNotices/ucm393576.htm)
8. AAGL report: Morcellation During uterine tissue extraction, May 2014 (http://www.aagl.org/wp-content/uploads/2014/05/Tissue_Extraction_TFR.pdf)
9. Cohen SL, Greenberg JA, Wang KC, Srouji SS, Gargiulo AR, Pozner CN et al (2014) Risk of leakage and tissue dissemination with various contained tissue extraction techniques: an in vitro pilot study. J Minim Invasive Gynecol 21:935–939
10. Cohen SL, Einarsson JI, Wang KC, Brown D, Boruta D, Scheib SA, Fader AN, Shibley T (2014) Contained power morcellation within an insufflated isolation bag. Obstet Gynecol 124(3):491–497

2

Anxiety at outpatient hysteroscopy

Pietro Gambadauro[1,2] · Ramesan Navaratnarajah[3] · Vladimir Carli[1,4]

Abstract This review summarises current understanding and research on the association between anxiety and outpatient hysteroscopy. Women undergoing hysteroscopy suffer from significant levels of anxiety, with repercussions on pain perception, success rates and satisfaction. Using validated tools such as the Spielberger State-Trait Anxiety Index (STAI) or the Hospital Anxiety and Depression Scale (HADS) in the outpatient hysteroscopy setting, average state anxiety scores similar or greater than those measured before more invasive procedures under general anaesthesia have been consistently reported. This clearly suggests a significant gap between our clinical viewpoint of what is "minimally invasive" and patients' expectations. In spite of its potential role of confounder in studies on pain-reduction interventions, we found that patient anxiety was evaluated in only 9 (13 %) out of a sample of 70 randomised controlled trials on outpatient hysteroscopy published since 1992. Factors such as trait anxiety, age, indication and the efficiency of the clinic can be correlated to state anxiety before hysteroscopy, but more robust data are needed. Promising non-pharmacological interventions to reduce anxiety at hysteroscopy include patient education, communication through traditional or multimedia approaches, interaction and support during the procedure and music listening.

Keywords Hysteroscopy · Anxiety · Pain · Outpatient hysteroscopy · Mental health · Patient-centred care

Introduction

During the last decades, enormous progress in technique and instruments has turned hysteroscopy into a common outpatient procedure, with both diagnostic and therapeutic potential, and increasing patient compliance [1, 2]. The assumption of the minimal invasiveness of hysteroscopy is based on facts such as the miniaturisation of scopes, the uncommon need of anaesthesia and the progressive simplification of the technique [3, 4]. This is certainly true, also when considering the burden of predecessors such as dilatation and curettage (D&C) or laparotomy. However, the common professional interpretation of what is "minimally invasive" does not take into account a patient's emotional experience while many women undergoing hysteroscopy suffer from significant levels of anxiety [5, 6].

The aim of this review was to summarise the current understanding and research on the association between anxiety and outpatient hysteroscopy. A secondary objective was to determine whether published randomised trials reporting pain at hysteroscopy to date have considered anxiety as a confounding factor.

✉ Pietro Gambadauro
gambadauro@gmail.com; pietro.gambadauro@ki.se

1   Karolinska Institutet, LIME/NASP-C7, 17177 Stockholm, Sweden

2   Res Medica Sweden, Uppsala, Sweden

3   St. Bartholomew's and the Royal London Hospital, Bart's Health NHS Trust, Queen Mary University of London, London, UK

4   WHO Collaborating Centre for Research, Training and Methods Development, and National Centre for Suicide Research and Prevention of Mental Ill-Health, Karolinska Institutet, Stockholm, Sweden

Methods

We searched scientific literature on anxiety related to hysteroscopy from PubMed, Scopus and PsychINFO online databases, using the keywords "anxiety" and "hysteroscopy" including thin word variants. We then searched reference lists of known systematic reviews [7–14] and PubMed for randomised controlled trials reporting pain at outpatient hysteroscopy. On PubMed we used a query based on the keyword "hysteroscopy" and the filter "randomized controlled trial [ptype]". This simple query has got high sensitivity (93.7 %; 95 %CI 92.5–94.9) and specificity (97.6 %; 95 %CI 97.4–97.7) for the identification of randomised trials on PubMed [15].

A total of 304 abstracts were considered for a general review on various specific aspects of anxiety at outpatient hysteroscopy, such as prevalence, intensity, risk factors and management. When the material found on hysteroscopy was deemed insufficient, general literature on preoperative anxiety in gynaecology, or other surgical disciplines, was reviewed.

We also conducted a targeted analysis aimed at investigating whether published trials on pain at hysteroscopy control for patient anxiety levels. The articles included in this analysis were selected according to the following criteria: being a RCT, hysteroscopies performed in an outpatient setting and pain as a primary or secondary outcome. Exclusion criteria were the following: trials where hysteroscopy was compared to other procedures such as operative hysteroscopy or ultrasound, pain not measured as an outcome and patients receiving general anaesthesia. Data were extracted regarding year of publication, study intervention (e.g. anaesthetic agent, instrumentation or distension media), assessment of patient anxiety and, in the latter case, tools used for measurement.

The findings of this comprehensive review are presented through the following three paragraphs, dealing respectively with the relevance of pre-hysteroscopy anxiety, its prevalence and intensity and possible management. A narrative format was chosen as a result of very heterogeneous data.

Findings

Anxiety at hysteroscopy: irrelevant or underestimated?

Anxiety is defined as an "abnormal and overwhelming sense of apprehension and fear often marked by physiological signs, doubt concerning the reality and nature of the threat, and by self-doubt about one's capacity to cope with it" [16]. Some anxiety connected to stress situations is in many cases inevitable. However, intense symptoms of anxiety might be related to personality characteristics and interfere with everyday activities, with negative health-related consequences.

Patient anxiety in association with a medical encounter, is a well-known phenomenon whose possibly most recognised and studied manifestation is the "white coat effect" [17]. Within healthcare, surgery represents the archetypal invasive method of managing disease, which reflects on the well-known high levels of preoperative anxiety commonly reported in the literature [18]. Surgery-related anxiety is an important problem that has also got negative repercussions and consequences before and after the procedure. Sleep disturbances, for instance, are common before gynaecological endoscopic

surgery, regardless of the nature and extent of the operations [19]. Anxiety is a possible risk factor for postoperative nausea and vomiting [20]. Preoperative anxiety prior to gynaecological surgery is associated with increased and persistent postoperative pain [21, 22]. Anxiety before major procedures can be triggered by the intrinsic invasiveness and risks of surgery and by an understandable fear of the loss of control linked to anaesthesia. One would expect lower anxiety levels before minimally invasive or outpatient procedures, which are very well represented in gynaecology. Hysteroscopy is one of the most emblematic minimal access gynaecological procedures. Initially, it replaced other more invasive techniques to become a routine outpatient procedure performed with minimal or no anaesthetic requirements [4, 23]. Paradoxically, despite the evolution of scope technology, intense preoperative anxiety has been reported in earlier [24] as well as in recent years of hysteroscopic development [25]. This suggests that the patient's perception of this common procedure induces anxiety, regardless of how patient-friendly hysteroscopy has become.

Anxiety can have consequences which are specific to hysteroscopy when performed in an outpatient setting on conscious patients, above all pain [5, 6]. Patients might experience pain as a result of physical stimuli such as cervical dilatation, intrauterine pressure and manipulation. However, pain is subjective and multifactorial, and its perception is modulated by mood and emotional states such as anxiety [26]. This explains why similar physical stimuli lead to great differences in pain perception and justify the finding that non-organic factors such as anxiety predict pain at hysteroscopy [5, 6].

In this context, we would expect that patient anxiety levels would be assessed in clinical trials on pain reduction interventions at outpatient hysteroscopy. In order to test this hypothesis, we have systematically reviewed relevant literature with the aim to assess whether published RCTs on outpatient hysteroscopy considered patients' anxiety as a variable. As summarised in Table 1, through our search strategy, we have identified 70 RCTs published from 1992 to 2013. Pre-hysteroscopy anxiety levels were evaluated in only 9 studies (13 %). Interestingly, a single research group (Adam Magos, London, UK) authored almost half of those articles (4/9). Therefore, published research on pain at hysteroscopy has not taken anxiety as a potential confounding factor until now, and this might constitute a significant bias.

Obviously, diagnostic hysteroscopy is a relatively short procedure, and the possibility of undergoing a quick, outpatient procedure is preferred by most patients, who might accept experiencing some pain or discomfort instead of waiting for an anachronistic procedure under general anaesthesia [27]. Nonetheless, pain is not just a problem in itself since it correlates to the success of outpatient hysteroscopy, both diagnostic and operative [28, 2].

Table 1 How often is anxiety assessed in RCTs on pain reduction interventions at outpatient hysteroscopy?

		Number	Percentage
RCTs included in analysis		70	100
Period	1992–2002	25	35.7
	2003–2013	45	64.3
Intervention	Anaesthesia/analgesia	32	45.7
	Instruments	9	12.9
	Cervical preparation	9	12.9
	Distension media	9	12.9
	Technique	8	11.4
	Others	3	4.3
Pain as main endpoint	Yes	57	81.4
	No	13	18.6
Anxiety assessment		9	13
	Method of assessment		
	Single question[a]	2	22
	VAS	4	44
	POMS[b]	1	11
	STAI	1	11
	Unclear	1	11

[a] Yes/no or quiet/anxious?

[b] Profile of Mood States

Anxiety, apart from increasing pain perception and the risk of failure of an outpatient hysteroscopy, also seems to determine lower patient satisfaction [29]. As previously reported, patients with higher level of anxiety would be more likely to choose general anaesthesia if they needed to undergo a new hysteroscopy in the future [29]. We believe that this information is extremely relevant since patient satisfaction is crucial in the context of modern patient-centred care. We could not find any data on the long-term effects of anxiety on satisfaction after hysteroscopy, but experiences on patients undergoing insertion of intrauterine devices show that women with higher pre-procedural anxiety still remember the procedure as a painful experience after 6 months [30].

Prevalence and intensity of anxiety at hysteroscopy

Elevated levels of anxiety in patients waiting for hysteroscopy have been reported in the last decades. In a large Italian study published in 2007, 65 % of 533 women interviewed by a physician before office hysteroscopy reported preoperative anxiety, defining it as "an unpleasant state of uneasiness or tension" [6]. However, measuring anxiety by answering a direct question (e.g. "do you feel anxious?") might lack validity, and therefore, other authors have attempted to measure pre-hysteroscopic anxiety by other structured, validated methods.

Dickson and Depares, back in 2000, published their measurements of anxiety levels among 30 women before outpatient hysteroscopy [24]. The Spielberger State-Trait Anxiety Index (STAI) was used, and an average anxiety level of 46.07 (±11.39 SD) was detected. The STAI is a self-administered, 40-item questionnaire consisting of two parts (S as state, and T as trait), which was first introduced in the 1970s, and revised in 1983 [31, 32]. One of its peculiarities is the ability to differentiate a present anxiety state (STAI-s; 20 items) from a long-standing trait anxiety (STAI-t; 20 items). Scores range from 20 (minimum anxiety) to 80 (maximum anxiety). It is relatively quick to complete (around 10 min) and is available in many languages. A short version of the STAI-s (6 items) is available [33].

The STAI has often been used as a measure of anxiety in patients undergoing hysteroscopy.

A study from 2004 reported STAI-measured state anxiety levels in 240 women attending an outpatient see-and-treat hysteroscopy clinic and compared them to women in other clinical situations [29]. The mean anxiety levels measured were 45.7 (median 45) at a full, 20-item STAI, and 47.3 at a reduced, 6-item STAI. Anxiety levels before hysteroscopy were significantly higher than those measured among 73 women attending a general gynaecology clinic (median 39, $p=.004$), while similar levels were detected among 36 women seen at a chronic pelvic pain clinic (median 46).

More recently, similarly high anxiety levels before hysteroscopy were confirmed by other authors. Carta et al. reported median STAI-s values of 41.50 (range 20–73) in a sample of 94 women [34]. In this study, 80 % of the women had moderate to severe anxiety state, defined by the authors as a STAI-s value ≥ 34. In the context of an RCT on the effect of music on pain, STAI-s scores of 39.45 were measured in a study population of 356 women undergoing office hysteroscopy [25]. In a very recent study evaluating the impact of anxiety on pain at hysteroscopy, the mean pre-procedural STAI-s score of 148 women was 44.8 ± 10.0 (SD) [5].

High anxiety levels have also been reported few days before outpatient hysteroscopy, outside the hospital environment. Tarling et al. used a 6-item STAI-s to assess anxiety in 18 postmenopausal patients receiving a priority referral to diagnostic hysteroscopy in the context of an urgent assessment of postmenopausal bleeding [35]. Eighteen patients were mailed the questionnaire home 4 days after the first encounter with the specialists, hence while waiting for hysteroscopy. These women had mean anxiety levels of 43.89 ± 17.98 (SD) compared to levels of 38.96 ± 9.79 (SD) among 16 women undergoing the same urgent assessment, but not referred to hysteroscopy.

The Hospital Anxiety and Depression Scale (HADS) is another validated tool which was designed to specifically screen patients for anxiety and depression. It can be self-administered. Its A component (HADS-A) focuses on anxiety and consists of 7 items. Scores might range between 0 and 21, with values below eight interpreted as normal (no anxiety).

Within the setting of endometrial and ovarian cancer screening in 26 women with family history of hereditary non-polyposis colorectal cancer, Wood et al. reported mean values of 6.8± 4.2 (95 %CI 5.2–8.5) at HADS anxiety subscale, before combined assessment with hysteroscopy and biopsy, transvaginal ultrasound and blood sampling for CA125 [36]. In this study, the patients were asked to fill the questionnaire at home and then bring it to the visit. Although the recorded scores are considered within the normal range (<8), they are higher than in women before laparoscopic tubal ligation (HADS-A median score 4) and similar to those before hysterectomy (HADS-A median score 7) [37, 22].

A simple 1 to 10 visual analog scale (VAS) has also been used by some authors. As we found in our review of RCTs on pain at hysteroscopy, the VAS was the most used tool to verify that anxiety levels between cases and controls were not statistically different (Table 1). In a cohort of 77 women undergoing hysteroscopy, Mc Gurgan et al. reported VAS measured anxiety scores of 3.5–4 (range 0.5–10), which, however, is a finding of difficult interpretation since scarce control data are found in the literature [38]. For instance, a 100-mm VAS has been validated for preoperative anxiety in the field of dental care, where authors have found a significant correlation with STAI scores, with a reference threshold for anxiety around 50 mm (corresponding to STAI-s 40) [39]. In gynaecology, Hong et al. found mean VAS of 4.7±2.3 among women undergoing egg collection, and the corresponding STAI-s scores in the same population were 40.0±9.7 [40].

Table 2 summarises the results of measurements that have been used to evaluate anxiety before outpatient hysteroscopy together with reference values obtained by published literature in the field of gynaecological surgery. Interestingly, women undergoing outpatient hysteroscopy appear to have higher levels than women undergoing laparoscopic tubal ligation [37] (Table 2; footnotes). On the contrary, the anxiety experienced before hysteroscopy is comparable to that by women undergoing gynaecological surgery under general anaesthesia [22, 41] (Table 2; footnotes). This clearly suggests a significant gap between our clinical viewpoint of what is minimally invasive and the patient's expectation about an outpatient hysteroscopy procedure.

Can anxiety before hysteroscopy be predicted or reduced?

We have documented the high levels of pre-hysteroscopy anxiety in the previous paragraphs and their potential impact on patient well-being and the success of the procedure. On the basis of this background, efforts should be made in order to identify predictors or interventions that could help respectively in identifying subjects at higher risk for anxiety and in preventing/limiting anxiety and its consequences.

Which factors are correlated to anxiety before hysteroscopy?

We will first summarise the knowledge we have about factors associated to anxiety. It would be logical to expect people with a trait anxiety to be more vulnerable to preoperative stress and therefore likely to experience higher levels of state anxiety before hysteroscopy. State anxiety is correlated to situations such as waiting for an invasive procedure like hysteroscopy. Trait anxiety predisposes some individuals to experience more anxiety states than others, both in frequency and intensity [42]. It also appears to be associated with ethnic and racial factors [43]. This knowledge would justify using both STAI

Table 2 Measuring anxiety before outpatient hysteroscopy

Measurement	Scoring range	Author	Number	Age	Values
Patient interview	Yes or no	Cicinelli et al. 2007 [6]	533	n/a	65 %[a]
VAS	1–10	Mc Gurgan et al. 2001 [38]	77	48[b]	3.5–4[b]
HADS-A	0–21	Wood et al. 2008 [36]	26	42.27[c]	6.8[c]
STAI-s	20–80	Dickson & Depares 2000 [24]	30	n/a	46.07[c]
		Gupta et al. 2004 [29]	240	n/a	45[b]
		Carta et al. 2012 [34]	94	48[b]	41.5[b]
		Angioli et al. 2014 [25]	356	56.05[c]	39.45[c]
		Kokanali et al. 2014 [5]	148	43.6[c]	44.8[c]
6-item STAI-s	20–80	Gupta et al. 2004 [29]	240	n/a	47.3[c]
		Tarling et al. 2013 [35]	18	63[c]	43.15[c]

Values were obtained on the day of hysteroscopy in all studies except for two of them [35, 36] where patients were sent the questionnaire by post. HADS-A median score before laparoscopic tubal ligation, 4 (59 women) [37]; before hysterectomy, 7 (186 women) [22]. STAI-s median score before laparoscopic tubal ligation, 29 (59 women) [37]; before gynaecological surgery, 42 (45 women) [41]

[a] Percentage of women answering "yes"

[b] Median score

[c] Mean score

questionnaires in order to control for trait anxiety. Interestingly, in one of the largest studies on pre-hysteroscopy anxiety reviewed here, the authors decided not to measure trait anxiety, stating that "there was no reason to think that these people were more anxious than any others in a general population" [29]. This assumption, albeit reasonable, does not seem to be unequivocally confirmed by the available literature (Table 3). Trait anxiety among women undergoing office hysteroscopy appears to be common, and it also independently predicts pain during the procedure as well as 60 min after, as recently reported by Kokanali et al. [5]. Further studies would be needed to verify whether women referred to hysteroscopy are more likely to have anxiety traits and whether an anxiety trait is directly correlated to state anxiety in the same women.

Age is another factor potentially correlated with anxiety. Although hysteroscopy may be needed at almost any age, it is more common in middle-aged women (see column "age" in Table 2). The frequent association of perimenopause with abnormal uterine bleeding should be taken into account when studying anxiety in these patients. As a matter of fact, recent research shows that women with previous low levels of anxiety become susceptible to higher levels of anxiety once transiting through the menopause [44].

As hysteroscopy is a gynaecological procedure, gender cannot be used as an independent variable when studying preoperative anxiety. Nevertheless, it is worth mentioning that anxiety is more common among women [45]. This also reflects on situational anxiety before surgery. Several studies have demonstrated that preoperative anxiety, regardless of the operation or the anaesthetic strategy, is significantly more frequent as well as more intense among women [46–48]. When it comes to the specific case of outpatient hysteroscopy, the gender of the gynaecologist has been studied in relation to patient anxiety. Reassuringly, Mc Gurgan et al. did not find any statistical difference in anxiety levels in women, whether they were attended by male (VAS 4; range 0.5–10) or female (VAS 3.5; 0.5–9) gynaecologists [38].

The indication to hysteroscopy can certainly correlate with patient anxiety although this hypothesis has not been thoroughly tested. We could, for instance, postulate that women fearing a cancer diagnosis would be more anxious [49]. A study from 2008 failed to demonstrate significant anxiety levels in women undergoing gynaecological cancer screening for hereditary colorectal cancer [36]. More recently, Tarling et al. reported anxiety levels among women undergoing hysteroscopy within an urgent assessment of postmenopausal bleeding [35]. Although these women had high anxiety scores at a 6-item STAI questionnaire (43.15±18.35), those were not significantly higher than in women undergoing the same urgent assessment, but exempted from hysteroscopy (38.96± 9.79) [35].

An operative hysteroscopy could have a greater impact on anxiety compared to a diagnostic procedure. Nevertheless, no significant differences in pre-hysteroscopy anxiety were reported by an Italian group of researchers comparing patients undergoing diagnostic and operative office hysteroscopy [25]. The authors, however, did not report whether the procedures were planned or performed according to a see-and-treat protocol. In the case of see-and-treat procedures, the patients would not have had awareness of the operative nature of the upcoming hysteroscopy at the time anxiety was measured.

Interestingly, a higher grade of concern before hysteroscopy has been reported among infertile women [50]. In that study, pain was also more frequent among the same infertile women, although a formal assessment of their anxiety levels was not performed.

Factors not directly linked to the patients can cause anxiety before hysteroscopy. Carta et al. found that having to wait 60 min or more for the procedure is associated to a higher likelihood of pain (OR 5.67; 95 %CI 1.48–37.39) [34]. Although the waiting time in that study seemed to be exceptionally long (median 100 min; range 20–420), similar findings were more recently confirmed by Kokanali et al., who found in-hospital waiting time to be significantly correlated to pain scores during hysteroscopy as well as 60 min after [5]. Long waiting lists before the procedure may also interfere with patients' experience. This has not been reported for hysteroscopy, but it is suggested by studies in other settings. For instance, a shorter waiting list for prostate biopsy appears to increase patient tolerance of the procedure, particularly in the case of higher anxiety [51]. The cited experiences support the idea that a good healthcare organisation improves patient experience.

How would anxiety before hysteroscopy be managed best?

In the inpatient surgery setting, preoperative anxiety is commonly managed by means of pharmacological interventions such as the use of anxiolytics and sedatives. Some authors describe the routine administration of anxiolytics in the setting of outpatient hysteroscopy under local anaesthesia [52, 53]. However, in view of the commonly short duration of the procedure, and the possible side effects of oral medication, non-pharmacological tools would be preferable and more in line

Table 3 Trait anxiety in women undergoing outpatient hysteroscopy

Author	Year	Number	Age	STAI-t average score
Carta et al. [34]	2012	94	48[a]	38[a]
Angioli et al. [25]	2014	356	56.05[b]	35.9[b]
Kokanali et al. [5]	2014	148	43.6[b]	38.4[b]

STAI-s median score before laparoscopic tubal ligation, 30 (59 women) [37]; before gynaecological surgery, 39 (45 women) [41]

[a] Median

[b] Mean

with the minimalistic philosophy of modern office hysteroscopy.

Communication and patient education have been proved as effective tools to reduce preoperative anxiety, and their role should be increasingly acknowledged, now that many patients are active consumers of unfiltered and largely unreliable information through the Internet. It has been demonstrated that preoperative anxiety is effectively reduced by the ability of doctors to answer patients' questions, which also increases patients' satisfaction [54]. Clarity is more important than the amount of information in order to reduce perceived anxiety before gastrointestinal endoscopy [55]. This might explain why standard written information is appreciated by patients, and it does not increase their anxiety [56]. Multidisciplinary strategies, involving psychological interventions, have been advocated in order to reduce anxiety in complex cases with high preoperative anxiety [57]. The difficulty of an effective preoperative communication could be overcome by multimedia approaches which seem to improve patient understanding and satisfaction, although a significant effect on preoperative anxiety has not been yet confirmed [58].

Since women are awake at outpatient hysteroscopy, communication is not just limited to preoperative setting but can continue during the procedure. Morgan et al. have studied the experiences and attitudes of women undergoing hysteroscopy [27]. According to their results, patients are positive about receiving continuous information on the progress of the procedure and on what they should expect. Many women also chose to follow the hysteroscopy on the screen because they were either interested or thought that watching could help them focus on something else. But almost half of the women chose not to look at the screen [27]. This might justify the results reported by authors who found that watching the screen during hysteroscopy is not beneficial to patients [59]. Interestingly, in the neighbouring field of colposcopy, recorded and live videos can significantly reduce patient anxiety [60–62]. Considering both the available literature and our own experience with surgical-video-mediated patient education, we would argue that the possibility to follow one's own hysteroscopy live on a screen might improve the interaction between patient and caregivers in many cases, although the choice of whether to look or not should be left to the patient [63, 64].

An improvement in pain thresholds and vaginal birth rates has been reported in obstetric research as a result of patient support by friends or "doulas" [65]. Similarly, some evidence shows that a relevant role in surgery-related anxiety reduction is played by nurses and nurse practitioners [66]. It would be useful to attempt replicating those findings in the hysteroscopic setting.

Finally, an interesting and possibly cost-effective tool to reduce preoperative anxiety is represented by music listening. Music interventions are known to have a general positive effect on anxiety reduction in medical patients [67]. A recent systematic review has demonstrated how effective listening to music can be in terms of preoperative anxiety reduction [68]. This has also been shown in the specific setting of day surgery, endoscopy and colposcopy [62, 69–71]. A recent randomised trial in office hysteroscopy has shown that listening to music during hysteroscopy might reduce pain, possibly as a consequence of a reduction of anxiety [25]. The question whether music might also reduce anxiety when listened prior to hysteroscopy remains open.

Conclusions

Women undergoing outpatient hysteroscopy suffer from significant levels of preoperative anxiety, comparable to those experienced before major surgery under general anaesthesia.

This can have repercussions on pain perception, success of the procedure as well as on overall patient experience and satisfaction. Anxiety, to date, has rarely been evaluated as a confounding factor in published RCTs reporting pain at outpatient hysteroscopy. In the future, similar randomised trials should measure preoperative anxiety with validated tools, in order to reduce the risk of significant bias. Factors such as trait anxiety, age, indication and the efficiency of the clinic can be correlated to state anxiety before hysteroscopy, but more robust data are needed. Promising non-pharmacological interventions to reduce anxiety at hysteroscopy include patient education, communication through traditional or multimedia approaches, interaction and support during the procedure and music listening.

Acknowledgments This work was conducted within eMeRGE, an interdisciplinary research platform for Mental health in Reproduction, Gynaecology and Endometriosis. Parts of this paper were presented by Pietro Gambadauro as an invited lecture at the European Society for Gynaecological Endoscopy (ESGE) 23rd Annual Congress, Brussels, Belgium, on the 24th of September, 2014.

Author contributions PG conceived and designed this review, conducted the literature searches, analysed and interpreted the findings and drafted the article. He is the lead and corresponding author. RN and VC agreed on the design, contributed to analysis and interpretation of the findings and critically revised the paper for intellectual content. All authors have read and approved the final version of the article.

References

1. Di Spiezio Sardo A, Taylor A, Tsirkas P, Mastrogamvrakis G, Sharma M, Magos A (2008) Hysteroscopy: a technique for all? Analysis of 5000 outpatient hysteroscopies. Fertil Steril 89(2):438–443

2. Gambadauro P, Martínez-Maestre MA, Torrejón R (2014) When is see-and-treat hysteroscopic polypectomy successful? Eur J Obstet Gynecol Reprod Biol 178:70–73

3. Sharma M, Taylor A, di Spiezio Sardo A et al (2005) Outpatient hysteroscopy: traditional versus the 'no-touch' technique. BJOG 112(7):963–967

4. Gambadauro P, Magos A (2010) Pain control in hysteroscopy. Finesse, not local anaesthesia. BMJ 340:c2097

5. Kokanali MK, Cavkaytar S, Guzel Aİ, Topçu HO, Eroğlu E, Aksakal O, Doğanay M (2014) Impact of preprocedural anxiety levels on pain perception in patients undergoing office hysteroscopy. J Chin Med Assoc 77(9):477–481

6. Cicinelli E, Rossi AC, Marinaccio M, Matteo M, Saliani N, Tinelli R (2007) Predictive factors for pain experienced at office fluid minihysteroscopy. J Minim Invasive Gynecol 14(4):485–488

7. Cooper NA, Khan KS, Clark TJ (2010) Local anaesthesia for pain control during outpatient hysteroscopy: systematic review and meta-analysis. BMJ 340:c1130

8. Cooper NAM, Smith P, Khan KS, Clark TJ (2010) Vaginoscopic approach to outpatient hysteroscopy: a systematic review of the effect on pain. BJOG 117(5):532–539

9. Munro MG, Brooks PG (2010) Use of local anesthesia for office diagnostic and operative hysteroscopy. J Minim Invasive Gynecol 17(6):709–718

10. Ahmad G, O'Flynn H, Attarbashi S, Duffy JM, Watson A (2010) Pain relief for outpatient hysteroscopy. Cochrane Database Syst Rev 11, CD007710

11. Cooper NAM, Smith P, Khan KS, Clark TJ (2011) A systematic review of the effect of the distension medium on pain during outpatient hysteroscopy. Fertil Steril 95(1):264–271

12. Cooper NAM, Smith P, Khan KS, Clark TJ (2011) Does cervical preparation before outpatient hysteroscopy reduce women's pain experience? A systematic review. BJOG 118(11):1292–1301

13. Mercier RJ, Zerden ML (2012) Intrauterine anesthesia for gynecologic procedures: a systematic review. Obstet Gynecol 120(3):669–677

14. Kaneshiro B, Grimes DA, Lopez LM (2012) Pain management for tubal sterilization by hysteroscopy. Cochrane Database Syst Rev 8, CD009251

15. McKibbon KA, Wilczynski NL, Haynes RB, Hedges Team (2009) Retrieving randomized controlled trials from MEDLINE: a comparison of 38 published search filters. Health Info Libr J 26(3):187–202

16. Anxiety (2014) In Merriam-Webster.com. Retrieved June 21st, 2014, from http://www.merriam-webster.com/dictionary/anxiety

17. Ogedegbe G, Pickering TG, Clemow L, Chaplin W, Spruill TM, Albanese GM, Eguchi K, Burg M, Gerin W (2008) The misdiagnosis of hypertension: the role of patient anxiety. Arch Intern Med 168(22):2459–2465

18. Mitchell M (2003) Patient anxiety and modern elective surgery: a literature review. J Clin Nurs 12(6):806–815

19. Sheizaf B, Almog B, Salamah K, Shehata F, Takefman J, Tulandi T (2011) A pragmatic evaluation of sleep patterns before gynecologic surgery. Gynecol Surg 8(2):151–155

20. Gan TJ (2006) Risk factors for postoperative nausea and vomiting. Anesth Analg 102:1884–1898

21. Carr E, Brockbank K, Allen S, Strike P (2006) Patterns and frequency of anxiety in women undergoing gynaecological surgery. J Clin Nurs 15(3):341–352

22. Pinto PR, McIntyre T, Nogueira-Silva C, Almeida A, Araújo-Soares V (2012) Risk factors for persistent postsurgical pain in women undergoing hysterectomy due to benign causes: a prospective predictive study. J Pain 13(11):1045–1057

23. Cooper MJ, Broadbent JA, Molnár BG, Richardson R, Magos AL (1995) A series of 1000 consecutive out-patient diagnostic hysteroscopies. J Obstet Gynaecol (Tokyo 1995) 21(5):503–507

24. Dickson MJ, Depares JC (2000) Anxiety and outpatient hysteroscopy. J Obstet Gynaecol 20(1):81

25. Angioli R, De Cicco Nardone C, Plotti F, Cafa EV, Dugo N, Damiani P et al (2014) Use of music to reduce anxiety during office hysteroscopy: prospective randomized trial. J Minim Invasive Gynecol 21(3):454–459

26. Tracey I, Mantyh PW (2007) The cerebral signature for pain perception and its modulation. Neuron 55(3):377–391

27. Morgan M, Dodds W, Wolfe C, Raju S (2004) Women's views and experiences of outpatient hysteroscopy: implications for a patient-centered service. Nurs Health Sci 6(4):315–320

28. Campo R, Molinas CR, Rombauts L, Mestdagh G, Lauwers M, Braekmans P, Brosens I, Van Belle Y, Gordts S (2005) Prospective multicentre randomized controlled trial to evaluate factors influencing the success rate of office diagnostic hysteroscopy. Hum Reprod 20(1):258–263

29. Gupta JK, Clark TJ, More S, Pattison H (2004) Patient anxiety and experiences associated with an outpatient "one-stop" "see and treat" hysteroscopy clinic. Surg Endosc 18(7):1099–1104

30. Murty J (2003) Use and effectiveness of oral analgesia when fitting an intrauterine device. J Fam Plann Reprod Health Car 29(3):150–151

31. Spielberger CD, Gorsuch RL, Lushene R, Vagg PR, Jacobs GA (1983) Manual for the state-trait anxiety inventory. Consulting Psychologists Press, Palo Alto

32. Julian LJ (2011) Measures of anxiety: State-Trait Anxiety Inventory (STAI), Beck Anxiety Inventory (BAI), and Hospital Anxiety and Depression Scale-Anxiety (HADS-A). Arthritis Care Res (Hoboken) 63(Suppl 11):S467–S472

33. Marteau TM, Bekker H (1992) The development of a six-item short-form of the state scale of the Spielberger State-Trait Anxiety Inventory (STAI). Br J Clin Psychol 31(Pt 3):301–306

34. Carta G, Palermo P, Marinangeli F, Piroli A, Necozione S, De Lellis V et al (2012) Waiting time and pain during office hysteroscopy. J Minim Invasive Gynecol 19(3):360–364

35. Tarling R, Gale A, Martin-Hirsch P, Holmes L, Kanesalingam K, Dey P (2013) Experiences of women referred for urgent assessment of postmenopausal bleeding (PMB). J Obstet Gynaecol 33(2):184–187

36. Wood NJ, Munot S, Sheridan E, Duffy SR (2008) Does a "one-stop" gynecology screening clinic for women in hereditary nonpolyposis colorectal cancer families have an impact on their psychological morbidity and perception of health? Int J Gynecol Cancer 18(2):279–284

37. Rudin A, Wölner-Hanssen P, Hellbom M, Werner MU (2008) Prediction of post-operative pain after a laparoscopic tubal ligation procedure. Acta Anaesthesiol Scand 52(7):938–945

38. Mc Gurgan P, O'Donovan P, Jones SE (2001) The effect of operator gender on patient satisfaction: does the "Y" in outpatient hysteroscopy matter? Gynaecol Endosc 10(1):53–56

39. Facco E, Stellini E, Bacci C, Manani G, Pavan C, Cavallin F et al (2013) Validation of visual analogue scale for anxiety (VAS-A) in preanesthesia evaluation. Minerva Anestesiol 79(12):1389–1395

40. Hong JY, Kang IS, Koong MK, Yoon HJ, Jee YS, Park JW et al (2003) Preoperative anxiety and propofol requirement in conscious sedation for ovum retrieval. J Korean Med Sci 18(6):863–868

41. Gras S, Servin F, Bedairia E, Montravers P, Desmonts JM, Longrois D et al (2010) The effect of preoperative heart rate and anxiety on

the propofol dose required for loss of consciousness. Anesth Analg 110(1):89–93

42. Meijer J (2001) Stress in the relation between trait and state anxiety. Psychol Rep 88:947–964

43. Weisenberg M, Kreindler ML, Schachat R, Werboff J (1975) Pain: anxiety and attitudes in black, white and Puerto Rican patients. Psychosom Med 37(2):123–135

44. Bromberger JT, Kravitz HM, Chang Y, Randolph JF Jr, Avis NE, Gold EB, Matthews KA (2013) Does risk for anxiety increase during the menopausal transition? Study of women's health across the nation. Menopause 20(5):488–495

45. Pigott TA (2003) Anxiety disorders in women. Psychiatr Clin North Am 26(3):621–672, **vi-vii**

46. Mitchell M (2013) Anaesthesia type, gender and anxiety. J Perioper Pract 23(3):41–47

47. Mavridou P, Dimitriou V, Manataki A, Arnaoutoglou E, Papadopoulos G (2013) Patient's anxiety and fear of anesthesia: effect of gender, age, education, and previous experience of anesthesia. A survey of 400 patients. J Anesth 27(1):104–108

48. Badner NH, Nielson WR, Munk S, Kwiatkowska C, Gelb AW (1990) Preoperative anxiety: detection and contributing factors. Can J Anaesth 37(4):444–447

49. Heyer CM, Thüring J, Lemburg SP, Kreddig N, Hasenbring M, Dohna M, Nicolas V (2015) Anxiety of patients undergoing CT imaging—an underestimated problem? Acad Radiol 22(1):105–112

50. Caprilli S, Baiocco F, Zanetti H, Medina MC (2000) Psychological reactions to outpatient hysteroscopy. [Italian]. Medicina Psicosomatica 45(1):11–21

51. Saraçoğlu T, Unsal A, Taşkın F, Sevinçok L, Karaman CZ (2012) The impact of pre-procedural waiting period and anxiety level on pain perception in patients undergoing transrectal ultrasound-guided prostate biopsy. Diagn Interv Radiol 18(2):195–199

52. Al-Sunaidi M, Tulandi T (2007) A randomized trial comparing local intracervical and combined local and paracervical anesthesia in outpatient hysteroscopy. J Minim Invasive Gynecol 14(2):153–135

53. Kabli N, Tulandi T (2008) A randomized trial of outpatient hysteroscopy with and without intrauterine anesthesia. J Minim Invasive Gynecol 15(3):308–310

54. Lim L, Chow P, Wong CY, Chung A, Chan YH, Wong WK et al (2011) Doctor-patient communication, knowledge, and question prompt lists in reducing preoperative anxiety: a randomized control study. Asian J Surg 34(4):175–180

55. Eberhardt J, Van Wersch A, Van Schaik P, Cann P (2006) Information, social support and anxiety before gastrointestinal endoscopy. Br J Health Psychol 11:551–559

56. Felley C, Perneger TV, Goulet I, Rouillard C, Azar-Pey N, Dorta G et al (2008) Combined written and oral information prior to gastrointestinal endoscopy compared with oral information alone: a randomized trial. BMC Gastroenterol 8:22

57. Granziera E, Guglieri I, Del Bianco P, Capovilla E, Dona B, Ciccarese AA et al (2013) A multidisciplinary approach to improve preoperative understanding and reduce anxiety: a randomised study. Eur J Anaesthesiol 30(12):734–742

58. Nehme J, El-Khani U, Chow A, Hakky S, Ahmed AR, Purkayastha S (2013) The use of multimedia consent programs for surgical procedures: a systematic review. Surg Innov 20(1):13–23

59. Ogden J, Heinrich M, Potter C, Kent A, Jones S (2009) The impact of viewing a hysteroscopy on a screen on the patient's experience: a randomised trial. BJOG 116(2):286–292

60. Walsh JC, Curtis R, Mylotte M (2004) Anxiety levels in women attending a colposcopy clinic: a randomised trial of an educational intervention using video colposcopy. Patient Educ Couns 55(2):247–251

61. Freeman-Wang T, Walker P, Linehan J, Coffey C, Glasser B, Sherr L (2001) Anxiety levels in women attending colposcopy clinics for treatment for cervical intraepithelial neoplasia: a randomised trial of written and video information. BJOG 108(5):482–484

62. Galaal K, Bryant A, Deane KH, Al-Khaduri M, Lopes AD (2011) Interventions for reducing anxiety in women undergoing colposcopy. Cochrane Database Syst Rev 12, CD006013

63. Papadopoulos N, Polyzos D, Gambadauro P, Papalampros P, Chapman L, Magos A (2008) Do patients want to see recordings of their surgery? Eur J Obstet Gynecol Reprod Biol 138(1):89–92

64. Gambadauro P, Magos A (2009) Watching the screen during hysteroscopy: a patient choice. BJOG 116(7):1006–1007

65. Arendt KW, Tessmer-Tuck JA (2013) Nonpharmacologic labor analgesia. Clin Perinatol 40(3):351–371

66. Lin LY, Wang RH (2005) Abdominal surgery, pain and anxiety: preoperative nursing intervention. J Adv Nurs 51(3):252–260

67. Bradt J, Dileo C, Potvin N (2013) Music for stress and anxiety reduction in coronary heart disease patients. Cochrane Database Syst Rev 12, CD006577

68. Bradt J, Dileo C, Shim M (2013) Music interventions for preoperative anxiety. Cochrane Database Syst Rev 6, CD006908

69. Ni CH, Tsai WH, Lee LM, Kao CC, Chen YC (2012) Minimising preoperative anxiety with music for day surgery patients—a randomised clinical trial. J Clin Nurs 21(5-6):620–625

70. Rudin D, Kiss A, Wetz RV, Sottile VM (2007) Music in the endoscopy suite: a meta-analysis of randomized controlled studies. Endoscopy 39(6):507–510

71. Chan YM, Lee PW, Ng TY, Ngan HY, Wong LC (2003) The use of music to reduce anxiety for patients undergoing colposcopy: a randomized trial. Gynecol Oncol 91(1):213–217

3

Low-cost total laparoscopic hysterectomy by single-incision laparoscopic surgery using only reusable standard laparoscopic instruments

Anneleen Reynders · Jan Baekelandt

Abstract The purpose of this study was to demonstrate the feasibility and safety of total laparoscopic hysterectomy (TLH) by single-incision laparoscopic surgery (SILS) with conventional, reusable laparoscopic instruments, inserted through an inexpensive, self-constructed single-port device. Between June 2013 and April 2014, 15 TLHs by SILS were performed by a single surgeon (BJ). Only conventional, reusable laparoscopic instruments were used. The self-constructed single-port device was made by assembling a surgical glove, a wound protector, one reusable 10-mm trocar, and four reusable 5-mm trocars. The vaginal cuff was closed by intracorporeal suturing. Patient and perioperative data were analysed. Fifteen patients underwent TLH by SILS, and no conversion to standard laparoscopy or laparotomy was necessary. Mean operation time was 97 min (55–135 min), and mean drop in haemoglobin level was 1.2 g/dl (0–2.4 g/dl). There were no operative complications. Postoperative pain scores were low. The mean weight of the removed uterus was 118 g (50–208 g). TLH by SILS is feasible even when performed with reusable, conventional laparoscopic instruments. An inexpensive, self-constructed single-port device allows every surgeon worldwide to accomplish single-incision surgery without the need to invest in expensive ports, disposable instruments, sealing devices, or auto-locking sutures.

Keywords Laparoscopy · Single incision · Total hysterectomy · Standard reusable instruments · Frugal innovation · Self-constructed single-port device

A. Reynders · J. Baekelandt (✉)
Department of Obstetrics and Gynaecology, Imelda Hospital, Imeldalaan 9, 2820 Bonheiden, Belgium
e-mail: jan.baekelandt@imelda.be

Background

The advantages of laparoscopy in gynaecological surgery, when compared with open surgery, have been accepted worldwide since the early 1980s [1]. Hysterectomies have thus been increasingly performed by laparoscopic approach. Even less invasive procedures, such as single-incision laparoscopic surgery (SILS), are now being introduced. This approach makes use of a single incision of skin and fascia, usually at the umbilicus, to introduce a trocar through which all instruments are inserted. This procedure produces a better cosmetic result and less port-related complications can be expected.

In this study, we aimed to demonstrate the feasibility of total laparoscopic hysterectomy (TLH) by SILS with the use of conventional, reusable laparoscopic instruments, and an inexpensive, self-constructed single-port device that can easily be assembled by every surgeon worldwide. We wanted to demonstrate that there is no need for expensive, commercially available disposable SILS ports, other disposable instruments, sealing devices or auto-locking sutures, to perform a safe and equally time efficient TLH by SILS.

Materials and methods

Patients

Between June 2013 and April 2014, a single surgeon (BJ) performed 15 total laparoscopic hysterectomies by SILS. All patients were selected for TLH because of benign or premalignant gynaecologic disease. The following patient and perioperative data were collected and retrospectively analysed: patient age, body mass index (BMI), general health status, total operating time, serum haemoglobin (Hb) drop (change between the preoperative Hb and postoperative Hb 1 day after surgery), (peri-)operative complications, postoperative pain score, and weight of the removed uterus.

The duration of surgery was defined as the time from umbilical incision to the end of skin closure. Bowel, bladder, ureteral or vascular injuries, as well as blood loss >500 ml, were considered as intraoperative complications. Short-term postoperative complications were classified as urinary tract infection, postoperative ileus, wound infection, vaginal vault bleeding, or hematuria.

Postoperative pain was assessed using the visual analogue pain scale (VAS) (scoring from 0=no pain, to 10=worst imaginable pain). The VAS score was evaluated immediately after surgery in the recovery and at 6, 24, and 48 h postoperatively. All patients received the same intraoperative analgesia: intravenous paracetamol (1000 mg) and ketorolac trometamol (20 mg). Postoperative pain was managed by tramadol hydrochloride 300 mg and alizapride hydrochloride 100 mg, administered intravenously over the first 24 h, together with intramuscular diclofenac 2×75 mg the first day. Over the next 24 h, intravenous tramadol 200 mg and alizapride hydrochloride 100 mg was infused. As long as there was no oral diet intake, intravenous paracetamol 4×1000 mg was associated. When the patient started diet intake, oral analgesics (paracetamol 1000 mg) were administered on patient's demand.

Prophylactic intravenous antibiotic therapy, cefazolin 2 g and metronidazole 500 mg, was administrated during surgery (this was a standard protocol for TLH in our centre at the time of the study, and recently it has been altered to cefazolin 2 g) [2].

Surgical technique

The procedure began with the patient in lithotomy position and placement of a reusable Hohl uterine manipulator (Karl Storz, Tuttlingen, Germany). A single intra-umbilical skin incision of 1–2 cm and a 2- to 3-cm fasciotomy was performed to insert the self-constructed single port device (Fig. 1). The device was constructed using an Alexis Wound Protector/Retractor (Applied Medical, Rancho Santa Margarita, CA, USA) attached to a size 8 surgical glove. One finger of the surgical glove was incised to place a 10-mm reusable trocar for CO_2 insufflation and laparoscope insertion. A maximum of 15 mmHg intra-abdominal CO_2 pressure was achieved to prevent the glove from overdistending. Four 5-mm reusable trocars were placed through the other fingers for insertion of the reusable laparoscopic instruments. We used a standard rigid 0° 10-mm laparoscope. The reusable conventional laparoscopic instruments were a bipolar forceps, a pair of cold scissors, an atraumatic forceps, a monopolar hook, a laparoscopic needle holder, and a suction-irrigation cannula. The

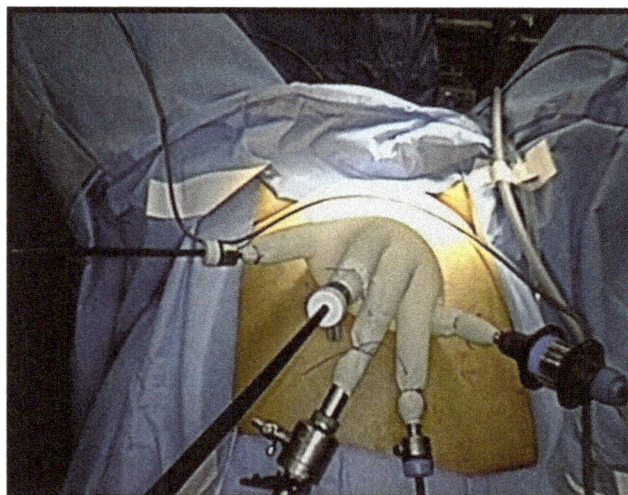
Fig. 1 Low cost self-constructed single port device

laparoscope and two laparoscopic instruments were inserted through the trocars, into the abdomen, together at one time. One or two additional laparoscopic instruments were inserted through the trocars but left outside the abdomen. Alternating instruments was done without the need to insert or withdraw them through the trocars.

The colpotomy was made using a reusable monopolar hook to incise the vagina circumferentially onto the vaginal cup of the uterine manipulator. After laparoscopic resection of the uterus, the uterus was extracted transvaginally. The vaginal vault was closed laparoscopically by three interrupted and intracorporeally knotted figure of eight sutures using a Vicryl-1 V-34 with 36-mm round-bodied needle (Ethicon, Piscataway, NJ, USA). After haemostasis, the abdomen was desufflated, the single-port device was removed, and the umbilical fascia and subcutaneous tissue were closed respectively with 1 Vicryl V-34 and 3–0 Monocryl PS-2 sutures (Ethicon, Piscataway, NJ, USA).

Table 1 Overview of patient and perioperative characteristics

Data	Mean	Range
Age (years)	52	42–64
BMI (kg/m^2)	25.0	16.8–37.1
Total operating time (min)	97	55–135
Serum haemoglobin drop (g/dl)	1.2	0–2.4
Postoperative pain score		
Immediate postoperative	1.8	0–4
6 h	2.5	2–4
24 h	2	1–5
48 h	2.2	1–6
Weight of removed uterus	118	50–208

Table 2 Patient and perioperative characteristics of consecutive patients

Patient no.	Age	BMI (kg/m^2)	Parity	Previous abdominal surgery	Type of surgery	Total operating time (min)	Serum haemoglobin drop	(Peri-)operative complications	Postoperative pain score		Uterus weight (g)
									6 h	48 h	
1	54	24.8	P2	–	TLH+BSO	135	2	–	2	2	146
2	52	24.7	P2	CE	TLH	110	1	–	4	4	157
3	52	26.4	P1	CS, LS	TLH+BSO	130	1.2	–	2	6	139
4	60	21.6	P2	LS	TLH+BSO	105	0.7	–	3	1	130
5	44	24.5	P2	CCE, CS	TLH	90	1.4	–	2	2	119
6	45	16.8	P0	Diagnostic laparoscopy	TLH	80	0	–	2	1	57
7	53	23.4	P1	Adhesiolysis	TLH	85	1.3	–	2	1	75
8	64	30.5	P3	CS, LS	TLH+BSO	110	0.7	–	3	1	152
9	42	24.8	P0	–	TLH	85	2.2	Cystitis	3	2	143
10	53	29.1	P3	–	TLH+BSO	105	0.8	–	2	3	153
11	50	24.2	P3	–	TLH	90	2.4	–	2	2	118
12	63	37.1	P2	–	TLH+BSO	100	0.6	–	2	2	50
13	50	26.1	P1	LS, AE	TLH	100	1.3	–	2	1	208
14	53	20.5	P3	CS, AE	TLH	55	1.2	–	2	2	51
15	43	21.2	P1	–	TLH	70	1.3	–	4	3	77

CE cystectomy, *CS* caesarean section, *LS* laparoscopic sterilisation, *CCE* cholecystectomy, *AE* appendectomy, *TLH* total laparoscopic hysterectomy, *BSO* bilateral salpingo-oophorectomy

Results

Between June 2013 and April 2014, 15 procedures were successfully performed by single-incision laparoscopic surgery using conventional, reusable laparoscopic instruments. No conversion to standard multi-incision laparoscopy or laparotomy was necessary. Nine patients underwent only a hysterectomy. In six patients, a simultaneous prophylactic bilateral salpingo-oophorectomy was performed.

Table 1 presents an overview of patient and perioperative data. Individual patient details are presented in Table 2. Mean operation time was 97 min. Nine patients had had previous abdominal surgery. There were no intraoperative complications, and only one patient had a postoperative cystitis for which oral antibiotic therapy was administered. The mean drop in haemoglobin level was 1.2 g/dl. Most patients scored a low postoperative pain score (range 0–4). Only one patient mentioned a score of 6/10 48 h after surgery. This was due to referred shoulder pain caused by intra-abdominal CO_2. Mean weight of the removed uterus was 118 g.

Each patient was examined 6 weeks after surgery. They were all in a good health, the umbilical scar was almost invisible due to its intra-umbilical position (Fig. 2), and there were no patients with port-site hernias.

Discussion

In this study, TLH by SILS with intracorporeal suturing of the vaginal vault was performed with conventional, reusable laparoscopic instruments, within a reasonable operation time and with a low complication rate.

We used an inexpensive, self-constructed single-port device that can be made by every surgeon worldwide. This port

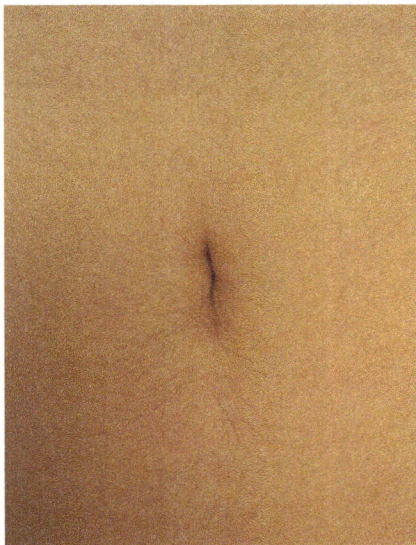

Fig. 2 Umbilical scar six weeks after surgery

device has been proven to be safe and effective previously [3–9]. Combining this poor man's single-port device with easily available, conventional, and reusable laparoscopic instruments, this study shows that TLH by SILS can be performed worldwide without increasing the cost of laparoscopic surgery. Even in a third-world setting, where only standard basic laparoscopic equipment is available, TLH can be performed with this SILS technique.

A self-constructed port using a surgical glove has advantages when compared to commercial ports. It is less costly, it has flexible material that enables greater manipulation of instruments, and a greater number and size of instruments can be passed through the incision. Assembling five trocars into the glove before starting the procedure allows to leave all instruments inserted through the trocars during surgery. This makes alternating between instruments less time consuming.

Suturing and knot tying for closure of the vaginal vault can be the most difficult part of TLH by SILS due to problems of collision between instruments, laparoscope, and trocars, and because of limited triangulation and traction of tissue [10, 11]. This study demonstrates that intracorporeal suturing and knot tying are feasible via SILS. The technical challenge of suturing via SILS can be reduced by practising on an endotrainer.

Our data on surgical outcomes and perioperative complications seem to be in line with those of other larger studies that evaluated the feasibility and safety of TLH by SILS [11–16].

There are several limitations of our study. To evaluate the feasibility of TLH by SILS with the use of a low cost single-port device and conventional, reusable laparoscopic instruments, this study was designed as a case series with no control group. Other limitations are its small sample size, its lack of generalizability, limited follow-up, and all procedures being performed by one surgeon.

A meta-analysis by Murji et al. [17] showed that there is no significant difference in overall complications between single-incision versus conventional laparoscopy. Operation time was significantly longer for adnexal surgery by SILS, but no significant difference in operation time for hysterectomy by SILS could be demonstrated. However, current evidence is not strong enough to make any conclusion on surgical approach based on operation time. A meta-analysis for postoperative pain, change in haemoglobin, length of hospital stay, and cosmetics was not possible because of inconsistent data in literature [17].

A review of the literature showed that there is no difference in length of hospitalization [17]. One randomized controlled trial reported no difference in postoperative pain scores; however, two other RCTs found statistically lower postoperative pain with SILS compared to conventional laparoscopy [18–20]. Regarding cosmetic results, patients who underwent SILS seem to be more satisfied compared to patients after conventional laparoscopy or open surgery [21].

Single-incision surgery is feasible in selected cases and may provide benefits when compared with conventional laparoscopy; however, one should be cautious by interpreting conclusions as the current evidence is derived from a limited number of small studies.

Conclusion

TLH by SILS with intracorporeal suturing and knot tying is feasible and can be performed by surgeons worldwide with the use of a low-cost single-port device and conventional, reusable laparoscopic instruments. Less postoperative pain and better cosmesis seem to be an advantage of SILS; however, larger cohort studies are necessary to encourage or discourage this minimally invasive procedure.

References

1. Nieboer TE, Johnson N, Lethaby A et al (2009) Surgical approach to hysterectomy for benign gynaecological disease. The Cochrane Database of Systematic Reviews, Issue 3. Art No: CD003677. DOI: 10. 1002/14651858. CD003677.pub4
2. Brummer TH, Keikkinen AM, Jalkanen J et al (2013) Antibiotic prophylaxis for hysterectomy, a prospective cohort study: cefuroxime, metronidazole, or both? BJOG 120:1269–1276
3. Lee YY, Kim TJ, Kim CJ et al (2009) Single-port access laparoscopic-assisted vaginal hysterectomy: a novel method with a wound retractor and a glove. J Minim Invasive Gynecol 16:450–453
4. Livraghi L, Berselli M, Bianchi V, Latham L, Farassino L, Cocozza E (2012) Glove technique in single-port access laparoscopic surgery: results of an initial experience. Minim Invasive Surg 2012:415–430
5. Elbert K, Iheule N, Partha P, Santanu M (2011) Improvised transumbilical glove port: a cost effective method for single port laparoscopic surgery. Indian J Surg 3:142–145
6. Barband A, Fakhree MB, Kakaei F, Daryani A (2012) Single-incision laparoscopic cholecystectomy using glove port in comparison with standard laparoscopic cholecystectomy SILC using glove port. Surg Laparosc Endosc Percutan Tech 22:17–20
7. Kim TJ, Lee YY, Kim MJ et al (2009) Single port access laparoscopic adnexal surgery. J Minim Invasive Gynecol 16:612–615
8. Choi YS, Shin KS, Choi J, Park JN, Oh YS, Rhee TE (2012) Single-port access laparoscopy-assisted vaginal hysterectomy: our initial experiences with 100 cases. Minim Invasive Surg 2012:543–627
9. Yang YS, Oh KY, Hur MH, Kim SY, Yim HS (2015) Laparoendoscopic single-site surgery using conventional laparoscopic instruments and glove port technique in gynecology: a single surgeon's experience. J Minim Invasive Gynecol 22:87–93
10. Peak J, Kim SW, Lee SH et al (2011) Learning curve and surgical outcome for single-port access total laparoscopic hysterectomy in 100 consctive cases. Gynecol Obstet Invest 72:227–233
11. Phongnarisorn C, Chinthakanan O (2011) Transumbilical single-incision laparoscopic hysterectomy with conventional laparoscopic instruments in patients with symptomatic leiomyoma and/or adenomyosis. Arch Gynecol Obstet 284: 893–900
12. Jung YW, Kim YT, Lee DW et al (2010) The feasibility of scarless single-port transumbilical total laparoscopic hysterectomy: initial clinical experience. Surg Endosc 24: 1686–1692
13. Fanfani F, Fagotti A, Rositto C et al (2012) Laparoscopic, minilaparoscopic and single-port hysterectomy: perioperative outcomes. Surg Endosc 26:3592–3596
14. Fanfani F, Fagotti A, Gagliardi ML et al (2013) Minilaparoscopic versus single-port total hysterectomy: a randomized trial. J Minim Invasive Gynecol 20:192–197
15. Yim GA, Jung YW, Peak J et al (2010) Transumbilical single-port access versus conventional total laparoscopic hysterectomy: surgical outcomes. Am J Obstet Gynecol 203:26.e1–6
16. Wang T, Chong GO, Park NY, Hong DG, Lee YS (2012) Comparison study of single-port (Octoport^{TM}) and four-port total laparoscopic hysterectomy. Eur J Obstet Gynecol Reprod Biol 161:215–218
17. Murji A, Patel VI, Leyland N, Choi M (2013) Single-incision laparoscopy in gynecologic surgery. Obstet Gynecol 121:818–829
18. Jung YW, Lee M, Yim GW et al (2011) A randomized prospective study of single-port and four-port approaches for hysterectomy in terms of postoperative pain. Surg Endosc 25: 2462–2469
19. Chen YJ, Wang PH, Ocampo EJ et al (2011) Single-port compared with conventional laparoscopic-assisted vaginal hysterectomy: a randomized controlled trial. Obstet Gynecol 117:906–912
20. Fagotti A, Bottoni C, Vizzielli G et al (2011) Postoperative pain after conventional laparoscopy and laparoendoscopic single site surgery (LESS) for benign adnexal disease: a randomized trial. Fertil Steril 96:255.e2–259.e2
21. Bradford LS, Boruta DM (2013) Laparoendoscopic single-site surgery in gynecology: a review of the literature, tools, and techniques. Obstet Gynecol Surv 68:295–304

4

Feasibility of laparoendoscopic single-site surgery in supracervical hysterectomy: technique and retrospective case-control comparison

Per Istre · Lars Franch Andersen ·
Henrik Halvor Springborg

Abstract One recent innovation in the field of gynecology is laparoendoscopic single-site surgery (LESS). It is associated with reduced postoperative pain and better cosmetic outcome. The present paper aims to explain techniques and instrumentations associated with single-port hysterectomies. A retrospective case-control study is included, comparing LESS with conventional four-port hysterectomies to highlight the feasibility of LESS. This study involved literature search and personal experience regarding single-port hysterectomy and a retrospective case-control study of 34 patients who underwent supracervical hysterectomy between April 2011 and November 2012. Operating time, blood loss, and length of hospital stay were similar in the two groups. Patient's evaluation of the cosmetic result was in favor of LESS, however not significant. LESS represents a new frontier in minimally invasive surgery. New instrumentation and recommendations have been developed which are expected to make the technique more feasible. This study demonstrates that LESS supracervical hysterectomy has comparable operative outcomes to conventional laparoscopic hysterectomy and is a feasible approach for supracervical hysterectomy. Based on the literature and our experience, a feasible step by step technique for surgeons who are interested in performing supracervical LESS hysterectomy is described. Comparative data and prospective trials are required in order to determine the clinical utility and impact of LESS in treatment of gynecological conditions in the future.

Keywords LESS · Single-port laparoscopy±hysterectomy · Conventional laparoscopy±hysterectomy · Single-port laparoscopy versus conventional laparoscopic hysterectomy

Introduction

Hysterectomy is among the most commonly performed gynecologic surgeries. The method of hysterectomy has evolved during the recent years from laparotomy to laparoscopic procedures which continuously are being improved [1]. The advantages of a minimally invasive laparoscopic approach compared to traditional laparotomy are reduced postoperative pain, reduced perioperative bleeding, reduced risk of infection, faster recovery, better cosmetic results, and shorter hospital stay [2, 3]. Current efforts aim to reduce perioperative morbidity associated with laparoscopic surgery. One of the more recent innovations in the field of minimally invasive surgery is laparoendoscopic single-site surgery (LESS). This technique allows the surgeon to perform the abdominal intervention through a single incision in the navel, as compared to the traditional multiport laparoscopic surgical technique, which requires three or more abdominal incisions [4]. Each working port has an inherent risk of bleeding, infection, organ damage, hernia formation, and decreased cosmetics; the ideal goal of laparoscopy is to reduce port number and port size [5].

LESS technique has been implemented in urology, gastrointestinal surgery, and gynecology in an attempt to reduce abdominal wall trauma [6]. Evidence suggests that single-port laparoscopic hysterectomy (LESSH) is a feasible and safe

P. Istre (✉)
Department of Gynecology/Obstetrics, Hvidovre University
Hospital, Kettegård Allé 30, 2650 Hvidovre, Denmark
e-mail: pistre@gmail.com

L. F. Andersen
Department of Gynecology/Obstetrics, Nordsjællands Hospital
Hillerød, Dyrehavevej 29, 3400 Hillerød, Denmark
e-mail: lars.franch.andersen@dadlnet.dk

H. H. Springborg
Department of Gynecology, Aleris-Hamlet Private Hospital,
Gyngemose Parkvej 66, 2860 Søborg, Denmark
e-mail: halvor-springborg@tdcadsl.dk

approach [1, 4, 5, 7, 8]. However, it remains to be seen whether there are significant benefits of LESSH compared to conventional laparoscopic hysterectomy (CLH).

The technical challenges of LESSH include limited triangulation and compromised retraction due to the limitation of the instruments through a single axis. Due to instrumental angulation, surgeons may encounter difficulty with suturing, requiring a greater level of surgical expertise. One significant finding has been the extended operation time performing LESSH [4, 9]. However, studies show that with increasing operator experience, operative time can be reduced [1, 4].

In gynecology, supracervical hysterectomy has been attractive for patients with fibroids or abnormal bleeding and the absence of a specific indication for removal of the cervix, citing lower complication rates (less bleeding, fewer infections/abscesses and vaginal cuff hematomas, trauma to urinary tract), shorter operative times, less postoperative pain, faster recovery, and a less complicated procedure. Arguments against the supracervical procedure are the potential for bleeding from residual endometrium in the cervical stump, absence of using the vagina as a port for specimen removal, the need for a continued cervical screening program, and the potential risk of future cervical pathology [10–14].

Subjective and objective outcomes such as less postoperative pain and improved cosmetic results have been associated with single-port surgery. It has been suggested that these findings can be partly explained by avoidance of the secondary ports penetrating abdominal muscles [15–17]. The present paper aims to explain techniques and instrumentations associated with single-port hysterectomies. A retrospective case-control study is included, comparing LESS with conventional four-port hysterectomies to highlight the feasibility of LESS (Fig. 1).

Material and methods

Methods

Patients were recruited from the primary health care sector by specialists in gynecology and were referred to the Minimal Invasive Gynecological Surgery (MIGS) unit at Aleris-Hamlet Hospital in Copenhagen, Denmark. All patients underwent pelvic examination and transvaginal ultrasound in the outpatient clinic. Patients were then scheduled for surgery within 3 weeks. Inclusion criteria for the LESSH procedure were BMI<35, ultrasound-estimated uterine weight<300 g, no suspicion of malignancy and periumbilical adhesions, and American Society of Anesthesia (ASA) I–II. If a patient met the inclusion criteria for the LESSH procedure, she was offered a choice between the two types of laparoscopic procedures: LESSH or CLH. The patients were informed that CLH was the standard procedure at the department and that the LESSH technique was a new but feasible technique, where studies indicated that the safety was comparable to CLH. The patients were further informed that the LESSH procedure

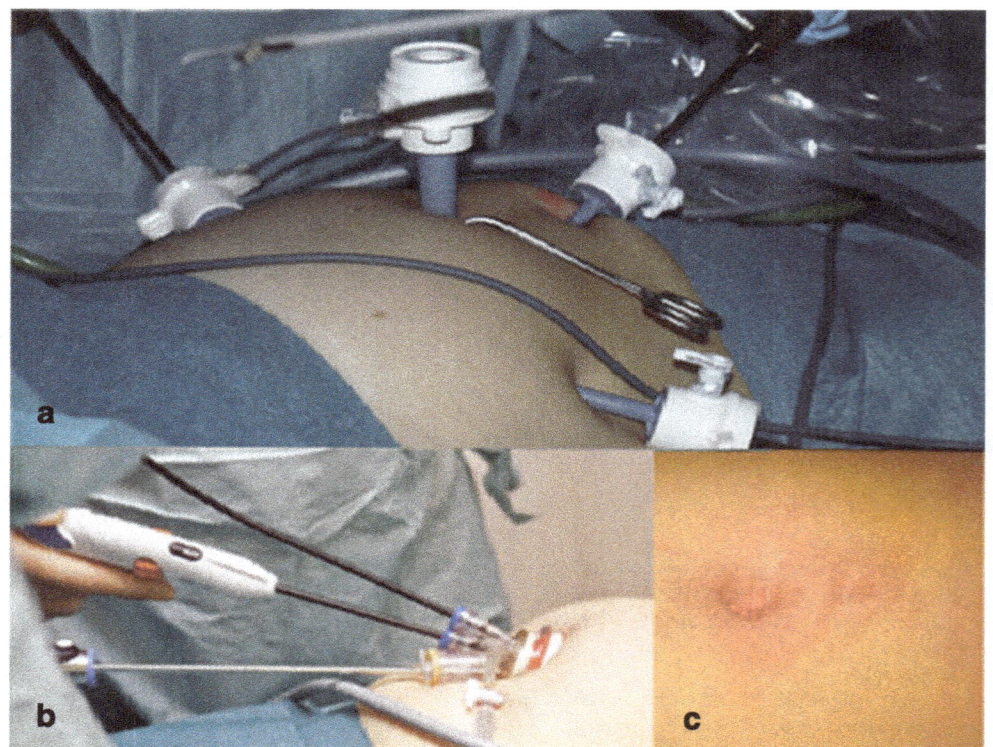

Fig. 1 a Conventional laparoscopy, using four ports. b Camera, cutting forceps, and grasper in three different ports during single-port laparoscopy. c Cosmetic result immediately after a single-port laparoscopy

might have cosmetic advances since the scar is partly hidden in the umbilicus.

To make the two procedures LESSH and CLH as comparable as possible for this study, only supracervical operations were included.

Study design

A case-control study including 34 performed supracervical hysterectomies between April 4, 2011, and November 16, 2012, was conducted. Based on the surgeon's explanation and preoperative discussion, the patients freely chose their preferred operation. Each corresponding CLH which met given LESSH inclusion criteria was picked after each selected LESSH, in order to make the two groups comparable. All operations were performed by the department's two experienced surgeons.

The primary endpoint of this retrospective study was to compare operative details, operation time, blood loss, and length of hospital stay between the two groups, as well as the technical difficulties with the procedures. Secondary endpoint was to evaluate patient satisfaction using a questionnaire sent out to the patients. The questionnaire focused on the time interval before returning to everyday activities and work and also the patient's evaluation of the performed operative procedure and cosmetic outcome.

Data collection

Clinical characteristics age, BMI, ASA, and indication for surgery and surgical characteristics operation time, blood loss, uterine weight, and length of hospital stay were recorded for each patient. Among the 34 patients, 27 completed the questionnaire in which they assessed the cosmetic result, overall satisfaction with the performed surgery, and whether they would recommend it to others. The excluded seven patients had either moved from the country, had an invalid telephone number, or were unreachable after repeated attempts to contact them during 1 month's time.

Statistics

Data were collected and processed using IBM SPSS v20®. Descriptive analytics included percentage, median, and range. Differences between the two groups were analyzed using the Mann-Whitney U test for nonparametric distribution. A p value <0.05 was considered to indicate statistical significance.

Results

A total of 34 supracervical laparoscopic hysterectomies were included in this study, with 17 patients in each group: LESSH

and CLH. Indication for hysterectomy included uterine fibroids, $n=20$ (58 %); lower abdominal pain from hematometra after endometrial resection, $n=4$ (11 %); dysmenorrhea, $n=4$ (11 %); menorrhagia, $n=3$ (8 %); and metrorrhagia, $n=2$ (6 %). Age, BMI, and ASA-value showed no statistical differences between the two groups. No LESSH operation was converted to CLH or laparotomy, and no CHL procedure was converted to laparotomy (Table 1).

Surgical outcomes are shown in Table 2: median operation time of 70 min, blood loss of 30 mL, and uterine weight of 140 g in the LESSH group compared to 70 min, 30 mL, and 130 g in the CLH group, respectively. Six patients from the LESSH group were discharged from hospital on the day of operation, compared with two patients from the CLH group. The majority of patients, 10 patients in the LESSH group and 15 in the CLH group, were discharged the next day. One patient in the LESSH group stayed more than 1 day because of postoperative nausea. There were no significant differences between the two groups in any of the parameters: duration of surgery, blood loss, and uterus weight. Reviewing LESSH, the median duration of surgery, blood loss, and uterus weight showed no significant difference between the first eight patients, compared to the next nine patients (Table 3).

Median time before returning to work was 14 days for patients in LESSH group and 10 for the CLH group. The median scores for cosmetic result, overall assessment, and if they were to recommend surgery for others were 10, 10, and 10, respectively, in the LESSH group against 9, 9, and 10 in the CLH group. No significant difference was found between the two groups for any of these parameters (Table 4).

Table 1 Demographic and clinical characteristics of patients who underwent either single-port laparoscopic hysterectomy (LESSH) or conventional laparoscopic hysterectomy (CLH), both supracervical hysterectomies for various benign gynecological diseases

Characteristics	LESSH (N=17)	CLH (N=17)	Total (N=34)
Age, years	45 (39–53)	45 (39–72)	45 (39–72)
Body mass index, kg/m^2	24 (19–32)	24 (19–34)	24 (19–34)
ASA grading			
1	14 (82)	11 (71)	25 (76)
2	3 (18)	6 (29)	9 (24)
Indication of surgery			
Lower abdominal pain	0 (0)	1 (5)	1 (3)
Dysmenorrhea	1 (5)	3 (17)	4 (11)
Uterine fibroid	9 (52)	11 (64)	20 (58)
Menorrhagia	3 (17)	0 (0)	3 (8)
Metrorrhagia	1 (5)	1 (5)	2 (6)
Hematometra	3 (17)	1 (11)	4 (11)

Data presented as median (range) or n (%) patients

ASA American Society of Anesthesia

Table 2 Surgical outcomes for patients who underwent either single-port laparoscopic hysterectomy (LESSH) or conventional laparoscopic hysterectomy (CLH), as supracervical hysterectomies for various benign gynecological diseases

Parameter	LESSH (N=17)	CLH (N=17)	p value[a]
Duration of surgery, min	70 (45–100)	70 (40–105)	0.375
Blood loss, mL	30 (10–200)	30 (5–150)	0.946
Uterus weight, g	140 (50–290)	130 (63–300)	0.760
Postoperative hospital stay, days			
Same day	6	2	
1 day	10	15	
More than 1 day	1	0	

Data is presented as median (range) or numbers

[a] Mann-Whitney U test.

Discussion

Recent advances in laparoscopic equipment and improvements in surgical skills have further enhanced the advantages of laparoscopic surgery. Many surgeons have attempted to reduce abdominal wall trauma by minimizing the number of ports and the size of instruments. A limited number of studies suggest that using a single-port entrance is associated with fewer days of immobilization and higher rates of patient satisfaction [1, 18]. This study may indicate likewise, as many patients who underwent the LESS procedure were discharged from hospital the same day as the operation.

LESSH patients' median score in this study on the questions concerning patient satisfaction, including cosmetic outcome, was 10, whereas CLH patients' median score was 9. This difference was not statistically significant; however, the score suggests that LESS might be advantageous cosmetically. A cross-sectional study done by Eom et al. [3] and a more recent randomized study by Song et al. [17] showed better cosmetic result and overall satisfactory rate by patients undertaking the LESS procedure compared to the conventional procedure.

The LESSH procedure has the disadvantage of restricted movements of surgical instruments due to the proximity of the instruments [2]. One of the indicators found to be significant in the majority of earlier studies was prolonged operation

Table 3 Surgical outcomes of the first eight patients who underwent single-port laparoscopic hysterectomy (LESSH), compared with the next nine patients who underwent the same procedure

Parameter	First 8 patients	Next 9 patients	p value[a]
Duration of surgery, min	67.5 (57–95)	70 (45–100)	0.673
Blood loss, mL	30 (15–200)	30 (10–100)	0.673
Uterus weight, g	140 (70–251)	135 (50–290)	0.743

Data is presented as median (range)

[a] Mann-Whitney U test

Table 4 Questionnaire outcome from the patients of the two different groups: LESSH and CLH

Parameter	LESSH (N=12)	CLH (N=15)	p value[a]
Everyday activities, days	6 (2–14)	4 (1–14)	0.277
Resuming to work, days	14 (3–42)	10 (2–21)	0.516
Overall assessment, score (1–10)	10 (8–10)	9 (2–10)	0.399
Cosmetic outcome, score (1–10)	10 (9–10)	9 (3–10)	0.167
Recommend surgery, score (1–10)	10 (9–10)	10 (8–10)	0.427

In the scoring procedure, 1 indicates unsatisfactory, while 10 satisfactory. Data is presented as median (range)

[a] Mann-Whitney U test

time. Lack of surgical experience and the need for new instruments with more flexibility have been suggested as the causes for the extended operating times with the single-port technique [1, 4, 9]. In this study, no difference in operation time was found, even when comparing the first eight patients with the next nine patients (Table 3), indicating that the learning curve was steep.

The steep learning curve may suggest the importance of following the technical recommendations from the literature. Additionally, the surgeons had experience with less complicated adnexal single-port operations on women as well as previous training in pig labs before performing hysterectomy. Lab training before performing LESSH operations is highly recommended, and simple adnexal operations are most feasible when LESSH is introduced.

The rate of complications in this study is, like in larger randomized controlled studies, low in laparoscopic hysterectomy [2, 3]. Even though the incision in the umbilicus with LESS in several procedures is larger than in traditional multiport laparoscopy, recent literature indicates that the risks of herniation are comparable [19]. In supracervical hysterectomy involving morcellator use as in this study, the length of the incision in the umbilical fascia is comparable to traditional multiport laparoscopic hysterectomy.

Recently, there have been concerns and discussions about possible remnants of the rare but serious sarcoma fibroid tissue left behind in the abdominal cavity after power morcellation (FDA Issues Safety Communication on Laparoscopic Uterine Power Morcellation in Hysterectomy and Myomectomy 2014). The LESSH procedure may contribute to a reduction of the risk of leaving morcellated tissue behind in the abdominal cavity, as this technique facilitates morcellation of uterus inside a plastic bag in combination with the LESS triport.

The design of this retrospective case-control study implies risks of bias. Patients who met the inclusion criteria for LESSH were informed about the procedure. Patients choosing the LESSH procedure were probably more motivated to receive the most minimal surgery possible, while patients choosing the standard procedure (CLH) probably were less concerned about the cosmetic outcome and preferred to undergo a procedure already well established.

To confirm the feasibility and safety of LESSH, including the risk of more rare complications and the safety of general implementation of the procedure, will require large randomized controlled studies.

Conclusion

LESSH represents a new frontier in minimally invasive surgery. New instrumentation and recommendations have been developed, which are expected to make the technique more feasible. This study demonstrates that LESSH has comparable operative outcomes to conventional laparoscopic hysterectomy and probably improved cosmetics. It is a feasible approach for supracervical hysterectomy when following recommendations from experienced surgeons in the field of LESS. Comparative data and prospective trials are required in order to determine the clinical utility and impact of LESS in treatment of gynecological conditions in the future.

Equipment and technical recommendations for performing LESS supracervical hysterectomy

The following recommendations are based on a combination of recommendations from leading surgeons in the field of LESS in the literature and lectures on conferences [20].

Recommended equipment

1. Access device of good quality like TriPort 15™ (Olympus®, Hamburg, Germany) or GelPoint™ (Applied Medical, Rancho Santa Margarita, CA) allowing an instrument of minimum of 12 mm for morcellation.
2. Five mm 30° rotable or flex tip optics, preferably with light cable in line with the shaft of the telescope. If not available, a 90° adaptor for the light cable can be used to minimize interference with the light cord.
3. Curved and/or straight grasper and straight active instrument (where the angle of the working instrument can be rotated). In order to reduce the number of instrument exchanges, a combined grasping, coagulation, and cutting instrument is recommended.
4. Uterine manipulator of good quality with a ring to delineate the vaginal fornix for better presentation of the uterine vessels.
5. For supracervical hysterectomy, no suturing is required; however, a monopolar/bipolar hook or loop (Lina loop, Lina medical®, Copenhagen, Denmark) facilitated amputation of the uterus at the cervical-isthmic level.

6. A 12–15-mm morcellator, preferably mechanical, to avoid formation of smoke during morcellation.

Recommended procedures and techniques

It is recommended to perform several simple adnexal LESS procedures before performing hysterectomy. Training in "Pig Lab" is an advantage, and performing the first LESS hysterectomies with a trained LESS surgeon is highly recommended.

1. Access technique (Hasson)—1.5–2-cm longitudinal transumbilical skin incision and opening of the subcutaneous fat. With two Kocher clamps, the fascia is elevated and an incision is made. A blunt retractor is inserted through the peritoneum into the peritoneal cavity. The access device is placed in accordance with the manufacturer's instructions for use.
2. General procedure—after insufflation, the optic is placed in the most cephalic port with the tip close to the abdominal wall looking down and the camera head close to the chest. Then, the straight or curved grasper is inserted. Consider whether the active instrument has to pass over or under the grasper before it is introduced. It is important to maintain the laparoscope and surgical instruments in different horizontal planes in order to avoid instrument clashing. To reduce the problem of instrument clashing on the outside, the instrument handles can be kept horizontal and parallel to the floor "gangsta". Multifunctional instruments, with grasp, coagulation, and cut, reduce the number of instrument movements and exchanges and are especially helpful in LESS surgery.
3. Hysterectomy step by step (the primary surgeon on the left side of the patient and will begin the hysterectomy on the left).

    a. After the camera is inserted as mentioned above, the uterus is positioned upward and toward the right by the uterine manipulator.
    b. The assistant instrument (curved or straight grasper) is then inserted through the left canula and can be used to augment the positioning of the uterus to present the left utero-ovarian and broad ligaments.
    c. The electrosurgical instrument is then inserted through the right canula and the utero-ovarian ligament and broad ligament including the round ligament can be sealed and transected. (When exposure is better when lateral tension on the left ovary is created, the grasper is inserted through the right canula and the active instrument through the left canula.)
    d. The broad ligament is opened and the bladder peritoneum is opened from the left to the midline, and

the peritoneum on the left side is pushed downwards. During this procedure, the uterus is positioned to the back with the uterine manipulator to expose the bladder peritoneum.

e. The left uterine vessels are sealed on the edge of the ring of the uterine manipulator in the vagina. During this procedure, the uterus is positioned upward and against the right by grasper and manipulator in order to reduce the risk of injury to the ureter.

f. The right side of the hysterectomy is performed by positioning the uterus toward the left. The grasper is positioned through the right canula and the operating instrument through the left canula. The same procedure is performed (c to e) on the right side, and the bladder is pushed down and the uterine vessels in both sides is sealed and transected.

g. The sealed uterine vessels are cut bilaterally and hemostasis ensured.

h. The loop is placed around the cervix, and it is visually secured that no bowel is close to the cutting edge. After removing the uterine manipulator, the cervix is pulled forward and away from the bowel using the loop and corpus uteri is amputated. The amputation can alternatively be performed with an electrical hook.

i. The endocervix is coagulated to reduce the risk of persisting endometrial tissue.

j. The uterus is morcellated by a 12- or 15-mm morcellator through the 15-mm port (or the GelPoint). During morcellation, it is of utmost importance that the morcellator is kept away from the bowel and close to the abdominal wall. The tip of the morcellator must at all time during morcellation be visible. A laparoscope with flexible tip is an advantage during this procedure.

k. If problems occur, including during morcellation, an additional port should always be considered.

l. The umbilical fascia is closed with delayed absorbable suture and the skin as a separate layer with consideration of perfect adaption of skin edges to avoid secretion and achieve perfect cosmetic appearance.

On the basis of the quite substantial and promising results in the literature and by following these recommendations, we find it feasible for experienced surgeons to initiate studies and, in protocol, perform LESS supracervical hysterectomies.

References

1. Li M, Han Y, Feng YC (2012) Single-port laparoscopic hysterectomy versus conventional laparoscopic hysterectomy: a prospective randomized trial. J Int Med Res 40(2):701–708

2. Jung YW et al (2011) A randomized prospective study of single-port and four-port approaches for hysterectomy in terms of postoperative pain. Surg Endosc 25(8):2462–2469

3. Eom JM et al (2013) A comparative cross-sectional study on cosmetic outcomes after single port or conventional laparoscopic surgery. Eur J Obstet Gynecol Reprod Biol 167(1):104–109

4. Wang T et al (2012) Comparison study of single-port (Octoport) and four-port total laparoscopic hysterectomy. Eur J Obstet Gynecol Reprod Biol 161(2):215–218

5. Choi YS et al (2013) Single-port vs. conventional multi-port access laparoscopy-assisted vaginal hysterectomy: comparison of surgical outcomes and complications. Eur J Obstet Gynecol Reprod Biol 169(2):366–369

6. Springborg H, Istre O (2012) Single port laparoscopic surgery: concept and controversies of a new technique. Acta Obstet Gynecol Scand 91(10):1237–1240

7. Park HS et al (2011) Single-port access (SPA) laparoscopic surgery in gynecology: a surgeon's experience with an initial 200 cases. Eur J Obstet Gynecol Reprod Biol 154(1):81–84

8. Puntambekar S et al (2012) Single-incision total laparoscopic hysterectomy with conventional laparoscopy ports. Int J Gynaecol Obstet 117(1):37–39

9. Ichikawa M et al (2011) Evaluation of laparoendoscopic single-site gynecologic surgery with a multitrocar access system. J Nippon Med Sch 78(4):235–240

10. Harmanli OH et al (2009) A comparison of short-term outcomes between laparoscopic supracervical and total hysterectomy. Am J Obstet Gynecol 201(5):536 e1–7

11. Mueller A et al (2009) Comparison of total laparoscopic hysterectomy (TLH) and laparoscopy-assisted supracervical hysterectomy (LASH) in women with uterine leiomyoma. Eur J Obstet Gynecol Reprod Biol 144(1):76–79

12. Cipullo L et al (2009) Laparoscopic supracervical hysterectomy compared to total hysterectomy. JSLS 13(3):370–375

13. Lieng M et al (2008) Long-term outcomes following laparoscopic supracervical hysterectomy. BJOG 115(13):1605–1610

14. Lieng M et al (2005) Outpatient laparoscopic supracervical hysterectomy with assistance of the lap loop. J Minim Invasive Gynecol 12(3):290–294

15. Kim TJ, Lee YY, An JJ, Choi CH, Lee JW, Kim BG, Bae DS (2012) Does single-port access (SPA) laparoscopy mean reduced pain? A retrospective cohort analysis between SPA and conventional laparoscopy. Elsevier Ireland Ltd, Ireland

16. Chen YJ, Wang PH, Ocampo EJ, Twu NF, Yen MS, Chao KC (2011) Single-port compared with conventional laparoscopic-assisted vaginal hysterectomy: a randomized controlled trial. Obstet Gynecol 117(4):906–912

17. Song T et al (2013) Cosmetic outcomes of laparoendoscopic single-site hysterectomy compared with multi-port surgery: randomized controlled trial. J Minim Invasive Gynecol 20(4):460–467

18. Yim GW et al (2010) Transumbilical single-port access versus conventional total laparoscopic hysterectomy: surgical outcomes. Am J Obstet Gynecol 203(1):26 e1–6

19. Gunderson CC et al (2012) The risk of umbilical hernia and other complications with laparoendoscopic single-site surgery. J Minim Invasive Gynecol 19(1):40–45

20. Fader AN et al (2010) Laparoendoscopic single-site surgery in gynecology. Curr Opin Obstet Gynecol 22(4):331–338

5

Pictorial blood loss assessment chart for quantification of menstrual blood loss: a systematic review

Sherif A. El-Nashar[1,2] · Sherif A. M. Shazly[1,2] · Abimbola O. Famuyide[1]

Abstract To evaluate the diagnostic accuracy of pictorial blood loss assessment chart (PBLAC) compared to objective measurements of menstrual blood loss (MBL), a systematic search of MEDLINE, EMBASE, Cumulative Index to Nursing & Allied Health Literature (CINAHL), Web of Science, and EBM Reviews-Cochrane Central Register of Controlled Trials from inception until September 30, 2014 was performed. Terms referring to "pictorial blood loss assessment chart," "menstrual blood loss evaluation," and "alkaline hematin" were used. The ability of PBLAC to predict significant blood loss, compared to alkaline hematin as a standard objective method, represents our primary outcome. Out of 255 reports identified by the primary search, seven reports were included in the review. Quality of these reports was assessed. Compared to alkaline hematin, PBLAC sensitivity and specificity ranged from 58 to 98 % and 7.5 to 97 %, respectively, with likelihood ratios (LR) for positive ranging from 1.1 to 7.8 and LR for negative tests ranging from 0.04 to 0.48. Diagnostic odds ratio ranged from 2.6 to 86.9. Although diagnostic testing was not always supportive in terms of sensitivity, specificity, and LRs, most studies support the use of PBLAC as a semi-objective method that can be implemented in research and clinical practice.

Keywords Menstruation · Menorrhagia · Heavy menstrual bleeding · Pictorial chart · Diagnostic accuracy · Systematic review

Background

Evaluation of menstrual blood loss (MBL) has evoked an insisting debate for gynecologic researchers and clinicians since the early twentieth century. One of the first reports dates back to 1904, when Hoppe-Seyler and colleagues reported on the use of acid hematin in quantifying MBL [1]. In 1936, Barer and Fowler from the University of Iowa reported the results of assessment of MBL in 100 women and performed a review of the literature in which they identified 32 publications reporting on the previously proposed amount for "normal" MBL [2]. Despite this early interest, to date, there is no tool in current clinical practice that is easy to use, has good correlation with patient complaint, and can detect change in menstruation after treatment [3].

The pictorial blood assessment chart (PBLAC) is a semi-quantitative method for evaluation of MBL that was first published by Higham and Shaw in 1990 and improved and validated by Janssen and colleagues in 1995 [4–6] (Fig. 1). Recently, PBLAC has been increasingly used in clinical research especially pivotal trials that evaluated the effectiveness of non-hysteroscopic-dependent endometrial ablation devices [7]. Nonetheless, there is conflicting evidence about its accuracy [4, 5, 8–12]. The objective of this systematic review is to

This manuscript was presented in the Thirty-Eighth Annual Society of Gynecological Surgeon (SGS) Meeting on April 13–15, 2012, Baltimore, Maryland.

✉ Sherif A. M. Shazly
   sherify2k2@gmail.com

[1] Department of Obstetrics and Gynecology, Mayo Clinic, Rochester, MN, USA

[2] Department of Obstetrics and Gynecology, Assiut University, Assiut, Egypt

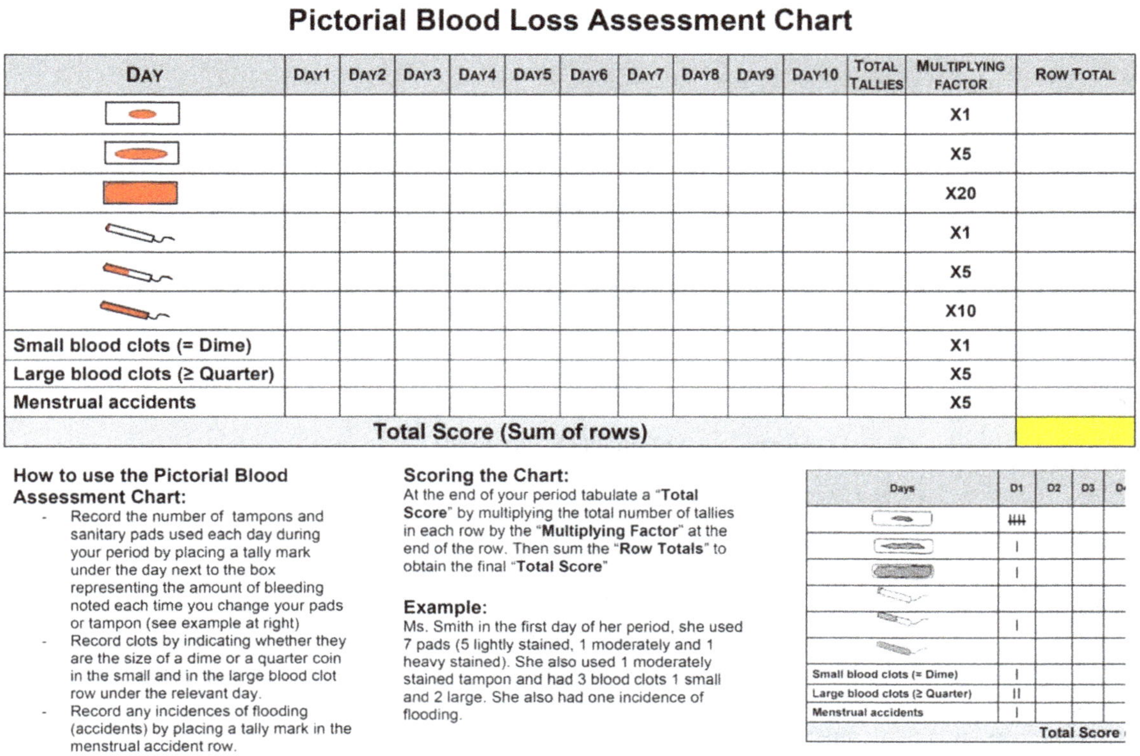

Pictorial Blood Loss Assessment Chart

DAY	DAY1	DAY2	DAY3	DAY4	DAY5	DAY6	DAY7	DAY8	DAY9	DAY10	TOTAL TALLIES	MULTIPLYING FACTOR	ROW TOTAL
▭												X1	
▭												X5	
▬												X20	
╱												X1	
╱												X5	
╱												X10	
Small blood clots (= Dime)												X1	
Large blood clots (≥ Quarter)												X5	
Menstrual accidents												X5	
Total Score (Sum of rows)														

How to use the Pictorial Blood Assessment Chart:
- Record the number of tampons and sanitary pads used each day during your period by placing a tally mark under the day next to the box representing the amount of bleeding noted each time you change your pads or tampon (see example at right)
- Record clots by indicating whether they are the size of a dime or a quarter coin in the small and in the large blood clot row under the relevant day.
- Record any incidences of flooding (accidents) by placing a tally mark in the menstrual accident row.

Scoring the Chart:
At the end of your period tabulate a "Total Score" by multiplying the total number of tallies in each row by the "Multiplying Factor" at the end of the row. Then sum the "Row Totals" to obtain the final "Total Score"

Example:
Ms. Smith in the first day of her period, she used 7 pads (5 lightly stained, 1 moderately and 1 heavy stained). She also used 1 moderately stained tampon and had 3 blood clots 1 small and 2 large. She also had one incidence of flooding.

Days	D1	D2	D3	D
▭	||||			
▬	I			
▬	I			
╱				
╱	I			
╱				
Small blood clots (= Dime)	I			
Large blood clots (≥ Quarter)	II			
Menstrual accidents	I			
Total Score				

Fig. 1 Pictorial blood assessment chart [modified with permission from John Wiley and Sons (Figure 1 in 4)]

evaluate the diagnostic accuracy of PBLAC in evaluating MBL.

Methods

This systematic review was reported in accordance with the Meta-analysis of Observational Studies in Epidemiology recommendation and the *Standards for Reporting of Diagnostic Accuracy initiatives* and the guidelines for conducting systematic reviews of diagnostic studies [13, 14].

Systematic search strategy and study selection

A systematic search of MEDLINE, EMBASE, Cumulative Index to Nursing & Allied Health Literature (CINAHL), Web of Science, and EBM Reviews-Cochrane Central Register of Controlled Trials from inception until September 30, 2014 was performed. The objective of the search was to identify all published reports on the evaluation of menstrual blood loss in humans. No language restriction was applied. In this search, terms referring to "menorrhagia," "menstrual blood loss evaluation," and "pictorial chart" were used. Only studies that compared PBLAC to alkaline hematin were included in the review. The search was designed and conducted with the help of an experienced librarian. In addition, the

bibliographies of the retrieved articles and recent reviews were used to identify additional studies.

Outcome of interest

The primary outcome was the diagnostic accuracy of PBLAC compared to objective measurements of MBL. The intention was to pool the results of identified studies using meta-analysis.

PBLAC is a chart that works by recording a count for each type of sanitary pad used and its degree of soaking as depicted in a pictorial example along with the count and size of blood clots. Menstrual accidents are also captured in a separate row. A *row score* is calculated by multiplying total count of each row by the "Multiplying factor" at the end of each row. Then, a "total score" is calculated by adding the row totals (Fig. 1). On the other hand, objective measurements of MBL are conducted by several spectrophotometric and radioisotopic methods, which directly measure the amount of blood in sanitary products based on hemoglobin content (alkaline hematin).

Data collection and evaluation of the quality of included studies

A sheet was designed for data collection; it included the number of patients in each study and the number who had subjective complaints. MBL in excess of 80 mL was used as the cutoff for the objective definition of excessive menstrual blood loss. Data about the range or variation of estimated MBL in each study were also included. The requisite data were extracted from the text, tables, or figures. Evaluation of the included reports using the *Standards for Reporting of Diagnostic Accuracy (STARD) guidelines* was planned [15].

Statistical analysis

For evaluation of the diagnostic accuracy of PBLAC score, sensitivity, specificity, likelihood ratios of a positive and negative test (LR+ and LR−), diagnostic odds ratio (DOR), and area under the curve (AUC) for receiver operator characteristic (ROC) curve were calculated. Likelihood ratio is the probability of a given level of a test result for patients with the disease divided by the probability of that same result for patients without the disease. Likelihood ratio of a positive test (LR+) equals sensitivity/(1−specificity); while, LR of a negative test (LR−) equals (1−sensitivity)/specificity. Diagnostic odds ratio ranges from zero to infinity, with higher values indicating better discriminatory test performance. Area under the curve ranges from zero to one with better accuracy with values towards 1.0 [15]. Receiver operator characteristic plot was done for studies which evaluated the diagnostic accuracy of pictorial blood assessment chart compared to alkaline hematin using statistical software program Meta-DiSc version 1.1.1 (Ramón y Cajal Hospital, Madrid, Spain). No pooling of data was attempted given the wide heterogeneity and variations between the included studies in the method used and the cutoffs for defining excessive menstrual blood loss. Analysis was done using JMP version 9.0 (SAS Institute Inc, Cary, NC, USA).

Findings

Our systematic search identified 295 reports. After exclusions, seven studies that evaluated the accuracy of PBLAC compared to alkaline hematin (gold standard) in the detection of MBL>80 mL were included for analysis (Fig. 2). Evaluation of the quality of the included reports was performed (Table 1) [4, 5, 8–12]. Apart from blinding to reference and index tests, the parameters of quality of these studies seemed satisfactory.

A total of 1152 women represented the pooled population of the seven studies. Of these, women who experienced MBL>80 mL ranged from 12 to 61 % (average 38.71 %). Five studies assigned "100 mL" as a cutoff point for assessment of PBLAC score accuracy including the first study that was conducted by Higham. Other cutoff points (50, 80, and 150 mL) were used in individual studies. Sanitary products that were utilized in PBLAC score assessment are listed in Table 2.

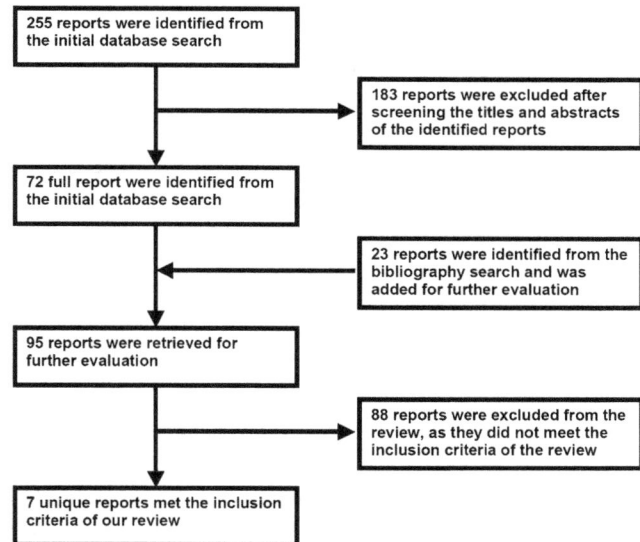

Fig. 2 Flow chart for study selection

The sensitivity of PBLAC ranged from 58 to 98 %, and the specificity from 7.5 to 97 % with likelihood ratios (LR) for positive ranging from 1.1 to 7.8 and LR for negative tests ranging from 0.04 to 0.48. The range of diagnostic odds ratio was from 2.6 to 86.9 (Table 2). However, the high level of variability among these studies precluded pooling of those estimates. Summary receiver operator characteristic (SROC) plot of the accuracy of PBLAC compared to alkaline hematin among recruited studies was illustrated in Fig. 3.

Discussion

MBL has been an issue of debate in both clinical practice and research work. Since PBLAC was introduced in the literature, validation of the chart has been a primary objective in several studies that were conducted in the last 25 years. In this systematic review, we described the diagnostic accuracy of PBLAC in these studies. Despite their heterogeneity, PBLAC seems to be a satisfactory alternative to objective methods that are difficult to implicate.

Objective methods for assessment of MBL

In the beginning of the twentieth century, several spectrophotometric and radioisotopic methods were developed to measure the amount of blood loss from sanitary products directly. The measurement of blood depended on either the measurement of hemoglobin content (e.g., acid hematin and alkaline hematin) or iron content (e.g.,

Table 1 Methodological quality evaluation with the quality assessment of diagnostic accuracy studies questionnaire

Quality	Question no. and primary characteristic	Study						
		Higham [4]	Janssen [3]	Deeny [8]	Barr [9]	Reid [10]	Wyatt [11]	Zakherah [12]
Generalizability	Q1: spectrum of patients	−	+	+	+	−	+	+
Clarity	Q2: selection criteria	+	+	+	+	+	+	+
	Q8: index test	+	+	+	+	+	+	+
	Q9: reference test	+	+	+	+	+	+	+
	Q13: uninterruptible/intermediate test results	+	+	+	+	−	+	+
	Q14: withdrawals	+	+	+	+	+	+	+
Validity	Q3: reference test	+	+	+	+	+	+	+
	Q4: time between reference test and index test	+	+	+	+	+	+	+
	Q5: verification using reference test	+	+	+	+	+	+	+
	Q6: reference standard regardless of index test results	+	+	+	+	+	+	+
	Q7: reference standard independent of the index test	+	+	+	+	+	+	+
	Q10: blinding to reference test	−	−	−	−	−	−	−
	Q11: blinding to index test	−	−	−	−	−	−	−
	Q12: same data available before interpretation of both index and reference tests	+	+	+	+	+	+	+

The information is from Whiting et al. [13]. In the questionnaire, plus sign indicates "yes," minus sign indicates "no," and question mark indicates "unclear."

iron-labeled isotopes and chemical extraction of iron) [1, 2, 16–19]. Methods that depend on iron chemical extraction were limited by the low extraction rates and systematic underestimation of blood loss. The use of

Table 2 Diagnostic accuracy parameters of pictorial blood assessment chart (PBLAC) in the diagnoses for objective heavy menstrual bleeding (MBL 80 mL)

Study	Number	PBLAC cutoff point (in mL)	Sanitary product	MBL>80 mL (%)	Sensitivity (%)	Specificity (%)	+LR	−LR	DOR
Higham et al. [4]	122	100	Tampax Fems super plus tampons and Kotex Simplicity size 2 towels	50	86	89	7.8	0.16	50.1
Janssen et al. [3]	288	100	Kotex Maxi Long Pads (Kimberly Clark, Veenendaal, Holland), Tampax super tampons (Unicura, Zoetermeer, Holland)	31	98	64	2.7	0.04	76.7
Deeny et al. [8]	53	100	Women used their customary sanitary material	47	88	52	1.8	0.23	8.0
Barr et al. [9]	281	50	Sanitary wear not specified	12	58	88	4.8	0.48	10.1
Reid et al. [10]	103	100	Tampax super (Tambrands, Havant, UK) and Kotex Simplicity size 2 (Kimberly Clark, Aylesford, Kent, UK)	61	97	7.5	1.1	0.40	2.6
Wyatt et al. [11]	108	80[a]	Tampax regular, super, or super plus and Kotex Maxi super or Maxi nighttime napkins	16	86	88	7.2	0.16	45.3
Zakherah et al. [12]	197	100	Always Ultra, Proctor & Gamble, Cairo, Egypt	54	99	39	1.6	0.02	86.9
	197	150		54	83	77	3.5	0.22	15.7

+LR likelihood ratio for a positive test, LR− likelihood ratio for a negative test, DOR diagnostic odds ratio

[a] In Wyatt report, the unit of score was an estimated milliliter unlike the original PBLAC by Higham, which included absolute values

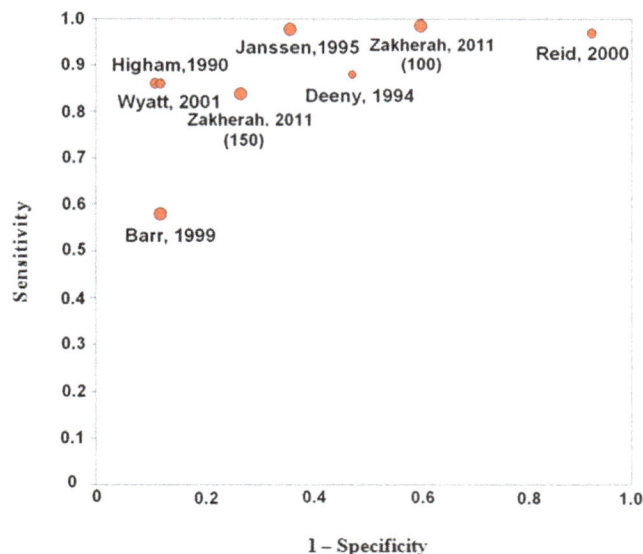

Fig. 3 Summary receiver operator characteristic (SROC) plot for studies which evaluated the diagnostic accuracy of pictorial blood assessment chart compared to alkaline hematin. Heterogeneity among study population and the use of various cutoff precluded pooling of the diagnostic accuracy measures in those studies

labeled isotopes conveyed some radiation exposure hazards and did not provide higher accuracy compared to spectrophotometric methods [20].

Because direct methods were sophisticated and were not suitable for implementation among general population, another approach was to indirectly calculate hemoglobin contents by weighing sanitary product before and after use [21]. Despite being simpler, the accuracy of this method is limited by the variability in the blood content of menstrual fluid which ranges between 30 and 50 % of total menstrual fluid volume and which differs from day to day during menstrual period [22, 23]. This method was refined by Fraser and colleagues in 2001; however, complexity of proper collection of the sanitary pads precluded its use in clinical and research settings [24].

In most objective methods, extensive efforts are needed by patients to collect their sanitary products along with the inconveniences and difficulties that often adversely impact the accuracy of collection of sanitary pads [4, 6]. In addition, the measuring technique is lab intensive and impractical in the clinical settings [24]. Another concern is the inability to measure extraneous blood loss which can affect the total amount of MBL especially in cases of severe bleeding [25]. Finally, the recovered amounts of alkaline hematin are influenced by the variability of absorption of different sanitary products, a problem that could not be overcome unless a sanitary product is standardized or a reference is set for different sanitary products. All these factors precluded the use of extraction-based quantitative methods in clinical settings [26].

Accuracy of pictorial blood assessment chart

Given the inaccuracies of the subjective evaluation of MBL and the limitations of the objective methods that preclude their use in clinical practice, other methods have been developed. The most widely used is the PBLAC. While the score in the original PBLAC was not measured with actual blood loss, another chart was developed by Wyatt and colleague in 2001 [25]. The PBLAC is a practical method for quick evaluation of MBL in women that can be helpful in diagnosis and follow-up of treatment in women with heavy menstrual bleeding [27]. According to our review, although sensitivity, specificity, and LRs were not sufficient to support the accuracy of PBLAC in some studies, the diagnostic odds ratio generally ranged from 2.6 to 86.9 which is a satisfactory range for a good diagnostic test. However, the high level of variability in the accuracy of those studies precluded pooling of their estimates.

It remains one of the most questionable points related to the accuracy of PBLAC that there is no standard sanitary product for assessment of the score; products there were used to test and validate the score were not exactly those that are used nowadays. Accordingly, it has been a serious concern that modern superabsorbent polymer-containing sanitary products in comparison with old products, that were available when PBLAC was created, can confound current interpretation of the chart. Nevertheless, when women were encouraged to use the brands they commonly used, PBLAC was still significantly correlated to their perception of MBL with low intraindividual variation. Accordingly, standardization of sanitary product was not found to grossly impact the applicability of PBLAC [28]. In this review, it does not seem that the type of sanitary product contributes to the heterogeneity of results. SROC showed that studies that used the same products did not necessarily reveal comparable results and vice versa. However, Magnay et al. presented a new version of the traditional menstrual pictogram (the superabsorbent polymer-c or SAP-c version) which was designed to measure MBL on these widely used products (Always Ultra slim feminine towels "Proctor & Gamble"). A validation study of this version yielded promising results when MBL was tested against alkaline hematin method and total menstrual fluid loss (MFL) against fluid weight [29, 30]. Although initial results seem promising, implementation of this version among larger cohorts could help to recognize its feasibility, accuracy, and pitfalls and identify whether this version could be superior to the traditional PBLAC.

Limitations

The need to accurately document the amount of MBL in women as a prerequisite for offering treatment, which is the function of the PBLAC, has been questioned. Indeed, some authors have suggested that any amount of bleeding that adversely impacts a woman's quality of life requires intervention regardless of whether or not specific bleeding criteria are met [27]. Nevertheless, this pitfall is not specific and is associated with any objective estimation of MBL. Also, PBLAC seems to be the most reliable approach for researches that generally require a feasible quantitative method to evaluate and compare therapeutic approaches in women with HMB. It is also suitable for patient follow-up in concordance with clinical evaluation. In certain clinical circumstances when patient's symptomatology may be contributed to by a variety of clinical issues, objective assessment of MBL may be helpful to evaluate the rule of HMB. Another potential limitation in this review was the variability in alkaline hematin assessment methods and the lack of a standard to perform that method.

This review is also limited by the lack of meta-analysis for identification of pooled diagnostic accuracy of PBLAC compared to alkaline hematin for assessment of MBL due to the high level of heterogeneity in the methods and the estimated MBL. In addition, there is lack of information about the reliability of the test when used in the same patients repeatedly and if used after treatment. There is lack of consistency in reporting various endpoints and absence of many demographic characteristics and reliability measurements. This was mainly due to inclusion of many early reports, which had missing information, and the time gap did not help contacting authors. Finally, the diagnostic accuracy of PBLAC was limited in some studies; the range of positive LR was as low as 1.1 and negative LR was as high as 0.48 which indicates careful interpretation of current evidence. However, the diagnostic odds ratio was generally encouraging in most studies.

Conclusions

Despite highlighted limitations, studies that were conducted over 25 years retrieved satisfactory diagnostic outcomes that support the accuracy of PBLAC as a semi-objective method with acceptable diagnostic accuracy compared to objective measurement of MBL.

Authors' contribution SAE carried out study search and selection and retrieval of data and participated in writing the manuscript. SAMS participated in writing the manuscript. AOF planned and supervised all these steps and revised the manuscript.

References

1. Hoppe-Seyler G, Brodersen A, Rudolph A (1904) About the loss of blood during menstruation. Z Physiol Chem 42:545–553
2. Barer AP, Fowler WM (1936) The blood loss during normal menstruation. Am J Obstet Gynecol 31:979–986
3. Janssen CA (2005) Menorrhagia: the 80 mL criterion and the usefulness in clinical practice. Am J Obstet Gynecol 192(6):2093
4. Higham JM, O'Brien PM, Shaw RW (1990) Assessment of menstrual blood loss using a pictorial chart. Br J Obstet Gynaecol 97(8):734–739
5. Janssen CA, Scholten PC, Heintz AP (1995) A simple visual assessment technique to discriminate between menorrhagia and normal menstrual blood loss. Obstet Gynecol 85(6):977–982
6. Janssen CAH (1996) A simple visual assessment technique to discriminate between menorrhagia and normal menstrual blood loss. Eur J Obstet Gynecol Reprod Biol 70(1):21–22
7. American College of Obstetrics and Gynecology (2007) ACOG practice bulletin no. 81: endometrial ablation. Obstet Gynecol 109(5):1233–1248
8. Deeny M, Davis JA (1994) Assessment of menstrual blood loss in women referred for endometrial ablation. Eur J Obstet Gynecol Reprod Biol 57(3):179–180
9. Barr F, Brabin L, Agbaje O (1999) A pictorial chart for managing common menstrual disorders in Nigerian adolescents. Int J Gynaecol Obstet 66(1):51–53
10. Reid PC, Coker A, Coltart R (2000) Assessment of menstrual blood loss using a pictorial chart: a validation study. Br J Obstet Gynaecol 107(3):320–322
11. Wyatt KM, Dimmock PW, Hayes-Gill B, Crowe J, O'Brien PMS (2002) Menstrual symptometrics: a simple computer-aided method to quantify menstrual cycle disorders. Fertil Steril 78(1):96–101
12. Zakherah MS, Sayed GH, El-Nashar SA, Shaaban MM (2011) Pictorial blood loss assessment chart in the evaluation of heavy menstrual bleeding: diagnostic accuracy compared to alkaline hematin. Gynecol Obstet Investig 71(4):281–284
13. Whiting P, Rutjes AW, Dinnes J, Reitsma J, Bossuyt PM, Kleijnen J (2004) Development and validation of methods for assessing the quality of diagnostic accuracy studies. Health Technol Assess 8(25):iii, 1–234
14. Stroup DF, Berlin JA, Morton SC, Olkin I, Williamson GD, Rennie D et al (2000) Meta-analysis of observational studies in epidemiology: a proposal for reporting. Meta-analysis Of Observational Studies in Epidemiology (MOOSE) group. JAMA 283(15):2008–2012
15. Bossuyt PM, Reitsma JB, Bruns DE, Gatsonis CA, Glasziou PP, Irwig LM et al (2003) Towards complete and accurate reporting of studies of diagnostic accuracy: the STARD initiative. Ann Intern Med 138(1):40–44
16. Hallberg L, Nilsson L (1964) Determination of menstrual blood loss. Scand J Clin Lab Invest 16:244–248
17. Baldwin RM, Whalley PJ, Pritchard JA (1961) Measurements of menstrual blood loss. Am J Obstet Gynecol 81:739–742
18. Price DC, Forsyth EM, Cohn SH, Cronkite EP (1964) The study of menstrual and other blood loss, and consequent iron deficiency, by Fe59 whole-body counting. Can Med Assoc J 90:51–54
19. Tauxe WN (1962) Quantitation of menstrual blood loss: a radioactive method utilizing a counting dome. J Nucl Med 3:282–287
20. Hallberg L, Hogdahl AM, Nilsson L, Rybo G (1966) Menstrual blood loss—a population study. Variation at different ages and attempts to define normality. Acta Obstet Gynecol Scand 45(3):320–351
21. Pendergrass PB, Scott JN, Ream LJ (1984) A rapid, noninvasive method for evaluation of total menstrual loss. Gynecol Obstet Invest 17(4):174–178

22. Fraser IS, McCarron G, Markham R, Resta T (1985) Blood and total fluid content of menstrual discharge. Obstet Gynecol 65(2): 194–198

23. Levin RJ, Wagner G (1986) Absorption of menstrual discharge by tampons inserted during menstruation: quantitative assessment of blood and total fluid content. Br J Obstet Gynaecol 93(7):765–772

24. Fraser IS, Warner P, Marantos PA (2001) Estimating menstrual blood loss in women with normal and excessive menstrual fluid volume. Obstet Gynecol 98(5 Pt 1):806–814

25. Wyatt KM, Dimmock PW, Walker TJ, O'Brien PM (2001) Determination of total menstrual blood loss. Fertil Steril 76(1): 125–131

26. O'Flynn N, Britten N (2000) Menorrhagia in general practice— disease or illness. Soc Sci Med 50(5):651–661

27. National Collaborating Center for Women's and Children Health. Heavy menstrual bleeding: Clinical Guidelines January, 2007. Welsh A, editor. London: RCOG Press; 2007. 152 p

28. Hald K, Lieng M (2014) Assessment of periodic blood loss: inter-individual and intraindividual variations of pictorial blood loss assessment chart registrations. J Minim Invasive Gynecol 21(4):662– 668

29. Magnay JL, Nevatte TM, O'Brien S, Gerlinger C, Seitz C (2014) Validation of a new menstrual pictogram (superabsorbent polymer-c version) for use with ultraslim towels that contain superabsorbent polymers. Fertil Steril 101(2):515–522

30. Magnay JL, Nevatte TM, Seitz C, O'Brien S (2013) A new menstrual pictogram for use with feminine products that contain superabsorbent polymers. Fertil Steril 100(6):1715–1721, e1-4

6

Large ovarian cysts assumed to be benign treated via laparoscopy

J. L. Herraiz Roda[1] · J. A. Llueca Abella[1] · C. Catalá Masó[1] ·
Y. Maazouzi[1] · M. Colecha Morales[1] · A. Serra Rubert[1] ·
D. Piquer Simó[1] · C. Oliva Martí[1] · E. Calpe Gómez[1]

Abstract The aim of this study was to assess the feasibility and outcome of laparoscopic surgery in the management of large ovarian cysts in patients treated at a university hospital. Twelve patients with large (diameter >10 cm) ovarian cysts were managed laparoscopically from November 2009 to July 2014. The cystic masses were not associated with ascites or enlarged lymph nodes on ultrasound. Serum CA-125 levels were within the normal range (35 U/ml). Preoperative evaluation included history, clinical examination, sonographic images, and serum markers. The management of these ovarian cysts included aspiration, cystectomy, or salpingo-oophorectomy, depending on the patient's age, obstetric history, and desire for future fertility. Five patients presented with abdominal pain and two with abdominal distension and discomfort. In the five patients, the cyst was an incidental finding on a routine review. The average maximum diameter of the ovarian cysts was 25 cm (range 13–41 cm). The mean duration of the operation was 87 min. The postoperative hospital stay was 1–4 days. No intraoperative complications occurred, and the hospital course of all patients was uncomplicated. In no case was laparoscopy converted to laparotomy. With proper patient selection, the size of an ovarian cyst is not necessarily a contraindication for laparoscopic surgery.

Keywords Laparoscopy · Large ovarian cyst · Minimally invasive surgery · Ovarian neoplasms

✉ J. L. Herraiz Roda
sgo.herraiz@gmail.com

[1] Department of Obstetrics and Gynecology, General University Hospital of Castellón, Avenida Benicassim, 12004 Castellas, Spain

Introduction

Ovarian neoplasms are a common clinical problem, affecting females of all age groups. In the USA, it has been estimated that approximately 10 % of the female population will undergo a surgical procedure for a suspected ovarian neoplasm during her lifetime [1].

Laparoscopy is considered as the gold standard approach to manage benign ovarian cysts. Treatment strategies of ovarian cysts are determined by the patient's age, menstrual status, symptoms, and the size and structure of the cyst [2]. The advantages of a laparoscopic approach over a laparotomy include better cosmetic results, less blood loss, less pain and analgesic requirement, faster recovery, and shorter hospitalization time [3].

A major factor affecting the gynecological surgeon's decision to perform a laparotomy is the size of the ovarian mass. The laparoscopic approach to large ovarian cysts extending to the umbilicus may be difficult because of the risk of cyst rupture and the small working space [4, 5]. The laparoscopic management of very large ovarian cysts has been described [6–14], but most patients are managed by laparotomy.

The aim of this study was to evaluate the safety, effectiveness, and feasibility of laparoscopy in the management of ovarian cysts extending above the umbilicus. The results of the 12 patients with large ovarian cysts managed laparoscopically are reported herein.

Materials and methods

Twelve patients with very large ovarian cysts were included in the study. All of the patients underwent laparoscopy at the General University Hospital of Castellón, Spain, between November 2009 and July 2014.

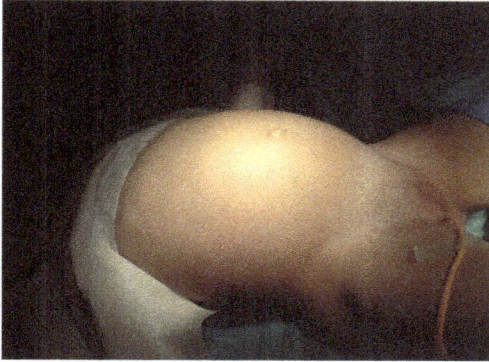

Fig. 1 Patient under general anesthesia

The cystic masses were not associated with ascites or enlarged lymph nodes on ultrasound. Serum CA-125 levels were within the normal range (35 U/ml) in all patients. Preoperative evaluation included history, clinical examination, sonographic images, and serum markers. No cases were excluded solely based on the cyst's size, only those suspected of malignant pathology. Therefore, out of all the cases, three patients with gigantic cysts did not undergo the laparoscopic procedure due to an elevated risk of malignancy. Two other cases were excluded due to high levels of serum markers and one due to the presence of ascites. Informed consent was obtained for possible conversion to laparotomy in case of technical difficulties or an incidental finding of malignancy. All surgeries were performed with the patients under general anesthesia (Fig. 1).

The Hasson method (open-entry laparoscopic technique) was used to avoid puncturing the cyst prior to its intraoperative evaluation. The cyst wall was inspected prior to drainage. If there were no signs of malignancy, three additional trocars were inserted. The cyst was then drained under laparoscopic guidance using a suction irrigation device. If the size of the cyst was too large for this approach, a 3-cm umbilical incision was made that extended into the peritoneal cavity. An incision was made on the surface of the cyst, through which a Hasson trocar was then inserted. The cyst's content was then aspirated through the Hasson trocar in order to avoid spillage. Once the cyst was emptied, the Hasson trocar was removed and the cystic capsule was released into the abdominal cavity. The Hasson trocar was once again inserted in the abdominal wall in the usual manner. Three accessory trocars were then inserted, and the laparoscopic adnexectomy was performed using the usual method (Fig. 2). The cyst was decompressed, with careful attention to avoid spillage of its contents, prior to the placement of accessory trocars. Laparoscopic oophorectomy was then performed in the usual manner. The cystic mass was removed via a laparoscopic bag through the umbilical incision (Fig. 3). In no case was laparoscopy converted to laparotomy.

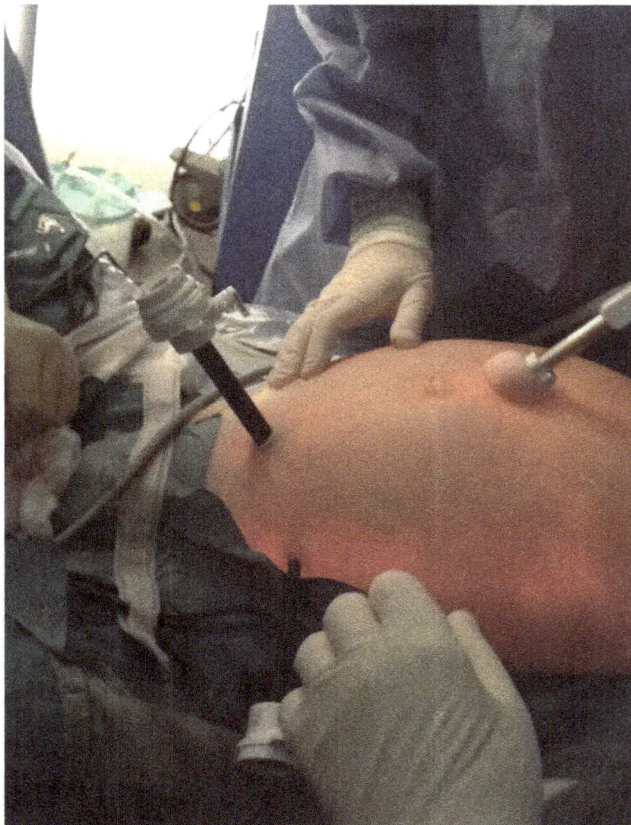

Fig. 2 The Hasson method (open-entry laparoscopic technique) in which three accessory trocars are inserted in the abdominal wall

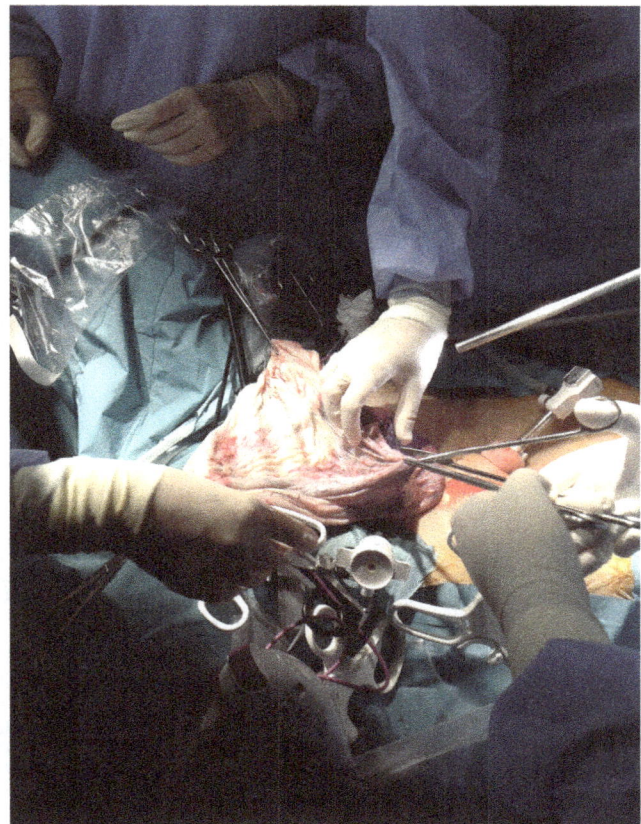

Fig. 3 Removal of a cystic mass

Table 1 Patient characteristics and operative details

Patient	1	2	3	4	5	6	7	8	9	10	11	12	Mean
Age (years)	62	62	82	18	49	59	11	61	17	19	48	53	45
Maximum cyst diameter (cm)	34	16	25	26	32	33	20	13	18	41	25	17	25
Tumor markers	Normal	Normal	Normal	Ca 125: normal Ca 19.9:256	Normal	Normal	Normal	Normal	Normal	Normal	Normal	Normal	
Family history	No	No	No	No	No	No	No	No	No	No	No	No	
CT scan	Yes	Yes	No	No	Yes	Yes	Yes	No	Yes	Yes	No	No	
Clinical presentation	Pain	Pain	Pain	Pain	Abdominal distension	Abdominal distension	Incidental finding	Incidental finding	Pain	Incidental finding	Incidental finding	Incidental finding	
Operation time (min)	110	105	70	115	60	50	100	90	90	80	75	95	87
Fluids drained	8000	2500	3200	3500	15,000	7000	3000	1900	2700	12,000	3400	2600	5400
Number of ports	4	4	4	4	4	4	4	4	4	4	4	4	
Pathology	Mucinous borderline tumor	Serous borderline tumor	Serous cystadenoma	Mucinous cystadenoma	Mucinous cystadenoma	Mucinous cystadenoma	Mature cystic teratoma	Serous cystadenoma	Mature cystic teratoma	Cystadenofibroma	Mucinous borderline tumor	Cystadenofibroma	
Procedure performed	Adnexectomy	Adnexectomy	Adnexectomy	Adnexectomy	Adnexectomy	Adnexectomy	Adnexectomy	Adnexectomy	Adnexectomy	Adnexectomy	Adnexectomy	Adnexectomy	
Postoperative discharge day	3	1	3	3	1	2	1	1	2	4	2	2	

Results

All the patients had similar, non-specific presentations, including pain, abdominal distention, and discomfort. The mean age was 45 years (range 11–82 years) (Table 1). Three patients had previously undergone surgery for non-related causes. The family history was negative for ovarian cancer in all patients. The tumor markers CA-125, CA-19.9, and carcinoma embryonic antigen were normal in all patients, except in one patient with a CA-19.9 of 256 (Table 1). Transabdominal ultrasound scans performed in the 12 patients revealed a large unilocular cyst, some with fine septations, but no solid components or ascites. At our institution, neither computed tomography (CT) nor magnetic resonance imaging (MRI) is performed if the ultrasound findings are highly suggestive of a benign cyst—that is, a unilocular cyst with no solid areas or thick septations and no ascites. However, some patients were referred with a CT scan (Fig. 4) and one with MRI. The mean size of the cysts as measured by preoperative ultrasound scans was 25 cm (range 13–41 cm).

The mean operative time was 87 min (range 50–115 min). The mean volume of fluid drained from the cysts was 5400 mL (range 1900–15,000 mL). Adnexectomy was performed in all patients. Histopathology revealed serous cystadenoma in two patients, mucinous cystadenoma in three, mature cystic teratoma in two, cystadenofibroma in two, serous borderline tumor in one, and mucinous borderline tumor in two.

Four trocars were used in each procedure, which were well tolerated by the 12 patients. There were no intraoperative or postoperative complications. All patients were discharged the next 1 to 4 days postoperatively.

Discussion

Very large ovarian cysts are traditionally managed using a full midline laparotomy [15]. Minimally invasive surgical techniques have been applied, but only a few cases have been reported. All reported techniques include decompression of the cyst to provide an adequate working space, facilitate manipulation of the cyst, and prevent inadvertent perforation and spillage.

Fifteen adult patients with giant (>10 cm) ovarian cysts as described by Salem underwent laparoscopic procedures. All of the cysts were benign, and the cyst fluid was aspirated after puncturing the cyst wall, after which the cyst was removed as usual. No conversions or other complications were recorded. Nine of the cysts were mucinous, and six were serous cystadenomas [16].

Other authors suggest drainage of these cysts via a minilaparotomy to allow for a more controlled approach to minimizing spillage than is possible with percutaneous

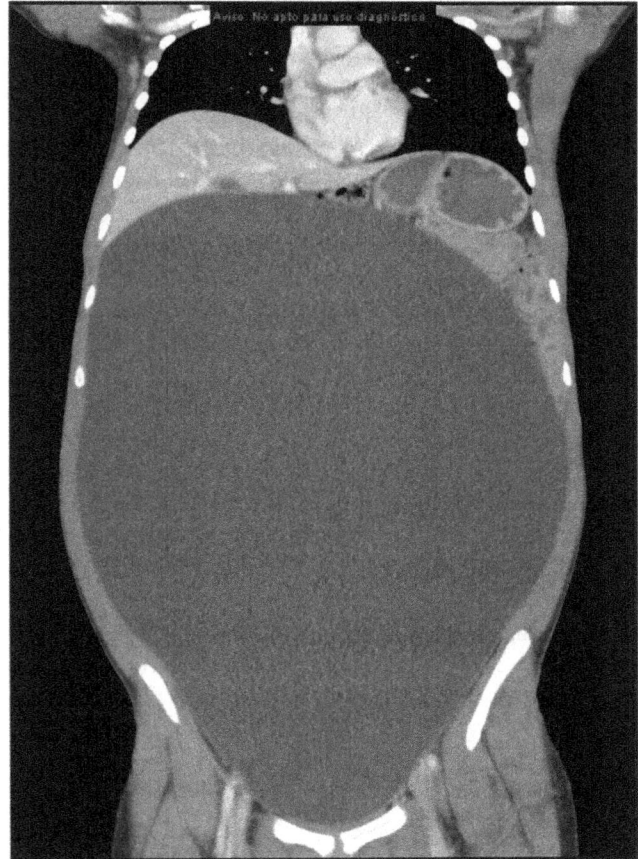

Fig. 4 CT scan of a patient with a large unilocular cyst

techniques; in addition, prelaparoscopic decompression is necessary to allow the establishment of a pneumoperitoneum for highly voluminous cysts [17].

Giant ovarian cysts can be drained before the laparoscopic approach to establish sufficient working space. Nagele [6] drained a large ovarian cyst with a Veress needle under ultrasonographic guidance before laparoscopy. Cevrioglu [18] performed a laparoscopic cyst excision after ultrasound-guided drainage with a spinal needle in a patient with a giant paraovarian cyst.

The use of laparoscopy in the management of ovarian cysts is determined by patient factors, including a history of previous abdominal surgery and premorbid conditions. However, this approach should provide all the benefits typically associated with laparoscopic techniques, i.e., decreased blood loss, less pain, shorter hospital stay, and a significantly better cosmetic result [5, 17].

The use of a laparoscopic approach for ovarian cysts with suspicious features is controversial owing to concerns related to potential spillage of the cyst contents into the peritoneal cavity. Spillage of dermoid cyst material can lead to an extensive inflammatory reaction, resulting in the formation of peritoneal adhesions, while spillage from a mucinous cyst may result in pseudomyxoma peritonei [19]. In the case of a malignant cyst, spillage of its contents can result in the intraperitoneal dissemination of malignant cells and thereby advance the stage of the disease [20].

It is uncommon to encounter an unexpected malignant ovarian mass. Nezhat intraoperatively discovered only four ovarian cancers in 1011 surgically managed patients [21]. There is no established guideline on the optimal timing of rescheduling the staging operation. A complete management plan based on accurate staging is more beneficial to patients in terms of long-term survival than under-treatment due to poor or no staging [22].

The literature data on the prognostic significance of intraoperative or surgical spill in the case of a malignant cyst are conflicting. In a meta-analysis of the effect of intraoperative rupture of the ovarian capsule on prognosis, Kim et al. [23] screened 518 studies and selected nine retrospective studies comprising 2382 patients. They found that preoperative rupture increased the recurrence rate when compared with intraoperative rupture (hazard ratio, 2.63; 95 % confidence interval, 1.11–6.20). Patients with preoperative rupture had a poorer overall survival than those with no or intraoperative rupture.

Animal studies have shown that laparoscopy may accelerate the dissemination of malignant cells [24], but this has yet to be proven in humans. Childers et al. [25] commented that laparoscopy itself is not the cause of the problem for these patients and that surgical mismanagement can occur with any surgical approach.

Conclusions

With proper patient selection, minimally invasive surgery is a feasible and safe treatment of large ovarian cysts, demonstrating that size is not necessarily a consideration in the laparoscopic management of very large ovarian cysts. When performed by experienced endoscopic surgeons, laparoscopy may decrease the rate of unnecessary laparotomies for benign cysts.

Author's contribution JL Herraiz was responsible for project development, data collection, and manuscript writing; Y Maazouzi for manuscript writing/editing; A Llueca for protocol development; C Catala, M Colecha, D Piquer, A Serra, and C Oliva for data collection; and E Calpe for protocol development.

References

1. Hilger WE, Magriña JF, Magtibay PM (2006) Laparoscopic management of the adnexal mass. Clin Obstet Gynecol 49:535–548
2. Helmrath MA, Shin CE, Warner BW (1998) Ovarian cysts in the pediatric population. Semin Pediatr Surg 7:19–28
3. Yuen PM, Yu KM, Yip SK et al (1997) A randomized prospective study of laparoscopy and laparotomy in the management of unending ovarian masses. Am J Obstet Gynecol 177:109–114
4. Knudsen UB, Tabor A, Mosgaard B et al (2004) Management of ovarian cysts. Acta Obstet Gynecol Scand 83:1012–1021
5. Ma KK, Tsui PZ, Wong WC et al (2004) Laparoscopic management of large ovarian cysts: more than cosmetic consideration. Hong Kong Med J 10:139–141
6. Nagele F, Magos AL (1996) Combined ultrasonographically guided drainage and laparoscopic excision of a large ovarian cyst. Am J Obstet Gynecol 175(5):1377–1378
7. Jeong EH, Kim HS, Ahn CS et al (1997) Successful laparoscopic removal of huge ovarian cysts. J Am Assoc Gynecol Laparosc 4:609–614
8. Postma VA, Wegdam JA, Janssen IM (2002) Laparoscopic extirpation of a giant ovarian cyst. Surg Endosc 16(2):361
9. Sagiv R, Golan A, Glezerman M (2005) Laparoscopic management of extremely large ovarian cysts. Obstet Gynecol 105:1319–1322
10. Eltabbakh GH, Charboneau AM, Eltabbakh NG (2008) Laparoscopic surgery for large benign ovarian cysts. Gynecol Oncol 108(1):72–76
11. Ate O, Karakaya E, Hakgüder G, Olguner M, Seçil M, Akgür FM (2006) Laparoscopic excision of a giant ovarian cyst after ultrasound-guided drainage. J Pediatr Surg 41(10):e9–e11
12. Goh SM, Yam J, Loh SF, Wong A (2007) Minimal access approach to the management of large ovarian cysts. Surg Endosc Interv Techn 21(1):80–83
13. Yi SW (2012) Minimally invasive management of huge ovarian cysts by laparoscopic extracorporeal approach. Minim Invasive Ther Allied Technol 21(6):429–434
14. Lim S, Lee KB, Chon SJ, Park CY (2012) Is tumor size the limiting factor in a laparoscopic management for large ovarian cysts? Arch Gynecol Obstet 285(5):1227–1232
15. Westfall CT, Andrassy RJ (1982) Giant ovarian cyst: case report and review of differential diagnosis in adolescents. Clin Pediat (Phila) 21:228–230
16. Salem AFH (2002) Laparoscopic excision of large ovarian cysts. J Obstet Gynaecol Res 28:290–294
17. Dolan MS, Boulanger SC, Salameh JR (2006) Laparoscopic management of giant ovarian cyst. JSLS 10:252–256
18. Cevrioglu AS, Polat C, Fenkc V et al (2004) Laparoscopic management following ultrasonographic-guided drainage in a patient with giant paraovarian cyst. Surg Endosc 18:346
19. Morrow CP (1998) Tumors of the ovary: classification: the adnexal mass. In: Morrow CP, Curtin J (eds) Synopsis of gynecologic oncology. Churchill Livingstone, Philadelphia, pp 215–232
20. Berek J (2000) Epithelial ovarian cancer. In: Berek J, Hacker N (eds) Practical gynecologic oncology. Lippincott Williams & Wilkins, Philadelphia, pp 457–522
21. Nezhat F, Nezhat C, Welander CE, Benigno B (1992) Four ovarian cancers diagnosed during laparoscopic management of 1011 women with adnexal masses. Am J Obstet Gynecol 167(3):790–796
22. Alvarez RD, Kilgore LC, Partridge EE, Austin JM, Shingleton HM (1993) Staging ovarian cancer diagnosed during laparoscopy: accuracy rather than immediacy. South Med J 86:1256–1258
23. Kim HS, Ahn JH, Chung HH, Kim JW, Park NH, Song YS et al (2013) Impact of intraoperative rupture of the ovarian capsule on prognosis in patients with early-stage epithelial ovarian cancer: a meta-analysis. Eur J Sug Oncol 39:279–289

7

Total laparoscopic hysterectomy with previous cesarean section using a standardized technique: experience of Pontificia Universidad Catolica de Chile

C. Celle[1] · C. Pomés[1] · G. Durruty[1] · M. Zamboni[1] · M. Cuello[1]

Abstract Total laparoscopic hysterectomy (TLH) in the presence of patients with previous cesarean section (CS) is becoming increasingly common. When performing TLH in these patients, bladder adhesions to the uterus may make dissection much more difficult with higher complication rates. The aim of this study was to assess the safety of TLH in patients with previous CS in an OBGYN residence program. Retrospective study of all TLH performed at our center for either benign or malignant conditions. Of our study cohort, 40 % had undergone one or more previous CS. Average surgical time was 128 min for patients without previous CS and 136 min for patients with previous CS ($p = $ NS). Conversion to laparotomy was required in 1 % of cases showing no variation between the CS and non-CS groups. The overall complication rate among patients undergoing TLH was 3.5 %. Major complication rate was of 3 % ($n=14$), 5 cases with previous CS and 9 cases with no previous CS ($p = $ NS). Urologic lesion was the most common major complication, accounting for 1.5 % ($n=7$) of all cases, 3 cases with previous CS and 4 with no previous CS ($p = $ NS). Of urologic complications, three were cystotomies, 1 with no previous CS and 2 with previous CS ($p = $ NS). TLH in patients with 1 or more previous CS is technically feasible. In the hands of thoroughly trained laparoscopic surgeons using a standardized technique, it is a safe procedure with minimal complication rates and may be even performed by OBGYN residents ensuring the same success rates.

Keywords Total laparoscopic hysterectomy · Cesarean section

Introduction

Hysterectomy is the most common gynecologic surgery performed worldwide [1]. More than 70 % of hysterectomies are indicated for benign pathologies, mainly uterine fibroids [2]. Three approaches exist to perform hysterectomy: vaginal, abdominal, and laparoscopic. To date, vaginal hysterectomy (VH), when feasible, is the preferred and recommended route for most of cases, especially in an unscarred uterus. A recent Cochrane review stated that VH should be performed in preference of abdominal hysterectomy (AH) when possible given the significant advantages that the vaginal approach offers [3]. They also concluded that laparoscopic hysterectomy (LH) is associated with less bleeding, similar surgical times, and shorter hospital stays when compared to AH, and therefore, LH should be the preferred route when VH is not possible [3].

Currently, hysterectomy constitutes the second most common operation performed in women after cesarean section (CS) [1], which accounts for up to 60 % of deliveries in some countries as estimated by the recent CORONIS trial [4]. In Chile, the current average rate of cesarean section has reached almost 40 %, and it has shown an increasing tendency during recent years [4, 5]. Moreover, health system statistics show that even as high as a 70 % of pregnancies are delivered through cesarean section in the private clinical setting [5–7]. This rate leaves us as the third country with the highest cesarean rate, among The organization for Economic Co-operation and Development (OECD) members, only preceded by Mexico and Turkey [5]. Thus, the estimated number of patients undergoing hysterectomy with a previous cesarean section is expected to be higher every year.

✉ C. Celle
claudiacelle@gmail.com

[1] Division of Obstetrics and Gynecology, UC-Christus Health Network, Pontificia Universidad Católica de Chile, Lira 85, 5th floor, Santiago 8330074, Chile

All patients undergoing hysterectomy, or any gynecologic surgery, are in risk of suffering complications during and after surgery. In patients with previous CS, these risks are much higher and principally related to major blood loss or urologic injuries [8]. Surgical adhesions caused by previous CS may cause distortion of pelvic anatomy, making the vaginal approach technically difficult and therefore an unsafe procedure. This is of outmost importance when mobilizing the bladder off the cervix, a critical step during any hysterectomy. Thus, making the abdominal route a safer alternative for gynecologic surgeons who have been better trained with open surgery. In fact, surgeons tend to prefer the access route with which they feel more confident and exprienced. Surgical innovation, against a well known and dominated technique, is always considered less safe and guilty of any adverse event observed when introducing the new technique. In addition, no publication has addressed the impact of introducing a standardized laparoscopic technique to evaluate the confidence acquired by surgeons and see how they decide to change their prefered access route for total hysterectomy in patients with previous scar.

With the progressive improvement of instrumentation, the reduction in costs associated to laparoscopy, and the gain of expertise among surgeons, LH has started to replace AH for several indications [3, 9]. A major advantage of laparoscopy is the magnified view and detailed exposure of pelvic anatomy that allows the surgeon to easily recognize and access pelvic structures (for example, vascular pedicles, ureters, and pelvic spaces) reducing the risk of bleeding and inadvertently damaging them during dissection [10]. Thus, the laparoscopic approach should constitute a good alternative for cases with previous CS particularly for surgeons who have become well trained in the technique. Besides offering a better view, the laparoscopic approach also offers advantages in terms of operative time, hospital stay, use of analgesia, and short-term patient satisfaction. Therefore, the safety of this approach for hysterectomy in patients with previous CS should be taken into account and evaluated.

No matter what route is chosen by the surgeon, hysterectomy will be a great challenge in patients with previous pelvic or abdominal surgeries, particularly with previous CS. Technical difficulties will be higher, and so will be the complications. Alternatively, surgeons could prefer to perform a subtotal laparoscopic hysterectomy (STLH) instead of total laparoscopic hysterectomy (TLH) to reduce the risk of urological injuries. So far, there is no evidence to support the election of STLH over TLH in patients with previous CS.

Aware of the importance of an adequate training in laparoscopy before performing any advanced laparoscopic procedure, such as TLH, the obstetrics and gynecology residence program in the school of medicine at Pontificia Universidad Católica de Chile has implemented a progressive and supervised laparoscopic training program. All residents must approve the basic and advanced modules before performing any laparoscopic procedure, especially a TLH. In addition, to reduce intraoperative complications, our division has adopted a standardized technique that is applied to all cases undergoing surgery at our institution.

The aim of this study was to assess the safety of TLH in patients with one or more previous CS compared to those without previous surgery in an institution that has an obstetrics and gynecology (OBGYN) residence program and in which all residents perform a standardized technique under supervision.

Materials and methods

We conducted a retrospective study of all TLH performed at the Clinical Hospital of Universidad Catolica and San Carlos Clinic, both belonging to the UC-Christus health network. All patients included in the study signed an informed consent, IRB approved, before undergoing TLH based on their medical condition. The data was collected between January 2006 and April 2014.

There were no exclusion criteria based on the number of previous cesarean section deliveries or surgical indication.

As mentioned in the introduction, a standardized surgical technique was used in all cases, with or without previous CS. We performed a lateral approach as described by Sinha et al. since the bladder is not in direct contact with the cervix at this area [11]. Most of the surgery was carried out using only bipolar energy (35 W), and we restricted the use of monopolar energy (pure cut, 50 W) exclusively to perform the colpotomy in order to reduce thermal damage which has been associated to an increased risk of future vault dehisence [12]. The vaginal vault was then sutured with one single uninterrupted VICRYL-CT Suture (Polyglactin 910) including a uterosacral ligament plicature.

Simultaneously with patient data recollection, we reviewed the delivery database of the health network to register the cesarean rate of each year included in the study to build up the cesarean rate tendency of the period.

Patient demographics, diagnosis, operative time, conversion to laparotomy, uterine weight, and intraoperative and postoperative complications were analyzed. All hysterectomies were performed in a teaching setting, most of them operated by a third year resident assisted by an experienced surgeon who was actively participating of the residence program. All third year residents were required to complete and approve both basic and advanced laparoscopic training modules, during their first and second year residence, respectively, in order to be able to perform a TLH or any other laparoscopic procedure. In order to have an estímate on how many TLH were performed by each resident, they are asked to register every surgical procedure done as first surgeons throughout their complete residency.

Major complications included ureteric injuries, inadvertent cystostomy, vesicovaginal fistula, bowel injuries, sepsis, vault hematoma, vault abscess, and significant hemorrhage.

Statistical analysis included all patients. Differences between groups with and without previous CS were tested with Chi Square, Fisher's exact test, or Student's t test. A p value<.05 was considered statistically significant.

Results

From January 2006 through April 2014, a total of 458 total laparoscopic hysterectomies were identified. Medical record of prior mode of delivery was available in 454 patients. Forty percent of patients ($n=181$) had 1 or more previous CS (median 1, range 1–4). The number of previous CS is detailed in Table 1.

A benign condition was the indication for hysterectomy in 85 % of cases and a malignancy for the remaining 15 %. Fibroid (symptomatic leiomyoma) was the main indication for hysterectomy accounting for 41 % of cases. Indications for hysterectomy are summarized in Table 2.

The median age of patients was 47 years (median 47, range 30–83). The average surgical time was of 131 min (median of 120 min, range 50–360 min). For the group of patients without previous CS, the average surgical time was 128 min (median 120 min, range 55–360 min). For patients with previous CS, the average time was 136 min (median 120 min, range 70–360) (p = NS). In both groups, we registered cases with longer surgical time. All of them corresponded to complex cases such as uterine or ovarian cancers and extensive or deep infiltrating endometriosis where complete surgical staging or extensive adherence removal was performed, respectively, in addition to TLH. Conversion to laparotomy was required in 1 % of patients ($n=5$). Three of these patients had 1 or more previous CS (p = NS, compared to patients without CS). Reasons for conversion were unrecognizable access to the uterine pedicles (1 case with CS), inadequate hemostasis of uterine vessels (1 case with CS), inadequate access to pelvic spaces due to severe adhesions to safely perform nodal staging in a uterine cancer (1 case without CS), severe pelvic adhesions with

extensive attachment of the uterus to rectosigmoid colon (1 case without CS), and repair of a urological lesion (1 case in a patient with 3 previous CS).

The overall complication rate among patients undergoing TLH was 3.5 %. Major complication rate was of 3 % ($n=14$), 5 cases with previous CS and 9 cases with no previous CS (p = NS). Urologic lesion was the most common major complication, accounting for 1.5 % ($n=7$) of all cases (Table 3), 3 cases with previous CS and 4 with no previous CS (p = NS). Regarding urologic complications, three were cystotomies, 1 with no previous CS and 2 with previous CS (p = NS).

There were 9 intraoperative complications. Three patients with cystotomy diagnosed and repaired during surgery (two laparoscopically and one after conversion to laparotomy). One of these cases developed a vesicovaginal fistula that was diagnosed shortly after removing the Foley catheter. She was asymptomatic and was managed conservatively showing complete sealing after 2 months of follow-up. Other two patients experienced ureteral thermic lesions adverted during surgery that required double J stent installation, postoperatively. Two patients with uncontrollable bleeding required conversion to achieve adequate hemostasis. Another patient presenting extensive subcutaneous emphysema required to stop the surgery and complete it via vaginal access. Finally, a patient with a rectal lesion repaired uneventfully during the same

Table 2 Indications for TLH

Main diagnosis	Without CS % (n)	With CS % (n)	p
Myoma	44,3 (121)	35 (63)	0.054
Adenomiosis	15 (41)	30,4 (55)	0.0001
Endometrial cancer	11,4 (31)	3,3 (6)	0.004
Endometrial hyperplasia	5 (13)	6,6 (12)	0.52
Metrorrhagia	6 (16)	2,2 (4)	0.1
Endometriosis	2,2 (6)	5 (9)	0.18
Endometrial polyp	2,6 (7)	3,4 (9)	0.27
Prolapse	1 (3)	1,1 (2)	1.0
Others	12 (33)	11,6 (21)	0.99
Total	100 (273)	100 (181)	

Table 1 Previous CS in TLH

Previous CS	Number of patients	%
0	273	60 %
1	99	22 %
2	61	13 %
3	18	4 %
4	3	1 %
Total	454	100 %

Table 3 Major complications of TLH

Type of complicaction	Number
Ureteric injury	4
Inadvertent cystotomy	3
Bowel injury	1
Vesicovaginal fistula	2
Vault hematoma	1
Vault abscess	1
Significant hemorrhage	3
Total	14

intervention. No significant difference in terms of intraoperative complication rate was observed between the two groups (see Table 4).

There were 8 postoperative complications. Two were diagnosed immediately after surgery, at the recovery room. The first case, a patient with massive intra-abdominal bleeding and hypovolemic shock reoperated and recovered without further adverse events. The second case, a patient with an atrial fibrillation handled successfully with external cardioversion with no further intervention. Late postoperative complications are described later on. No significant difference in terms of postoperative complication rate was observed between the two groups (see Table 4).

The average postoperative hospital stay was of 3 days (range 2–6 days) interchangeably between patients with or without previous CS. No difference in hospital stay was observed between groups.

Pathologic analysis demonstrated similar distribution of diagnosis between groups. The average uterine weight was 155 g for both groups (range 30–1170 g). No difference was observed in uterine weight between groups.

There were 9 (2 %) readmissions. Four of them were due to postoperative fever. In three cases, a vault abscess was diagnosed, and all were discharged in good conditions after completion of their antibiotic treatment. The remaining patient presented with fever of unknown origin, with normal blood tests and normal abdomen/pelvis CT scan, who was discharged in good conditions after completing her antibiotic treatment. Two cases corresponded to inadvertent ureteral lesions that presented with acute abdomen due to uroperitoneum (approximately 2 weeks after surgery). Both cases were successfully managed with ureteral reimplantation. Another readmission corresponded to a patient with vaginal discharge, starting 1 week after surgery, who was diagnosed with a vesicovaginal fistula. She was initially managed with permanent Foley catheter, and after 2 months of use, she underwent successful surgical repair of her fistula. Worth mentioning, we had 1 more case of vesicovaginal fistula that originated from a cystotomy repaired during TLH surgery. This case was successfully managed, in an ambulatory setting, with prolonged bladder catheterization until complete fistula sealing with no further need of surgery. Finally, the last two readmission cases corresponded to a case of acute pyelonephritis (treated with

antibiotic regimen) and a case of vault hematoma (managed with oral analgesia).

In this study, we also included patient data from the San Carlos Clinic where normally, residents do not carry out clinical rotations. This center covers 12 to 15 % of all our TLH procedures. Overall, once accounting for the total number of TLH perfomed by each resident, we estimated that about 85–90 % of our TLH were performed by a third year resident as first surgeon, and the remaining 10–20 % performed exclusively by 2 experienced laparoscopic surgeons.

Discussion

In the present paper, we demonstrated that laparoscopic approach for total hysterectomy in patients with previous cesarean section is a safe procedure and that our results are comparable to other series already published (see Table 5) [11, 13]. The use of a standardized technique accelerates the learning curve and minimizes surgical risks, thus allowing us to offer the best surgical intervention possible indistinctively to all patients, regardless of the previous number of CS. This is important, especially in a country like Chile where the rate of CS is one of the highest reported to date worldwide and where local health authorities have not been yet able to find a solution in order to revert this worrisome tendency.

It is a fact that TLH in the presence of patients with previous CS is becoming increasingly common since the number of cesarean deliveries is increasing worldwide [5]. This might pose a higher difficulty for surgeons approaching TLH since bladder adhesions to the uterus may make dissection much more difficult and might even preclude bladder mobilization off the cervix. In our series, all TLH were successfully performed with the lateral approach to the space. Of these, only 13 % (n=54) were vaginally assisted due to surgeon expertise. When adjusting by year, more than 60 % of these cases were performed before year 2010 supporting the learning curve of the laparoscopic technique. The inclusion of standardized techniques in the learning process of TLH, or any surgery for that matter, accelerates the learning curve. This only puts to evidence that our surgeons have acquired the necessary

Table 4 Surgery characteristics and postoperative stay

Characteristics	Without CS	With CS	p
Surgical time (min)	128	136	1.0
Intraoperative complications (n)	4	5	0.494
Postoperative complications (n)	7	1	0.15
Postoperative hopital stay (days)	2,5	2,5	0.61

Table 5 Complication comparisson between publications

Publications	TLH with CS (%)	Inadvertent cystotomy with CS (%)	Total major complication with CS (%)
Wang et al.	141 (24,4)	7 (5)	20 (14,2)
Sinha et al.	261 (100)	2 (0,8)	n/a
Celle et al.	181 (40)	2 (1,1)	5 (2,8)
Total	583	11 (2)	n/a

n/a data not available

Table 6 Major complications of TLH according to number of previous CS

Type of complicaction	1 CS (*N*=99)	2 CS (*N*=61)	≥3 CS (*N*=21)	NO CS (*N*=273)	Total
Ureteric injury	1	0	0	3	4
Inadvertent cystotomy	1	0	1	1	3
Bowel injury	0	0	0	1	1
Vesicovaginal fistula	1	0	0	1	2
Vault hematoma	0	0	0	1	1
Vault abscess	0	1	0	0	1
Significant hemorrhage	1	0	0	2	3
Total					14

skills in order to feel confident completing the totality of this procedure through the laparoscopic access, having no further need of assistance through the vaginal approach thus reducing surgical times, risks, and costs of adding further surgical equipment (vaginal and laparoscopic). In our center, the use of this standardized technique has determined that the number of previous CS has no detrimental influence in the surgical outcome (see Table 6). In fact, no difference was observed in the number of major complications when comparing TLH carried out in patients with 1 versus ≥3 previous CS. Accordingly, before year 2010, around 20–30 % of our TLH had 1 or more previous CS, whereas to date, 40 to 50 % of our patients have one or more previous CS, and yet, our TLH procedures have not diminished. Figure 1 shows the percentage of previous CS for every TLH performed each year. In addition, for the same period of time, a sustained reduction in the number of abdominal hysterectomies and subtotal

hysterectomies has taken place. More importantly, surgeons that used to prefer a subtotal or total abdominal hysterectomy for this type of patients currently choose TLH as first option after learning the standardized technique. Nowadays, there is no longer contraindication for TLH based on number of previous CS in our institution; we just ask to have a well-trained team.

Urinary tract injuries are the most feared complications in gynecologic surgery. They account for 1 % of all gynecologic procedures [8]. The series by Donnez et al. shows a 0.56 % of urinary tract injuries and a 1.59 % of overall complications [14]. Our overall complication rate was of 3.5 % with a 1.5 % of urologic lesions. As we mentioned earlier, no statistical difference was observed between groups. A major concern for surgeons, when performing TLH in patients with one or more previous CS, would be the risk of bladder injury. Rooney et al. demonstrated that previous cesarean section is

Fig. 1 Evolution in the number of TLH with or without previous CS and the percentage of cesarian section per year at the Pontificia Universidad Catolica de Chile between 2006 and 2014

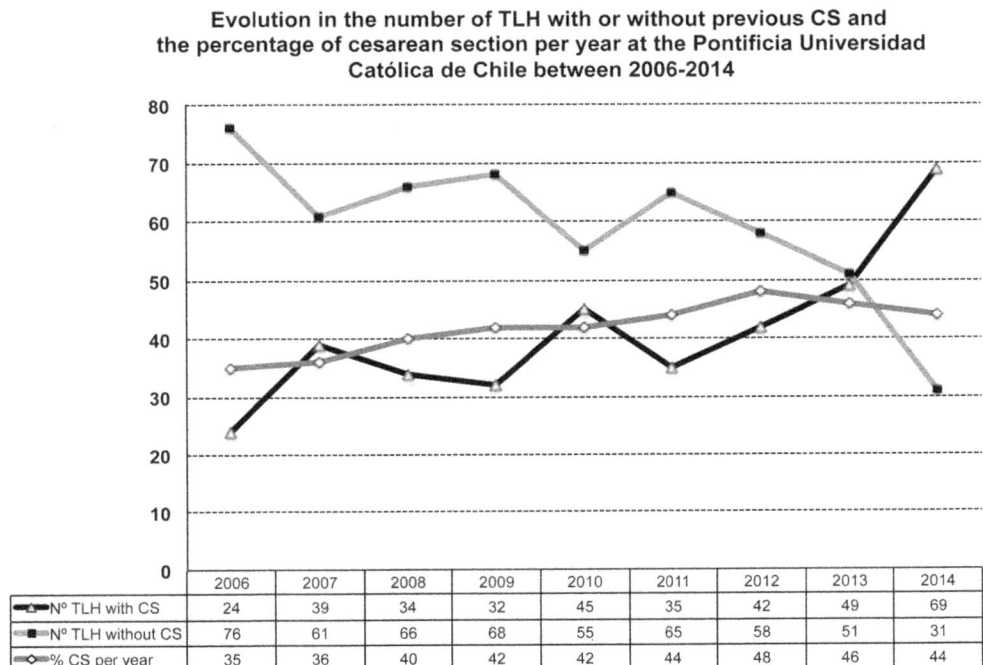

Evolution in the number of TLH with or without previous CS and the percentage of cesarean section per year at the Pontificia Universidad Católica de Chile between 2006-2014

	2006	2007	2008	2009	2010	2011	2012	2013	2014
N° TLH with CS	24	39	34	32	45	35	42	49	69
N° TLH without CS	76	61	66	68	55	65	58	51	31
% CS per year	35	36	40	42	42	44	48	46	44

a significant independent risk factor for lower urinary tract damage, reporting a 1 % incidental cystotomy rate [15]. Pillet et al. also reported a 1 % rate of bladder injury in their TLH series and found that previous CS as well as previous laparotomy were the main risk factors associated to bladder injury [16]. We had a 0.7 % (*n*=3) of cystotomies, all of them repaired in the same surgical act.

Assuming then that the risk of cystotomy should be higher in patients with increasing number of previous CS, we further analyzed major complication rate occurrence in the subgroup of patients with 1, 2, and 3 or more previous CS. We observed that the number of previous scars had no relation to the number or type of complication (Table 6). Under this same assumption, surgical operative time should be longer due to the major surgical challenge associated to numerous scars. Average surgical time was of 140 min in patients with 1 previous CS, 130 min with 2, and 136 min for patients with 3 or more previous CS showing that this was not a conditioning factor regarding operative time.

Based in our results and others, we believe that there is no justification for subtotal hysterectomy, in most of cases, as an alternative to TLH in order to reduce urological complications. Technically speaking, for many surgeons, subtotal laparoscopic hysterectomy (STLH) could be easier to perform since no bladder dissection and descent are required to remove the uterine corpus. Thus, a reduced complication rate should be expected with this approach. However, the evidence has showed that retaining the cervix does not offer advantages in regards to complication rate, bladder symptoms or incontinence, improvement of libido, and bowel dysfunction [1, 17]. More importantly, we must recall that by preferring TLH, where the cervix is removed, there is no risk of future bleeding as seen occasionally in subtotal hysterectomy cases [17].

We believe that a major determinant of our complication rate is based on the training program and the standardized technique that we have incorporated at our institution. All our residents, fellows, and teaching surgeons have completed the same laparoscopic training program and perform the same hysterectomy technique. Completion of the training program and learning curve, adequate case selections for our trainees to start operating, and the appropriate supervision through a gradual increase in difficulty guarantee the success rate. In fact, following this educational strategy, about 90 % of TLH are currently operated by a third year fellow with the assistance of a teaching surgeon and with low complication rate.

However, some limitations exist to the analysis reported in our study. First, although we tried to control for all patient and surgical variables that could potentially increase surgical difficulty, this was a retrospective study, and as such, we were unable to recollect information on patient BMI and uterine size, two known factors that could independently increase the difficulty of hysterectomy. Second, our data included cases where the learning curve was taking place. The fact that almost all our procedures are performed at a teaching institution by a third year resident might have influenced on surgical timing and complications despite the fact that they were not statistically significant between groups. In a private clinical setting, bladder adhesions secondary to previous CS might pose much less of a challenge to an experienced surgeon comfortable using sharp dissection regularly.

To date, the current published literature on TLH in patients with previous CS is scarce and limited. To our knowledge, this is the first study that evaluates the feasibility of performing TLH in patients with previous CS performed predominantly by fellows in their OBGYN residence program. We firmly believe that TLH offers multiple advantages over any other approach. Our findings support the safety of TLH in patients with previous CS. The use of a standardized technique allows trainees to perform this surgery safely with minimal complication rates.

References

1. Sutton C (2010) Past, present, and future of hysterectomy. J Minim Invasive Gynecol 17:421–435. doi:10.1016/j.jmig.2010.03.005
2. Whiteman MK, Hillis SD, Jamieson DJ et al (2008) Inpatient hysterectomy surveillance in the United States, 2000–2004. Am J Obstet Gynecol 198:34.e1–7
3. Nieboer TE, Johnson N, Lethaby A, Tavender E, Curr E, Garry R et al (2009) Surgical approach to hysterectomy for benign gynaecological disease. Cochrane Database Syst Rev. doi:10.1002/14651858.CD003677.pub1
4. The CORONIS Collaborative Group (2013) Caesarean Section surgical techniques (CORONIS): a fractional, factorial, unmasked, randomised controlled trial. Lancet 382:234–248. doi:10.1016/S0140-6736(13)60441-9
5. OECD. Health Statistics 2013. OECD Publishing, 10.1787/health-data-en
6. Departamento de Estadística e Informática del Ministerio de Salud, Instituto Nacional de Estadísticas, Atenciones del sector privado, REMSAS 2011. http://intradeis.minsal.cl/reportesremsas/2011/partos_abortos/partos_abortos.aspx. Published 2011. Accessed 19 Aug 2014
7. Guzmán E (2012) Epidemiological profile of caesarean section in Chile in the decade 2000–2010. Medwave 12(3), e5331. doi:10.5867/medwave.2012.03.5331
8. Bai SW, Huh EH, Jung DJ, Park JH, Kim SK, Park KH (2006) Urinary tract injuries during pelvic surgery: incidence rates and predisposing factors. Int Urogynecol J 17:360–364
9. Jacoby VL, Autry A, Jacobson G, Domush R, Nakagawa S, Jacoby A (2009) Nationwide use of laparoscopic hysterectomy compared with abdominal and vaginal approaches. Obstet Gynecol 114:1041–1048. doi:10.1097/AOG.0b013e3181b9d222
10. Walsh CA, Walsh SR, Tang TY, Slack M (2009) Total abdominal hysterectomy versus total laparoscopic hysterectomy for benign disease: a meta-analysis. Eur J Obstet Gynecol Reprod Biol 144:3–7. doi:10.1016/j.ejogrb.2009.01.003

11. Sinha R, Sundaram M, Lakhotia S, Hedge A, Kadam P (2010) Total laparoscopic hysterectomy in women with previous caesarean sections. J Minim Invasive Gynecol 17:513–517. doi:10.1016/j.jmig.2010.03.018

12. Cronin B, Sung V, Matteson K (2012) Vaginal cuff dehiscence: risk factors and management. Am J Obstet Gynecol 206(4):284–288. doi:10.1016/j.ajog.2011.08.026

13. Wang L, Merkur H, Hardas G, Soo S, Lujic S (2010) Laparoscopic hysterectomy in the presence of previous caesarean section: a review of one hundred forty-one cases in the Sydney West Advanced Pelvic Surgery Unit. J Minim Invasive Gynecol 17:186–191. doi:10.1016/j.jmig.2009.11.007

14. Donnez O, Jadoul P, Squifflet J, Donnez J (2009) A series of 3190 laparoscopic hysterectomies for benign disease from 1990 to 2006: evaluation of complications compared with vaginal and abdominal procedures. BJOG 16(4):492–500. doi:10.1111/j.1471-0528.2008.01966.x

15. Rooney CM, Crawford AT, Vassallo BJ, Kleeman SD, Karram MM (2005) Is Previous cesarean section a risk for incidental cystotomy at the time of hysterectomy?: A case-controlled study. J Minim Invasive Gynecol 193:2041–2044. doi:10.1016/j.ajog.2005.07.090

16. Lafay Pillet MC, Leonard F, Chopin N, Malaret JM, Borghese B, Foulot H, Fotso A, Chapron C (2009) Incidence and risk factors of bladder injuries during laparoscopic hysterectomy indicated for benign uterine pathologies: a 14.5 years experience in a continuous series of 1501 procedures. Hum Reprod 24:842–849. doi:10.1093/humrep/den467

17. Lethaby A, Mukhopadhyay A, Naik R (2012) Total versus subtotal hysterectomy for benign gynaecological conditions. Cochrane Database Syst Rev. doi:10.1002/14651858.CD004993.pub3

8

Conservative laparoscopic electrocoagulation adenomyolysis for the management of symptomatic adenomyosis

Hosam Abdel-Fattah[1] · Nasser El-Lakkany[1] · Adel Saad Helal[1] · Alaa Mosbah[1] ·
El-Said Abdel-Hady[1] · Mahmoud Abdel-Shaheed[2]

Abstract The objective of the study was to assess the safety
and efficacy of conservative laparoscopic electrocoagulation
adenomyolysis (CLEA) in the management of women with
symptomatic adenomyosis. The study design is prospective
observational study. The setting was Department of Obstetrics
and Gynecology, Mansoura University Hospital. Thirty-nine
premenopausal women, complaining of chronic pelvic pain
and/or menorrhagia, were diagnosed to have adenomyosis
by transvaginal ultrasonography (TVS) and/or magnetic resonance imaging (MRI), between June 2008 and June 2011.
They were subjected to laparoscopic multiple uterine unipolar
electrocoagulation diathermy punctures aiming at
adenomyolysis. Women were evaluated before and at 3, 6,
and 12 months after the procedure. Main outcome is the magnitude of pain by using the visual analog scale (VAS) and the
overall patient self satisfaction as assessed by short form 36
(SF-36) questionnaires; secondary outcome is the uterine volume as measured by TVS. At 3-, 6-, and 12-month follow-up
visits, there was a gradual, yet a significant, reduction in the
median VAS scoring system of pain ($p<0.01$), a significant
improvement in every scale of the SF-36 ($p<0.01$), and also a
significant reduction ($p<0.01$) in the median uterine volume
as assessed by TVS. Conservative laparoscopic
electrocoagulation adenomyolysis may be an effective and
safer minimal invasive procedure for the management of
symptomatic adenomyosis in premenopausal women.

✉ Adel Saad Helal
adelsaadhelal@yahoo.com

1 Department of Obstetrics and Gynecology,
Mansoura University, Mansoura, Egypt

2 Department of Diagnostic Radiology,
Mansoura University, Mansoura, Egypt

Keywords Adenomyosis · Pain · Laparascopy ·
Adenomyolysis

Introduction

Adenomyosis is a benign gynecological disease in which the
endometrial stroma invades the uterine myometrium.
Adenomyosis is divided into diffuse and localized forms according to the extent of the lesion. Localized adenomyosis is
also known as adenomyoma [1].

The incidence of the disease varies between 5 and 70 %.
Generally, it occurs in women aged between 40 and 50 years,
with a prevalence rate of 70–80 %. Adenomyosis was found
in 23 % of uteri that were removed due to fibroids [2].

The etiology of this disease has not been clearly elucidated.
However, several pathophysiological mechanisms have been
proposed, such as damage of endometrial-myometrial border
due to trauma and high estrogen biosynthesis associated with
increased activities of aromatase enzyme [3]. The clinical
manifestations include dysmenorrhea, chronic pelvic pain,
and menorrhagia. It is usually combined with pelvic endometriosis, endometrial cysts of the ovary, uterine fibroids, or other estrogen-dependent diseases [4].

The diagnosis of adenomyosis was based on clinical symptoms. In recent years, the development of imaging techniques
has made diagnosis more accurate. It has been reported that
the sensitivity of diagnosis by vaginal ultrasound was 80–
86 % and the specificity was 74–86 %. The sensitivity of
magnetic resonance imaging (MRI) was 80–86 % and the
specificity was 74–86 % [5].

The myometrium has three distinct sonographic layers: the
outer, middle, and inner layers. The middle layer is the most
echogenic and is separated from the outer layer by the arcuate
venous and arterial plexus. The inner layer (the

subendometrial halo) is composed of longitudinal and circular closely packed smooth muscle fibers. The inner layer (archimyometrium or stratum subvasculare, e.g., the subendometrial halo) is hypoechogenic at transvaginal ultrasonography (TVS) but at MRI, it is readily and more distinctly seen as a low-signal intensity (SI) band referred to as the JZ [6].

The sonographic findings of adenomyosis, best obtained by transvaginal sonography, include the following [7]:

1. Uterine enlargement—globular uterine enlargement that is generally up to 12 cm in uterine length and that is not explained by the presence of leiomyomata is a characteristic finding (Fig. 1).
2. Cystic anechoic spaces or lakes in the myometrium—the cystic anechoic spaces within the myometrium are variable in size and can occur throughout the myometrium. The cystic changes in the outer myometrium may on occasion represent small arcuate veins rather than adenomyomas. The application of color Doppler imaging at low velocity scales may help in this differentiation (Fig. 2).
3. Uterine wall thickening—the uterine wall thickening can show antero-posterior asymmetry, especially when the disease is focal (Fig. 3).
4. Subendometrial echogenic linear striations—invasion of the endometrial glands into the subendometrial tissue induces a hyperplastic reaction, which appears as echogenic linear striations fanning out from three endometrial layer (Fig. 4).
5. Heterogeneous echo texture—there is a lack of homogeneity within the myometrium with evidence of architectural disturbance (Fig. 5). This finding has been shown to be the most predictive of adenomyosis.
6. Obscure endometrial/myometrial border—invasion of the myometrium by the glands also obscures the normally distinct endometrial/myometrial border (Fig. 6).
7. Thickening of the transition zone—this zone is a layer that appears as a hypoechoic halo surrounding the endometrial layer. A thickness of 12 mm or greater has been shown to be associated with adenomyosis.

Doppler sonography may facilitate the differentiation between myomas and adenomyosis (Fig. 7). Vessels around myomas produce a well-defined rim with a few vessels entering the body of the mass. In contrast, in adenomyosis, vessels follow their normal perpendicular course in myometrial areas [8].

Adenomyosis typically presents as either diffuse or focal thickening of the inner myometrium or an ill-defined myometrial nodule of low SI on MRI T2-WIs (Figs. 8, 9, and 10). In healthy women of reproductive age, the inner myometrium, which is also called the JZ, appears as the band

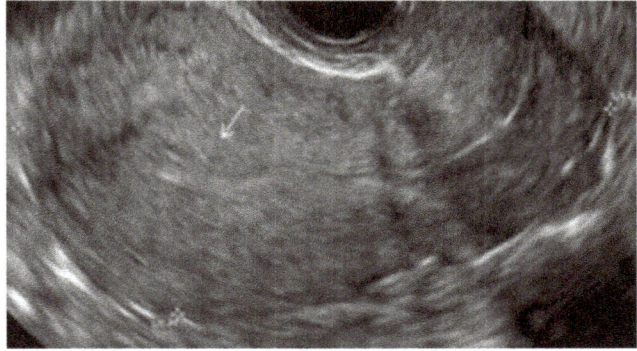

Fig. 1 Globular uterine enlargement with an obscure endometrialmyometrial border (arrow)

of low SI between the endometrium of high SI and the outer myometrium of intermediate SI. Although adenomyosis can be readily suspected when it present as focal thickening of the JZ, diffuse thickening of the JZ should be carefully distinguished from physiological change since the thickness of the JZ varies considerably during the menstrual cycle [9].

The JZ is generally widest and most clearly visible in the late secretory phase. Generally, a maximal thickness of the JZ (>12 mm) is highly predictive of the presence of adenomyosis, while a uterus with the JZ (<8 mm) is unlikely to have adenomyosis. Since the JZ can frequently show thickness of >12 mm during menstruation, especially on cycle days 1 and 2 in our experience (Fig. 11), MR examination during the menstrual phase should be avoided for evaluating adenomyosis [10].

The decreased SI on T2-WIs represents smooth muscle hyperplasia associated with ectopic endometrium. Occasionally, the islands of ectopic endometrial tissue can be demonstrated as punctate foci of high SI on T2-WIs (Fig. 12a). When menstrual hemorrhage occurs within these ectopic endometrial glands, cystically dilated glands are presented as foci of high SI on T1-WIs (Fig. 12b). Less commonly, benign invasion of the basal endometrium into the myometrium can manifest as "linear striations" of high SI radiating out from the

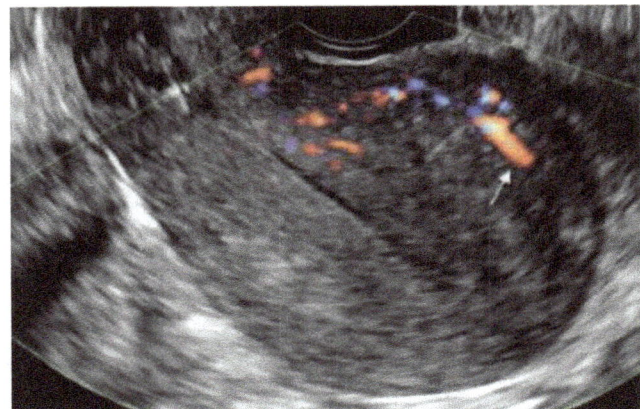

Fig. 2 The application of color Doppler imaging at low velocity scales

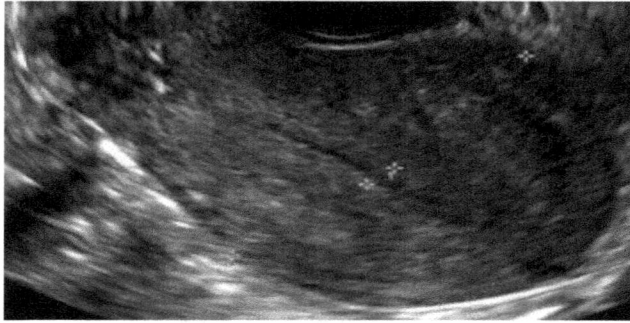

Fig. 3 Uterine wall thickening which shows antero-posterior asymmetry

endometrium on T2-WIs, resulting in "pseudowidening" of the endometrium (Fig. 13) [11].

Variation in MR features of adenomyosis

Adenomyoma

Adenomyoma is a localized and well-circumscribed form of adenomyosis. Recognition of this entity is of clinical importance because adenomyomas are frequently confused with leiomyomas, not only on MRI but also at pathological examination. On MRI, myometrial adenomyomas typically exhibit low SI on T2-WIs, which may closely simulate leiomyoma. When the lesion is accompanied by hyperintense foci representing ectopic endometrium on T2-WIs, MRI can allow correct diagnosis of this entity (Fig. 14). Unlike the ordinary form of adenomyosis, myometrial adenomyoma can be treated surgically with myomectomy [12].

Adenomyomatous polyp (polypoid adenomyoma)

Adenomyomatous polyp (polypoid adenomyoma) presents as a pedunculated or sessile polypoid mass in the lower uterine endometrium or endocervix, and accounts for about (2 %) of all endometrial polyps. It typically affects premenopausal women, presenting as abnormal genital bleeding. On MRI, the lesion typically presents as a hypointense polypoid mass representing myometrial tissue, associated with hyperintense

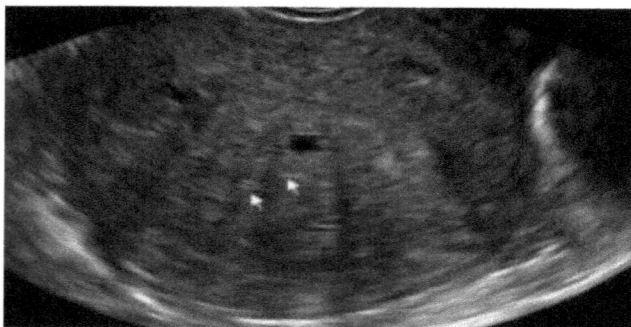

Fig. 4 Subendometrial echogenic linear striations

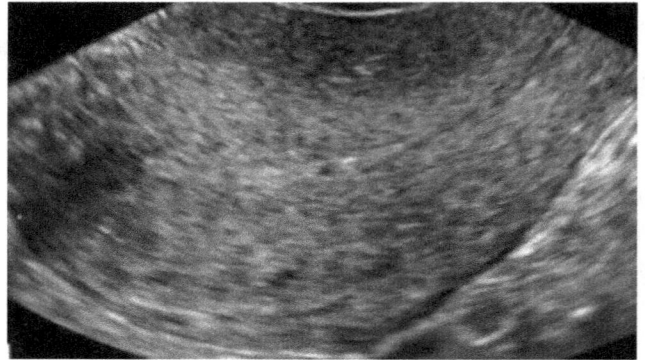

Fig. 5 Heterogeneous echo texture

foci on T2-WIs. The recognition of the attachment site of the polypoid lesion and the typical signal pattern on MRI may allow preoperative diagnosis of polypoid adenomyoma. Atypical polypoid adenomyoma is a rare variant of a polypoid adenomyoma, microscopically characterized by architectural and cytologic atypia. MR findings are similar to those an ordinary polypoid adenomyoma and may reveal a hemorrhagic cyst within the lesion (Fig. 15) [10].

Adenomyotic cyst (cystic adenomyosis)

Adenomyotic cyst is a rare variant of adenomyosis characterized by the presence of a large hemorrhagic cyst resulting from extensive menstrual bleeding in the ectopic endometrial gland. The lesion can be entirely within the myometrial, submucosal, or subserosal tissue. On MRI, fluid content exhibits high SI on T1-WIs, and the surrounding solid wall exhibits a distinct low SI on T2-WIs (Fig. 16). Occasionally, the solid wall may consist of an inner zone of low SI that resembles a JZ and an outer zone of a relatively increased intensity; an adenomyoma with this finding can be called a "miniature uterus" [10].

Different strategies for the management of adenomyosis have been tried [13]; for patients who prefer conservative measures, medical therapy may be the least invasive and most acceptable strategy and includes the use of prostaglandin inhibitors, oral contraceptive pills, progestogens, danazol,

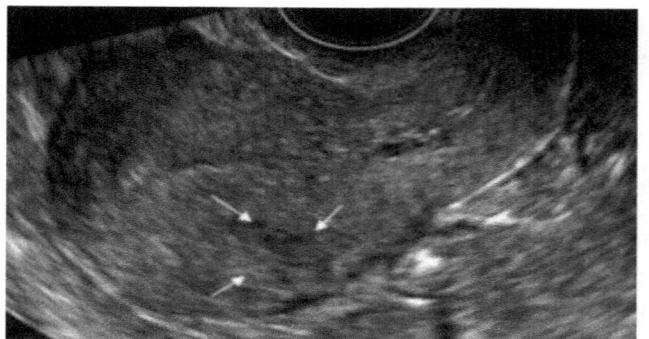

Fig. 6 Obscure endometrial/myometrial border

Fig. 7 a, b Doppler sonography
may facilitate the differentiation
between myomas and
adenomyosis

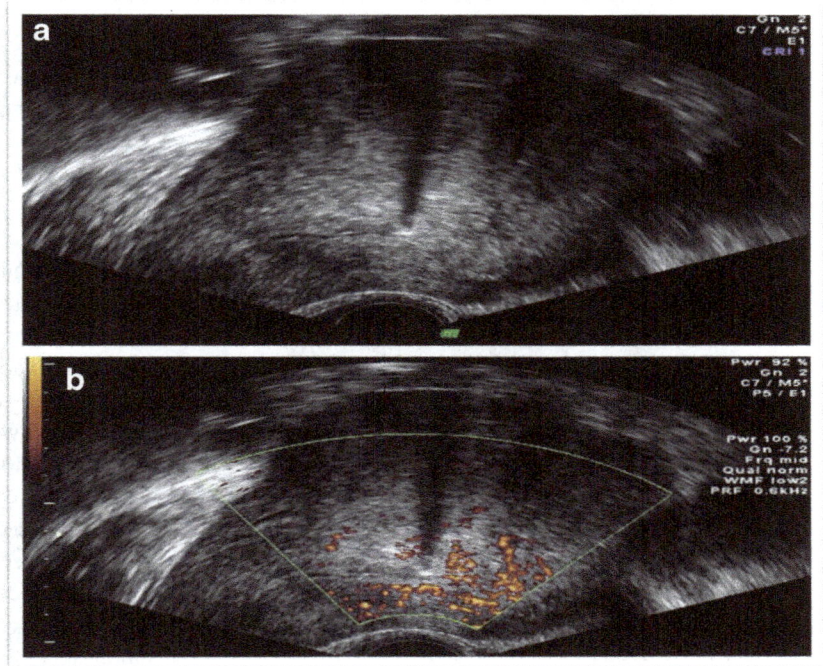

Fig. 7 **a, b** Doppler sonography may facilitate the differentiation between myomas and adenomyosis

gestrinone, and gonadotropin-releasing hormone (GnRH) agonists. Unfortunately, the effect of these medical treatments is often transient, and the symptoms (especially pain) usually reappear after discontinuing medication [14].

The surgical approach for preserving the uterus can be considered when dysmenorrhea does not respond to drug treatment; these include excision of the myometrial adenomyoma through a laparotomy. Less invasive conservative surgical approaches, including endomyometrial ablation, laparoscopic myometrial electrocoagulation, and laparoscopic surgery, have been attempted [15]. All conservative surgical treatments

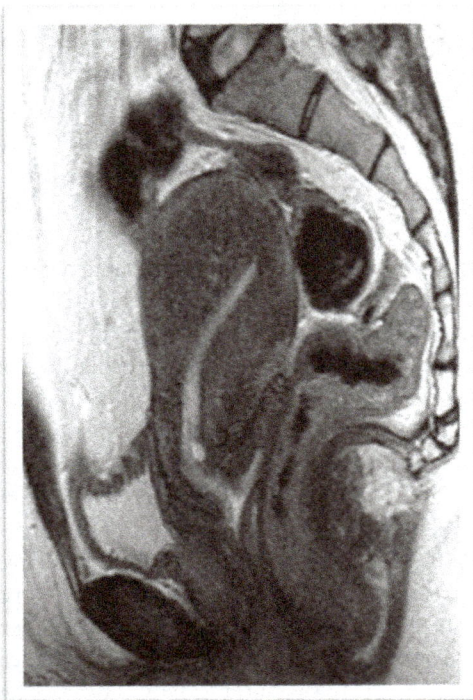

Fig. 8 Adenomyosis presenting as diffuse thickening of the JZ. MRI Sagittal T2-WI shows an enlarged uterus with diffusely thickened JZ which measures >12 mm in thickness

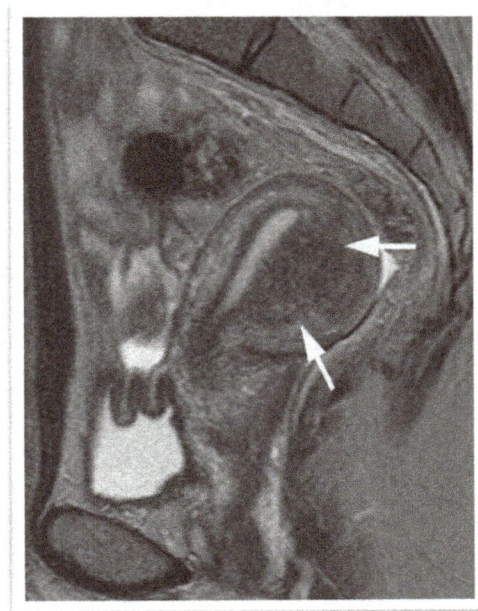

Fig. 9 Adenomyosis presenting as focal thickening of the JZ. MRI Sagittal T2-WI shows focal thickening of the JZ in the posterior wall of the uterus (*arrows*)

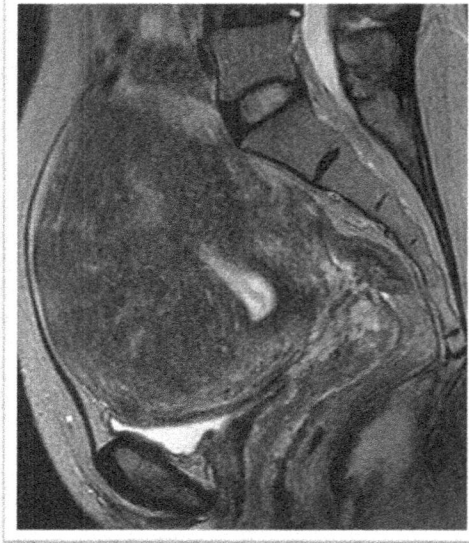

Fig. 10 Diffuse adenomyosis presenting as an ill-defined myometrial mass. MRI Sagittal T2-WI shows a diffusely enlarged uterus with indistinct zonal anatomy. There is an ill-defined mass of decreased SI in the myometrium of the anterior wall and the fundus

have proven effective in up to 50 % of patients; however, the follow-up assessment periods have been of short duration [16].

The conventional and definitive management of symptomatic adenomyosis is hysterectomy [17]. Phillips et al. [18] studied laparoscopic bipolar coagulation for conservative treatment of adenomyomata with preoperative GnRH analog and concluded that further evaluation of this technique is necessary to determine its definitive role.

Wood's study [16] showed that endometrial ablation, myometrial electrocoagulation, or laparoscopic excision were effective in >50 % of patients. Laparoscopic resection versus myolysis in the management of symptomatic uterine

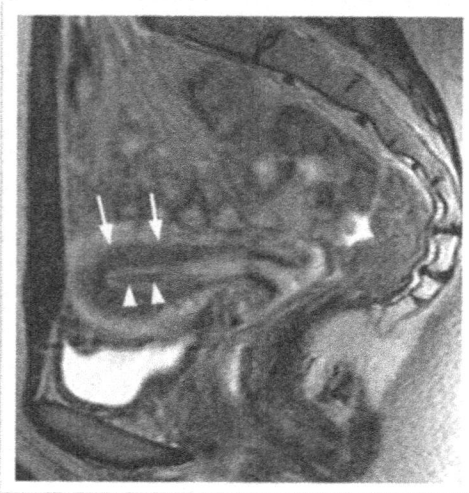

Fig. 11 JZ can frequently show thickness of >12 mm during

adenomyosis was also studied before [2]; no significant differences were found in the median reduction of menorrhagia and dysmenorrhea scores between the resection and the myolysis groups.

Patients and methods

This study included 39 women admitted to the Department of Obstetrics and Gynecology, Mansoura University Hospital, between June 2008 and June 2011. They complained of chronic pelvic pain and/or menorrhagia with a provisional diagnosis of adenomyosis. The inclusion criteria included premenopausal women (40–50 years), who had completed their families and were not willing to undergo hysterectomy; other pelvic pathology was excluded. Diagnosis of adenomyosis was established by TVS, color Doppler, and MRI. Laparoscopy was decided, and the intended procedure was explained; a written consent was signed by the patient and her husband. Also, the procedure was approved by Mansoura Medical Ethical Committee. Usual preoperative investigations and preparations including 400 μg prostaglandin E$_1$ analog, misoprostol (Misotac Sigma) per rectum were immediately placed before laparoscopy. Laparoscopy was performed under general anesthesia in the neutral-lithotomy position. Patients were catheterized and vaginally prepared, and uterine manipulator was inserted. Pneumo-peritoneum was done with Veress needle through the umblicus. For the primary puncture, 10-mm port was inserted through the umblical incision with a video laparoscope introduced. For the second puncture, 5-mm port was placed laterally on Pfannenstiel line for uterine manipulation. For the third puncture, 5-mm port was inserted in the middle of Pfannenstiel line for adenomyolysis diathermy needle. A unipolar diathermy needle was introduced for puncture and cauterization of the anterior and posterior uterine wall, as well as the fundus. An average of 6–10 punctures was placed through the anterior uterine wall and 4–6 punctures for the fundus; the latter was brought perpendicular to the needle axis by extreme anteflexion by an instrument through second port. The posterior wall was approached perpendicularly by the diathermy needle introduced in a 5-mm reducer through the primary port, and the procedure was monitored by 5-mm scope through the suprapubic incision (changing entry) and 6–10 punctures were done in posterior wall. The needle punctures were 1–2 cm using 100-W current; the depth of punctures was about 10–15 mm; saline wash was done. Finally, intaperitoneal drain was left in place for 24 h. Women were advised to use condoms for contraception, to avoid the effects of hormonal therapy and the intra uterine device. Patients were followed up at 3, 6, and 12 months. At each visit, patients were evaluated as regards (a) chronic pelvic pain, which was assessed by the visual analog score (VAS), (b) quality of life scales which was assessed by the short form 36 (SF-36), and (c) the uterine volume which was evaluated by TVS.

Fig. 12 a The islands of ectopic endometrial tissue can be demonstrated as punctate foci of high SI and **b** when menstrual haemorrhage occurs within ectopic endometrial glands, cystically dilated glands are presented as foci of high SI on T1- WIs

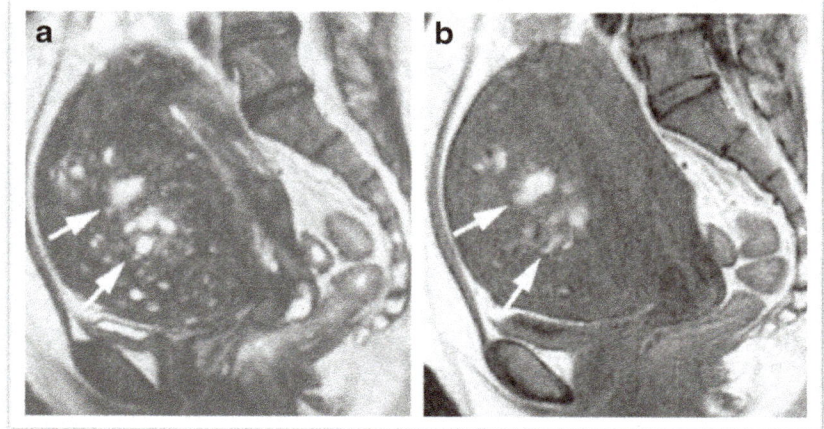

Fig. 13 a, **b** Benign invasion of the basal endometrium into the myometrium can manifest as "linear striations" of high SI radiating out from the endometrium on T2-WIs, resulting in "pseudowidening" of the endometrium

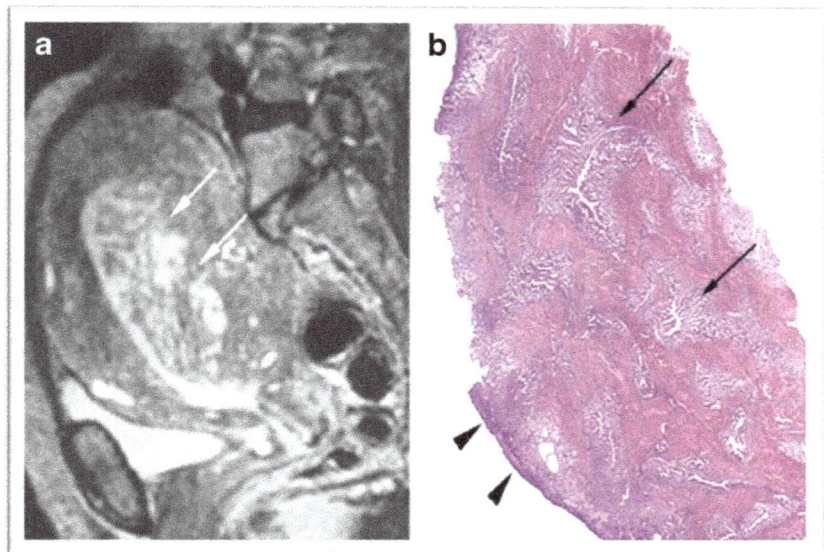

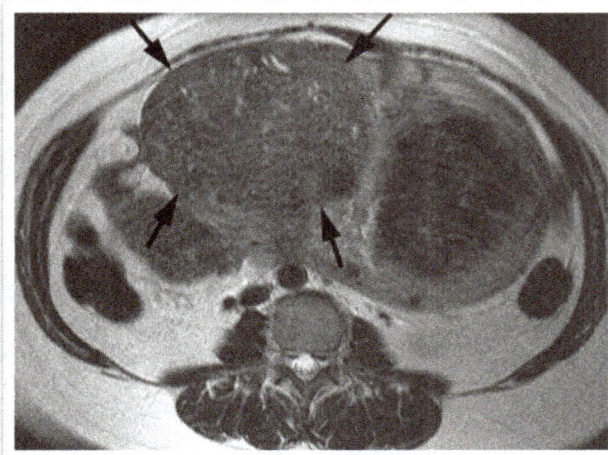

Fig. 14 When the lesion is accompanied by hyperintense foci representing ectopic endometrium on T2-WIs, MRI can allow correct diagnosis of this entity

Statistical analysis used SPSS (version 11) with median values and SD, and Student's t test was used to compare between preoperative and follow-up visits. The difference was considered significant when p value was less than 0.05.

Results

The magnitude of pelvic pain was significantly improved ($p<0.01$), following the procedure and at 3, 6, and 12 months as assessed by the visual analog score as given in Table 1. The quality of life scores showed significant improvement as assessed by the SF-36 scores. By 12 months following the procedure, a significant improvement was observed in each item of the SF-36 scores ($p<0.01$) as given in Table 2.

The uterine volume as assessed by transvaginal ultrasound showed a gradual, yet a significant, reduction in the mean

Fig. 15 a, b Haemorrhagic cyst
within the lesion

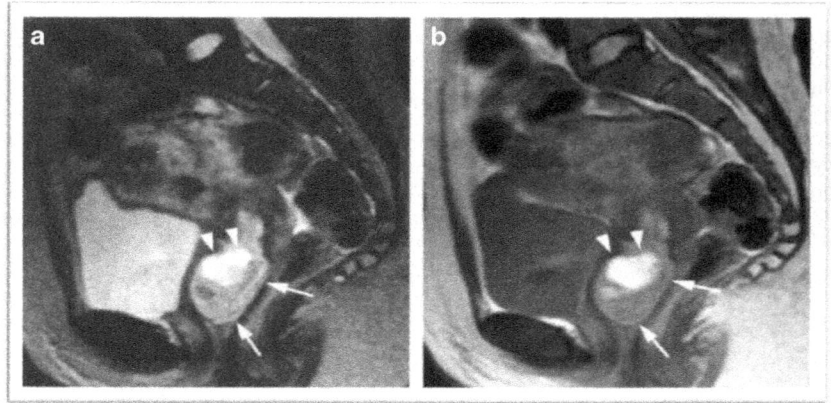

Fig. 16 a, b On MRI, fluid
content exhibits high SI on T1-
WIs and the surrounding solid
wall exhibits a distinct low SI on
T2-WIs

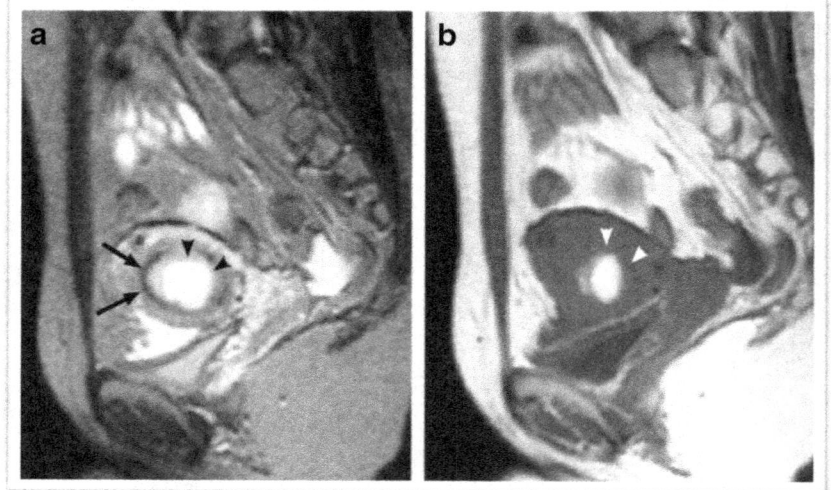

uterine volume with an average reduction of volume by 43 %
at 12 months following the procedure ($p<0.01$) as given in
Table 3. The procedure was not associated with significant
complication apart from any routine laparoscopic procedure.
Patients' requirements for analgesics were comparable to any
routine laparoscopic procedure.

Discussion

This study includes 39 women with symptomatic
adenomyosis aged between 40 and 50 years who were subjected to conservative laparoscopic adenomyolysis from the
period of June 2008 to June 2011, as shown in Fig. 1. And
they were followed up for 12 months. Many patients in such
an age group especially in early 1940s may prefer a rather
minimally invasive technique to improve their symptoms.
Hysterectomy, as a standard surgical procedure for the

management of symptomatic adenomyosis, may not be an
accepted modality option by many premenopausal women.
Simple random unipolar electrocauterization of adenomyotic
uteri was tried in this study, assuming that necrosis of
adenomyotic implants will improve the symptoms.

Main findings

A recoded significant improvement at 3-, 6-, and 12-month
follow-up include the severity of pain as assessed by the VAS
as well as the quality of life as assessed by SF-36 scores
following conservative laparoscopic electrocoagulation
adenomyolysis (CLEA) procedure as given in Tables 1 and
2. Also, the assessment of the uterine volume by TVS revealed
a significant reduction, average 43 %, by the end of 1 year as
given in Table **3** as a secondary outcome. There were no recorded significant complications following the procedure.

Table 1 Assessment of pain by VAS: visual analog score was significantly improved at 3, 6, and 12 months after the procedure ($p<0.01$)

VAS	N	Median±	SD	p value
Preoperative	39	69.0000	6.6176	
3 months	36	59.6667	9.8027	<0.01
6 months	30	41.0000	14.7040	<0.01
12 months	30	40.0333	14.7028	<0.01

VAS visual analog scale

Table 3 Assessment of the uterine volume by TVS: there was a gradual, yet a significant, reduction in the mean uterine volume as assessed by TVS, by an average of 43 % at 12 months following the procedure ($p<0.01$)

	Preoperative (mean) (cm^3)	Postoperative (mean) (cm^3)		
		3 months	6 months	12 months
Uterine volume	435.3	262.5	247.4	247.5
p		0.01	0.01	0.01

TVS transvaginal ultrasonography

Strength and limitations

Small sample size represents the main limitation in this study as the use of unipolar diathermy was the first trial and also no preceding adjuvant medical treatment.

Interpretation

The use of unipolar diathermy needle in our study was intended to ensure better speed of current through the tissues, rather than the use of bipolar needle. The latter was tried by others [2, 18], on a smaller number of cases. In these studies, either pre- or postoperative adjuvant GnRH therapy was used. In this study, CLEA was attempted only with no added adjuvant medical treatment. Two unplanned pregnancies occurred in this series within the follow-up period. One pregnancy ended in a spontaneous miscarriage at 8 weeks, and the other pregnancy continued with no adverse effects up to 38 weeks and the baby was born by an elective cesarean section; a healthy baby weighing 3 kg was born (data not shown).

Table 2 Assessment of quality of life scales by short form (SF-36 scores): there was a gradual improvement in each item of the SF-36 scores and by 12 months following the procedure; a significant improvement was observed in each item of the SF-36 scores ($p<0.01$)

Scale	Pre	12 months	p value
Physical functioning	13±1.6	39±14	<0.01
Role limitations due to physical health	27±16	48±24	<0.01
Role limitations due to emotional problems	36.3±21.8	36.5±22.1	<0.01
Energy/fatigue	39±4.9	54±13	<0.01
Emotional well-being	58±6.7	69±12	<0.01
Social functioning	28±5.6	52±16.5	<0.01
Pain	30±3.7	62±18.8	<0.01
General health	31±5.3	59±15.9	<0.01

Conclusions

Laparoscopic electrocoagulation adenomyolysis is recommended as an effective and safer minimal invasive procedure for the management of symptomatic adenomyosis.

Yet, more studies and larger number of patients are recommended to assess the effectiveness and side effects of this procedure.

Acknowledgments The authors thank all the staff members in the Department of Obstetrics and Gynecology, the operating room staff members, and all the patients who shared information and experiences in this research. This research is approved by local ethical research committee of Mansoura University, Faculty of Medicine on May 2008.

Funding None.

Authors' contributions Hossam abd elfatah, Nasser Allakany, and Adel Saad Helal made the design and did the operations. Alaa mesbah performed the preoperative and postoperative TVS evaluation of all patients. Mahmoud abd elshahied did the preoperative and postoperative Doppler study of all patients. Elsaid M. Abd elhady wrote the paper and helped in statistical analysis.

References

1. Ai-jun SUN, Min LUO, Wei WANG, Rong CHEN, Jing-he LANG (2011) Characteristics and efficacy of modified adenomyomectomy in the treatment of uterine adenomyoma. Chin Med J 124(9):1322–1326
2. Wachyu H, Dewi Anggraeni T (2006) Laparoscopic resection versus myolysis in the management of symptomatic uterine adenomyosis: alternatives to conventional treatment. Med J Indones 15(1):9–17
3. Ota H, Igarashi S, Hatazawa J, Tanaka T (1998) Is adenomyosis an immune disease? Hum Reprod Update 4:360–367
4. Reinhold C, McCarthy S, Bret PM (1996) Diffuse adenomyosis: comparison of endovaginal UA and MR imaging with histopathologic correlation. Radiology 199:151–158
5. Ascher SM, Arnold LL, Patt RH (1994) Adenomyosis: prospective comparison of MR imaging and transvaginal sonography. Radiology 190:803–806
6. Gilks CB, Clement PB, Hart WR et al (2000) Uterine adenomyomas excluding atypical polypoid adenomyomas and

adenomyomas of endocervical type: a clinicopathologic study of 30 cases of an underemphasized lesion that may cause diagnostic problems with brief consideration of adenomyomas of other female genital tract sites. Int J Gynecol Pathol 19:195–205

7. Tanaka YO, Tsunoda H, Kitagawa Y et al (2004) Functioning ovarian tumors: direct and indirect findings at MR imaging. Radiographics 24(supplement 1):S147–S166

8. Ascher SM, Imaoka I, Lage JM (2000) Tamoxifen-induced uterine abnormalities: the role of imaging. Radiology 214:29–38

9. Masui T, Katayama M, Kobayashi S et al (2003) Pseudolesions related to uterine contraction: characterization with multiphase-multisection T2-weighted MR imaging. Radiology 227:345–352

10. Tamai K, Togashi K, Ito T et al (2005) MR imaging findings of adenomyosis: correlation with histopathologic features and diagnostic pitfalls. Radiographics 25:21–40

11. Tamai K, Koyama T, Umeoka S (2006) Spectrum of MR features in adenomyosis. Best Pract Res Clin Obstet Gynaecol 20(4):583–602

12. Kinkel K, Frei KA, Balleyguier C, et al (2005) Diagnosis of endometriosis with imaging: a review. Eur Radiol

13. Yen MS, Yang TS, Yu KJ, Wang PH (2004) Comments on laparoscopic excision of myometrial adenomyomas in patient with adenomyosis uteri and main symptoms of severe dysmenorrhea and hypermenorrhea. J Am Assoc Gynecol Laparosc 11:441–442

14. Wang P-H, Liu W-M, Fuh J-L, Cheng M-H, Chao H-T (2009) Comparison of surgery alone and combined surgical-medical treatment in the management of symptomatic uterine adenomyoma. Fertil Steril 92:876–885

15. Wang CJ, Yuen LT, Chang SD, Lee CL, Soong YK (2006) Use of laparoscopic cytoreductive surgery to treat infertile women with localized adenomyosis. Fertil Steril 86:462, **e5–8**

16. Wood C (1998) Surgical and medical treatment of adenomyosis. Hum Reprod Update 4:323–326

17. Atri M, Reinhold C, Mehio AR, Chapman WB, Bret PM (2000) Adenomyosis: US features with histologic correlation in an vitro study. Radiology 215:783–790

18. Phillips DR, Nathanson HG, Milim SJ, Haselkorn JS (1996) Laparoscopic bipolar coagulation for the conservative treatment of adenomyomata. J Am Assoc Gynecol Laparosc 4(1):19–24

9

Extensive peritoneal lavage decreases postoperative C-reactive protein concentrations: a RCT

Carlo De Cicco [1,2] · Ron Schonman [1,3] · Anastasia Ussia [4] · Philippe R. Koninckx [1,4,5]

Abstract Although extensive lavage is useful in peritoneal infections as diverticulitis, the extent of peritoneal lavage that should be used at the end of surgery is unclear. A randomised controlled trial comparing standard lavage with 0.5 litre (L) with extensive 8-L lavage was performed in 20 consecutive patients, following a full thickness resection of the rectum for deep endometriosis. Randomisation was done by the research nurse using sealed envelopes. Endpoints were C-reactive protein (CRP) concentration, white blood cell (WBC) count, temperature and the occurrence of complications. After lavage with 8 L, the CRP concentrations were consistently lower than that after lavage with 0.5 L and this from day 1 to day 7 after surgery ($P=0.01$). Rigorous peritoneal lavage seems preferable when a risk of pelvic contamination exists. Clinicaltrials.gov registration: NCT00930696

Keywords Peritoneal lavage · Bowel perforation · Peritonitis · Endometriosis · Laparoscopy · Adhesion formation

✉ Philippe R. Koninckx
pkoninckx@gmail.com

[1] Department of Obstetrics and Gynaecology, University Hospital Gasthuisberg, Katholieke Universiteit Leuven, Leuven, Belgium

[2] Department of Gynecology, Campus Bio-Medico University, Rome, Italy

[3] Department of Obstetrics and Gynecology, Tel Aviv University, Tel Aviv, Israel

[4] Gruppo Italo Belga, Villa del Rosario, Rome, Italy

[5] Vuilenbos 2, 3360 Bierbeek, Belgium

Introduction

Extensive peritoneal lavage was introduced 100 years ago [1] to decrease the mortality of diffuse peritonitis following appendicitis, and repeated lavage by laparotomy was introduced in 1990 for four-quadrant peritonitis [2]. Although lavage during laparoscopy is more efficient than during laparotomy [3], its usefulness remains controversial [4–7]. Over the last years, extensive peritoneal lavage during laparoscopy was reported to be useful for the treatment of complications following colorectal surgery and for diverticulitis [8–16]. In animal models, lavage decreases adhesion formation following peritonitis [17].

Peritoneal lavage, although widely used, is poorly defined. It is a good clinical practice to rinse the abdominal cavity at the end of surgery in order to remove blood and/or debris. It seems common sense that lavage should be more rigorous following massive contamination to treat or prevent peritonitis. There are no data, however, that document how extensive peritoneal lavage should be.

Peritoneal lavage thus has a series of effects, some of which can be assumed to be beneficial, whereas others might be detrimental. Lavage obviously decreases the microbial load of an infection, although bacteria sticking to the mesothelial cells are not removed [18]. The importance of removing debris and blood for the prevention of adhesion formation, although logic, has not been proven. Negative consequences of the removal of immunocompetent cells as macrophages, natural killer cells and neutrophils were not reported. Although saline is routinely used for historical and economic reasons, saline was demonstrated to be harmful to mesothelial cells [19].

Since it was unclear whether a more extensive lavage was useful for minimal contamination of the abdominal cavity,, we conducted a RCT in women following a full thickness resection of bowel endometriosis.

Materials and methods

Deep endometriosis surgery

The technique used for excision of deep endometriosis was described recently [20]. In summary, patients received a full bowel preparation with 6 L of Prepacol (Codali SA, Belgium). Endometriosis was excised completely. Following a full thickness resection, the bowel opening was sutured transversally in two layers with a running suture of poliglactyn 3/0. Leakage of the suture was controlled with 150 mL of methylene blue for rectal defects. Following lavage of the pelvis, a drain was left in the pouch of Douglas and another in the right paracolic gutter. Postoperative care consisted of full spectrum antibiotics and nil by mouth for seven days and daily monitoring of CRP concentrations and WBC count. Immediately after surgery, all surgical data were entered into our database.

Peritoneal lavage in deep endometriosis surgery

After excision of deep endometriosis, peritoneal lavage of the pelvis was performed with 200 to 400 mL of saline. In women with a late bowel perforation and a beginning peritonitis, extensive peritoneal lavage was performed [21]. Extensive peritoneal lavage was started in the upper abdomen with the patient in anti-Trendelenburg position; subsequently, the patient was put horizontally to rinse the bowels, and finally with the patient in slight Trendelenburg, lavage of the pelvis was performed. Lavage was continued until the liquid was transparent clear. This generally required 3 up to 5 L for the upper abdomen and 3 up to 5 L for the pelvis.

Randomised controlled trial

Management of full thickness resection of endometriosis still is a matter of debate, centred on the consequences of opening the bowel and pelvic contamination. Some groups prefer to do a bowel resection or a discoid excision with a circular or linear stapler. Some prefer to leave a rim of fibrosis or even some endometriosis in order not to open the bowel. Our standard surgery since the early 1990s has been complete excision resulting in some 10 % full thickness resections especially in larger nodules.

Since an open bowel is always associated with some bacterial contamination, more extensive lavage was considered.

Following IRB approval and registration (NCT00930696), a trial was performed in 20 women in whom a full thickness resection for deep endometriosis was performed at the University Hospital Gasthuisberg, University of Leuven, Belgium. The only exclusion criterion was concomitant diseases jeopardising the outcome of surgery. Following informed consent of the patient and randomisation by the trial nurse using sealed envelopes, lavage was performed either as done routinely or until the liquid was clear. In order to standardise lavage during this trial, either 0.5 or 8 L of warmed saline was used. Using CONSORT guidelines, all women scheduled to undergo deep endometriosis surgery consented to participate; 20 women were randomised during surgery; there were no losses to follow up, and all 20 women were analysed. The endpoints of the trial were CRP concentrations and white blood cell count, the clinical follow-up and eventual postoperative complications.

Statistics

Since full thickness resections of deep endometriosis are not that frequent, a larger sample size would have taken unrealistically long. Since the number of patients is small, median and ranges, are given for demographic data. CRP and WBC values were analysed for significance with repeated measurement ANOVA. For the figure, mean and SE are used for clarity.

Results

Both groups were comparable for age, weight, duration of surgery and size of deep endometriosis nodules. Women in the extensive lavage group and in the control group were 34.4 years (range, 28–47 years) and 34.8 years (range, 27–42 years) old, respectively. Duration of surgery was 273.5 min (range, 153–391 min) and 226.5 min (range, 83–354 min), respectively. The deep endometriosis nodules were big in both groups, with a mean diameter of 33.7 mm (range, 18–41 mm) and 26.8 mm (range, 10–40 mm), respectively.

Postoperative CRPs were systematically lower in the lavage group from day 1 onwards to day 7 ($P=0.01$) (Fig. 1). Moreover, in the lavage group, CRP declined faster, being less than 13 mg/L on day 5, whereas in the control group, CRPs

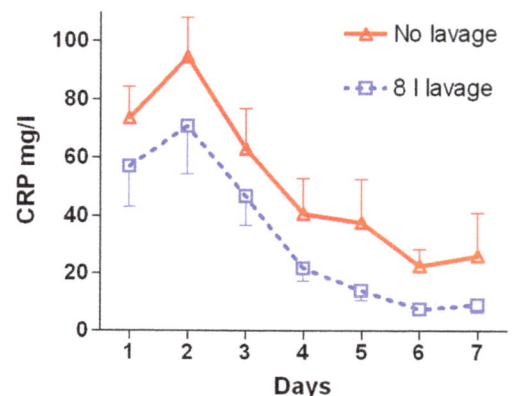

Fig. 1 Mean and standard error of CRP concentrations following full thickness resection of deep endometriosis of the rectum in case of extensive lavage with 8 or 0.5 L. Overall significance, $P=0.01$ (repeated measurement ANOVA)

still were markedly elevated on day 6 with a mean of 22 mg/L. WBC counts did not show any difference, being from day 1 to day 7, 13,330±3510, 11,650±3720, 10,140±3280, 8430± 2240, 7690±2300, 6370±830 and 8010±1810/mL in the lavage group and 10,450±3220, 9690±3280, 8170±2630, 7200±1600, 7640±1830, 6920±2530 and 7650±990/mL in the control group.

In the control group, 1/10 women had a late bowel perforation in comparison with 0/10 in the lavage group. Follow-up was uneventful in all.

Discussion

The treatment of deep endometriosis surgery penetrating the bowel wall varies from excision with a single suture of a muscularis lesion or a two-layer suture following a full thickness resection to a discoid excision with a circular or a linear stapler and to a bowel resection and anastomosis. The debate is still open, between those who consider that an open bowel should be avoided in any case and those who accept an open bowel with a suture if necessary. This trial was designed to evaluate whether more extensive lavage should be introduced to decrease the bacterial contamination when the bowel had been opened. The results that CRP concentrations are lower after extensive lavage suggest, at least, that more extensive lavage decreases the postoperative inflammatory reaction.

The risks and benefits of extensive peritoneal lavage should be balanced. Extensive lavage was reported not to have negative effects even up to 30 L. Also, the concern that macrophages and other immune-competent cells are removed is probably rather theoretical. Also in this series and in those patients undergoing extensive lavage for late bowel perforations, we never identified negative side effects or complications. A benefit of lavage is the decrease of the bacterial contamination in the peritoneal cavity. Lavage decreases mortality in animal models of peritonitis [22]. In observational studies, repeated lavage by laparotomy for four-quadrant peritonitis [2] decreased mortality and morbidity. Lavage reduced morbidity in peritonitis [7]. Recent evidence suggests that lavage could be used as a first line in treatment of diverticulitis, if not to cure the disease, at least to prevent a colostomy during subsequent surgery. Also for complications after bowel surgery, lavage is suggested [8–16]. RCTs to confirm the beneficial effect of lavage in diverticulitis have been initiated in the Netherlands [23] and in Scandinavia. In gynaecology, lavage has become a standard practice for PID [24] and for pelvic abscesses [25]. Although today, the evidence of a better outcome is scanty, it seems logic that lavage is performed with the concept that if it does not help, it does no harm.

It remains unclear how extensive peritoneal lavage should be done. It is unclear whether the upper abdomen should be included and whether lavage should be continued until the fluid is clear. The lower postoperative CRP concentrations after extensive lavage demonstrate, at least, that the postoperative inflammatory reaction is decreased in women who had a full thickness resection with an open bowel. It seems logic to postulate that the effect of extensive lavage will even be more pronounced when the abdominal bacterial load is more severe as in peritonitis. In the absence of negative side effects, we therefore suggest that more extensive peritoneal lavage should be considered to decrease the postoperative inflammatory reaction.

It is unclear whether the observed decrease in postoperative CRP concentrations is important in the absence of other demonstrated clinical benefits. A decreased postoperative inflammatory reaction, however, is associated with less adhesion formation in a laparoscopic mouse model [26] and in women [27]. Since lavage decreases adhesions following an infection in animal models [17], we suggest that a more rigorous and extensive lavage could also be beneficial in women.

The data on mesothelial damage [28], acute inflammation and enhanced adhesion formation by factors in peritoneal fluid shed new light on lavage [19, 22]. In addition to the removal of bacterial load, lavage is bound to affect the abdominal temperature. If the rinsing fluid is heated, care should be taken not to heat too much, since adhesion formation increases exponentially with temperature [29]. Since 80 % of the beneficial effect of lower temperatures upon adhesion formation is obtained at 31 °C, it is suggested to use a fluid around 31 °C. High volumes of fluid at a lower temperature indeed might affect the core body temperature. Considering that saline can be harmful to mesothelial cells, causing retraction and bulging [19, 30, 31], a richer solution, as Ringer's lactate, might be preferable. This also explains that adhesions increase after lavage with saline supplemented with 1 % povidone-iodine, 0.5 % povidone-iodine or 0.05 % chlorhexidine gluconate [32] probably through mesothelial cell trauma. The addition of antiseptics, antibiotics and substances affecting osmolality and pH anyway remains controversial [7]

In conclusion, more extensive lavage is suggested to be beneficial to remove bacterial load in diverticulitis, perforated appendicitis and severe PID or pelvic abscesses. Extensive lavage moreover decreases inflammation and CRP concentrations after surgery, which is important for reducing postoperative adhesion formation. Indirect evidence suggests that extensive lavage should be performed with a fluid around 30–31 °C, that a richer fluid as Ringer's might be preferable, and that antiseptics should be avoided.

Acknowledgments The authors wish to thank Marleen Craessaerts and Diane Wolput, Leuven, Belgium, for instrumental help.

Compliance with ethical standards All procedures performed were in accordance with the ethical standards of the institutional and/or national research committee and with the 1964 Helsinki declaration and its later amendments or comparable ethical standards.

Contributions of the authors Dr De Cicco, Dr Schonman, Dr Ussia and Prof Koninckx designed the trial. Surgery was performed by Koninckx with the help of Dr De Cicco or Dr Schonman. Dr Ussia helped in reviewing the literature.

References

1. Hotchkiss LW (1906) V. The treatment of diffuse suppurative peritonitis, following appendicitis. Ann Surg 44:197–208
2. Scholefield JH, Wyman A, Rogers K (1991) Management of generalized faecal peritonitis—can we do better? J R Soc Med 84:664–666
3. Linhares L, Jeanpierre H, Borie F, Fingerhut A, Millat B (2001) Lavage by laparoscopy fares better than lavage by laparotomy: experimental evidence. Surg Endosc 15:85–89
4. Kim DW (2014) Intraoperative peritoneal lavage: limitations of current evidence for clinical implementation. Ann Coloproctol 30:248–249
5. Cirocchi R, Trastulli S, Desiderio J, Listorti C, Boselli C, Parisi A et al (2013) Treatment of Hinchey stage III-IV diverticulitis: a systematic review and meta-analysis. Int J Colorectal Dis 28:447–457
6. Whiteside OJ, Tytherleigh MG, Thrush S, Farouk R, Galland RB (2005) Intra-operative peritoneal lavage—who does it and why? Ann R Coll Surg Engl 87:255–258
7. Platell C, Papadimitriou JM, Hall JC (2000) The influence of lavage on peritonitis. J Am Coll Surg 191:672–680
8. Cirocchi R, Trastulli S, Vettoretto N, Milani D, Cavaliere D, Renzi C et al (2015) Laparoscopic peritoneal lavage: a definitive treatment for diverticular peritonitis or a "bridge" to elective laparoscopic sigmoidectomy?: a systematic review. Medicine (Baltimore) 94, e334
9. Sorrentino M, Brizzolari M, Scarpa E, Malisan D, Bruschi F, Bertozzi S et al (2015) Laparoscopic peritoneal lavage for perforated colonic diverticulitis: a definitive treatment? Retrospective analysis of 63 cases. Tech Coloproctol 19:105–110
10. Hupfeld L, Burcharth J, Pommergaard HC, Rosenberg J (2014) The best choice of treatment for acute colonic diverticulitis with purulent peritonitis is uncertain. Biomed Res Int 2014:380607
11. Rade F, Bretagnol F, Auguste M, Di GC, Huten N, de CL (2014) Determinants of outcome following laparoscopic peritoneal lavage for perforated diverticulitis. Br J Surg 101:1602–1606
12. Welbourn HL, Hartley JE (2014) Management of acute diverticulitis and its complications. Indian J Surg 76:429–435
13. Edeiken SM, Maxwell RA, Dart BW, Mejia VA (2013) Preliminary experience with laparoscopic peritoneal lavage for complicated diverticulitis: a new algorithm for treatment? Am Surg 79:819–825
14. Afshar S, Kurer MA (2012) Laparoscopic peritoneal lavage for perforated sigmoid diverticulitis. Colorectal Dis 14:135–142
15. Toorenvliet BR, Swank H, Schoones JW, Hamming JF, Bemelman WA (2010) Laparoscopic peritoneal lavage for perforated colonic diverticulitis: a systematic review. Colorectal Dis 12:862–867
16. Favuzza J, Friel JC, Kelly JJ, Perugini R, Counihan TC (2009) Benefits of laparoscopic peritoneal lavage for complicated sigmoid diverticulitis. Int J Colorectal Dis 24:797–801
17. Sortini D, Feo CV, Maravegias K, Carcoforo P, Pozza E, Liboni A et al (2006) Role of peritoneal lavage in adhesion formation and survival rate in rats: an experimental study. J Investig Surg 19:291–297
18. Edmiston CE Jr, Goheen MP, Kornhall S, Jones FE, Condon RE (1990) Fecal peritonitis: microbial adherence to serosal mesothelium and resistance to peritoneal lavage. World J Surg 14:176–183
19. Breborowicz A, Oreopoulos DG (2005) Is normal saline harmful to the peritoneum? Perit Dial Int 25(Suppl 4):S67–S70
20. Koninckx PR, Ussia A, Adamyan L, Wattiez A, Donnez J (2012) Deep endometriosis: definition, diagnosis, and treatment. Fertil Steril 98:564–571
21. Koninckx PR, Timmermans B, Meuleman C, Penninckx F (1996) Complications of CO2-laser endoscopic excision of deep endometriosis. Hum Reprod 11:2263–2268
22. Sortini D, Feo CV, Maravegias K, Carcoforo P, Pozza E, Liboni A et al (2006) Role of peritoneal lavage in adhesion formation and survival rate in rats: an experimental study. J Investig Surg 19:291–297
23. Swank HA, Vermeulen J, Lange JF, Mulder IM, van der Hoeven JA, Stassen LP et al (2010) The ladies trial: laparoscopic peritoneal lavage or resection for purulent peritonitis and Hartmann's procedure or resection with primary anastomosis for purulent or faecal peritonitis in perforated diverticulitis (NTR2037). BMC Surg 10:29
24. Agresta F, Ciardo LF, Mazzarolo G, Michelet I, Orsi G, Trentin G et al (2006) Peritonitis: laparoscopic approach. World J Emerg Surg 1:9
25. Henry-Suchet J (2000) PID: clinical and laparoscopic aspects. Ann N Y Acad Sci 900:301–308
26. Corona R, Verguts J, Schonman R, Binda MM, Mailova K, Koninckx PR (2011) Postoperative inflammation in the abdominal cavity increases adhesion formation in a laparoscopic mouse model. Fertil Steril 95:1224–1228
27. Koninckx PR, Corona R, Timmerman D, Verguts J, Adamyan L (2013) Peritoneal full-conditioning reduces postoperative adhesions and pain: a randomised controlled trial in deep endometriosis surgery. J Ovarian Res 6:90
28. Volz J, Koster S, Spacek Z, Paweletz N (1999) Characteristic alterations of the peritoneum after carbon dioxide pneumoperitoneum. Surg Endosc 13:611–614
29. Binda MM, Molinas CR, Hansen P, Koninckx PR (2006) Effect of desiccation and temperature during laparoscopy on adhesion formation in mice. Fertil Steril 86:166–175
30. Polubinska A, Breborowicz A, Staniszewski R, Oreopoulos DG (2008) Normal saline induces oxidative stress in peritoneal mesothelial cells. J Pediatr Surg 43:1821–1826
31. Polubinska A, Winckiewicz M, Staniszewski R, Breborowicz A, Oreopoulos DG (2006) Time to reconsider saline as the ideal rinsing solution during abdominal surgery. Am J Surg 192:281–285
32. Roberts LM, Sanfilippo JS, Raab S (2002) Effects of laparoscopic lavage on adhesion formation and peritoneum in an animal model of pelvic inflammatory disease. J Am Assoc Gynecol Laparosc 9:503–507

10

Belgian consensus on adhesion prevention in hysteroscopy and laparoscopy

Verguts Jasper[1,2] · Bosteels Jan[3] · Corona Roberta[4] · Hamerlynck Tjalina[5] ·
Mestdagh Greet[6] · Nisolle Michelle[7] · Puttemans Patrick[8] · Squifflet Jean-Luc[9] ·
Van Herendael Bruno[10] · Weyers Steven[5]

Abstract Intrauterine and intraabdominal adhesions are a major cause for infertility. The most recent investigations have demonstrated the potential of intraperitoneal adhesion barriers combined with good surgical technique to reduce adhesion formation. For intrauterine adhesions we suggest to minimize unipolar and bipolar instrumentation whenever possible. We advocate the use of estrogens for 10 days after adhesiolysis: 2dd two tablets of estradiol 2 mg. Instillation of Hyalobarrier Gel Endo actually is not reimbursed but may have a beneficial effect after myomectomy or adhesiolysis. Concerning laparoscopic and laparotomic prevention of adhesion also, meticulous surgical technique is of the utmost importance. Residual blood should be avoided by careful hemostasis and rinsing with Ringer's lactate with heparin. Preferably braided sutures are not to be left in the abdominal cavity. We advise to avoid unipolar and bipolar cauterization when possible and to replace with ultrasonic or laser energy. The use of floatation barriers does not seem to add substantial benefit in the prevention of adhesions. Gel barriers (Hyalobarrier Gel Endo® or Intercoat®) are proven to have a significant effect on adhesion prevention. As for sheets, there is enough evidence that they prevent adhesions. The use of NSAID in the prevention of pain and/or corticosteroids in the prevention of postoperative nausea is already mainstay after surgery and can be further endorsed in the prevention of adhesions.

Keywords Adhesion prevention · Consensus · Hysteroscopy · Laparoscopy · Laparotomy

✉ Verguts Jasper
  Jasper.verguts@jessazh.be; Jasper.verguts@uzleuven.be

1   Department of Obstetrics and Gynecology, Jessa Hospital, Stadsomvaart 11, 3500 Hasselt, Belgium

2   UZ Leuven, Herestraat 49, 3000 Leuven, Belgium

3   Department of Obstetrics and Gynecology, Imelda Hospital, Bonheiden, Belgium

4   Unit of Reproductive Medicine, Department of Obstetrics and Gynecology, University Hospital Brussels, Brussels, Belgium

5   Department of Obstetrics and Gynaecology, Ghent University Hospital, Gent, Belgium

6   Department of Obstetrics and Gynecology, ZOL, Genk, Belgium

7   Department of Obstetrics and Gynecology, University of Liège, Liège, Belgium

8   Unit of Reproductive Medicine, Leuven Institute for Fertility and Embryology, Heilig Hart Hospital, Leuven, Belgium

9   Department of Obstetrics and Gynecology, Catholique de Louvain, Woluwe-Saint-Lambert, Belgium

10 Department of Obstetrics and Gynecology, ZNA Stuivenberg, Antwerp, Belgium

Introduction

Adhesions are fibrous bands between tissues and organs and are one of the most underestimated problems which may occur following surgery. Adhesions are not restricted to one type of organ or tissue but can involve any kind of tissue or even foreign material. A synonym of adhesions is synechias, coming from the Greek word synechia meaning continuation.

A study published in Digestive Surgery showed that adhesions developed in more than 90 % of patients who underwent open abdominal surgery and in 55–100 % of women who underwent pelvic surgery [1]. Adhesions from prior abdominal or pelvic surgery can decrease visibility and access at subsequent abdominal or pelvic surgery. In a very large study (29, 790 participants) published in The Lancet, 35 % of patients who underwent open abdominal or pelvic surgery were readmitted to the hospital on an average of two times after their surgery due to adhesion-related or adhesion-suspected complications [2]. Over 22 % of all readmissions occurred in the first year after the initial surgery and were linear over time. In the SCAR trial, it was demonstrated that the risk of readmission due to adhesions was 5 % over a 10-year period following an initial open surgical procedure for a gynecological condition [3]. Of the readmissions, about 40 % was readmitted between two and five times. This suggests that a great number of adhesions formed after surgery occur without symptoms.

Intrauterine adhesions (IUAs) are fibrous strings between opposing walls of the uterus. A randomized controlled trial reported the following incidences of postsurgical IUAs at second-look hysteroscopy: 3.6 % after polypectomy, 6.7 % after resection of uterine septa, and 31.3 % after myomectomy [4]. These adhesions are also referred to as Asherman syndrome when the endometrium is not functioning adequately (amenorrhea or painful menstruation due to hematometra).

The duration of the endometrial wound healing differs according to the type of pathology as reported by Yang and coworkers in a prospective cohort study of 163 women undergoing operative hysteroscopy [5]. At second-look hysteroscopy 1 month after operative hysteroscopy, more women achieved a full healing of the endometrial cavity after removal of endometrial polyps (32/37 women or 86 %) compared to adhesiolysis (30/45 women or 67 %), metroplasty (3/16 women or 19 %), or myomectomy (12/65 women or 18 %) (P<0.05). Significantly more women suffered from de novo IUAs at second-look hysteroscopy after metroplasty (14/16 women or 88 %) or adhesiolysis (34/45 women or 76 %) compared to removal of submucous fibroids (26/65 women or 40 %) or endometrial polyps (0/37 women or 0 %). Women with de novo IUAs were less likely to achieve full endometrial wound healing within 1 month compared with those without adhesions (23/74 women or 31 % versus 54/89 women or 61 %, P=0.0003). The authors conclude that the time needed for a complete recovery of the endometrium ranges from 1 to 3 months, following, respectively, the hysteroscopic removal of endometrial polyps and submucous fibroids.

With this consensus, we aim to help the gynecologist in discussing the problem of adhesions with their patients and in offering them easy and everyday care to prevent adhesions when possible.

Clinical significance of postoperative adhesions

Hysteroscopy

Significance depends on the degree and the location in the uterine cavity. Typical signs of IUAs such as menstrual abnormalities (irregular bleeding, hypomenorrhea, amenorrhea) can be masked by hormonal therapy, and dysmenorrhea or cyclic pelvic pain can be masked by use of oral contraceptives.

IUAs are associated with a poor reproductive outcome. Infertility rate has a prevalence as high as 43 % (922 of 2151 women) according to a large review of observational studies [6]. Recurrent miscarriage is increased ranging from 5 to 39 % in women with IUAs according to a review of observational studies [7]. Major and, at times, devastating obstetric complications may occur, e.g., placenta accreta/increta and higher risks for preterm delivery, uterine rupture, and peripartum hysterectomy [8].

Postabortion/retention: resection of placenta

Surgical treatment of placental remnants traditionally consists of dilation and curettage (D&C) using vacuum aspiration and/or a metal curette. In this context, it is well established that "blind" removal of tissue causes destruction or damage to healthy surrounding tissue, which may lead to IUAs. The interval after pregnancy at which trauma to the endometrium occurs is the most important factor in the risk of IUA formation [9]. In women undergoing secondary procedures to remove placental remnants after delivery or repeat curettage, IUAs are found in 40 % [10]. The results of a recent systematic review of IUA after miscarriage are in line with previous findings [11]. In a cohort study, hysteroscopic cold loop resection of placental remnants showed a lower rate (4.2 %) of IUAs at routine second-look hysteroscopy as compared with ultrasound-guided curettage using a metal curette (30.8 %) [12]. A similar rate of IUAs (4.4 %) was found in a retrospective series on hysteroscopic morcellation of placental remnants, where routine second-look hysteroscopy was performed in part of the patients [13]. Routine second-look hysteroscopy should be performed after surgical interventions for removal of placental remnants to further assess the risk of IUA formation [14]. Hysteroscopic treatment, allowing for selective removal of placental remnants and thus minimizing the risk of unnecessary trauma to the uterine cavity, may be the preferred surgical treatment [11].

Laparoscopy

Major complications of adhesions will depend on localization of the adhesion, causing chronic pelvic pain, bowel obstruction, or infertility [1–3]. Adhesion-related complexity at reoperation added significant risk to subsequent surgical procedures [15–17].

Pathophysiology of adhesion formation

Hysteroscopy

Any trauma to the basal layer of the endometrium may lead to the formation of de novo IUAs; nearly 90 % of all cases of

IUAs are associated with postpartum or postabortion dilatation and curettage [18]. The etiological role of infection in the formation of IUAs is, with the exception of genital tuberculosis, controversial [8]. IUA formation is the major long-term complication of hysteroscopic surgery in women of reproductive age.

The mechanisms of tissue repair in the human endometrium are poorly understood despite several hypotheses on the origin of cells for endometrial regeneration [19].

Laparoscopy–laparotomy

The classic model: a local phenomenon between opposing lesions

Adhesion formation is mediated through different mechanisms. Damage to peritoneal surfaces induces a response starting with an acute inflammatory reaction and a process involving mesothelial cells; macrophages; and exudate with cytokines and coagulation factors, neutrophils, and leukocytes [20]. Within hours, a peritoneal defect (i.e., caused by a trauma during surgery) is covered with macrophages and mesothelial cells [21].

If mesothelial cells are capable in covering the lesion, then fibrinolysis will be complete within a few days and reepithelialization will result in a smooth healed tissue surface.

If the normal repair fails or when repair is delayed, fibroblasts invading the fibrin scaffold start to proliferate, leading invariably to adhesion formation.

The updated model: the important role of the peritoneal cavity

The origin of the mesothelial cells involved in the repair of a serosal injury (cfr. supra) remains somehow unclear. Free-floating mesothelial cells are present at all times, and their number increases 12 times within 2 to 5 days after injury [22]. Also, these cells were demonstrated to implant and extensive lavage with removal of these free-floating cells slows down peritoneal healing [23].

The entire peritoneal cavity is exposed to the laparoscopic gas and to air during laparotomy, and the mesothelial cells are thus influenced as homeostasis is disrupted. The direct relation between CO_2 insufflation, acidification of the peritoneum, and decreased immunoprotection might thus result in an altered adhesion formation [24]. Identified so far are as follows: (1) hypoxia of the mesothelial cells due to the inner pressure of the CO_2 pneumoperitoneum, (2) desiccation of cells, and (3) tissue manipulation or combinations of these factors. Also, the CO_2 pneumoperitoneum itself has been demonstrated to increase adhesions and this increase is time- and pressure-dependent [25, 26].

Prevention of adhesions in hysteroscopy

IUD

There is no evidence on the effectiveness of any IUD in the prevention of intrauterine adhesions (IUAs) or on recolonization of the endometrial layers.

An IUD represents a physical barrier and might be helpful in separating the uterine walls and the endometrial layers. The ideal IUD for preventing adhesions should have a large surface; therefore, a simple T-shaped model is not ideal [27]. A Cu-IUD provokes a local inflammatory response and might thus even have a negative effect on the endometrial recolonization [28]. Progesterone IUDs have a suppressive effect on the endometrium and can therefore not be used. One small RCT showed no difference in reformation of adhesions between IUD plus hormone therapy and hormone therapy alone [29]. Moreover, introducing an IUD after adhesiolysis presents an extra risk of infection and perforation [30, 31].

Barriers

Five randomized studies have assessed the effectiveness of barriers (Hyalobarrier and Intercoat) in hysteroscopic surgery and were recently reviewed in a meta-analysis [32–37]. There is no evidence for an effect favoring the use of any barrier gel following operative hysteroscopy for the key outcomes live birth or clinical pregnancy (relative risk (RR) 3.0, 95 % confidence interval (CI) 0.35 to 26, $P=0.32$, one study, 30 women, very-low-quality evidence). The use of any gel following operative hysteroscopy decreases, however, the incidence of de novo adhesions at second-look hysteroscopy at 1 to 3 months (RR 0.65, 95 % CI 0.45 to 0.93, $P=0.02$, five studies, 372 women, very-low-quality evidence). After using any gel following operative hysteroscopy, there are more AFS 1988 stage I (mild) adhesions (RR 2.81, 95 % CI 1.13 to 7.01, $P=0.03$, four studies, 79 women) and less stage II (moderate) adhesions (RR 0.26, 0.09 to 0.80, $P=0.02$, three studies, 58 women) or stage III (severe) adhesions (RR 0.46, 95 % CI 0.03 to 7.21, $P=0.58$, three studies, 58 women) (all very-low-quality evidence).

Gynecologists might use any barrier gel following operative hysteroscopy for suspected uterine cavity abnormalities in infertile women: its use may decrease de novo adhesion formation [38] (very-low-quality evidence). If de novo adhesion formation occurs, there are less moderate or severe adhesions and more mild adhesions by using any anti-adhesion gel. Hyalobarrier is, for the moment, the only gel officially indicated for this purpose. Infertile women nevertheless should be counseled that there is, at present, no evidence for higher live birth or pregnancy rates by using any barrier gel following operative hysteroscopy (very-low-quality evidence); further randomized studies are needed to assess the direction and the magnitude of the treatment effect for these key reproductive outcomes.

Medical prevention

There is no evidence from randomized studies that the use of estrogen will prevent adhesion formation.

Since its first use in 1964, several regimens have been proposed to promote the reepithelialization of the endometrium after adhesiolysis [31, 39]. No data exists on the ideal dose and length of the therapy. Preoperative estrogen therapy has been suggested to optimize the endometrial growth before surgical intervention; however, evidence on its effectiveness is lacking [40]. Moreover, the possible adverse effects of hormonal therapy (nausea, thromboembolic disease) should be taken into account when considering its use.

There is no significant evidence from any published study to recommend the use of steroids (such as dexamethasone, hydrocortisone, and prednisolone) in humans, and several side effects still have to be ascertained [41, 42].

Some case reports describe the use of other medication (aspirin, sildenafil citrate, and nitroglycerin) to promote the perfusion of the endometrium [31]. At present, no evidence exists on its efficacy, and therefore, its use cannot be sustained.

Surgical aspects: technique/equipment

There are no randomized trials comparing the use of different surgical instruments regarding postoperative adhesions.

Cold scissors Mechanical separation is the most accessible mean of adhesiolysis. There are several possible advantages: direct view without destruction of the normal endometrium and easier insertion of a small barrel hysteroscope (3.8-mm outer diameter in median), without dilatation of the cervical canal allowing adhesiolysis without anesthesia or sedation.

Unipolar electrical energy Be aware that electrical energy engenders passage into the tissues to a depth of 0.6 mm in median causing a slower recuperation to *restitutio ad integrum*. The current has to travel to the recuperation plate where the patient remains within the circuit. An anionic distention medium is indispensable. Dilatation of the cervix up to Hegar 10.5 for the 27-French resectoscopes and up to Hegar 8 for the 25-French resectoscopes is needed as well as general anesthesia.

Bipolar electrical energy Bipolar electrical energy is in fact a monopolar cutting electrical current with the advantage that the current travels between two poles at some 8-mm distance from one another. The distention medium is ionic. There is direct view without passage of the energy into the tissues,

hence less destruction of the normal endometrium except for the endometrium in the immediate vicinity of the impact. Dilatation of the cervix up to Hegar 10.5 for the 27-French resectoscopes is also needed here. There are no small barrel resectoscopes available, thus necessitating general anesthesia. When using specific bipolar 4–5-French needle sounds (available in reusable or disposable versions), bipolar energy can be used through small barrel hysteroscopes of 3.8 mm with 5-French working channel. This way, it can be used without anesthesia or sedation.

Laser light The only available laser is the YAG laser where heat is diffused deep into the tissues causing thermal damage up to 1 cm in depth. The fibers are very fragile and expensive to replace. It can be used through small barrel scopes and can therefore be used without anesthesia or sedation [43].

Prevention of adhesion formation in laparoscopy and laparotomy

Surgical aspects

Surgical manipulation

Meticulous surgical technique is a means of preventing adhesions. The main approaches in preventing adhesions include adjusting surgical techniques to minimize trauma to intraabdominal structures, minimizing the risk of infection, avoiding contaminants and use of foreign materials, and achieving optimal hemostasis [44, 45]. Other foreign materials such as glove powder can cause a peritoneal inflammatory reaction. Controversy exists over the benefits of the use of sponges, as there are no randomized trials. When the bowel needs to be packed, an atraumatic bag might reduce injury to the serosa. Principles of gentle tissue handling and meticulous hemostasis prevent the presence of free blood and ischemic tissues [1]. Fibrin plays an important role in the pathophysiology of adhesions. When possible, a laparoscopic approach is generally preferred over laparotomy [45]. However, up till now, there is no evidence from randomized controlled trials to sustain this.

Blood

There are no randomized trials comparing the presence of blood to the formation of adhesions in the human. Animal experiments however showed that leaving blood in the abdominal cavity after surgery is a risk factor for adhesion formation [46]. It therefore is advised to clean the abdominal cavity with saline or Ringer's lactate. The addition of heparin (5000 IU/l) can be advised to keep the blood from clotting and making it easier to aspirate. In the absence of peritoneal injury, small clots did not contribute to adhesion formation in animal studies, while large clots did so [47].

Threads and meshes

There are no randomized trials comparing neither meshes nor threads to the formation of adhesions in the human. Leaving a mesh exposed to the abdominal cavity (not covered by peritoneum) will result in an increased risk of adherence to the mesh, with the risk of bowel obstruction. The presence of suture material and tightening the sutures to the point of ischemia promote adhesion formation [48].

Equipment

There is no evidence of any instrument causing fewer adhesions. Consensus is, however, to minimize tissue damage, which can possibly be achieved by using ultrasonic or laser energy rather than bipolar energy. Unipolar energy is likely to cause the most tissue damage.

Altering the peritoneal environment

The insufflation gas with carbon dioxide used for laparoscopy is known to have an effect on the total cavity resulting in inflammation. There is evidence from small trials in human that switching to a mixture of carbon dioxide with 10 % nitrous oxide and 4 % oxygen can decrease adhesions [49]. In a trial with 44 women undergoing laparoscopic resection of endometriosis, adhesions were significantly decreased ($P<0.0005$). Women in the study group also received dexamethasone, rinsing with heparin and control for humidity and temperature. No trials are available to support the use of the sole gas mixture in clinical practice regarding efficacy and safety [50].

Local products

Floatation barriers (Ringer's lactate, saline, Hartman's solution)

The instillation of such large-volume isotonic solutions (normal saline, Ringer's lactate, etc.) into the peritoneal cavity at the end of the surgery to produce a "hydroflotation" effect has represented the most popular and economic agent used for adhesion prevention in gynecological surgery. However, a meta-analysis of clinical trials has shown that crystalloids do not reduce the formation of postsurgical adhesions whether in laparoscopy or in laparotomy [51, 52]. This seems to be due to rapid absorption rate of the peritoneum (30–60 ml/h) which ensures a nearly complete assimilation of the fluid into the vascular system within 24–48 h, far too short to influence adhesion formation.

Adept® (4 % icodextrin solution, Baxter Biosurgery, Baxter International, Deerfield IL, USA) seemed to have a sufficient long intraperitoneal residence in animal and peritoneal dialysis patients [53]. It has to be used throughout the surgery, and 1.000 ml has to be left in the abdominal cavity [54, 55]. In a randomized, controlled pilot study, lavage plus instillation with 4 % isodextrin was well tolerated and reduced incidence, extent, and severity of adhesion formation and reforming after laparoscopic adnexal surgery even if the group sizes were not powered for statistical significance [56]. A recent randomized double-blind trial confirmed the previous results by demonstrating that icodextrin 4 % was effective and safe in reducing adhesions in patients undergoing gynecological laparoscopy involving adhesiolysis [57]. In a study by Trew et al., there was no evidence of a clinical effect, but various surgical covariates including surgery duration, blood loss, number and size of incisions, suturing, and number of knots were found to influence de novo adhesion formation [58]. Occasional adverse effects include vulvar edema, allergic reactions (allergy to starch-based polymers or maltose and isomaltose intolerance), fluid leakage through the wounds, and some abdominal distention and discomfort [59].

Gel barriers

Hyaluronic acid In a large multicenter randomized trial, Intergel® (ferric hyaluronate, Ethicon–J&J, Somerville, NJ, USA) was effective in reducing the extension and severity of postoperative adhesions in comparison with Ringer's solution in patients undergoing peritoneal cavity surgery by laparotomy with a planned second-look laparoscopy [60]. But, due to unacceptable postoperative complications, the gel is no longer available [61].

Auto-cross-linked hyaluronic acid gels (ACP gel, Hyalobarrier® Gel Endo, Nordic Pharma) are particularly suitable for preventing adhesion formation because of their higher adhesivity and prolonged residence time on the injured surface than unmodified HA. A prospective randomized controlled study showed that in 36 patients treated by laparoscopic myomectomy, application of the ACP gel reduced the rate of patients who developed postoperative adhesions significantly [62]. The same authors also demonstrated that the application of ACP in infertile patients undergoing a laparoscopic myomectomy was associated with an increased pregnancy rate [63]. The favorable safety profile and the efficacious antiadhesive action of the adjunct following laparoscopic myomectomy have been confirmed in a blinded, controlled, randomized, multicenter study [64]. Hyalobarrier is fairly easy to use in laparoscopic surgery and should be used at the end of surgery, as further rinsing can remove the gel.

Solution of hyaluronic acid, Sepracoat® coating solution (HAL-C; Genzyme Corporation, Cambridge, USA), is a liquid composed of 0.4 % sodium hyaluronate in phosphate buffered saline and is applied intraoperatively, prior to dissection, to protect peritoneal surfaces from indirect surgical trauma or postoperatively to separate surfaces after they are traumatized. No studies evaluating Sepracoat® in preventing adhesions following laparoscopic gynecological procedures are available in the literature, although efficacy in laparotomy was well established [65].

Hydrogel, Spraygel®, or SprayShield® (Covidien, Dublin, Ireland) consist of two synthetic liquid precursors that, when mixed, rapidly cross-link to form a solid, flexible, absorbable hydrogel. The solid polymer should be applied by laparoscopy, but the abdomen should be inflated with air which may cause air embolisms. It is sprayed over the affected area and remains for approximately 5 to 7 days. After that period, it is degraded and absorbed. One of the components contains a blue food colorant, so there is an intraoperative visualization where the SprayShield® was used. The currently available evidence does not support the use of SprayShield® neither by decreasing the extent of adhesion nor in reducing the proportion of women with adhesions. Mettler et al. randomized 64 women undergoing a myomectomy by laparoscopy or laparotomy. Only 22 returned for a second-look laparoscopy. Although the treated patients were more adhesion-free at second-look laparoscopy compared with the control group, the difference was not significant [66]. Further research is needed to evaluate the efficacy of SprayShield in multicenter randomized controlled trials.

Other gel barriers Intercoat® (Ethicon–J&J, Somerville, NJ, USA) is a viscoelastic absorbable gel composed of polyethylene oxide and carboxymethylcellulose stabilized by calcium chloride. Functioning as a mechanical barrier during the healing process, Intercoat is applied as a single layer at the end of the procedures. Lundorff et al. published the results of a randomized third-party blinded multicenter European trial showing that viscoelastic gel did significantly reduce adnexal adhesions in patients undergoing gynecological laparoscopic surgery [67]. Simultaneously, Young et al. (2005) performed a prospective randomized study evaluating the efficacy of Oxiplex® gel (FzioMed, San Luis Obispo, CA) and reported that the gel was safe, was easy to use with laparoscopy, and produced a reduction of adnexal adhesions [68].

There is considerable experience with CoSeal® (resorbable hydrogel polyethylene glycol polymer solutions, Baxter Biosurgery, Deerfield, IL, USA) in vascular reconstruction over 200,000 patients since 2002. When used together with good surgical technique in both open and laparoscopic surgery, the agent reduces significantly the incidence, severity, and extent of postoperative adhesions [69].

Sheets

Expanded polytetrafluorethylene nonabsorbable barrier Gore-Tex surgical membrane (Gore-Tex surgical membrane; W. L. Gore & Associates, Inc., Flagstaff, USA) has a microscope structure preventing cellular growth. It is noninflammatory and nonabsorbable. In patients undergoing gynecological surgery by laparotomy for adhesions or myoma, Gore-Tex surgical membrane was shown to decrease the severity, extent, and incidence of adhesions in treated areas [70]. Its usefulness is limited by the nature of the product: it must be sutured in place, and in most cases, it should be removed at a subsequent surgery. It is very difficult to apply at laparoscopy.

Oxidized regenerated cellulose (Interceed®, Ethicon–J&J, Somerville, NJ, USA) is the most widely used adhesion prevention agent and has been shown to reduce adhesion formation in both animal and human studies. It works by transforming into a gelatinous mass covering the damaged peritoneal surfaces and forming a barrier, physically separating the adjacent raw peritoneal surfaces. The efficacy of Interceed® has been studied in more than 13 clinical trials that included 600 patients. A meta-analysis of ten randomized, controlled studies reported a 24.2 % reduction in adhesion formation on the side treated with Interceed [71]. Despite this report, concerns about Interceed® continue, especially regarding its efficacy in preventing adhesions and its apparent ineffectiveness in the presence of blood. In this setting, Interceed® may aggravate rather than prevent adhesion formation.

Sodium hyaluronate and carboxymethylcellulose (Seprafilm®, Genzyme Genzyme Biosurgery, Bridgewater, USA) is a hyaluronate–carboxymethylcellulose membrane, which is placed over a suture or an injured area without stitches and remains in place for 7 days. In contrast to Interceed®, no loss of efficacy in the presence of blood has been reported. Several studies have demonstrated the efficacy of Seprafilm® mainly in general surgery. It is one of the most widely studied adhesion barriers, with more than 20 published studies that included over 4600 patients [70]. In gynecological surgery, the efficacy of Seprafilm® has also been demonstrated for some procedures, but it is not easy to use in all procedures. Seprafilm is fragile and, therefore, difficult to handle particularly in laparoscopy.

Drugs

Ketorolac is an NSAID that has shown some evidence in animals to prevent adhesions [72]. Dexamethasone was tested in 126 patients who have been operated upon by microsurgery and by second-look laparoscopy 3 to 6 months later [73]. Mean improvement on adhesion score was 23.2 in the corticosteroid group and 10.2 in the control group. Forty percent of patients in the corticosteroid group versus 19 % in the control group ($P<0.02$) became pregnant. No adverse effect has been noted.

Conclusion—general recommendations

Intrauterine and intraabdominal adhesions are a major cause for infertility. The most recent investigations have demonstrated the potential of intraperitoneal adhesion barriers combined with good surgical technique to reduce adhesion formation. The reduction of postoperative adhesions may be associated with clinically significant benefits such as improved fertility, reduction in pelvic pain, and improved quality of live.

Regarding adhesion prevention, available data show some improvement with different approaches. Taking into account data with strong and weak evidence, we have reached the following consensus:

For IUAs, we suggest to minimize unipolar and bipolar instrumentation whenever possible (i.e., cutting uterine septum with scissors). We advocate the use of estrogens for 10 days after adhesiolysis: 2dd two tablets of estradiol 2 mg. Instillation of Hyalobarrier Gel Endo may have a beneficial effect after myomectomy or adhesiolysis.

Concerning laparoscopic and laparotomic prevention of adhesion also, meticulous surgical technique is of the utmost importance. Residual blood should be avoided, and this can be obtained by careful hemostasis and rinsing with Ringer's lactate with heparin. The proper sutures should be used, and preferably braided sutures are not to be left in the abdominal cavity. Regarding instruments, we advise to avoid unipolar and bipolar cauterization when possible and to replace with ultrasonic or laser energy. The use of floatation barriers does not seem to add substantial benefit in the prevention of adhesions. Gel barriers (Hyalobarrier Gel Endo® or Intercoat®) based on hyaluronic acid are proven to have a significant effect on adhesion prevention and are reimbursed in some procedures. We advocate the proper use of these barriers. As for sheets, there is enough evidence that they prevent adhesions. The use of NSAID in the prevention of pain and/or corticosteroids in the prevention of postoperative nausea is already mainstay after surgery and can be further endorsed in the prevention of adhesions.

Altering the laparoscopic gas to a mixture of carbon dioxide +10 % nitrous oxide+4 % oxygen may be a future option, as this is an easy way to prevent adhesions, but further studies are needed to provide stronger data regarding efficacy and safety.

Our consensus is not a systematic review and does not provide guidelines with strengths of recommendation according to level of evidence. This consensus is intended as a supporting tool for gynecologists to give them a broad range of possible actions to be taken to reduce postoperative adhesions.

References

1. Liakakos T, Thomakos N, Fine PM, Dervenis C, Young RL (2001) Peritoneal adhesions: etiology, pathophysiology, and clinical significance—recent advances in prevention and management. Dig Surg 18:260–273
2. Ellis H, Moran BJ, Thompson JN et al (1999) Adhesion-related hospital readmissions after abdominal and pelvic surgery: a retrospective cohort study. Lancet 353:1476–1480
3. Lower AM, Hawthorn RJ, Ellis H, O'Brien F, Buchan S, Crowe AM (2000) The impact of adhesions on hospital readmissions over ten years after 8849 open gynaecological operations: an assessment from the Surgical and Clinical Adhesions Research Study. BJOG 107:855–862
4. Taskin O, Sadik S, Onoglu A, Gokdeniz R, Erturan E, Burak F (2000) Wheeler JM Role of endometrial suppression on the frequency of intrauterine adhesions after resectoscopic surgery. J Am Assoc Gynecol Laparosc 7(3):351–354
5. Yang JH, Chen MJ, Chen CD, Chen SU, Ho HN, Yang YS (2013) Optimal waiting period for subsequent fertility treatment after various hysteroscopic surgeries. Fertil Steril 99(7):2092-6-e3
6. Schenker JG, Margalioth EJ (1982) Intrauterine adhesions: an updated appraisal. Fertil Steril 37:593–610
7. Kodaman PH, Arici A (2007) Intra-uterine adhesions and fertility outcome: how to optimize success? Curr Opin Obstet Gynecol 19(3):207–214
8. Deans R, Abbott J (2010) Review of intrauterine adhesions. J Minim Invasive Gynecol 17:555–569
9. Al-Inany H (2001) Intrauterine adhesions. An update. Acta Obstet Gynecol Scand 80(11):986–993
10. Westendorp IC, Ankum WM, Mol BW, Vonk J (1998) Prevalence of Asherman's syndrome after secondary removal of placental remnants or a repeat curettage for incomplete abortion. Hum Reprod 13(12):3347–3350
11. Hooker AB, Lemmers M, Thurkow AL, Heymans MW, Opmeer BC, Brölmann HA, Mol BW, Huirne JA (2014) Systematic review and meta-analysis of intrauterine adhesions after miscarriage: prevalence, risk factors and long-term reproductive outcome. Hum Reprod Update 20(2):262–278
12. Rein DT, Schmidt T, Hess AP, Volkmer A, Schöndorf T, Breidenbach M (2011) Hysteroscopic management of residual trophoblastic tissue is superior to ultrasound-guided curettage. J Minim Invasive Gynecol 18(6):774–778
13. Hamerlynck TW, Blikkendaal MD, Schoot BC, Hanstede MM, Jansen FW (2013) An alternative approach for removal of placental remnants: hysteroscopic morcellation. J Minim Invasive Gynecol 20(6):796–802
14. Hrazdirova L, Svabik K, Zizka Z, Germanova A, Kuzel D (2012) Should hysteroscopy be provided for patients who have undergone instrumental intrauterine intervention after delivery? Acta Obstet Gynecol Scand 91(4):514–517
15. Menzies D, Ellis H (1990) Intestinal obstruction from adhesions—how big is the problem? Ann R Coll Surg Engl 72:60–63
16. van Goor H (2007) Consequences and complications of peritoneal adhesions. Color Dis 9:25–34
17. van der Krabben AA, Dijkstra FR, Nieuwenhuijzen M, Reijnen MMPJ, Schaapveld M, van Goor H (2000) Morbidity and mortality of inadvertent enterotomy during adhesiotomy. Br J Surg 87:467–471

18. Nappi C, Di Spiezio Sardo A, Greco E, Guida M, Bettocchi S, Bifulco G (2007) Prevention of adhesions in gynaecological endoscopy. Hum Reprod Update 13(4):379–394

19. Revaux A, Ducarme G, Luton D (2008) Prevention of intrauterine adhesions after hysteroscopic surgery. Gynecol Obstet Fertil 36(3): 311–317

20. diZerega GS (1997) Biochemical events in peritoneal tissue repair. Eur J Surg Suppl 10–16

21. diZerega GS, Campeau JD (2001) Peritoneal repair and post-surgical adhesion formation. Hum Reprod Update 6(7):547–555

22. Fotev Z, Whitaker D, Papadimitriou JM (1987) Role of macrophages in mesothelial healing. J Pathol 151:209–219

23. Tolhurst Cleaver CL, Hopkins AD, Kee Kwong KC, Raftery AT (1974) The effect of postoperative peritoneal lavage on survival, peritoneal wound healing and adhesion formation following fecal peritonitis: an experimental study in the rat. Br J Surg 61:601–604

24. Corona R, Verguts J, Schonman R, Binda MM, Mailova K, Koninckx PR (2011) Postoperative inflammation in the abdominal cavity increases adhesion formation in a laparoscopic mouse model. Fertil Steril 95(4):1224–1228

25. Molinas CR, Tjwa M, Vanacker B, Binda MM, Elkelani O, Koninckx PR (2004) Role of CO(2) pneumoperitoneum-induced acidosis in CO(2) pneumoperitoneum-enhanced adhesion formation in mice. Fertil Steril 81(3):708–711

26. Corona R, Verguts J, Koninckx R, Mailova K, Binda MM, Koninckx PR (2011) Intraperitoneal temperature and desiccation during endoscopic surgery. Intraoperative humidification and cooling of the peritoneal cavity can reduce adhesions. Am J Obstet Gynecol 205(4):392.e1–7

27. March CM, Israel R (1981) Gestational outcome following hysteroscopic lysis of adhesions. Fertil Steril 36(4):455–459

28. Vesce F, Jorizzo G, Bianciotto A, Gotti G (2000) Use of the copper intrauterine device in the management of secondary amenorrhea. Fertil Steril 73(1):162–165

29. Sanfilippo JS, Fitzgerald MR, Badawy SZ, Nussbaum ML, Yussman MA (1982) Asherman's syndrome. A comparison of therapeutic methods. J Reprod Med 27(6):328–330

30. Orhue AA, Aziken ME, Igbefoh JO (2003) A comparison of two adjunctive treatments for intrauterine adhesions following lysis. Int J Gynaecol Obstet 82(1):49–56

31. Deans R, Abbott J (2010) Review of intrauterine adhesions. J Minim Invasive Gynecol 17(5):555–569

32. Acunzo G, Guida M, Pellicano M, Tommaselli GA, Di Spiezio SA, Bifulco G, Cirillo D, Taylor A, Nappi C (2003) Effectiveness of auto-cross-linked hyaluronic acid gel in the prevention of intrauterine adhesions after hysteroscopic adhesiolysis: a prospective, randomized, controlled study. Hum Reprod 18(9):1918–1921

33. De Iaco PA, Muzzupapa G, Bovicelli A, Marconi S, Bitti SR, Sansovini M, Bovicelli L (2003) Hyaluronan derivative gel (Hyalobarrier gel) in intrauterine adhesion (IUA) prevention after operative hysteroscopy. Ellipse 19(1):15–18

34. Di Spiezio SA, Spinelli M, Bramante S, Scognamiglio M, Greco E, Guida M, Cela V, Nappi C (2011) Efficacy of a polyethylene oxide–sodium carboxymethylcellulose gel in prevention of intrauterine adhesions after hysteroscopic surgery. J Minim Invasive Gynecol 18(4):462–469

35. Guida M, Acunzo G, Di Spiezio SA, Bifulco G, Piccoli R, Pellicano M, Cerrota G, Cirillo D, Nappi C (2004) Effectiveness of auto-crosslinked hyaluronic acid gel in the prevention of intrauterine adhesions after hysteroscopic surgery: a prospective, randomized, controlled study. Hum Reprod 19(6):1461–1464

36. Pansky M, Fuchs N, Ben Ami I, Tovbin Y, Halperin R, Vaknin Z, Smorgick N (2011) Intercoat (Oxiplex/AP Gel) for preventing intrauterine adhesions following operative hysteroscopy for suspected retained products of conception—a pilot study. J Minim Invasive Gynecol 18(S21):68

37. Bosteels J, Weyers S, Mol B, D'Hooghe T (2014) Anti-adhesion barrier gels following operative hysteroscopy for treating female subfertility: a systematic review and meta-analysis. Gynecol Surg 11:113–127

38. Bosteels J, Kasius JC, Weyers S, Broekmans FJ, Mol BWJ, D'Hooghe TM (2014) Anti-adhesion therapy following operative hysteroscopy for treating female subfertility. The Cochrane Library, Cochrane Database of Systematic Reviews, 5

39. Wood J, Pena G (1964) Treatment of traumatic uterine synechias. Int J Fertil 9:405–410

40. Magos A (2002) Hysteroscopic treatment of Asherman's syndrome. Reprod Biomed Online 4(Suppl 3):46–51, Review

41. Watson A, Vandekerckhove P, Lilford R (2000) Liquid and fluid agents for preventing adhesions after surgery for subfertility. Cochrane Database Syst Rev 3, CD001298

42. Metwally M, Watson A, Lilford R, Vandekerckhove P (2006) Fluid and pharmacological agents for adhesion prevention after gynaecological surgery. Cochrane Database Syst Rev 2, CD001298

43. Haimovich S, Mancebo G, Alameda F, Agramunt S, Solé-Sedeno JM, Hernández JL, Carreras R (2013) Feasibility of a new two-step procedure for office hysteroscopic resection of submucous myomas: results of a pilot study. Eur J Obstet Gynecol Reprod Biol 168(2):191–194

44. Risberg B (1997) Adhesions: preventive strategies. Eur J Surg Suppl 577:32–39

45. Robertson D, Lefebvre G, Leyland N, Wolfman W, Allaire C, Awadalla A, Best C, Contestabile E, Dunn S, Heywood M, Leroux N, Potestio F, Rittenberg D, Senikas V, Soucy R, Singh S (2010) Society of Obstetricians and Gynaecologists of Canada. SOGC clinical practice guidelines: adhesion prevention in gynaecological surgery: no. 243, June 2010. Int J Gynaecol Obstet 111(2):193–197

46. Corona R, Binda MM, Mailova K, Verguts J, Koninckx PR (2013) Addition of nitrous oxide to the carbon dioxide pneumoperitoneum strongly decreases adhesion formation and the dose-dependent adhesiogenic effect of blood in a laparoscopic mouse model. Fertil Steril 100(6):1777–1783

47. Diamond MP, Decherney AH (1987) Pathogenesis of adhesion formation/reformation: application to reproductive pelvic surgery. Microsurgery 8(2):103–107, Review

48. Luijendijk RW, de Lange DC, Wauters CC, Hop WC, Duron JJ, Pailler JL, Camprodon BR, Holmdahl L, van Geldorp HJ, Jeekel J (1996) Foreign material in postoperative adhesions. Ann Surg 223(3):242–248

49. Koninckx PR, Corona R, Timmerman D, Verguts J, Adamyan L (2013) Peritoneal full-conditioning reduces postoperative adhesions and pain: a randomised controlled trial in deep endometriosis surgery. J Ovarian Res 6(1):90

50. Mynbaev OA, Biro P, Eliseeva MY, Tinelli A, Malvasi A, Kosmas IP, Medvediev MV, Babenko TI, Mazitova MI, Simakov SS, Stark M. A surgical polypragmasy: Koninckx PR, Corona R, Timmerman D, Verguts J, Adamyan L. Peritoneal full-conditioning reduces postoperative adhesions and pain: a randomised controlled trial in deep endometriosis surgery. J Ovarian Res. 2013 Dec 11;6(1):90. J Ovarian Res. 2014 Mar 10;7(1):29

51. Wiseman DM, Trout JR, Diamond MP (1998) The rates of adhesion development and the effects of crystalloid solutions on adhesion development in pelvic surgery. Fertil Steril 70(4)

52. Ahmad G, Mackie FL, Iles DA, O'Flynn H, Dias S, Metwally M, Watson A (2014) Fluid and pharmacological agents for adhesion prevention after gynaecological surgery. Cochrane Database Syst Rev 7, CD001298

53. Harris ES, Morgan RF, Rodehaver GT (1995) Analysis of the kinetics of peritoneal adhesion formation in the rat an evaluation of potential antiadhesive agents. Surgery 117:663–669

54. Hart R, Magos A (1996) Laparoscopically instilled fluid: the rate of absorption and the effect on patient discomfort and fluid balance. Gynaecol Endosc 5:287–291

55. Verco SJS, Peers EM, Brown CB, Rodgers KE, Roda N, diZerega GS (2000) Development of a novel glucose polymer solution (icodextrin) for adhesion prevention: pre-clinical studies. Hum Reprod 15:1764–1772

56. diZerega GS, Verca SJS, Young P, Kettel M, Kobak W et al (2002) A randomized, controlled pilot study of the safety and efficacy of 4% icodextrin solution in the reduction of adhesions following laparoscopic gynecological surgery. Hum Reprod 17:1031–1038

57. Brown CB, Luciano AA, Martin D, Peers E, Scrimgeour A (2006) diZerega GS. On behalf of the Adept Adhesion Reduction Study Group. Adept® (icodextrin 4% solution) reduces adhesions after laparoscopic surgery for adhesiolysis: a double-blind, randomized, controlled study. Fertil Steril 88:1413–1426

58. Trew G, Pistofidis G, Pados G, Lower A, Mettler L, Wallwiener D, Korell M, Pouly JL, Coccia ME, Audebert A, Nappi C, Schmidt E, McVeigh E, Landi S, Degueldre M, Konincxk P, Rimbach S, Chapron C, Dallay D, Röemer T, McConnachie A, Ford I, Crowe A, Knight A, Dizerega G, Dewilde R (2011) Gynaecological endoscopic evaluation of 4% icodextrin solution: a European, multicentre, double-blind, randomized study of the efficacy and safety in the reduction of de novo adhesions after laparoscopic gynaecological surgery. Hum Reprod 26(8):2015–2027

59. Douplis D, Majeed GS, Sieunarine K, Richardson R, Smith JR (2007) Adverse effects related to icodextrin 4%. Our experience. Gynaecol Surg 4:97–100

60. Johns DB, Keyport GM, Hoehler F, diZerega GS (2001) Intergel Adhesion Prevention Study Group Reduction of postsurgical adhesions with Intergel adhesion prevention solution: a multicenter study of safety and efficacy after conservative gynecologic surgery. Fertil Steril 76(3):595–604

61. Tang CL, Jayne DG, Seow-Choen F, Ng YY, Eu KW, Mustapha N (2006) A randomized controlled trial of 0.5% ferric hyaluronate gel (Intergel) in the prevention of adhesions following abdominal surgery. Ann Surg 243(4):449–455

62. Pellicano M, Bramante S, Cirillo D, Palomba S, Bifulco G, Zullo F, Nappi C (2003) Effectiveness of autocrosslinked hyaluronic acid gel after laparoscopic myomectomy in infertile patients: a prospective, randomized, controlled study. Fertil Steril 80(2):441–444

63. Pellicano M, Guida M, Bramante S, Acunzo G, Di Spiezio SA, Tommaselli GA, Nappi C (2005) Reproductive outcome after autocrosslinked hyaluronic acid gel application in infertile patients who underwent laparoscopic myomectomy. Fertil Steril 83(2):498–500

64. Mais V, Bracco GL, Litta P, Gargiulo T, Melis GB (2006) Reduction of postoperative adhesions with an auto-crosslinked hyaluronan gel in gynaecological laparoscopic surgery: a blinded, controlled, randomized, multicentre study. Hum Reprod 21(5):1248–1254

65. Diamond MP (1998) Reduction of de novo postsurgical adhesions by intraoperative precoating with Sepracoat (HAL-C) solution: a prospective, randomized, blinded, placebo-controlled multicenter study. The Sepracoat Adhesion Study Group. Fertil Steril 69(6):1067–1074

66. Mettler L, Audebert A, Lehmann-Willenbrock E, Schive-Peterhansl K, Jacobs VR (2004) A randomized, prospective, controlled, multicenter clinical trial of a sprayable, site-specific adhesion barrier system in patients undergoing myomectomy. Fertil Steril 82(2):398–404

67. Lundorff P, Donnez J, Korell M, Audebert AJM, Block K, diZerega GS (2005) Clinical evaluation of a viscoelastic gel for reduction of adhesions following gynaecological surgery by laparoscopy in Europe. Hum Reprod 20:514–520

68. Young P, Johns A, Templeman C, Witz C, Webster B, Ferland R, Diamond MP, Block K, diZerega G (2005) Reduction of postoperative adhesions after laparoscopic gynecological surgery with Oxiplex/AP Gel: a pilot study. Fertil Steril 84(5):1450–1456

69. Mettler L, Hucke J, Bojar B, Tinneberg HR, Leyland N, Avelar A (2008) A safety and efficacy study of the resorbable hydrogel for reduction of post-operative adhesions following myomectomy. Hum Reprod 23:1093–1100

70. Farquhar C, Vandekerckhove P, Watson A, Vail A, Wiseman D (2000) Barrier agents for preventing adhesions after surgery for subfertility. Cochrane Database Syst Rev 2, CD000475

71. Wiseman DM, Trout JR, Franklin RR, Diamond MP (1999) Metaanalysis of the safety and efficacy of an adhesion barrier (Interceed TC7) in laparotomy. J Reprod Med 44(4):325–331

72. Montz FJ, Monk BJ, Lacy SM, Fowler JM (1993) Ketorolac tromethamine, a nonsteroidal anti-inflammatory drug: ability to inhibit post-radical pelvic surgery adhesions in a porcine model. Gynecol Oncol 48(1):76–79

73. Querleu D, Vankeerberghen-Deffense F, Boutteville C (1989) Adjuvant treatment of tubal surgery. Randomized prospective study of systemically administered corticoids and noxythiolin. J Gynecol Obstet Biol Reprod (Paris) 18(7):935–940

11

Patient satisfaction and amenorrhea rate after endometrial ablation by ThermaChoice III or NovaSure: a retrospective cohort study

I. Muller · J. van der Palen · D. Massop-Helmink ·
R. Vos-de Bruin · J. M. Sikkema

Abstract Heavy menstrual bleeding poses an important health problem, which can be managed, besides other treatments, with endometrial ablation. Nowadays, the bipolar radio frequency device (NovaSure) is the most commonly used device for endometrial ablation, followed by the thermal balloon device (ThermaChoice III). Thus far, studies looking at treatment outcomes have mainly been done comparing NovaSure with the older ThermaChoice (I–II) devices. The aim of this study is to compare the effectiveness of the improved ThermaChoice III with NovaSure. Patients treated with ThermaChoice III at the Ziekenhuisgroep Twente hospital and NovaSure at the Medisch Spectrum Twente hospital were included in the study. The primary outcome measure was patient satisfaction after treatment, measured by the condition-specific menorrhagia multi-attribute scale (MMAS). The secondary outcome measure was effectiveness of the treatment, measured by the amenorrhea rate and the hysterectomy rate. Five hundred fourteen patients were included in this study; of these, 216 patients were treated with ThermaChoice III and 289 patients with NovaSure. The score on the condition-specific MMAS was high for both groups, without a significant difference between the groups (88.8 vs 86.5, $p=0.183$). The amenorrhea rate was significantly higher in the NovaSure group (45 vs 27 %, $p=0.001$). The hysterectomy rate was slightly higher in the ThermaChoice III group, without a significant difference between the groups (19 compared to 13 %, $p=0.066$). Patient satisfaction is comparable in patients treated with ThermaChoice III or NovaSure. However, NovaSure endometrial ablation leads to a significantly higher amenorrhea rate.

Keywords Heavy menstrual bleeding · Treatment ·
Endometrial ablation · NovaSure · ThermaChoice III

I. Muller
Faculty of Medical Sciences, University of Groningen,
Groningen, The Netherlands

J. van der Palen
Faculty of Behavioral Sciences, University of Twente,
Enschede, The Netherlands

D. Massop-Helmink
Department of Obstetrics and Gynaecology, Medisch Spectrum
Twente hospital, Enschede, The Netherlands

R. Vos-de Bruin · J. M. Sikkema (✉)
Department of Obstetrics and Gynaecology, Ziekenhuisgroep
Twente hospital, Zilvermeeuw 1, 7609 PP Almelo/
Hengelo, The Netherlands
e-mail: j.sikkema@zgt.nl

Background

Heavy menstrual bleeding (HMB) is an important health problem [1]. HMB has an incidence of 25 % among menstruating women, with the highest incidence between the ages of 45 and 54 years (27.8 %) [2].

Women with HMB without an organic cause can be treated with various drugs. However, 73 % of the women are not satisfied after this treatment and frequently resort to a hysterectomy as a solution [3, 4]. Hysterectomy is fully effective in the treatment of HMB, but it is expensive and can cause severe complications [5].

A less invasive treatment option for women suffering HMB is endometrial ablation. Endometrial ablation techniques intend to destroy the entire endometrial tissue. The first-generation devices for endometrial ablation were introduced in 1989 and subsequent years [6]. Nowadays, the bipolar radio frequency device (NovaSure) is the most commonly used device, followed by the thermal balloon device (ThermaChoice III). A network meta-analysis that compared second-generation endometrial ablation techniques showed a significantly higher satisfaction and amenorrhea rate 1 year after ablation for NovaSure when compared to ThermaChoice I [7, 8].

In contrast to the latex balloon of the ThermaChoice I, the ThermaChoice III uses a tear-shaped silicon balloon with an internal propeller, resulting in a better heat distribution in the whole uterine cavity. Varma et al. [9] showed higher amenorrhea (35 and 23 %) and satisfaction rates (84 and 69 %) after ThermaChoice III treatment when compared to ThermaChoice I.

Only one small study ($n=81$) compared ThermaChoice III with NovaSure. This study found an amenorrhea rate of 39 % in the NovaSure group and 21 % in the ThermaChoice III group, without a significant difference between the groups ($p=0.100$). The quality of life was significantly improved in both groups, without a difference between the groups ($p=0.100$). The lack of significant findings could be due to the relatively small study size [10].

We performed a larger retrospective cohort study within women who were treated with ThermaChoice III or NovaSure. The aim of the study was to compare the effectiveness of ThermaChoice III versus NovaSure with regard to patient satisfaction, amenorrhea rate, and hysterectomy rate. Safety aspects were also taken into account.

Methods

The study was performed in two similar teaching hospitals in the eastern part of the Netherlands: the Ziekenhuisgroep Twente (ZGT) hospital in Almelo/Hengelo, and the Medisch Spectrum Twente (MST) hospital in Enschede. Patients treated with ThermaChoice III or NovaSure between January 2010 and November 2012 were included in the study. Depending on the hospital, the patients were treated with the ThermaChoice III (ZGT) or NovaSure (MST). Women who were born before 1961 or who were treated with either device within 6 months before the start of the study were excluded.

The endometrial ablations were performed according to the manufacturer's instructions. In short, ThermaChoice III (Gynecare) device uses a probe with an attached silicon balloon. The silicon balloon is inserted into the uterine cavity via the probe. The balloon is expanded to a pressure of 160 to 220 mmHg with 5 % dextrose in water. The fluid is heated to 87 °C, and ablation requires 8 min. The procedure was performed in day care setting. The ThermaChoice III patients underwent spinal or general anesthesia.

The NovaSure (Hologic) device is inserted into the uterine cavity, and the mesh is expanded until it comes into contact with the endometrium. The system delivers a radiofrequency current until a tissue impedance of 50 Ω of resistance is achieved or after a total treatment time of 2 min. The procedure was performed in office. The NovaSure patients were administered 1 to 2 ml alfentanil intravenously and a paracervical block.

A failed ThermaChoice III procedure was defined as a shutdown of the system before the 8-min treatment time was reached; the system was shut down because either the fluid failed to reach the target temperature or the balloon failed to properly pressurize. A failed NovaSure procedure was defined as a shutdown of the system before a tissue impedance of 50 Ω of resistance was reached, unless the maximum treatment time of 2 min was reached. An inability to insert the device was also defined as failed procedure for both procedures. In case of a failed procedure, the levonorgestrel-intrauterine system (LNG-IUS), medical treatment, or hysterectomy were offered to the patient.

A retrospective cohort study was performed. In June 2013, data about patient characteristics, the surgery, and re-interventions were collected from the patient files and a questionnaire was administered. Patients were asked to return the questionnaire by mail or complete the questionnaire online with a personal login code. In the case of non-response, patients received a reminder telephone call.

The first section of the questionnaire addressed complaints patients had before and after the treatment and measured the satisfaction rate regarding the whole procedure. The second section of the questionnaire consisted of the condition-specific menorrhagia multi-attribute scale (MMAS). The questionnaire included questions about the consequences of HMB in six different domains: practical difficulties, social life, psychological health, physical health and well-being, work/daily routine, and family life/relationships. The sum of these domains gives a score between 0 (severely affected) and 100 (not affected) [11]. The condition-specific MMAS has a high face validity, good convergent, and discriminant validity and test-retest reliability with high internal consistency [12].

The primary outcome measure of the study was patient satisfaction after treatment, measured by validated condition-specific MMAS. The secondary outcome measure was effectiveness of the treatment. The effectiveness was determined by the rate of amenorrhea and the time until amenorrhea, together with the rate of hysterectomies and time until hysterectomy. Safety aspects were also evaluated. Safety was determined by the number and type of complications during and after treatments.

Analyses were performed using SPSS (SPSS Statistics for Windows, version 20.0. Armonk, NY; IBM Corp.). For all analyses, a p value <0.05 was considered significant.

The baseline characteristics of the patients and outcome variables were compared between the two groups. Continuous variables were compared with the independent t test if normally distributed and with the Mann-Whitney U test if not normally distributed. Categorical variables were compared with the χ^2 test or with Fisher's exact test, as appropriate. The Wilcoxon signed-rank test was used to compare two related continuous, not normally distributed variables, and a scatter plot was constructed to visually inspect the linear association between two continuous variables. Time to hysterectomy and time to amenorrhea after treatment were compared using a Kaplan-Meier analysis and the log rank test. Women who underwent a hysterectomy after the endometrial ablation were analyzed as non-amenorrhoeic. Variables that were different between the two groups and were also related to the outcomes of interest (both at $p<0.10$) were considered to be potential confounders. Subsequently, the relationship between the intervention and the outcomes of interest were corrected for these potential confounders using logistic regression analysis, and adjusted odds ratios (OR) are presented.

Findings

A total of 514 patients were included in the cohort: 216 patients in the ThermaChoice III group and 298 patients in the NovaSure group (Fig. 1). Table 1 shows the characteristics of the two groups. The parity was slightly higher in the ThermaChoice III group (2.3 vs 2.0, $p=0.001$) as well as the number of previous treatments (81 vs 71 %, $p=0.010$). There was no significant difference in sound length (mean 9.0 cm, range 5–13 cm) or age of the patient (mean 42.5 and

Table 1   Characteristics of the patients included in the cohort

	NovaSure 298 patients	ThermaChoice III 216 patients	*p* value
Age (years)	42.5±4.9	42.3±5.1	*0.567*
Parity	2.0±1.0	2.3±1.3	*0.001*
Previous treatment for HMB	212 (71)	175 (81)	*0.010*
>1 previous treatments	85 (29)	85 (39)	*0.010*
LNG-IUS	109 (37)	97 (45)	*0.057*
Oral contraceptives	143 (48)	106 (49)	*0.808*
Other drugs	61 (21)	59 (27)	*0.070*
Endometrial ablation	2 (1)	12 (6)	*0.010*
Number of myomata	0.3±0.7	0.3±0.7	*0.213*
Size of myoma (mm)	24.0±11.2	23.3±10.4	*0.810*
Subsereus	11 (4)	10 (5)	*0.554*
Intramural	32 (11)	29 (14)	*0.305*
Submuceus	5 (2)	2 (1)	*0.705*
Sound length (cm)	9.0±1.0	9.0±1.9	*0.787*
Filling balloon (ml)		20.4±10.3	
Power (W)	98.7±27.1		
Duration of current (s)	98.9±19.9		

Mean±standard deviation or frequency (%). Other drugs = goserelin, leuprorelin, lynestrenol, medroxyprogesteron, norethisterone, and transexamic acid

HMB heavy menstrual bleeding, *LNG-IUS* levonorgestrel-intrauterine system

p-value <0.05 was considered significant

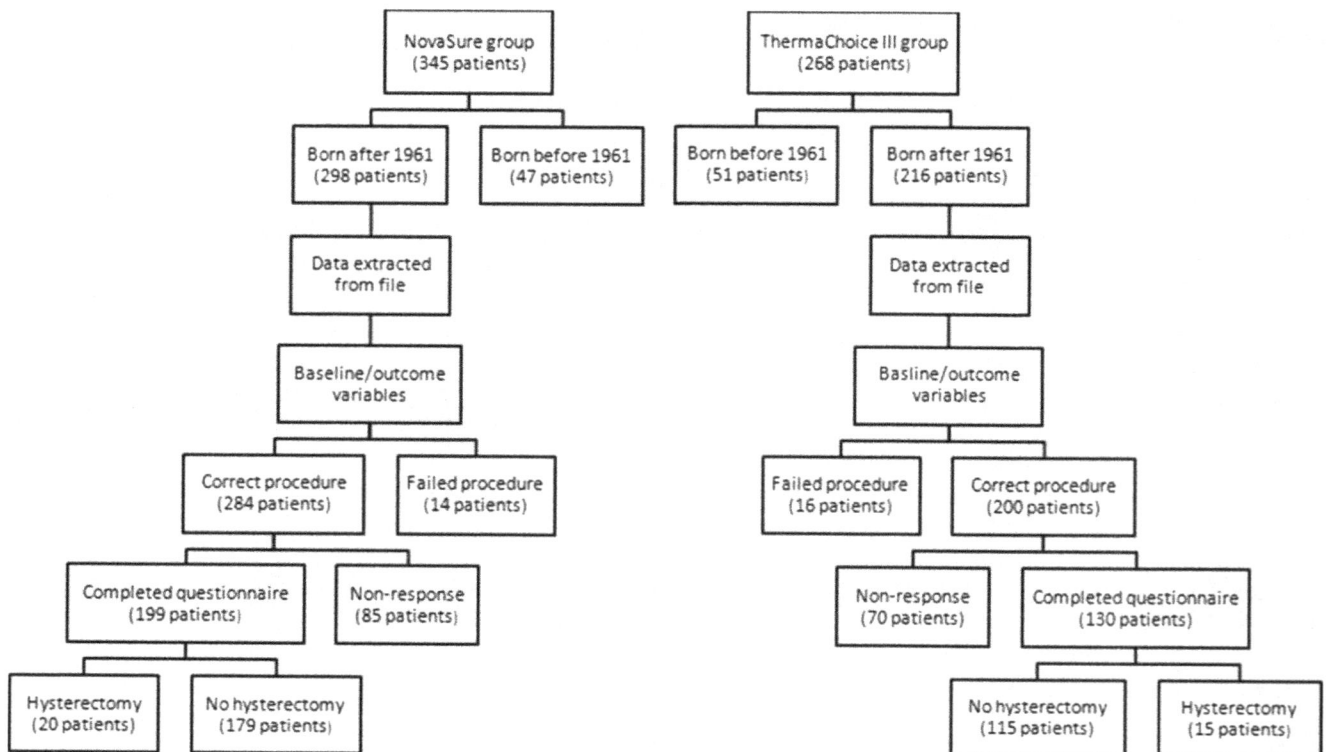

Fig. 1   Flowchart of the cohort

42.3 years, range 27–52 years) between the treatment groups. Myomata were noted in 19 % of the patients (ThermaChoice III 21 %, NovaSure 17 %). There were no differences in number, size, or type of the myomata.tgroup

The mean duration of ThermaChoice III procedure was 24.4 min, while the mean duration of NovaSure procedure was 10.5 min. However, during treatment with ThermaChoice III, other treatments were performed concomitantly more often. The most commonly performed procedures during ThermaChoice III were removal of a LNG-IUD and laparoscopic sterilization. However, the duration of the treatment with ThermaChoice III was still significantly longer if patients who had undergone concomitant treatments were excluded (Table 2).tgroup

The procedures were completed successfully in 93 % of the ThermaChoice III patients and 95 % of the NovaSure patients. The complications during and after the treatment were divided into five groups: infection, bleeding, perforation, cervical stenosis, and failed procedure. Besides the failed procedure, the other complications were very rare (Table 2).

A total of 329 patients returned the questionnaire: 199 patients (70 %) in the NovaSure group and 130 patients (65 %) in the ThermaChoice III group (Fig. 1). There was a slightly higher parity (2.3 vs 1.9, $p=0.008$), more previous treatments (81 vs 69 %, $p=0.021$), and more coagulopathies (5 vs 1 %, $p=0.007$) in the ThermaChoice III group. There were no

significant differences in age, body mass index, flushes, myomata, or sound length between the groups (Table 3).tgroup

The score on the condition-specific MMAS was high after both techniques, without a significant difference between the groups (88.8 vs 88.6, $p=0.183$). The NovaSure only gave a significant better score in the domain work/daily routine (16.4 vs 15.4, $p=0.031$) (Table 4). It should be noted that women who had undergone a hysterectomy did not complete the condition-specific MMAS questionnaire; consequently, women with a hysterectomy are excluded in Table 4. The amenorrhea rate was significantly higher in the NovaSure group (45 vs 27 %, $p=0.001$) (Table 5).tgrouptgroup

Of the two differences between the groups (i.e., parity and previous treatment for HMB, Table 1), parity was a potential confounder in the relationship between intervention and amenorrhea ($p=0.061$). However, after correction for parity, the relationship between intervention and amenorrhea remained significant ($p=0.001$, OR 2.46). The survival analysis shows the time until amenorrhea after NovaSure and

Table 2 Outcome variables extracted from the patient files

	NovaSure 298 patients	ThermaChoice III 216 patients	p value
Duration of entire procedure (min)	10.5±6.1	24.4±12.8	<0.001
Other procedure in the same session	14 (5)	40 (19)	<0.001
Duration if only ablation performed (min)	9.9±5.1	22.2±7.8	<0.001
Complications	19 (6)	19 (9)	0.154
Infection	4	1	
Bleeding	1	0	
Uterus perforation	0	2	
Cervical stenosis	0	2	
Failed procedure	14	16	
Re-intervention	59 (20)	58 (27)	0.060
Hysterectomy	40 (13)	42 (19)	0.066
Re-ablation	0 (0)	5 (2)	0.013
LNG-IUS	4 (1)	7 (3)	0.216
Non-surgical	27 (9)	12 (6)	0.139

Mean±standard deviation or frequency (%). Non-surgical = oral contraceptive pill, goserelin, leuprorelin, lynestrenol, medroxyprogesteron, norethisterone, and transexamic acid

LNG-IUS levonorgestrel-intrauterine system

p-value <0.05 was considered significant

Table 3 Characteristics of the patients who completed the questionnaire

	NovaSure 199 patients	ThermaChoice III 130 patients	p value
Age (years)	43.1±4.5	42.2±4.6	0.081
Parity	1.9±1.1	2.3±1.3	0.008
Body mass index (kg/m²)	26.0±4.4	26.5±5.7	0.366
Anticoagulantia	13 (7)	7 (5)	0.670
Coagulopathie	1 (1)	7 (5)	0.007
Flushes	51 (26)	32 (25)	0.901
Previous treatments for HMB	138 (69)	105 (81)	0.021
>1 previous treatments	53 (27)	50 (39)	0.024
LNG-IUS	65 (33)	57 (44)	0.040
Oral contraceptives	99 (50)	63 (49)	0.819
Other drugs	34 (17)	39 (30)	0.006
Endometrial ablation	1 (1)	7 (5)	0.005
Number of myomata	0.3±0.8	0.3±0.7	0.909
Size of myoma (mm)	22.2±10.1	21.8±10.5	0.884
Subsereus	10 (5)	7 (5)	0.859
Intramuraal	22 (11)	16 (13)	0.701
Submuceus	5 (3)	1 (1)	0.410
Sound length (cm)	9.1±1.0	8.9±1.1	0.236
Filling balloon (ml)		20.3±11.4	
Power (W)	98.9±27.9		
Duration of current (s)	97.6±19.9		

Mean±standard deviation or frequency (%). Other drugs = goserelin, leuprorelin, lynestrenol, medroxyprogesteron, norethisterone, and transexamic acid

HMB heavy menstrual bleeding, *LNG-IUS* levonorgestrel-intrauterine system

p-value <0.05 was considered significant

Table 4 Outcome of the patients who completed the questionnaire without hysterectomy

	NovaSure 179 patients	ThermaChoice III 115 patients	p value
Condition-specific MMAS	88.8±18.1	86.5±18.6	0.183
Practical problems	13.0±2.6	12.6±2.9	0.114
Social life	9.3±1.7	9.0±2.1	0.324
Psychological health	12.3±3.4	12.4±3.5	0.828
Physical health and well-being	17.9±5.9	17.7±5.5	0.342
Work/daily routine	16.4±3.3	15.4±4.1	0.031
Family life	20.0±4.8	19.3±5.1	0.211

Mean±standard deviation

MMAS menorrhagia multi-attribute scale

p-value <0.05 was considered significant

ThermaChoice III treatment, with a significant difference between the groups (log rank test *p*=0.001) (Fig. 2).

The experienced complaints related to the amount of monthly blood loss and dysmenorrhea significantly decreased in both treatment groups. Patients in the NovaSure group had significantly less complaints about menstrual blood loss and dysmenorrhea after treatment compared to those in the ThermaChoice III group (2.3 vs 3.1, *p*=0.009; 3.4 vs 3.1, *p*=0.014) (Table 5).

Many patients would recommend the treatment to a friend, and this percentage was significantly higher in the NovaSure group (93 vs 83 %, *p*=0.005). On the other hand, there was no

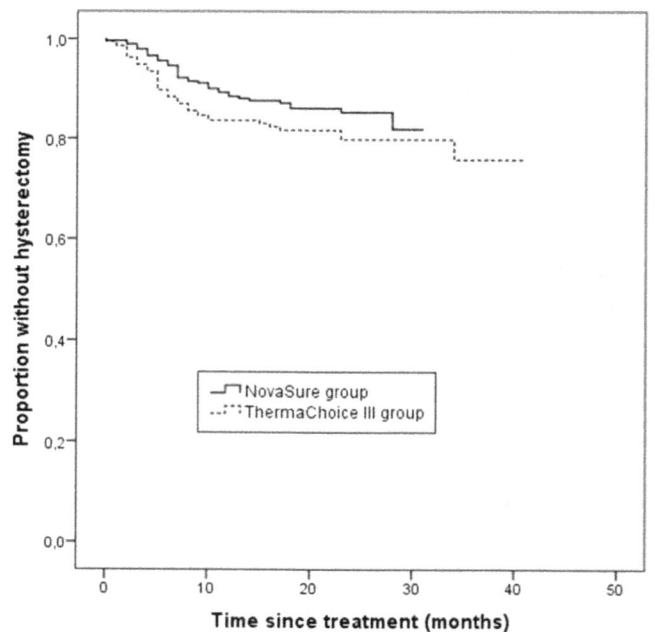

Fig. 2 Kaplan-Meier one minus survival curves showing the cumulative amenorrhea rate after NovaSure and ThermaChoice III ablation (log rank 0.001)

difference in satisfaction rate between the groups (8.1 vs 7.8, *p*=0.598) (Table 5).

Re-interventions (hysterectomy, re-ablation, LNG-IUS, non-surgical) were performed in 27 % of the patients in the ThermaChoice III group and in 20 % of the patients in the NovaSure group (*p*=0.060). There were slightly more

Table 5 Outcome variables of the patients who completed the questionnaire

	NovaSure 199 patients	ThermaChoice III 130 patients	p value
Amenorrhea	89 (45)	35 (27)	0.001
Months until amenorrhea	2.9±4.3	4.8±5.4	0.059
Experienced amount of monthly blood loss			
Before treatment	8.8±1.2	8.7±1.5	0.670
After treatment	2.3±2.9	3.1±3.1	0.009
Experienced dysmenorrhea (abdominal/back pain, headache)			
Before treatment	7.2±2.6	7.0±2.7	0.297
After treatment	3.4±3.0	4.2±3.0	0.014
Pain after treatment	4.0±3.0	4.4±3.2	0.217
Satisfaction	8.2±2.5	7.9±2.8	0.598
Recommendation of the treatment to a friend	174 (93)	105 (83)	0.011

Mean±standard deviation or frequency (%)

p-value <0.05 was considered significant

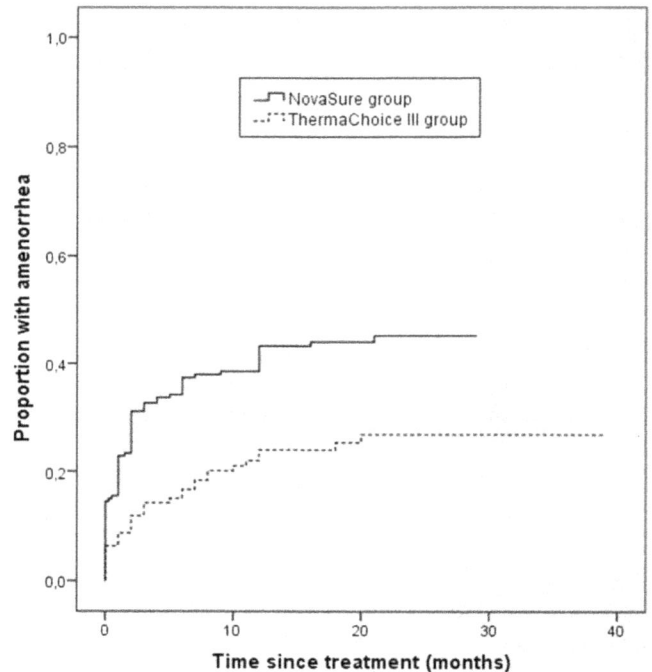

Fig. 3 Kaplan-Meier survival curves showing the cumulative hysterectomy rate after NovaSure ablation and ThermaChoice III ablation (log rank 0.124)

hysterectomies in the ThermaChoice III group compared to the NovaSure group, although this difference was not significant (19 vs 13 %, $p=0.066$). Previous treatment was a potential confounder for the relationship between intervention and hysterectomy ($p=0.080$). After correction for previous treatment for HMB, there was still no significant relationship between intervention and hysterectomy ($p=0.100$, OR 1.49). After exclusion of patients with failed procedures, there was still no significant difference in hysterectomy rate between the groups (ThermaChoice III 18 %, NovaSure 12 %, $p=0.063$) (Table 2). The survival analysis (Fig. 3) shows no difference in hysterectomy rate between the groups, not even after correction for the differences between the groups (parity and previous treatments).

Significantly more patients underwent re-ablation in the ThermaChoice III group. Two of the five re-ablations were performed because of failure of the first ablation procedure. The frequencies of the other re-interventions were comparable between the groups. Non-surgical re-interventions were the oral contraceptive pill, goserelin, leuprorelin, lynestrenol, medroxyprogesteron, norethisterone, and transexamic acid.

Conclusions

This study compared two second-generation endometrial ablation devices for the treatment of HMB. While ThermaChoice III and NovaSure performed comparably in terms of score on the condition-specific MMAS and hysterectomy rate, NovaSure gave a significantly higher amenorrhea rate. The number of complications was very low, which indicates that both techniques are safe and feasible.

We compared this study's outcomes with previous comparison studies of ThermaChoice III and NovaSure/ThermaChoice I [9, 10]. The scores on the condition-specific MMAS were notably higher for both NovaSure and ThermaChoice III in our study [10]. This could be due to the fact that dissatisfied women in our study might already have undergone a hysterectomy and therefore did not complete the questionnaire. As a result, our mean score on the condition-specific MMAS was too high to be representative for the whole group. However Varma et al. [9] found a score of 87 on the condition-specific MMAS, which is comparable with the 86.5 points we found. The amenorrhea rates in our study (27 vs 45 % for ThermaChoice III and NovaSure, respectively) were similar to those found in previous studies (21–35 vs 39 %) [9, 10]. The hysterectomy rate was higher in our study for both groups [10]. This is probably due to the longer mean follow-up time in our study.

The major limitation of the study is the retrospective study design, which renders randomization impossible. The non-randomized study design could explain the difference in previous treatments between the groups.

Patients treated with ThermaChoice III had more previous treatments (LNG-IUS, oral contraceptives, other drugs, endometrial ablation) than patients treated with NovaSure. An explanation may be that patients treated with ThermaChoice III underwent spinal/general anesthesia, rendering a higher threshold to treat a patient with endometrial ablation. Moreover, it is likely that the relatively higher number of previous treatments in the ThermaChoice III group resulted in a higher incidence of therapy resistance, which could partly account for the lower amenorrhea rates and higher hysterectomy rates in that group.

Another limitation is the large variation in time between treatment and completion of the questionnaire, which ranged from 6 to 41 months. As a result of this variation in follow-up time, some women would not yet have experienced the full treatment effect, while others could have experienced a relapse. However, the survival analysis solved this issue for amenorrhea rate and hysterectomy rate. In addition, there was no relationship between time since treatment and the condition-specific MMAS.

No cost-effectiveness studies have been done to compare ThermaChoice III and NovaSure treatments. In our study, the main cost difference will likely have been caused by the need for a day care setting for ThermaChoice procedures compared to the outpatient setting in NovaSure. Due to the fear of pain, the outpatient setting in ThermaChoice III has not been implemented in many hospitals.[13] Recently Kumar and Gupta demonstrated that ThermaChoice ablation was feasible in an outpatient setting using local anesthesia in a large cohort [14].

Overall, our results suggest that NovaSure gives slightly better results than ThermaChoice III, especially with regard to amenorrhea rate. It is possible that a certain technique would be advantageous for a particular patient group. Further research is needed to identify the best ablation technique based on patient characteristics such as presence of myomata, age, and dysmenorroea.

Authors' contributions I Muller: Concept and design of the protocol, execution of the study, data collection, data analysis, statistical processing, manuscript writing, and manuscript editing

J van der Palen: Data analysis, statistical processing, and manuscript editing

D Massop-Helmink: Manuscript editing

R Vos-de Bruin: Manuscript editing

JM Sikkema: Concept and design of the protocol and manuscript editing

Statement of responsibility The corresponding author confirms that (1) every author has agreed to allow the corresponding author to serve as the primary correspondent with the editorial office, to review the edited typescript and proof; (2) that each author has given final approval of the submitted manuscript; and (3) that each author has participated sufficiently in the work to take public responsibility for all of the contents, their individual roles being further specified in the text, which entitles the qualification for co-authorship.

References

1. Lukes AS, Baker J, Eder S, Adomako TL (2012) Daily menstrual blood loss and quality of life in women with heavy menstrual bleeding. Womens Health (Lond Engl) 8(5):503–511
2. Shapley M, Jordan K, Croft PR (2004) An epidemiological survey of symptoms of menstrual loss in the community. Br J Gen Pract 54(502):359–363
3. Marjoribanks J, Lethaby A, Farquhar C (2006) Surgery versus medical therapy for heavy menstrual bleeding. Cochrane Database Syst Rev (2):CD003855
4. Cooper KG, Parkin DE, Garratt AM, Grant AM (1997) A randomised comparison of medical and hysteroscopic management in women consulting a gynaecologist for treatment of heavy menstrual loss. Br J Obstet Gynaecol 104(12):1360–1366
5. Pinion SB, Parkin DE, Abramovich DR, Naji A, Alexander DA, Russell IT et al (1994) Randomised trial of hysterectomy, endometrial laser ablation, and transcervical endometrial resection for dysfunctional uterine bleeding. BMJ 309(6960):979–983
6. Lethaby A, Hickey M, Garry R, Penninx J (2009) Endometrial resection / ablation techniques for heavy menstrual bleeding. Cochrane Database Syst Rev (4):CD001501
7. Bongers MY, Bourdrez P, Mol BWJ, Heintz AP, Brölmann HAM (2004) Randomised controlled trial of bipolar radio-frequency endometrial ablation and balloon endometrial ablation. BJOG 111(10):1095–1102
8. Daniels JP, Middleton LJ, Champaneria R, Khan KS, Cooper K, Mol BWJ et al (2012) Second generation endometrial ablation techniques for heavy menstrual bleeding: network meta-analysis. BMJ 344: e2564
9. Varma R, Soneja H, Samuel N, Sangha E, Clark TJ, Gupta JK (2010) Outpatient Thermachoice endometrial balloon ablation: long-term, prognostic and quality-of-life measures. Gynecol Obstet Invest 70(3):145–148
10. Clark TJ, Samuels N, Malick S, Middleton L, Daniels J, Gupta J (2011) Bipolar radiofrequency compared with thermal balloon endometrial ablation in the office: a randomized controlled trial. Obstet Gynecol 117(5):1228
11. Shaw RW, Brickley MR, Evans L, Edwards MJ (1998) Perceptions of women on the impact of menorrhagia on their health using multi-attribute utility assessment. Br J Obstet Gynaecol 105(11): 1155–1159
12. Pattison H, Daniels JP, Kai J, Gupta JK (2011) The measurement properties of the menorrhagia multi-attribute quality-of-life scale: a psychometric analysis. BJOG 118(12):1528–1531
13. Marsh F, Thewlis J, Duffy S (2007) Randomized controlled trial comparing Thermachoice III* in the outpatient versus daycase setting. Fertil Steril 87(3):642–650
14. Kumar V, Gupta JK (2013) The effectiveness of outpatient Thermachoice endometrial balloon ablation: a long-term 11-year outcome study. Gynecol Surg 10(4):261–265

12

Total laparoscopic hysterectomy for non-puerperal uterine inversion: anatomical and operative considerations

Vasileios Minas[1] · Antonios Anagnostopoulos[1] · Nahid Gul[1]

Abstract The diagnosis and management of non-puerperal uterine inversion can be challenging. The majority of cases are caused by benign leiomyomas, but 15 % are related to a malignant mass. Published case reports can guide gynaecologists who encounter this rare condition and provide valuable insight in its management. We present a case of non-puerperal uterine inversion in a pre-menopausal woman treated by total laparoscopic hysterectomy. We discuss the challenges we encountered due to the distorted pelvic anatomy and conclusions drawn from a literature review. The article is accompanied by relevant video material. A high level of suspicion is required for the diagnosis of non-puerperal uterine inversion. Morcellation techniques should be avoided due to the potential for malignancy. Where myomectomy is performed vaginally, the possibility of uterine rupture should be taken into account. Management by total laparoscopic hysterectomy has not been reported previously, but appears to be feasible. The technique should be meticulous and aim to identify by dissection important structures.

Keywords Total laparoscopic hysterectomy · Uterine inversion · Uterine myoma · Laparoscopy

✉ Vasileios Minas
  billminas@gmail.com

[1] Minimal Access Centre, Department of Obstetrics & Gynaecology, Wirral University Teaching Hospital, Upton, UK

Introduction

Uterine inversion can occur either in the third stage of labour, when it is usually an iatrogenic complication due to premature traction of the umbilical cord, or in non-pregnant women as a result of a uterine mass which can be benign or malignant [1]. The majority of cases of non-puerperal uterine inversion occur in women over 45 years old. It is a rare clinical condition, and high level of suspicion is required to diagnose it [2]. The most common presenting symptom is abnormal vaginal bleeding. The patients may also complain of pelvic pain, presence of a mass in their vagina or protruding through the vagina, or acute urine retention. Although imaging can be of help, the diagnosis is often reached intra-operatively. Hysterectomy is recommended for women who have completed their families [2]. Here, we describe a case of a 47-year-old woman with non-puerperal uterine inversion associated with a large uterine myoma managed by total laparoscopic hysterectomy.

Case report

A 47-year-old patient presented to her primary care physician with a recent onset history of heavy vaginal bleeding and symptoms of anaemia. Physical examination raised the suspicion of a vaginal/cervical mass, and she was referred to secondary care as an emergency. She was reviewed by the resident on-call gynaecologist in our unit the same day. Besides a raised body mass index (BMI of 35), her medical history was uncomplicated. Recent cervical cytology was normal. She was significantly anaemic and was transfused 3 units of packed red blood cells. Pelvic examination revealed a 6–8-cm mass occupying the vagina in its entity. The mass was friable and bled on palpation. A fibroid protruding through the cervix was suspected; however, malignancy could not be excluded. An MRI was therefore arranged, and the patient was referred as an outpatient to a consultant gynaecologist with expertise in oncology and laparoscopic surgery on an urgent basis. The MRI suggested absence of pelvic lymphadenopathy and myometrial or parametrial invasion and supported the diagnosis of a fibroid. Fertility preservation was not an issue; therefore, the patient was consented for a hysterectomy.

On examination under general anaesthetic, vaginal access was limited due to the presence of the large fibroid. Its base appeared to be broad rather than pedunculated; therefore, a vaginal myomectomy was not attempted. Standard four-port laparoscopy was performed (video). It was not feasible to insert a uterine manipulator or a vaginal fornix delineator. Partial uterine inversion was diagnosed. The pelvic anatomy was distorted by the inward traction of the proximal part of the round and ovarian ligaments and fallopian tubes within the inverted uterine fundus. Bilateral salpingectomies were performed, and the ovaries were preserved. Bilateral ureterolysis was performed to identify the ureters which were seen drawn proximal to the uterus. Dissection of the ureters was continued down to the level of the uterine arteries which were clipped with Luger clips. Colpotomy was performed by digitally identifying the anterior vaginal vault above the invaginated fibroid. A total laparoscopic hysterectomy with bilateral salpingectomies and conservation of the ovaries was completed, and the specimen was extracted vaginally without the need for morcellation. The vaginal cuff was closed laparoscopically with four interrupted polyglactin absorbable sutures and extracorporeal knots. The estimated blood loss was less than 50 ml. The operating time was 146 min. Recovery was uneventful, and histological examination proved a benign leiomyoma.

Discussion

Non-puerperal uterine inversion is usually caused by a benign leiomyoma. Malignancy accounts for 15 % of the cases [2]. The diagnosis can be challenging and is often established intra-operatively. Gomez-Lobo et al. reported 150 cases of non-puerperal uterine inversions documented from 1887 to 2006 [3]. The majority have been managed by either vaginal or abdominal hysterectomy [3, 4]. There is one case report which described a combined laparoscopic and vaginal approach to perform a total hysterectomy for a 40-year-old patient with non-puerperal uterine inversion resulting from a 7-cm leiomyoma attached to the uterine fundus [1]. To our knowledge, the case presented here is the first case of non-puerperal uterine inversion managed by total laparoscopic hysterectomy.

Uterine preservation following extirpation of the mass has been described for women who wish to retain their fertility.

Rathod et al. adopted Kustner's method to manage a massive leiomyoma causing uterine inversion in a 28-year-old woman [5]. Kustner's method involves anterior and posterior transection to the cervix by vaginal approach to replace the uterine fundus and has been used mainly in cases of peri-partum uterine inversion. The authors still had to perform a laparotomy to repair the uterine incision that occurred during vaginal myomectomy. De Vries et al. also encountered uterine rupture requiring laparotomy while performing a vaginal myomectomy for a pedunculated leiomyoma in a 19-year-old nulliparous woman with non-puerperal uterine inversion [6]. In another case, the Haultain's procedure was used successfully following vaginal myomectomy to replace the inverted uterus, by incising the cervical rim that entrapped the uterus [7].

In our case, we decided to avoid vaginal manipulation of the fibroid as we were concerned we might encounter significant haemorrhage due to its broad base. At laparoscopy, distortion of the pelvic anatomy required extensive ureterolysis and identification of the uterine arteries at the level where they cross the ureters to safely ligate them (video). Identification of the correct area to perform the colpotomy also proved difficult. Colpotomy was finally performed laparoscopically by inserting two fingers in the vagina above the fibroid and digitally palpating and applying tension onto the anterior vaginal vault. Indeed other authors have reported that the identification of the limit between the cervix and the vagina can be particularly laborious [8]. Auber et al. achieved complete devascularization of the uterus laparoscopically and thus identified the limit between the ischaemic reversed cervix and the normal vascularized vagina. They then used this limit to guide the colpotomy which they performed by vaginal route [1]. In retrospect, apart from the limited access, a vaginal approach to our case would place the ureters at risk due to the distorted pelvic anatomy; therefore, we recommend that the colpotomy can be performed laparoscopically with safety by the method described above.

Conclusions

In summary, non-puerperal uterine inversion is rare, and a high level of suspicion is required for diagnosis since both clinical examination and imaging can be misleading. Morcellation techniques should be avoided due to the potential for malignancy. Where myomectomy is performed vaginally, the possibility of uterine rupture should be taken into account. Management by total laparoscopic hysterectomy is feasible. The technique should be meticulous and aim to identify by dissection important structures, including the ureters and uterine arteries, as the anatomy can be distorted. We suggest digital palpation of the anterior vaginal fornix to guide the colpotomy.

Compliance with ethical standards On behalf of all authors, the corresponding author states that there is no conflict of interest.

All procedures followed were in accordance with the ethical standards of the responsible committee on human experimentation (institutional and national) and with the Helsinki Declaration of 1975, as revised in 2008.

Informed consent was obtained from all patients for being included in the study.

Authors' contribution A Anagnostopoulos is responsible for data collection and manuscript writing. N Gul is responsible for the patient's clinical care. V Minas is responsible for video and manuscript writing/editing.

References

1. Auber M, Darwish B, Lefebure A, Ness J, Roman H (2011) Management of nonpuerperal uterine inversion using a combined laparoscopic and vaginal approach. Am J Obstet Gynecol 204:e7–e9

2. Lupovitch A (2005) Non-puerperal uterine inversion in association with uterine sarcoma: case report in a 26-year-old and review of the literature. Gynecol Oncol 97:938–941

3. Gomez-Lobo V, Burch W, Khanna PC (2007) Non-puerperal uterine inversion associated with an immature teratoma of the uterus in an adolescent. Obstet Gynecol 110:491–493

4. Lascaride E (1968) Surgical management of nonpuerperal inversion of the uterus. Obstet Gynecol 32:376–381

5. Rathod S, Samal SK, Pallavee P, Ghose S (2014) Non puerperal uterine inversion in a young female- a case report. J Clin Diagn Res 8:OD01–OD02

6. de Vries M, Perquin DA (2010) Non-puerperal uterine inversion due to submucous myoma in a young woman: a case report. J Med Case Rep 4:21

7. Tibrewal R, Goswami S, Chakravorty PS (2012) Non puerperal uterine inversion. J Obstet Gynaecol India 62:452–453

8. Jones HW (1951) Non puerperal inversion of uterus. Am J Surg 81:492–495

13

A study to compare the pain, discomfort and tiredness between straight stick and single-incision laparoscopic surgery: an in vitro study

Debjani Mukhopadhyay[1] · Thomas E. J. Ind[2,3]

Abstract This study compares pain and tiredness experienced by a student and gynaecological surgeons of varying experience between straight sticks (SS) and single-incision laparoscopic surgery (SILS) in vitro. Data was collected prospectively with randomization of the mode sequence. Participants from two hospitals performed identical exercise of cutting circles using SS and SILS in vitro. Questionnaires (Borg CR10 scale scores) were completed at 0, 30 and 60 min, respectively. Wilcoxon's signed ranked tests were performed on matched pairs of SS and SILS on the number of circles cut and the mistakes between 0–30 and 30–60 min, respectively. There were significant differences between the two groups at 30 min in arm discomfort, hand and finger discomfort, shoulder girdle tiredness, arm tiredness and most significantly in wrist discomfort with a matched median difference of 1.83, confidence interval (CI) 1.00 to 2.67 and $P=0.003$. At 60 min, the significant differences between the two groups were in shoulder girdle pain, arm discomfort, hand and finger discomfort, neck tiredness, wrist tiredness, and hand and finger tiredness and the most significant was wrist discomfort with a matched median difference of 1.75, CI 0.50 to 3.25 and $P=0.011$. SS causes less tiredness and discomfort in an in vitro setting than with SILS.

Keywords Laparoscopy · In vitro training · Single port · Straight stick · Pain score · Fatigue score

Introduction

There are increasing numbers of complex operations performed laparoscopically [17]. Laparoscopic surgery reduces hospital stay and time to return to normal activity. However, it is also associated with prolonged operating times compared to open surgery which may challenge the surgeon's mental and physical stamina [8]. Single-incision laparoscopic surgery (SILS) has been advocated for gynaecological and other laparoscopic procedures [17, 20]. There is a direct co-relation between sustained low-level muscular activity and musculoskeletal pain in turn affecting the surgeon's efficiency [16]. Therefore, we have investigated the difference in discomfort, pain and tiredness between SILS and straight stick (SS) in vitro.

Methods

Ten subjects with varying grades of experience participated. This included one medical student, three junior registrars, one senior registrar, two sub-specialty fellows in gynaecological oncology and three consultants (Table 1). One of the participants, who was a junior registrar, completed only one of the exercises and was excluded from the analysis.

Each participant performed an identical exercise with both SILS and SS. The first mode performed was determined by the flip of a coin. The exercise consisted of cutting out a piece of gauze between two circles of 5 and 3.5 cm diameter [18]. Templates of the circles were printed with a rubber ink stamp on gauze. Borg CR10 scale was completed prior to

✉ Debjani Mukhopadhyay
 debjani_2008@yahoo.com

1 The Department of Gynaecology and Obstetrics, Ipswich Hospital NHS Trust, Heath Road, Ipswich, Suffolk IP4 5PD, UK

2 The Department of Gynaecological Oncology, St. George's Hospital NHS Trust, Blackshaw Road, London SW17 0QT, UK

3 The Department of Gynaecological Oncology, The Royal Marsden Hospital, Fulham Road, London SW3 6JJ, UK

commencing the exercise [4]. The circles were excised in an in vitro training set, using a grasper (Endo Grasp™ single use instrument Covidien, MA, USA) and scissors (Endo Shears™ laparoscopic scissors, Covidien, MA, USA) appropriate for SS. The grasper (Autosuture Roticulator™ Endo Dissect, Covidien, MA, USA) and scissors (Autosuture Roticulator™ Endo Mini-Shears™ Covidien, MA, USA) used for the SILS had an extension with a curve that could protrude or retract as per surgeon's choice using a circular knob on the handle. The exercises were performed on a bespoke laparoscopic trainer using the in-built single instrument ports for SS and in-built SILS port.

The instruments used were out of date instruments retrieved from the hospital store. Borg CR10 questionnaires were completed at 30 and 60 min. The number of circles cut were numbered, stacked in sequence and sealed in an envelope with the participant's number. Participants returned on a separate day to do the same exercise using the other mode. The participants also filled out questionnaires at the same intervals as for the first exercise mentioned above.

The data collected included the grade, gender, handedness, hospital, exercise and time of day they did the exercise, the number of circles they cut between 0–30 and 30–60 min and the number of mistakes on each circle they cut. A mistake was defined as a cut in the line marking the inner or outer circles. This was done for both SS and SILS.

In the absence of any data in the literature, a power analysis was not possible and the number of subjects selected in each arm was empirical. The Shapiro-Wilk test for normality showed that some variables significantly differed from a normal distribution. Therefore, variables were expressed as medians with interquartile ranges. The Wilcoxon signed rank test was used to compare SS and SILS matching for each subject.

Results

Among the participants, six of nine (66.7 %) were females and three (33.3 %) were males. One out of nine (11.1 %)

was left-handed, one (11.1 %) was ambidextrous and seven (77.8 %) were right-handed (Table 1).

At 30 min, there was no significant difference detected between SS and SILS for 'headaches', 'shoulder girdle pain' and 'general tiredness' (Table 2). In addition, at 30 min, there were significantly less 'neck pain', 'arm discomfort', 'wrist discomfort', 'hand and finger discomfort', 'neck tiredness', 'shoulder girdle tiredness', 'arm tiredness', 'wrist tiredness' and 'hand and finger tiredness' in SS compared to SILS (Table 2).

At 60 min, there was no significant difference detected between SS and SILS for 'headaches', 'neck pain' and 'general tiredness' in SS compared to SILS (Table 2). In addition, at 60 min, there were significantly less 'shoulder girdle pain', 'arm discomfort', 'wrist discomfort', 'hand and finger discomfort', 'neck tiredness', 'shoulder girdle tiredness', 'arm tiredness', 'wrist tiredness' and 'hand and finger tiredness' in SS compared to SILS.

More circles were cut and less mistakes made over the hour-long exercise when using straight stick compared to single incision (Table 3). This has been demonstrated at both 30 and 60 min for the number of circles completed but only at the first 30 min for mistakes (Table 3).

Discussion

The study demonstrates that participants experienced overall less discomfort, pain and tiredness using SS compared to SILS at both 30 and 60 min into the exercise irrespective of their experience with laparoscopy. There were no differences in 'headaches' and 'general tiredness' between SS and SILS. Also, there were no differences in 'shoulder girdle pain' in the first 30 min and no differences in 'neck pain' in the second 30 min (Table 2). This in part may be due to low numbers of participants in the study. The participants cut more circles and made fewer mistakes using SS than SILS (Table 3). However, the design was too small to enable an assessment between doctors of different grades.

Table 1 The demographics of participants

Participant	Grade	Gender	Handedness	Hospital	First mode
1	Medical student	Female	Right	SGH	SILS
2	Gynecological oncology consultant	Female	Left	RMH	SS
3	Clinical research fellow	Female	Right	RMH	SS
4	Gynecological oncology consultant	Male	Right	RMH	SS
5	Gynecological oncology sub-specialty trained fellow	Female	Right	RMH	SILS
6	Specialist trainee—year 4	Male	Ambidextrous	SGH	SILS
7	Clinical fellow	Female	Right	SGH	SILS
8	Specialist trainee—year 3	Female	Right	SGH	SILS
9	Consultant gynecologist	Male	Right	SGH	SS

Table 2 Comparison of tiredness and discomfort scores between straight stick and SILS surgery in vitro

		Straight stick	SILS	Matched median difference	
		MoBLS (IQ range)	MoBLS (IQ range)	MoBLS (95 % CI)	Wilcoxon P
Discomfort and pain					
Headache	After 30 min	1.00 (1.00–1.00)	1.00 (1.00–1.20)	NC	ns
	After 60 min	1.00 (1.00–1.00)	1.00 (1.00–1.20)	NC	ns
Neck pain	After 30 min	1.00 (1.00–1.00)	1.50 (1.33–2.00)	0.50 (0.00 to 1.00)	0.0938
	After 60 min	1.50 (1.00–1.67)	2.00 (1.33–3.00)	0.75 (−0.17 to 2.00)	0.2500
Shoulder girdle pain	After 30 min	1.00 (1.00–1.33)	1.50 (1.00–2.25)	0.46 (−0.25 to 1.21)	0.2188
	After 60 min	1.60 (1.00–2.00)	3.00 (2.00–3.50)	1.00 (0.00 to 2.00)	0.0391
Arm discomfort	After 30 min	1.33 (1.00–1.50)	3.00 (2.00–3.00)	1.42 (0.50 to 2.25)	0.0195
	After 60 min	1.00 (1.00–2.00)	4.00 (3.00–4.00)	2.50 (0.83 to 3.25)	0.0156
Wrist discomfort	After 30 min	1.50 (1.00–2.00)	4.00 (3.50–4.00)	1.83 (1.00 to 2.67)	0.0039
	After 60 min	2.00 (1.50–3.00)	4.00 (3.00–5.00)	1.75 (0.50 to 3.25)	0.0117
Hand and finger discomfort	After 30 min	3.00 (2.00–4.00)	4.00 (4.00–4.00)	1.50 (0.75 to 2.25)	0.0078
	After 60 min	3.00 (3.00–4.00)	5.00 (5.00–5.33)	1.75 (0.25 to 3.50)	0.0391
Tiredness					
General tiredness	After 30 min	1.00 (1.00–2.00)	1.33 (1.00–3.00)	0.92 (−0.17 to 2.00)	0.1563
	After 60 min	1.50 (1.00–2.00)	2.50 (1.00–4.00)	1.00 (−0.46 to 2.13)	0.1484
Neck tiredness	After 30 min	1.00 (1.00–1.33)	2.50 (1.50–3.00)	1.00 (0.33 to 2.00)	0.0156
	After 60 min	1.50 (1.00–2.00)	3.00 (2.00–4.00)	1.17 (−0.08 to 2.42)	0.0781
Shoulder girdle tiredness	After 30 min	1.33 (1.00–1.50)	3.67 (2.00–4.00)	1.50 (0.00 to 2.75)	0.0313
	After 60 min	1.80 (1.00–2.00)	4.00 (3.00–4.00)	2.00 (0.50 to 3.00)	0.0156
Arm tiredness	After 30 min	1.50 (1.00–1.67)	3.50 (3.00–4.00)	2.17 (0.75 to 2.75)	0.0078
	After 60 min	2.00 (2.00–3.00)	4.00 (4.00–5.00)	2.00 (0.75 to 3.00)	0.0117
Wrist tiredness	After 30 min	1.50 (1.50–1.67)	4.00 (3.00–4.00)	1.75 (0.50 to 3.00)	0.0117
	After 60 min	2.33 (1.50–3.00)	5.00 (4.00–5.00)	2.25 (1.00 to 3.33)	0.0039
Hand and finger tiredness	After 30 min	2.00 (1.50–3.00)	4.00 (4.00–4.50)	2.00 (0.75 to 3.00)	0.0195
	After 60 min	4.00 (1.5–4.00)	5.33 (4.00–6.00)	2.25 (0.50 to 3.58)	0.0234

MoBLS multiples of the baseline score at 0 min after addition of the value 1 to all scores to account for zeros, *IQ range* interquartile range, *NC* not calculated as number of non-zero differences less than 4, *ns* not significant

The limitation with the exercise is that it is performed in an in vitro setting. However, in vitro scoring is known to reflect well in real-life surgery, and there are studies that demonstrate there is good correlation with in vivo practice [12, 14]. It would be interesting to note if there are any differences in the scores as the exercises become more difficult or with more senior groups of participants.

Psychophysical scores have been studied extensively and have been applied implicitly to sports in order to assess physical activity and to optimize training [1]. Borg CR10 scores

Table 3 Comparison of the number of circles completed and number of mistakes per circle between SS and SILS exercises in-vitro

	SS Circles	SILS Circles	Median matched difference, N (95 % CI)	Wilcoxon P
	Number completed, N (IQ range)	Number completed, N (IQ range)		
First 30 min	11 (9–15)	4 (3–9)	6.5 (5.0 to 8.0)	0.0039
Second 30 min	12 (10–17)	5 (4–8)	6.5 (4.0 to 10.0)	0.0039
Total	23 (21–34)	8 (8–17)	13.0 (9.5 to 17.5)	0.0039
	Mistakes per circle, N (IQ range)	Mistakes per circle, N (IQ range)		
First 30 min	1.28 (0.69–1.50)	2.22 (1.70–4.00)	1.44 (0.31 to 2.87)	0.0391
Second 30 min	0.56 (0.33–2.10)	1.00 (0.50–5.00)	0.77 (−0.55 to 2.79)	0.1289
Total	0.96 (0.52–2.10)	1.59 (0.80–4.50)	0.97 (0.08 to 2.65)	0.0391

have a maximum value 10 and have been extensively in surgery [2, 10]. All surgery involves physical as well as mental activity. The port site can pose problems in optimal handling of laparoscopic instruments intra-operatively when the focus is intense. This may result in pain or fatigue owing to sustained muscular contractions, in turn, affecting the surgical ability. The port site contributes significantly to the surgeon's comfort during laparoscopic surgery [12].

The surgeon's experience is thought to influence the type and the time taken for a procedure, although it does not affect postoperative recovery [9]. Endoscopic surgical experience improves with repeated performance of the surgery over a period of time [3, 7, 19]. This study does not assess skills per se, yet experience would influence the psychophysical score. Engelmann et al. showed that breaks during complex laparoscopic surgery reduced psychological stress maintaining efficiency without prolonging operating time [5]. In athletics, Borg CR10 is used to score and plan the methodology of training [15]. This helps to decide the optimal time spent in training as low-level sustained muscular activity results in musculoskeletal pain [16]. Taking these factors into account, it would be possible to have personal scores to modify the ergonomics and understand the time limit for optimal performance, thus prevent future musculoskeletal problems. In laparoscopic surgery, this would help plan the route of surgery aiming to complete it within a personal optimal time frame.

Repetitive intermittent static movements cause muscle fatigue, and this correlates with discomfort scores [11]. A study to predict musculoskeletal discomfort using Borg CR10 scales showed that trunk inclination and handling frequency are the major determinants of musculoskeletal discomfort [13]. Video feedback to the participants may have helped improve the discomfort scores. A systematic review of single-incision laparoscopic colonic surgery gave a cautious conclusion that SILS should be restricted to highly selected group of patients and surgeons [6]. That study concluded that only experienced surgeons should perform SILS surgery, and our data would support this as in in vitro a group of less experienced surgeons had more pain and discomfort using SILS.

Conclusion

Laparoscopic surgery needs a unique skill set. This study demonstrates that surgeon's pain and tiredness scores are better in SS than SILS. There is need for further research to establish whether there are any differences between SS and SILS with more difficult exercises and in in vivo.

Funding   The authors received no funding for this study.

Authors' contribution   Debjani Mukhopadhyay contributed to the collection of data, literature search and drafting the manuscript. Thomas J. Ind conceived the idea, analysed the data, and critically revised and approved the final version for submission.

References

1. Bajaj P, Graven-Nielsen T, Arendt-Nielsen L (2001) Post-exercise muscle soreness after eccentric exercise: psychophysical effects and implications on mean arterial pressure. Scand J Med Sci Sports 11: 266–273
2. Bertolaccini L, Viti A, Terzi A (2014) Ergon-trial: ergonomic evaluation of single-port access versus three-port access video-assisted thoracic surgery. Surg Endosc. doi:10.1007/s00464-014-4024-6
3. Bock O, Schneider S, Bloomberg J (2001) Conditions for interference versus facilitation during sequential sensorimotor adaptation. Exp Brain Res 138:359–365
4. Borg G (1990) Psychophysical scaling with applications in physical work and the perception of exertion. Scand J Work Environ Health 16(Suppl 1):55–58
5. Engelmann C, Schneider M, Kirschbaum C, Grote G, Dingemann J, Schoof S, Ure BM (2011) Effects of intraoperative breaks on mental and somatic operator fatigue: a randomized clinical trial. Surg Endosc 25:1245–1250. doi:10.1007/s00464-010-1350-1
6. Fung AK-Y, Aly EH (2012) Systematic review of single-incision laparoscopic colonic surgery. Br J Surg 99:1353–1364. doi:10.1002/bjs.8834
7. Gallagher AG, Ritter EM, Champion H, Higgins G, Fried MP, Moses G, Smith CD, Satava RM (2005) Virtual reality simulation for the operating room: proficiency-based training as a paradigm shift in surgical skills training. Ann Surg 241:364–372
8. Glinatsis MT, Griffith JP, McMahon MJ (1992) Open versus laparoscopic cholecystectomy: a retrospective comparative study. J Laparoendosc Surg 2:81–86, discussion 87
9. Herrero A, Philippe C, Guillon F, Millat B, Borie F (2013) Does the surgeon's experience influence the outcome of laparoscopic treatment of common bile duct stones? Surg Endosc 27:176–180. doi: 10.1007/s00464-012-2416-z
10. Hubert N, Gilles M, Desbrosses K, Meyer JP, Felblinger J, Hubert J (2013) Ergonomic assessment of the surgeon's physical workload during standard and robotic assisted laparoscopic procedures. Int J Med Robot 9:142–147. doi:10.1002/rcs.1489
11. Iridiastadi H, Nussbaum MA (2006) Muscle fatigue and endurance during repetitive intermittent static efforts: development of prediction models. Ergonomics 49:344–360. doi:10.1080/00140130500475666
12. Kobayashi SA, Jamshidi R, O'Sullivan P, Palmer B, Hirose S, Stewart L, Kim EH Bringing the skills laboratory home: an affordable webcam-based personal trainer for developing laparoscopic skills. J Surg Educ 68(2):105–9. doi:10.1016/j.jsurg.2010.09.014.

13. Kruizinga C, Delleman N, Schellekens J (1998) Prediction of musculoskeletal discomfort in a pick and place task (a pilot study). Int J Occup Saf Ergon 4:271–286

14. McCluney AL, Vassiliou MC, Kaneva PA, Cao J, Stanbridge DD, Feldman LS, Fried GM (2007) FLS simulator performance predicts intraoperative laparoscopic skill. Surg Endosc 21:1991–1995. doi:10.1007/s00464-007-9451-1

15. Minganti C, Capranica L, Meeusen R, Amici S, Piacentini MF (2010) The validity of sessionrating of perceived exertion method for quantifying training load in teamgym. J Strength Cond Res 24:3063–3068. doi:10.1519/JSC.0b013e3181cc26b9

16. Østensvik T, Veiersted KB, Nilsen P (2009) A method to quantify frequency and duration of sustained low-level muscle activity as a risk factor for musculoskeletal discomfort. J Electromyogr Kinesiol 19:283–294. doi:10.1016/j.jelekin.2007.07.005

17. Pathiraja P, Tozzi R (2013) Advances in gynaecological oncology surgery. Best Pract Res Clin Obstet Gynaecol 27:415–420. doi:10.1016/j.bpobgyn.2013.01.002

18. Peters JH, Fried GM, Swanstrom LL, Soper NJ, Sillin LF, Schirmer B, Hoffman K (2004) Development and validation of a comprehensive program of education and assessment of the basic fundamentals of laparoscopic surgery. Surgery 135:21–27. doi:10.1016/S0039-6060(03)00156-9

19. Verdaasdonk EGG, Stassen LPS, van Wijk RPJ, Dankelman J (2007) The influence of different training schedules on the learning of psychomotor skills for endoscopic surgery. Surg Endosc 21:214–219. doi:10.1007/s00464-005-0852-8

20. Yang TX, Chua TC (2013) Single-incision laparoscopic colectomy versus conventional multiport laparoscopic colectomy: a meta-analysis of comparative studies. Int J Colorectal Dis 28:89–101. doi:10.1007/s00384-012-1537-0

14

Obesity and older age as protective factors for vaginal cuff dehiscence following total hysterectomy

Nicole M. Donnellan · Suketu Mansuria · Nancy Aguwa ·
Deirdre Lum · Leslie Meyn · Ted Lee

Abstract Studies have shown an increased risk of vaginal cuff dehiscence following total laparoscopic hysterectomy (TLH). Patient variables associated with dehiscence have not been well described. This study aims to identify factors associated with dehiscence following varying routes of total hysterectomy. This is a retrospective, matched, case-control study of women who underwent a total hysterectomy at a large, urban, university-based teaching hospital from January 2000 to December 2011. Women who underwent a total hysterectomy and had a dehiscence ($n=31$) were matched by surgical mode to the next five total hysterectomies ($n=155$). Summary statistics and conditional logistic regression were performed to compare cases to controls. Obese women (BMI≥30) were 70 % less likely than normal weight women (BMI<25) to experience a dehiscence ($p=0.02$). When stratified by hysterectomy route, obese women were 86 % less likely to have a dehiscence following robotic-assisted total hysterectomy (RAH) and TLH than normal weight women ($p=0.04$). Further, increasing age was protective of dehiscence in this subgroup of women ($p=0.02$). Older age and obesity were associated with a decreased risk of dehiscence following RAH and

TLH but not following other routes. Increased risk of dehiscence following TLH observed in previous studies may be partially due to patient characteristics.

Keywords Dehiscence · Hysterectomy · Laparoscopy ·
Robotic surgery · Obesity

Background

As the number of laparoscopic hysterectomies performed each year increases [1, 2], complications associated with this procedure are becoming more evident. One such complication, vaginal cuff dehiscence, has been studied extensively, and numerous reports have described rates of dehiscence to be higher in patients undergoing total laparoscopic hysterectomy (TLH) and robotic-assisted total hysterectomy (RAH) compared to the abdominal or vaginal route [3–9]. This complication is concerning for many gynecologists given the potential morbidity associated with dehiscence, such as peritonitis, sepsis, bowel evisceration, and need for further surgical intervention.

Surgical factors unique to laparoscopic hysterectomy, compared to the abdominal or vaginal route, have been postulated to contribute to the increased risk of dehiscence. Theories include increased tissue damage to the vagina from the use of thermal energy (i.e., monopolar and/or bipolar energy) for colpotomy creation and hemostasis as well as inferior cuff closure due to techniques of laparoscopic suturing [4, 10]. While attempts to investigate the relationship of these factors with dehiscence have been reported, results in the literature remain controversial [11–13] and confusion surrounding the etiology of vaginal cuff dehiscence persists.

N. M. Donnellan (✉) · S. Mansuria · T. Lee
Obstetrics, Gynecology and Reproductive Sciences, University of Pittsburgh, Magee-Womens Hospital of UPMC, 300 Halket Street, Pittsburgh, PA 15213, USA
e-mail: donnellann2@upmc.edu

N. Aguwa
School of Medicine, University of Texas Health Science Center at San Antonio, 7703 Floyd Curl Drive, San Antonio, TX 78229, USA

D. Lum
Obstetrics and Gynecology, Stanford University, 900 Blake Wilbur Drive, Palo Alto, CA 94304, USA

L. Meyn
Obstetrics, Gynecology and Reproductive Sciences, Magee-Womens Research Institute, 204 Craft Ave, Pittsburgh, PA 15213, USA

Despite overwhelming interest and investigation into the topic of vaginal cuff dehiscence, one variable that has not been well described in previous studies is the patient. Studies have shown that demographic factors such as obesity, smoking, and advanced age are associated with an increased risk of wound breakdown and wound infection; however, these studies focused on open abdominal incisions [14, 15]. The goal of our study was to evaluate if patient-related variables may play a role in the healing of the vaginal cuff. Through performing a retrospective, case-control study, we aimed to discern if, in addition to surgical factors, specific demographic and clinical variables predispose patients to vaginal cuff dehiscence following varying modes of total hysterectomy.

Methods

This study was a retrospective, matched, case-control study that examined demographic, clinical, and surgical characteristics of women who experienced a vaginal cuff dehiscence following total hysterectomy compared to women who did not experience this complication. Institutional review board approval was obtained from the University of Pittsburgh prior to initiation of the study. Pertinent *Physicians' Current Procedural Terminology Coding System*, 4th edition (CPT-4) procedure codes and *International Classification of Diseases*, 9th revision diagnostic codes were used to identify all women who had a repair of a vaginal cuff dehiscence at Magee-Womens Hospital, which is a large, urban, university-based teaching hospital, between January 2000 and December 2011. Surgeons included general gynecologists, gynecologic oncologists, urogynecologists, and gynecologists trained in minimally invasive gynecologic surgery. Patients were excluded if their primary surgery (hysterectomy) was not performed at our institution.

Cases of vaginal cuff dehiscence were matched 1:5 temporally and by route of hysterectomy. Thus, for each case of dehiscence, diagnostic codes were used to identify the next five uncomplicated hysterectomies performed at Magee by the same route as the case. We controlled for route of hysterectomy as previous studies have shown an increased risk of vaginal cuff dehiscence following TLH compared to a vaginal or abdominal approach [3–9]. Five controls per case were obtained to maximize study size while appreciating that minimal statistical power is gained by increasing this ratio beyond 1:4 or 1:5 [16].

Vaginal cuff dehiscence was defined as partial or complete separation of the vaginal cuff with or without evisceration. TLHs and robotic-assisted laparoscopic hysterectomies (RAHs) in our study were defined as hysterectomies performed entirely through a laparoscopic or robotic approach, including colpotomy and cuff closure [17]. Hysterectomies performed laparoscopically but with a vaginal colpotomy and/or cuff closure were categorized as laparoscopic-assisted vaginal hysterectomy (LAVH). As a separate diagnostic code

did not exist to distinguish TLH and RAH from LAVH for a majority of the study period, appropriate classification of hysterectomy type was confirmed by operative note review.

A chart review of paper and electronic medical records was performed to obtain demographic, clinical, and surgical characteristics of all cases and controls. Demographic information obtained included age, body mass index (BMI), and race. Clinical characteristics included parity, tobacco use, menopausal status, and diagnosis of hypertension or diabetes. Preoperative diagnoses, postoperative pathology, and intraoperative details, such as estimated blood loss (EBL), case length, uterine specimen weight, and techniques of colpotomy creation and cuff closure, were also recorded.

Statistical analyses were performed using Stata statistical software version 11.2 (StataCorp LP, College Station, Texas, USA), and statistical tests were evaluated at the two-sided 0.05 significance level. The association between vaginal cuff dehiscence and demographic, clinical, and surgical characteristics was assessed using conditional logistic regression to estimate odds ratios (OR) and 95 % confidence intervals (CI) both in univariable and multivariable models. A subanalysis was performed stratifying based upon route of hysterectomy.

Findings

From January 2000 through December 2011, there were 31 cases of vaginal cuff dehiscence that presented to Magee-Womens Hospital following a total hysterectomy initially performed at our institution. These cases were matched, as previously described, to 155 uncomplicated controls. Among the dehiscence cases, 13 (41.8 %) presented after TLH, 12 (38.7 %) after total abdominal hysterectomy (TAH), 2 (6.5 %) after total vaginal hysterectomy (TVH), 2 (6.5 %) after LAVH, and 2 (6.5 %) after RAH.

Vaginal cuff dehiscence cases had a mean age of 45.0 years (SD 13.4), mean BMI of 27.0 kg/m^2 (SD 6.7), and mean parity of 2.1 (SD 1.4). Controls had a mean age of 47.9 years (SD 12.5), mean BMI of 30.1 kg/m^2 (SD 7.4), and mean parity of 1.7 (SD 1.3). Seven cases (22.6 %) and 26 controls (16.8 %) had a preoperative diagnosis of cancer. Surgical characteristics of cases included a mean EBL of 258.4 cc (SD 426.6), mean operative length of 141 min (SD 51), and mean uterine weight of 182.8 g (SD 161.6). Controls had a mean EBL of 217 cc (SD 234.4), mean operative length of 141 min (SD 61), and mean uterine weight of 186.1 g (SD 172.5). Further demographic, clinical, and surgical characteristics are summarized in Table 1.

When comparing cases to controls, obese women (BMI≥ 30) were 70 % less likely than normal weight women (BMI< 25) to experience a dehiscence ($p=0.02$). All other demographic, clinical, and surgical factors examined were not associated with vaginal cuff dehiscence ($p>0.05$, Table 1).

Table 1 Association of demographic and clinical factors with vaginal cuff dehiscence following total hysterectomy

Factor	Cases (n=31)	Controls (n=155)	Unadjusted OR (95 % CI)	p value[a]
Age (years)	45.0±13.4	47.9±12.5	0.98 (0.95–1.01)	0.23
Body mass index (kg/m^2)				
<25	14 (45.2)	45 (29.2)	1.0 (referent)	
≥25 to <30	10 (32.3)	40 (26.0)	0.81 (0.33–1.99)	0.64
≥30	7 (22.6)	69 (44.8)	0.29 (0.10–0.83)	0.02*
Race				
African-American	6 (19.4)	20 (12.9)	1.69 (0.59–4.91)	0.33
Parity				
≥1	26 (83.9)	119 (78.3)	1.47 (0.50–4.30)	0.48
Tobacco	11 (35.5)	38 (24.7)	1.92 (0.76–4.88)	0.17
Menopause	9 (30.0)	50 (32.5)	0.83 (0.34–2.01)	0.68
Hypertension	8 (25.8)	39 (25.16)	1.03 (0.43–2.49)	0.94
Diabetes	3 (9.7)	10 (6.5)	1.58 (0.40–6.27)	0.52
Indication for surgery				
Pelvic pain	12 (38.7)	61 (39.4)	0.97 (0.43–2.20)	0.95
Abnormal uterine bleeding	14 (45.2)	70 (45.2)	1.00 (0.45–2.24)	>0.99
Fibroids	7 (22.6)	36 (23.2)	0.96 (0.34–2.65)	0.93
Endometrial cancer	4 (12.9)	24 (15.5)	0.81 (0.26–2.52)	0.71
Endometriosis	3 (9.7)	12 (7.7)	1.30 (0.32–5.13)	0.71
Prolapse	2 (6.5)	8 (5.2)	1.34 (0.22–8.05)	0.75
Malignant pathology	7 (22.6)	32 (20.8)	1.15 (0.42–3.16)	0.79
Monopolar colpotomy	16 (51.6)	75 (66.4)	1.33 (0.33–5.30)	0.69
Suture for cuff closure				
Polysorb	18 (78.3)	84 (65.6)	2.53 (0.58–11.09)	0.22
PDS	2 (8.7)	11 (8.6)	0.86 (0.13–5.53)	0.88
Barbed	1 (4.4)	8 (6.3)	0.47 (0.04–5.68)	0.56
Estimated blood loss (cc)				
≥200	14 (45.2)	64 (41.3)	1.28 (0.49–3.39)	0.62
Length of case (minutes)				
≥120	11 (35.5)	58 (37.4)	0.91 (0.40–2.10)	0.91
Uterine weight (g)				
≥200	9 (30.0)	37 (24.2)	1.35 (0.55–3.27)	0.51

Data presented as mean±SD for continuous variables or n (%) for dichotomous variables

OR odds ratio, CI confidence interval

*p<0.05, statistically significant

[a] p value from unadjusted conditional logistic regression model

A subanalysis was performed after stratifying cases and controls based upon route of surgery (TLH and RALH versus VH, LAVH, and TAH; Table 2). Following stratification, overweight (BMI 25–29) women were 80 % less likely than normal weight women (BMI<25) to have a dehiscence following RAHs and TLHs (p=0.04; Table 2). Obese women were 86 % less likely to have a dehiscence following RAHs and TLHs than normal weight women (p=0.04; Table 2). Further, increasing age was protective of a dehiscence event in this subgroup of women who underwent RAHs or TLHs (p=0.02; Table 2). Age and BMI were not significantly associated with dehiscence in the other routes (p>0.05, Table 2). Race was the only factor associated with dehiscence following LAVH, TVH, and TAH. In this hysterectomy subgroup, black women had a four-fold increased risk of dehiscence compared to other races (p=0.03; Table 2).

Conclusion

To our knowledge, this is the first study to demonstrate that patient characteristics of age, BMI, and race are significantly associated with vaginal cuff dehiscence following total hysterectomy. Recent literature has voiced concern regarding the increased risk of vaginal cuff dehiscence following TLH, with a reported incidence as high as 4.6 % [4]. A major shortcoming of these studies is the lack of information detailing the patients undergoing the various types of total hysterectomy. Thus, we designed a case-control study matched on mode of hysterectomy and found that obesity is associated with a significant decrease in dehiscence. After stratifying by hysterectomy type, we found that in the subpopulation of women undergoing a TLH or RAH, this association remains significant. In addition, being overweight and increasing age were also independently associated with a decrease in dehiscence following the laparoscopic and robotic modes.

Our findings suggest that the increased risk of vaginal cuff dehiscence following TLH and RAH may not be entirely explained by the surgical characteristics inherent to these procedures, as has been previously theorized in the literature. Instead, we have shown that patient characteristics may account for, at least partially, the increased rate of dehiscence following a laparoscopic approach. We hypothesize that obesity is protective against dehiscence following TLH and RALH secondary to both structural and physiologic properties. Act of first coitus following total hysterectomy has been a commonly identified inciting event for vaginal cuff dehiscence [4, 5, 8, 10, 11]. Physical forces at the apex of the vaginal cuff during intercourse may be decreased in more obese women, thus providing a protective effect. Similarly, positioning during intercourse may be different in obese patients as compared to normal weight individuals (i.e., as in pregnant patients), which may also confer decreased physical force along the healing vaginal cuff. Older women may experience decreased postoperative activity, including intercourse, which may explain the protective effect demonstrated in this study. However, such proposed theories need to be further examined

Table 2 Association of demographic factors with vaginal cuff dehiscence following total hysterectomy stratified by mode of hysterectomy

Factor	Cases	Controls	Unadjusted OR (95 % CI)	p value[a]	Adjusted[b] OR (95 % CI)	p value[a]
Total laparoscopic and robotic hysterectomy	N=15	N=75				
Age (years)	38.2±7.8	46.1±12.4	0.92 (0.86–0.99)	0.02*	0.90 (0.82–0.98)	0.02*
Body mass index (kg/m^2)						
<25	10 (66.7)	23 (30.7)	1.0 (referent)	–	1.0 (referent)	–
≥25 to <30	3 (20.0)	23 (30.7)	0.31 (0.08–1.23)	0.10	0.19 (0.04–0.90)	0.04*
≥30	2 (13.3)	29 (38.7)	0.16 (0.03–0.80)	0.03*	0.14 (0.02–0.92)	0.04*
Other routes of total hysterectomy	N=16	N=80				
Age (years)	51.4±14.5	49.7±12.5	1.01 (0.97–1.05)	0.62		
Body mass index (kg/m^2)						
<25	4 (25.0)	22 (27.9)	1.00 (referent)	–		
≥25 to <30	7 (43.8)	17 (21.5)	2.43 (0.57–10.41)	0.23		
≥30	5 (31.3)	40 (50.6)	0.62 (0.14–2.83)	0.54		
Race						
African-American	6 (37.5)	11 (13.8)	4.34 (1.16–16.27)	0.03*		

Data presented as mean±SD for continuous variables or n (%) for dichotomous variables

OR odds ratio, CI confidence interval

*p<0.05, statistically significant

[a] p value from conditional logistic regression model

[b] Adjusted for age and body mass index

through studies involving detailed patient questionnaires to better elucidate specific postoperative activity patterns.

Past studies demonstrating an increased risk of dehiscence following TLH have suggested that the technique of monopolar electrosurgery may predispose patients to dehiscence. While we did not demonstrate an association between dehiscence and technique of colpotomy, obesity may confer a protective effect through the physiologic property of increasing impedance in the monopolar circuit. With increased impedance owing to increased adipose tissue in the circuit, less total energy is delivered to a given area, which may lead to less tissue destruction at time of colpotomy. Further studies detailing the thermal effect of electrosurgery as it relates to tissue type are warranted.

Our findings of obesity and increasing age being associated with cuff dehiscence following TLH or RALH could have major implications on clinical practice patterns in minimally invasive gynecologic surgery. If surgeons at our institution had performed laparoscopic supracervical hysterectomies instead of TLHs on all patients with a BMI <25 kg/m^2 over the past 10 years, the dehiscence rate would be estimated to be 0.4 %, a greater than three-fold risk reduction from our most recent reported incidence of 1.4 % [8]. However, such a radical practice change does not take into account other clinical reasons and indications, in addition to economic factors, for performing a total versus a supracervical hysterectomy. Supracervical hysterectomy is not without associated morbidities and costs, including cervical stump bleeding and the need for continued cervical cancer screening [18–21]. Further, reoperation for trachelectomy has been reported to be as high as 22 % [21]. Such a

proposed practice change may simply reduce the incidence of one specific complication while giving rise to others and may not reduce overall patient morbidity.

Analysis of our stratified data also revealed that African-American race was associated with a greater than four-fold increased risk of dehiscence following vaginal and abdominal procedures. One must be cautioned prior to making any conclusions about this result, as less than 15 % of the entire study population identified themselves as African-American. This already low prevalence can lead to erroneous conclusions when attempting to further stratify and analyze data. Race may also be a marker for other demographic or behavioral risk factors. Analysis of a more heterogeneous population in regard to race is merited prior to forming definitive conclusions regarding the impact of race on vaginal cuff dehiscence.

A major limitation to this study is the difficulty in designing a feasible yet valid study focusing on an event with an extremely low incidence. At our institution, greater than 1000 total hysterectomies are performed each year, yet only 31 vaginal cuff dehiscences in an 11-year period were identified, producing a dehiscence rate of less than 0.3 % [5]. While a case-control design assists in studying rare events or conditions, such study designs have inherent biases including sampling and case ascertainment [22]. The rarity of a dehiscence event also makes stratification and statistical analysis by single mode of hysterectomy impossible with our current data set. Thus, while we have grouped similar modes of hysterectomy together and performed a subanalysis (TLH and RAH versus TAH, TVH, and LAVH), there may be intrinsic procedure-specific risks related to dehiscence on which we are unable to comment owing to the extremely low event rate. Another limitation to this chart review is the difficulty in providing accurate correction for rare, patient characteristics, such as prior pelvic radiation, which may confound dehiscence susceptibility. Further, a single laparoscopic radical hysterectomy was grouped with the TLHs as there were limitations in obtaining laparoscopic radical hysterectomy controls. Such a procedure with aggressive pelvic dissection may also have inherent surgical characteristic which could predispose a patient to dehiscence. In addition, although our study is from a high-volume, tertiary care facility, another limitation is the narrow geographic range and its generalizability to other patient populations (i.e., external validity). Overcoming such limitations underscores the importance of future multicenter collaborations in order to increase both absolute dehiscence event numbers as well as patient heterogeneity.

In addition to larger, multicentered collaborations, future studies should also focus on examining the proposed theories we have highlighted to explain the protective effect of obesity and older age on vaginal cuff dehiscence. Such studies should include patient-based investigations focusing on detailed postoperative activities and habits, as well as basic-science studies examining tissue strength and integrity. Until such studies are conducted, however, we present novel data that can assist the gynecologic surgeon to better preoperatively identify patients at increased risk of dehiscence and counsel them accordingly, with the ultimate goal of optimizing surgical outcomes.

Informed consent A waiver to obtain informed consent was obtained by the University of Pittsburgh IRB as the retrospective chart review study met the four following criteria mandated by Federal policy:

(1) The research involves no more than minimal risk to the subjects.
(2) The waiver or alteration will not adversely affect the rights and welfare of the subjects.
(3) The research could not practicably be carried out without the waiver or alteration.
(4) Whenever appropriate, the subjects will be provided with additional pertinent information after participation.

Authors' contributions The authors alone were responsible for the content and writing of the paper. ND, SM, DL, and TL were responsible for the concept/study design. The execution of the study and data collection were done by ND and NA. ND, SM, NA, DL, LM, and TL were responsible for the data analysis and manuscript editing. Statistical processing was performed by ND and LM. Manuscript writing was done by ND, SM, NA, and LM.

References

1. Uccella S, Cromi A, Bogani G et al (2013) Systematic implementation of laparoscopic hysterectomy independent of uterus size: clinical effect. J Minim Invasive Gynecol 20:505–516
2. Andryjowicz E, Wray T (2011) Regional expansion of minimally invasive surgery for hysterectomy: implementation and methodology in a large multispecialty group. Perm J 15:42–46
3. Uccella S, Ghezzi F, Mariani A et al (2011) Vaginal cuff closure after minimally invasive hysterectomy: our experience and systematic review of the literature. Am J Obstet Gynecol 205:119.e1–119.e12
4. Hur HC, Guido RS, Mansuria SM et al (2007) Incidence and patient characteristics of vaginal cuff dehiscence after different modes of hysterectomy. J Minim Invasive Gynecol 14:311–317
5. Kho RM, Akl MN, Cornella JL et al (2009) Incidence and characteristics of patients with vaginal cuff dehiscence after robotic procedures. Obstet Gynecol 114:231–235
6. Agdi M, Al-Ghafri W, Antolin R et al (2009) Vaginal vault dehiscence after hysterectomy. J Minim Invasive Gynecol 16:313–317
7. Rivlin ME, Meeks GR, May WL (2010) Incidence of vaginal cuff dehiscence after open or laparoscopic hysterectomy: a case report. J Reprod Med 55:171–174
8. Hur H, Donnellan N, Mansuria S et al (2011) Vaginal cuff dehiscence after different modes of hysterectomy. Obstet Gynecol 118:794–801
9. Chan W, Kong K, Nikam Y et al (2012) Vaginal vault dehiscence after laparoscopic hysterectomy over a nine-year period at Sydney West Advance Pelvic Surgery Unit—our experiences and current understanding of vaginal vault dehiscence. Aust N Z J Obstet Gynaecol 52:121–127
10. Cronin B, Sung V, Matteson K (2012) Vaginal cuff dehiscence: risk factors and management. Am J Obstet Gynecol 206:284–288
11. Iaco PD, Ceccaroni M, Alboni C et al (2006) Transvaginal evisceration after hysterectomy: is vaginal cuff closure associated with a reduced risk? Eur J Obstet Gynecol Reprod Biol 125:134–138
12. Siedhoff MT, Yunker AC, Steege JF (2011) Decreased incidence of vaginal cuff dehiscence after laparoscopic closure with bidirectional barbed suture. J Minim Invasive Gynecol 18:218–223
13. Uccella S, Ceccaroni M, Cromi A et al (2012) Vaginal cuff dehiscence in a series of 12,398 hysterectomies: effect of different types of colpotomy and vaginal closure. Obstet Gynecol 120:516–523
14. Turan A, Mascha EJ, Roberman D et al (2011) Smoking and perioperative outcomes. Anesthesiology 114:837–846
15. Pavlidis TE, Galatianos IN, Papaziogas BT et al (2001) Complete dehiscence of the abdominal wound and incriminating factors. Eur J Surg 167:351–354
16. Hennessy S, Bilker WB, Berlin JA et al (1999) Factors influencing the optimal control to case ratio for case-control studies. Am J Epidemiol 149:195–197
17. Olive DL, Parker WH, Cooper JM et al (2000) The AAGL classification system for laparoscopic hysterectomy. Classification committee of the American Association of Gynecologic Laparoscopists. J Am Assoc Gynecol Laparosc 7:9–15
18. Thakar R, Ayers S, Clarkson P et al (2002) Outcomes after total versus subtotal abdominal hysterectomy. N Engl J Med 347:1318–1325
19. Ghomi A, Hantes J, Loteze EC (2005) Incidence of cyclical bleeding after laparoscopic supracervical hysterectomy. J Minim Invasive Gynecol 12:201–205
20. American College of Obstetricians and Gynecologists (2012) ACOG practice bulletin no. 131: screening for cervical cancer. Obstet Gynecol 120:1222–1238
21. Okaro E, Jones K, Sutton C (2001) Long term outcome following laparoscopic supracervical hysterectomy. Br J Obstet Gynecol 108:107–120
22. Kopec J, Esdaile J (1990) Bias in case-control studies. J Epidemiol Community Health 44:179–186

15

The prevalence of occult leiomyosarcoma at surgery for presumed uterine fibroids: a meta-analysis

Elizabeth A. Pritts[1] · David J. Vanness[2] · Jonathan S. Berek[3] · William Parker[4] · Ronald Feinberg[5] · Jacqueline Feinberg[5] · David L. Olive[1]

Abstract There is a concern regarding the risk of occult leiomyosarcomas found at surgery for presumed benign fibroids. We sought to produce a comprehensive review of published data addressing this issue and provide high-quality prevalence estimates for clinical practice and future research. A comprehensive literature search using the PubMed/MEDLINE database and the Cochrane Library was performed. Inclusion criteria were human studies, peer-reviewed, with original data, involving cases for surgery in which fibroid-related indications were the primary reason for surgery, and histopathology was provided. Candidate studies (4864) were found; 3844 were excluded after review of the abstract. The remaining 1020 manuscripts were reviewed in their entirety, and 133 were included in the Bayesian binomial random effect meta-analysis. The estimated rate of leiomyosarcoma was 0.51 per 1000 procedures (95 % credible interval (CrI) 0.16–0.98) or approximately 1 in 2000. Restricting the meta-analysis to the 64 prospective studies resulted in a substantially lower estimate of 0.12 leiomyosarcomas per 1000 procedures (95 % CrI <0.01–0.75) or approximately 1 leiomyosarcoma per 8300 surgeries. Results suggest that the prevalence of occult leiomyosarcomas at surgery for presumed uterine fibroids is much less frequent than previously estimated. This rate should be incorporated into both clinical practice and future research.

Keywords Leiomyosarcoma · Fibroids · Surgery · Incidental malignancy · Prevalence

This information was presented at the Obstetrics and Gynecology Devices Panel of the Medical Devices Advisory Committee; FDA, July 10–11, 2014, Washington, D.C., and ESGE 23rd Annual Congress; September 24–27, 2014, Brussels, Belgium, and the 43rd AAGL Global Conference; November 17–21, Vancouver, B.C., Canada.

✉ Elizabeth A. Pritts
epritts@wisconsinfertilty.com

[1]   Wisconsin Fertility Institute, Middleton, WI, USA

[2]   University of Wisconsin School of Medicine and Public Health, Madison, WI, USA

[3]   Stanford University School of Medicine, Stanford, CA, USA

[4]   University of California, Los Angeles, Los Angeles, CA, USA

[5]   Reproductive Associates of Delaware, Newark, DE, USA

Introduction

Uterine fibroids, also known as leiomyomas or myomas, are a significant gynecologic problem, affecting 70–80 % of all women during their reproductive years. These tumors are often symptomatic, producing complaints of abnormal bleeding, pain, and infertility in many of those afflicted. The disease represents a large economic burden for the health care system and significantly affects the quality of life of many with these tumors [1].

Two primary procedures have been utilized over the last century to treat myomas: the hysterectomy, for those who do not wish to retain their uterus, and myomectomy for those who wish to maintain uterine structure and function, often for future reproduction. Traditionally, these procedures were performed via a large abdominal incision (laparotomy), often required by the large size of the fibroid uterus.

Less invasive surgical approaches have been advocated and performed for many years, although with much less frequency than laparotomy. The challenge for surgeons performing these less invasive operations is the usual requirement to remove large amounts of tissue through small apertures.

Manual morcellation via scalpel or other devices has been available for decades, allowing the completion of hysterectomies (and even myomectomies) involving quite large specimens through a vaginal or mini-laparotomy route. The advent of minimally invasive surgery (MIS) utilizing endoscopy initially provided a resurgence in morcellation. As MIS skills improved among surgeons and as equipment improved in concert with the enhanced surgical skills being developed, endoscopic procedures for both hysterectomy and myomectomy increased in number and popularity. A key innovation allowing the performance of these procedures endoscopically was the development and utilization of the electromechanical (or "power") morcellator.

The US Food and Drug Administration (FDA) first approved an electromechanical morcellation device in 1995, and a number now exist in the market. However, recently, the FDA issued a statement discouraging the use of such devices, citing safety concerns, chief among these being the inadvertent dissemination of occult uterine cancer in patients undergoing hysterectomy and myomectomy for presumed benign leiomyomata [2]. Their stated prevalence for unsuspected uterine sarcoma, based upon their review of the medical literature, was 1 in 352 for any sarcoma and 1 in 498 for leiomyosarcoma.

We and others were concerned that the FDA figures might not be the product of a comprehensive and systematic review. In response, our group decided to further investigate the prevalence of uterine leiomyosarcoma among women undergoing surgery for presumed fibroids with a thorough review of published studies of myomectomy or hysterectomy performed for the indication of symptomatic fibroids that included histopathologic analysis of all tissue removed.

Sources

A literature search was initially performed using the PubMed/MEDLINE database and the Cochrane Library. The search was performed for all manuscripts published after 1960 and all languages using the search terms "myoma," "leiomyoma," "fibroid," "hysterectomy," "incidental malignancy," "myomectomy," "neoplasm," "leiomyosarcoma," "incidence," "pathology," "histopathology," "morcellation," and "complication." These terms were used alone and in combination. All references found were evaluated for the inclusion and exclusion criteria listed below and their bibliographies handsearched for other potentially relevant publications. One author (EAP) conducted a preliminary review; all papers deemed to meet inclusion and exclusion criteria were then reviewed by at least one other author for categorization (RF, JF, DLO). If a disagreement was found between

reviewers, a conference involving multiple reviewers was used to reach a decision.

Study selection

Inclusion criteria encompassed publications involving humans that were peer-reviewed. All publications were required to contain original data. Papers were included if they involved cases for surgery (hysterectomy or myomectomy) in which fibroid-related indications were the primary reason for surgery. If this was the exclusive focus of the manuscript, then all cases in the publication were extracted. If, however, there were multiple indications for surgery, only those cases with a fibroid-related primary indication were extracted and included in the analysis. To avoid case reports, a minimum of five subjects from an individual study was necessary for inclusion in this review.

Only those manuscripts in which the postoperative histopathologic findings were provided for all extracted patients were included in the analysis. Manuscripts stating "all specimens were sent to pathology" without final reports were deemed inadequate for inclusion. If the histopathologic description of a leiomyosarcoma in any study was inconsistent with the current World Health Organization (WHO) diagnostic criteria, we noted this, but included it as a leiomyosarcoma in our evaluable data [3] (see below).

Studies that initially searched their databases for a pathologic diagnosis of fibroids, then worked backward to uncover the primary indications for surgery, were excluded. Similarly, all prospective analyses that a priori excluded any patient with malignancy were excluded from the review. All letters to the editor, abstracts, and all other non-peer-reviewed publications of data were omitted. In many cases, we found multiple reports based on a single patient cohort or overlapping cohorts. When this was encountered, we included only one of these papers, with selection based on the following hierarchy of priorities: the publication with the most comprehensive presentation of information with the most leiomyosarcomas, the largest number of patients, or the one that was the most recent. Studies in which "sarcomas" or "malignancies" were found but were not specified as "leiomyosarcoma" were excluded. The first study adequate for inclusion was published in July, 1984; the final was published in September, 2014.

After a thorough search of the literature, 4864 candidate studies were found. Of these, 3844 were excluded after review of the abstract. The remaining 1020 manuscripts were reviewed in their entirety. Of these, 887 were excluded after not meeting the inclusion and exclusion criteria above. One hundred thirty-three publications with 134 analyses (1 publication included both retrospective and prospective data) comprised our evidence base and were used in the final analysis as they contained postoperative histopathologic information for all reported patients (Fig. 1) (Supplemental Digital Content 1: Tables of all included studies and their characteristics).

Statistical methods

We conducted our meta-analysis using a Bayesian binomial random effect specification (R 3.1.1; JAGS 3.3; Supplemental Digital Content 2: Bayesian statistical details and model code). We estimated separate models for prospective and retrospective studies and a model combining both study types. Inference was performed directly on posterior samples generated by Markov chain Monte Carlo. We calculated the rate of leiomyosarcoma per 1000 cases using the posterior random effect mean and constructed 95 % credible intervals (CrIs) using the posterior 2.5 and 97.5 percentiles and on the probability scale by applying the logistic retransformation to the posterior mean of the random effect mean parameter. We assessed heterogeneity on the log-odds scale by calculating the posterior mean of the random effect variance parameter τ^2 and on the probability scale by applying the logistic transformation to the posterior mean of the random effect mean parameter $\mu_\alpha \pm 1.96\tau$.

For comparison with the FDA analysis, we used an unadjusted binomial mixed model with exact 95 % confidence intervals (CIs) (PROC GLIMMIX SAS 9.4).

Sensitivity analysis was conducted to determine whether the conclusions were robust in the presence of small numerical changes in events (leiomyosarcomas).

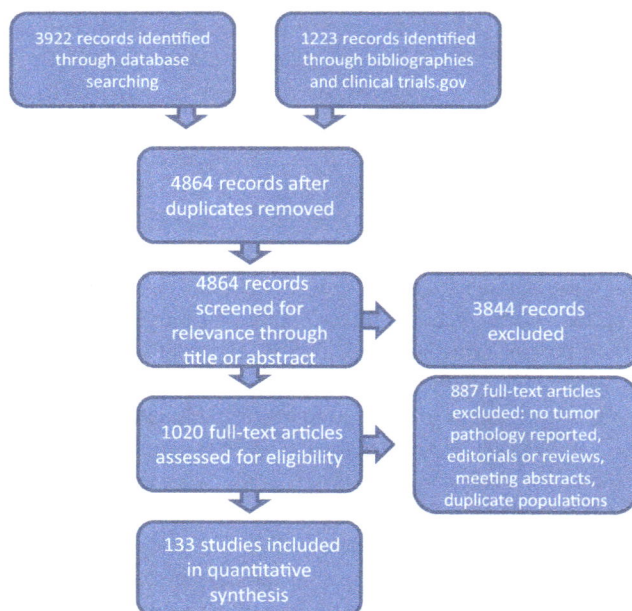

Fig. 1 PRISMA evaluation of studies

Results

a. Rate of occult leiomyosarcoma in surgery for presumed fibroids

Sixty-four published prospective analyses were included in this review: 38 as prospective cohorts [4–41] and 26 as part of a randomized clinical trial [42–67]. Thirteen studies contained more than 100 subjects, 34 included 25–99 subjects, and six had less than 25 subjects. Thirty-five studies were limited to myomectomies, 24 involved only hysterectomies, four studies included patients having either, and one did not state the type of surgery (Table 1). These analyses encompassed 5223 women, with three leiomyosarcomas being found. Only two prospective analyses found a leiomyosarcoma [34, 36].

Seventy published analyses with retrospective cohorts qualified for this review, encompassing a total of 24,970 patients [33, 68–136]. Forty-four cohorts contained more than 100 women, 19 had 25–99 subjects, and seven included less than 25 women. Twenty-five reports were limited to myomectomies, 33 involved only hysterectomies, and 12 included women undergoing either (Table 1). Of these, 29 were noted to have leiomyosarcomas postsurgically. The leiomyosarcomas were found in 13 of the 70 retrospective analyses [75, 79, 84, 98, 100, 101, 106, 114, 115, 124, 125, 128, 129].

Taken together, these 134 analyses reported 32 leiomyosarcomas in 30,193 women undergoing surgery (Supplemental Digital Content 3: Tables of all leiomyosarcomas, sources, and their histopathology). A forest plot of these studies can be seen in Fig. 2. The meta-analysis of the 64 prospective analyses provided an estimated prevalence of leiomyosarcoma to be 0.12 per 1000 surgeries (95 % credible interval <0.01–0.75) or approximately 1 leiomyosarcoma per 8300 surgeries. When restricted to the 70 retrospective analyses, the estimated prevalence was 0.57 per 1000 surgeries (95 % CrI

Table 1 The studies: number of patients and type of surgery

	Randomized controlled studies	Prospective studies	Restrospective studies
# of patients			
>100 patients	5	8	44
25–99 patients	15	19	19
<25 patients	6	11	7
Type of surgery			
Myomectomy	12	23	25
Hysterectomy	13	11	33
Both	1	3	12
Unknown		1	

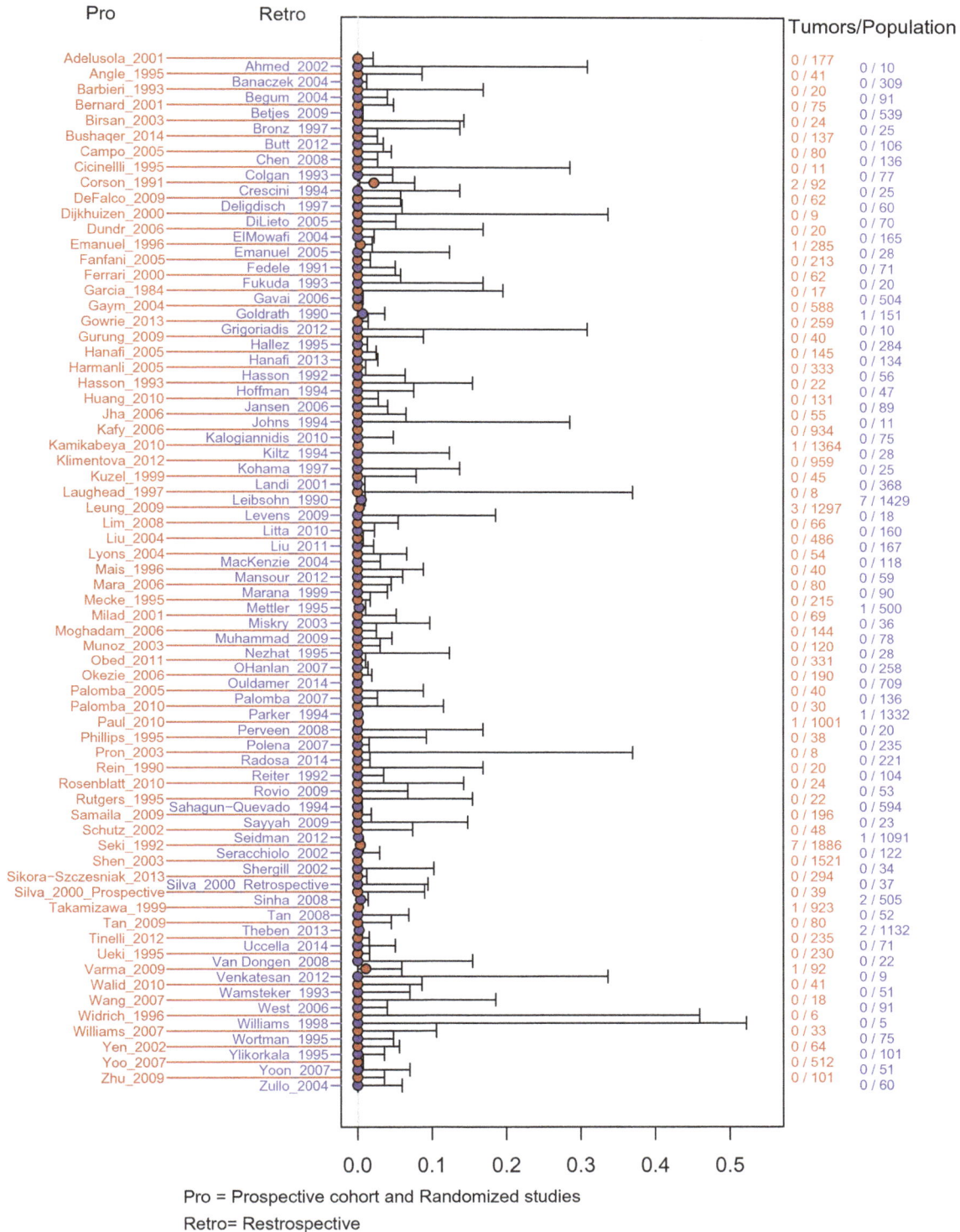

Fig. 2 Forest plot of included studies. *Pro* prospective cohort and randomized studies, *Retro* retrospective

0.17–1.13) or approximately 1 leiomyosarcoma per 1700 surgeries. Meta-analysis of all 134 analyses estimated prevalence to be 0.51 per 1000 surgeries (95 % CrI 0.16–0.98) or approximately 1 leiomyosarcoma for every 2000 procedures (Table 2). The posterior mean of the random effect variance parameter $\tau^2 = 1.375$, which

Table 2 Meta-analyses of evidence base Bayesian model generalized linear mixed model

Dataset	Number of studies	Posterior mean; rate per 1000 surgeries	95 % credible interval	Rate per 1000 surgeries	95 % confidence interval
All studies	133	0.51	0.16, 0.98	0.79	0.5, 1.26
Prospective studies	64	0.12	0, 0.75	0.48	0.14, 1.72
Retrospective studies	70	0.57	0.17, 1.13	0.87	0.52, 1.46
All studies, $N \geq 100$	57	0.55	0.17, 1.06	0.81	0.49, 1.33
Prospective studies, $N \geq 100$	13	0.06	0, 0.62	0.45	0.06, 3.15
Retrospective studies, $N \geq 100$	44	0.59	0.18, 1.15	0.85	0.5, 1.45
FDA dataset	9	1.86	0.7, 3.32	2.02	1.06, 3.84

implies that there is 95 % probability that the 134 underlying true study-specific rates of LMS ranged between 0.09 and 4.50 per 1000 surgeries.

b. Sensitivity analysis

Sensitivity of our analysis was tested in a variety of ways. First, seven leiomyosarcomas from three retrospective analyses uncovered in our search failed to meet current diagnostic criteria. We correctly classified these seven tumors as non-malignant and reran our analysis; the resulting prevalence estimate from our complete evidence base was essentially unchanged from the previous estimate (Table 3).

Secondly, we tested the robustness of the estimates by adding one leiomyosarcoma to either the largest or smallest study reporting no such malignancies. This maneuver changed the estimated rate per 1000 surgeries by 0.02–0.08 for the meta-analysis of all studies and by 0.01–0.24 per 1000 cases for the meta-analysis of prospective datasets only (Table 3).

Finally, we investigated the responsiveness of our Bayesian methodology to heterogeneity of observed rates among studies by reallocating the 32 observed leiomyomas to studies in proportion to their sample size (two each to the six largest studies and one each to the next 20 largest). This maneuver minimizes heterogeneity in observed rates and therefore should yield an estimate that approaches the crude calculated rate (number of leiomyosarcomas/number of surgeries). This was in fact the case (Table 3).

Discussion

This meta-analysis of the existing literature reveals an estimated prevalence of leiomyosarcomas in surgeries for presumed fibroids that is substantially less than that previously estimated. For this reason, it is important to take a close look at how the estimates were derived and what they mean clinically.

Rigorously conducted systematic review and meta-analysis is widely recognized as among the highest standards of evidence for informed medical decision-making [137]. When

Table 3 Sensitivity analyses

Dataset	Posterior mean rate per 1000	95 % credible interval
All studies	0.51	0.16, 0.98
All studies; add 1 LMS case to largest study	0.59	0.21, 1.08
All studies; add 1 LMS case to smallest study	0.53	0.16, 1.02
All studies; reclassification based on histopathology	0.53	0.16, 0.99
Prospective studies	0.12	0, 0.75
Prospective studies; add 1 LMS case to largest study	0.36	0, 1.27
Prospective studies; add 1 LMS case to smallest study	0.13	0, 0.89
All studies; crude test rate	1.03	0.69, 1.43
All studies; actual crude rate	1.06	0.75, 1.50

LMS leiomyosarcoma

See text for explanation of adding LMS cases and reclassification.

Crude test rate involved adding 32 LMS to 31 largest studies

Actual crude rate is (number of LMS/number of total surgeries) for all studies assessing the rate of rare events, formal meta-analysis may offer the only reliable and accessible approach. It is often asked why crude rates calculated by summing the total number of events (in this case leiomyosarcomas) across studies and dividing by the total number of observations (surgeries) is not adequate for estimating the prevalence. The answer lies in the fact that the aggregate of populations from multiple studies is not the same as a single large population undergoing sampling. The heterogeneity among studies for inclusion and exclusion, confounders, and even definitions of risk factors and outcomes leads to tremendous bias in calculating a crude prevalence [138, 139]. In statistical terms, crude calculations are only appropriate if [1] each study was an independent and identically distributed measure of the overall population, and [2] the variance of each study's estimate is known [140]. These conditions are rarely if ever met.

Heterogeneity among studies in a meta-analysis also dictates the type of analytic approach. When included studies investigate the same population with the same research questions and structure, a fixed effect model can be used. As the vast majority of studies in this analysis were not designed to estimate the prevalence of leiomyosarcomas in surgery for presumed fibroids, some degree of statistical heterogeneity is likely. Thus, a random effect meta-analysis, which assumes that design differences lead each study to produce rates that are different but related to the rate of the population of interest, was the approach used here [141]. The estimated random effect variance parameter $\tau^2 = 1.375$ suggests substantial heterogeneity between studies. However, a high degree of statistical variability between studies is to be expected in rare events random effect meta-analysis given the large number of studies with zero events (thus having arbitrarily negative log-odds).

Finally, there are a number of random effect models from which to choose. Our choice was to use a Bayesian binomial model, which has a number of advantages over classical meta-analysis techniques that are particularly important given the complexities of estimating rare event rates [141, 142] (for details, see supplemental digital content 2). Bayesian random effect meta-analysis has been used extensively under such conditions for clinical decision-making and policy analysis [143].

The best available estimate for the rate of occult leiomyosarcoma lies in the data collected prospectively: that gathered from randomized trials and prospective cohort studies. In these investigations, the data collection is begun at a predefined time point, consecutive cases are included avoiding selection bias and patient exclusion, and the data are uniformly collected for all surgeries throughout the duration of the study. In this review, the estimated prevalence of leiomyosarcoma using only data derived from prospective studies was 0.12 per 1000 surgeries, with a 97.5 % probability of being less than 0.75 per 1000 surgeries. Our sensitivity analysis suggests that this estimate is modestly sensitive to adding an incremental case of leiomyosarcoma to the largest study reporting zero events, as would be expected given the small number of prospective studies finding leiomyosarcomas.

Expanding the evidence to include retrospective studies yields an estimated rate of 0.51 per 1000 surgeries, with 97.5 % probability of being less than 0.98 per 1000. Retrospective data collection and analysis has a number of inherent biases, and these can affect the calculated prevalence in either direction. Data that cannot be found when doing chart reviews may not be representative of the entire study population but rather may represent an enriched sample. Prevalence would be underestimated if, for example, records of leiomyosarcomas were more frequently undiscovered because of being moved to hospital risk management files! Conversely, retrospective studies are often initiated after the discovery of an index case at an institution. If the ensuing study population then includes the index case, the resulting bias will uniformly overestimate rate of prevalence. In the case of leiomyosarcomas in fibroid surgery, this definitely occurred in at least two published studies [79, 100]. It is reasonable to suspect that other retrospective studies were also initiated in response to an index case but did not report this reason.

Our prevalence estimates differ substantially from that calculated in the FDA meta-analysis, which was 2.02 per 1000 surgeries. Our group has been asked why these differences are so profound. They can be attributed to both the base of evidence and the statistical methodology. To sort out the relative contribution of each, we applied our Bayesian methods to the FDA dataset and estimated a rate of 1.86 per 1000 surgeries (95 % CrI 0.70–3.32), which is about 8 % lower than the FDA's rate (Table 2). Thus, while differences in methodology accounted for some of the difference in estimated rates, differences in the evidence base accounted for a much larger share.

The evidence base used in this study differed from the studies utilized by the FDA in a number of significant ways. First, our search and screen protocol identified all papers where surgery was being performed for presumed fibroids and where histopathology results were explicitly provided for every subject in the study. This strategy yielded 134 analyses in 133 published studies.

In contrast, to obtain their evidence, the FDA performed a targeted search using the search terms "uterine cancer" AND "hysterectomy or myomectomy" AND "incidental cancer or uterine prolapse, pelvic pain, uterine bleeding, and uterine fibroids." Using uterine cancer as a required search term necessitates the presence of uterine cancer in the manuscripts available for analysis, while those studies without uterine cancers would be overlooked. Indeed, this was the case: 8/9 studies found in their search contained at least one leiomyosarcoma. Of the 133 published studies included in our review, 118 had no leiomyosarcomas and thus would not have appeared in the FDA's targeted search.

A second difference lies in the fact that only studies with more than 100 subjects were included in the evidence base compiled by the FDA; their reasoning was that this would reduce bias from smaller studies. Recognizing the arbitrary nature of any predefined size threshold, our preferred approach was to include eligible studies of all sizes, while allowing for the Bayesian model to weigh each study according to its size and degree of statistical heterogeneity.

Nevertheless, the number of studies included in our evidence base with 100 or more observations was 57, a number far greater than that of the FDA. Restricting our meta-analysis approach to just these 57 prospective and retrospective studies resulted in a prevalence estimate essentially unchanged from our analysis of all 134 studies and approximately one-fourth that of the FDA's estimates: 0.55 per 1000 (95 % CrI 0.17 to 1.06) (see Table 2). Applying the sample size restriction to our prospective-only dataset resulted in inclusion of 13 studies and an estimated rate of 0.06 per 1000 (95 % CrI <0.01 to 0.62). Thus, even utilizing the same arbitrary study size restriction as the FDA, our more comprehensive database significantly lowers the prevalence estimate from their original report.

Third, the FDA included only studies that exclusively examined procedures performed for presumed leiomyomas; if multiple indications were listed by the author of the study, it was excluded from their evidence base and was unavailable for analysis. However, many publications containing multiple indications for surgery contained unequivocal information about those women with a primary surgical indication of fibroids and the data were easily extractable. They were included in our evidence base if the patients undergoing hysterectomy or myomectomy for fibroids were clearly identified, if histopathology was performed on all cases, and if results were explicitly provided.

Fourth, the FDA excluded all non-English articles from consideration. We felt the inclusion of non-English publications made for a more comprehensive review of the subject and thus included studies regardless of the language of publication.

Fifth, the FDA included one non-peer-reviewed abstract [144] and one letter to the editor [145] in their dataset. We excluded these and other similar data, restricting our analysis to peer-reviewed publications containing five or more applicable subjects. Parenthetically, the letter to the editor included in the FDA evidence base was written in English [145]. The original data were reported in their entirety in a French language publication. We excluded the letter to the editor but found the original, peer-reviewed publication and included it in our evidence base. There were three leiomyosarcomas presented in this study [101].

Finally, we note that in the FDA's review of the nine studies referenced, eight were retrospective studies [98, 100, 101, 106, 114, 124, 128, 144] and one was a report from prospectively collected data [34]. Such a preponderance of retrospective reports raises concerns of significant ascertainment bias in the resulting prevalence rate. Our analysis contained a sufficient number of prospective studies to allow analysis restricted to only these, producing what we believe to be the most appropriate evidence base from which to calculate prevalence.

An additional bias may affect the analysis in both our study and that of the FDA. Many of the publications used were from referral centers, where patients are often sent for surgery because of an increased suspicion of additional pathology; without the ability to exclude such cases from the routine hysterectomy or myomectomy for presumed fibroids, the rate of sarcoma will be overstated. This could be compounded by the known bias of non-publication of negative results. A group looking for occult sarcomas with zero events in their study would be less likely to submit for or be accepted for publication.

Despite the comprehensiveness of this review, there are still potential shortcomings of this type of assessment. First, due to the large number of publications involving surgery for uterine fibroids from around the world, it is possible that some went undiscovered by our investigation. However, the large number of studies evaluated and the breadth of contexts considered suggest that such publications are few in number. Another related concern would be that if only a few leiomyosarcomas were overlooked, the calculated prevalence might change substantially. This is unlikely, however, due to the relatively small changes in prevalence seen with our sensitivity analysis.

It is also possible that leiomyosarcomas were missed in the surgeries performed due to incomplete removal of all fibroids or inadequate histopathologic examination. While we do not have evidence to estimate this rate, we believe this to be at most a relatively rare phenomenon. Nevertheless, our sensitivity analyses suggested robustness of our results, as there were relatively small changes in estimated rates from the addition of an incremental case of leiomyosarcoma to one large or small trial previously reporting no cases. There was also a relatively small change when correctly categorizing seven benign tumors that were originally diagnosed as leiomyosarcomas.

Concern might also be expressed that the vast majority of studies included in this analysis, including all prospective studies and randomized controlled trials, were not designed to address the issue of leiomyosarcoma prevalence in such surgeries. Thus, inclusion criteria may have inadvertently eliminated many subjects who would be at higher risk for such malignancies. While this is undoubtedly the case with some trials, the large number of studies and the widely varying reasons for study performance speak against a systematic bias. Age ranges were similar for all datasets and very few restricted patient inclusion a priori to premenopausal women (Table 4). Moreover, the wide-ranging study hypotheses suggest that the

Table 4 Age distributions by study type and histopathology

Dataset	Study number	Premenopausal only	Study mean ages	Age range
Randomized trials	26	10	35.8–53.4	20–70
Prospective	38	4	28.9–67.4	20–83
Retrospective	70	0	32.6–59.6	19–91
Studies with leiomyosarcomas	14	0	32.6–48.0	21–81
Leiomyosarcoma patients	–	–		30–63
				17≤50
				6>50
				9 unknown

information obtained is applicable to real-world clinical situations where surgery is performed for uterine fibroids.

We note that during data extraction, studies were excluded from our analysis when they stated that all specimens were sent for histopathologic analysis, but the results were not included in the publications. In these cases, we expect that the tumors were benign, as surely an event such as an occult leiomyosarcoma would warrant reporting. Excluding such studies potentially underestimated benign cases in our study, but we believe that our conservative approach and rigorous inclusion criteria increase the credibility of our prevalence rate.

A final issue worth noting is that of the criteria for the diagnosis of leiomyosarcoma. The criteria used today for leiomyosarcoma are those adopted by the World Health Organization in 2003 [3]. These criteria indicate that a malignant neoplasm composed of cells demonstrating uterine smooth muscle differentiation with coagulative tumor cell necrosis (not hyaline necrosis) is a leiomyosarcoma. If no such necrosis exists, then the diagnosis is made only if the mitotic index is ≥10 mitoses per 10 high-power fields and there is diffuse, moderate to severe cytologic atypia. The microscopic criteria to meet each of the three requirements are quite specific.

Many of the leiomyosarcomas found in our search provided histologic detail in the manuscript. Interestingly, 7 of the 32 "leiomyosarcomas" found in our search would, based on

current WHO criteria, not be so classified today (Table 5). Further validation of their non-malignant nature is found in the fact that none of the seven had recurrence following surgery. Despite convincing evidence that these seven tumors were not in fact leiomyosarcomas, we have maintained the original diagnosis in our calculations. Our sensitivity analysis suggests these mislabeled tumors had little impact on the estimated prevalence. Nevertheless, this factor highlights a potential bias in utilizing data from older or less highly scrutinized studies: the potential for overestimating prevalence of clinically relevant leiomyosarcomas via misinterpretation of histopathology. Our search for this review included manuscripts published after 1960, in an attempt to be as all-inclusive as possible. We found no studies that met inclusion criteria between 1960 and 1983. The FDA's inclusion dates for studies were between 1980 and 2014, making comparison of these two analyses justifiable. However, both reviews are likely to be overstating the number of actual leiomyosarcomas uncovered.

While we have found that the prevalence of occult leiomyosarcoma is less than previously estimated, this does not negate the fact that such occult malignancies can and do occur. Furthermore, a number of other malignancies have been found at these surgical procedures. It is ideal to diagnose a tumor accurately prior to deciding the type of surgery that is appropriate. The more common

Table 5 Tumors inconsistent with World Health Organization 2003 leiomyosarcoma criteria

Author/date type	Leiomyoma sub-type	Age (years)	Pathology	Recurrence
∞Leibsohn/1990 retro	Atypical	36	6 mitoses/10 HPF, "poorly demarcated," cellular atypia	NED 6 months
	Atypical	48	7 mitoses/10 HPF, cellular atypia	NED 16 months
∞Parker/1994 retro	Atypical	30	Irregular infiltrative borders, mild nuclear atypia, 5–8 mitoses/10 HPF	NED "years"
Seki/1992 retro	Mitotically active	33	6 mitoses/10 HPF, no cellular atypia	NED 11 months
	Mitotically active	34	5 mitoses/10 HPF, no cellular atypia	NED 57 months
	Mitotically active	43	8 mitoses/10 HPF, no cellular atypia	NED 61 months
	Mitotically active	43	9 mitoses/10 HPF, no cellular atypia	NED 72 months

HPF high-powered field

Retro retrospective

∞ included in FDA analysis

NED no evidence of disease

types of uterine cancers may be diagnosed preoperatively, but there is no accurate way to do so for leiomyosarcomas. Many uterine leiomyosarcomas, particularly in younger women, are diagnosed after the tumor has been removed surgically. It was beyond the scope of this analysis to detail or quantify the risk of other cancers in surgery for presumed fibroids, but investigation should continue for a more thorough elucidation of the risks of all such tumors as well as the relative benefits of different surgical approaches. We believe that such data will allow more meaningful research into the decision analysis required for this complex clinical issue.

Acknowledgments The authors express their profound gratitude to Robert Koehler, Chief Librarian, and Meghan Kasprzyk, Library Assistant, Meriter-Unity Point Health Medical Library, Madison, WI.

Authors contributions EA Pritts: protocol/project development, data collection and evaluation, data analysis, and manuscript writing/editing.
  DJ Vanness: data analysis and manuscript writing/editing.
  JS Berek: data analysis and manuscript writing/editing.
  W Parker: data analysis and manuscript writing/editing.
  R Feinberg and J Feinberg: project development, data collection, and evaluation.
  DL Olive: protocol development, data collection and evaluation, data analysis, and manuscript writing/editing.

Ethical statement All procedures performed in studies involving human participants were in accordance with the ethical standards of the institutional and/or national research committee and with the 1964 Helsinki Declaration and its later amendments or comparable ethical standards. For this type of study, formal consent is not required. This article does not contain any studies with animals performed by any of the authors.

References

1. Rowe MK, Kanouse D, Mittman BS, Bernstein SJ (1999) Quality of life among women undergoing hysterectomies. Obstet Gynecol 93:915–921
2. Quantitative assessment of the prevalence of unsuspected uterine sarcoma in women undergoing treatment of uterine fibroids-summary and key findings. http://www.fda.gov/downloads/AdvisoryCommittees/CommitteesMeetingMaterials/MedicalDevices/MedicalDevicesAdvisoryCommittee/ObstetricianandGynecologyDevices/UCM404148.pdf. Referenced July 25, 2014
3. WHO Classification of tumors. In: Tavassoli FA, Devilee P, editors. Pathology and genetics of tumors of the breast and female genital organs. Lyon: IARC Press; 2003. p. 233–38
4. Ahmed AA, Stachurski J, Abdel Aziz E et al (2002) Minilaparotomy-assisted vaginal hysterectomy. Int J Gynecol Obstet 76:33–39
5. Begum S, Khan S (2004) Audit of leiomyoma uterus at Khyber teaching hospital Peshawar. J Ayub Med Coll Abbottabad 16(2):46–49
6. Bernard JP, Rizk E, Camatte S et al (2001) Saline contrast sonohysterography in the preoperative assessment of benign intrauterine disorders. Ultrasound Obstet Gynecol 17:145–149
7. Birsan A, Deval B, Detchev R et al (2003) Vaginal and laparoscopic myomectomy for large posterior myomas: results of a pilot study. Eur J Obstet Gynecol Reprod Biol 110:89–93
8. Bronz L, Suter T, Rusca T (1997) The value of transvaginal sonography with and without saline instillation in the diagnosis of uterine pathology in pre-and postmenopausal women with abnormal bleeding or suspect sonographic findings. Ultrasound Obstet Gynecol 9:53–58
9. Campo S, Campo V, Gambadauro P (2005) Short-term and long-term results of resectoscopic myomectomy with and without pretreatment with GnRH analogs in premenopausal women. Acta Obstet Gynecol Scand 84:756–760
10. Chen S, Chang D, Sheu B et al (2008) Laparoscopic-assisted vaginal hysterectomy with in situ morcellation for large uteri. J Minim Invasive Gynecol 15:559–565
11. Cicinelli E, Romano F, Anastasio PS, Blasi N, Parisi C, Galantino P (1995) Transabdominal sonohysterography, transvaginal sonography, and hysteroscopy in the evaluation of submucous myomas. Obstet Gynecol 85:42–47
12. Crescini C, Amuso G, Cappato M et al (1994) Elettroresezione transcervicale dei miomi sottomucosi. Minerva Ginecol 46:395–402
13. Dijkhuizen F, De Vries LD, Mol B et al (2000) Comparison of transvaginal ultrasonography and saline infusion sonography for the detection of intracavitary abnormalities in premenopausal women. Ultrasound Obstet Gynecol 15:372–376
14. Fanfani F, Fagotti A, Bifulco G et al (2005) A prospective study of laparoscopy versus minilaparotomy in the treatment of uterine myomas. J Minim Invasive Gynecol 12:470–474
15. Fedele L, Bianchi S, Dorta M, Brioschi D, Zanotti F, Vercellini P (1991) Transvaginal ultrasonography versus hysteroscopy in the diagnosis of uterine submucous myomas. Obstet Gynecol 77:745–748
16. Garcia CR, Tureck RW (1984) Submucosal leiomyomas and infertility. Fertil Steril 42:16–19
17. Hoffman M, DeCesare S, Kalter C (1994) Abdominal hysterectomy versus transvaginal morcellation for the removal of enlarged uteri. Am J Obstet Gynecol 171:309–315
18. Jansen FW, de Kroon CD, van Dongen H, Grooters C, Louwe L, Trimbos-Kemper T (2006) Diagnostic hysteroscopy and saline infusion sonography: prediction of intrauterine polyps and myomas. J Minim Invasive Gynecol 13:320–324
19. Kalogiannidis I, Prapas N, Xiromeritis P et al (2010) Laparoscopically assisted myomectomy versus abdominal myomectomy in short-term outcomes: a prospective study. Arch Gynecol Obstet 281:865–870
20. Kiltz RJ, Rutgers J, Phillips J, Murugesapillai ML, Kletzky OA (1994) Absence of a dose-response effect of leuprolide acetate on leiomyomata uteri size. Fertil Steril 61(6):1021–1026
21. Kohama T, Hashimoto S, Ueno H, Terada S, Inoue M (1997) A technique of minilaparotomy-assisted vaginal hysterectomy. Obstet Gynecol 89:127–129

22. Kuzel D, Toth D, Fucikova Z, Cibula D, Hruskova H, Zivny J (1999) Hysteroscopic resection of submucous myomas in abnormal uterine bleeding: results of a four-year prospective study. Ces Gynek 64:363–367

23. Landi S, Zaccoletti R, Ferrari L, Minelli L (2001) Laparoscopic myomectomy: technique, complications, and ultrasound scan evaluations. J Am Assoc Gynecol Laparosc 8(2):231–240

24. Laughead MK, Stones LM (1997) Clinical utility of saline solution infusion sonohysterography in a primary care obstetric-gynecologic practice. Am J Obstet Gynecol 176:1313–1318

25. Liu L, Li Y, Xu H, Chen Y, Zhang G, Liang Z (2011) Laparoscopic transient uterine artery occlusion and myomectomy for symptomatic uterine myoma. Fertil Steril 95:254–258

26. Liu WC, Tzeng CR, Yi–Jen C, Wang PH (2004) Combining the uterine depletion procedure and myomectomy may be useful for treating symptomatic fibroids. Fertil Steril 82:205–210

27. Mara M, Fucikova Z, Kuzel D, Sosna O, Dundr P, Kriz P et al (2006) Enucleation of intramural uterine fibroids in women at fertile age: midterm results of prospective clinical trials. Ces Gynek 71:16–24

28. Milad MP, Morrison K, Sokol A, Miller D, Kirkpatrick L (2001) A comparison of laparoscopic supracervical hysterectomy vs laparoscopically assisted vaginal hysterectomy. Surg Endosc 15:286–288

29. Obed JY, Bako B, Usman J, Moruppa JY, Kadas S (2011) Uterine fibroids: risk of recurrence after myomectomy in a Nigerian population. Arch Gynecol Obstet 283:311–315

30. Palomba S, Zupi E, Falbo A, Russo T, Marconi D, Zullo F (2010) New tool (Laparotenser) for gasless laparoscopic myomectomy: a multicenter-controlled study. Fertil Steril 94:1090–1096

31. Phillips DR, Nathanson HG, Milim SJ, Haselkorn JS (1995) 100 laparoscopic hysterectomies in private practice and visiting professorship programs. J Am Assoc Gynecol Laparosc 3(1):47–53

32. Pron G, Mocarski E, Cohen M, Colgan T, Bennett J, Common A (2003) Hysterectomy for complications after uterine artery embolization for leiomyoma: results of a Canadian multicenter clinical trial. J Am Assoc Gynecol Laparosc 10(1):99–106

33. Silva BAC, Falcone T, Bradley L, Goldberg J, Mascha E, Lindsey R et al (2000) Case-control study of laparoscopic versus abdominal myomectomy. J Laparoendosc Adv S 10(4):191–197

34. Sinha R, Hegde A, Mahajan C, Dubey N, Sundaram M (2008) Laparoscopic myomectomy: do size, number, and location of the myomas form limiting factors for lapaorsopic myomectomy? J Minim Invasive Gynecol 15:292–300

35. Tinelli A, Hurst BS, Hudelist G, Tsin DA, Stark M, Mettler L et al (2012) Laparoscopic myomectomy focusing on the myoma pseudocapsule: technical and outcome reports. Hum Reprod 27(2):427–435

36. Varma R, Soneja H, Clark T, Gupta J (2009) Hysteroscopic myomectomy for menorrhagia using Versascope bipolar system: efficacy and prognostic factors at a minimum of one year follow up. Eur J Obstet Gynecol Reprod Biol 142:154–159

37. Venkatesan AM, Partanen A, Pulanic T, Dreher MR, Fischer J, Zurawin RK et al (2012) Magnetic resonance imaging-guided volumetric ablation of symptomatic leiomyomata: correlation of imaging with histology. J Vasc Interv Radiol 23:786–794

38. Wamsteker K, Emanuel MH, de Kruif JH (1993) Transcervical hysteroscopic resection of submucous fibroids for abnormal uterine bleeding: results regarding the degree of intramural extension. Obstet Gynecol 82:736–740

39. Wang CJ, Soong YK, Lee CL (2007) Laparoscopic myomectomy for large intramural and submucous fibroids. Int J Gynecol Obstet 97(3):206–207

40. Widrich T, Bradley LD, Mitchinson AR, Collins RL (1996) Comparison of saline infusion sonography with office

hysteroscopy for the evaluation of the endometrium. Am J Obstet Gynecol 174:1327–1334

41. Williams CD, Marshburn PB (1998) A prospective study of transvaginal hydrosonography in the evaluation of abnormal uterine bleeding. Am J Obstet Gynecol 179:292–298

42. Barbieri R, Dilena M, Chumas J, Rein MS, Friedman AJ (1993) Leuprolide acetate depot decreases the number of nucleolar organizer regions in uterine leiomyomata. Fertil Steril 60(3):569–570

43. De Falco M, Staibano S, Mascolo M, Mignona C, Improda L, Ciociola F et al (2009) Leiomyoma pseudocapsule after presurgical treatment with gonadotropin releasing hormone agonists: relationship between clinical features and immunohistochemical changes. Eur J Obstet Gynecol Reprod Biol 144:44–47

44. DiLieto A, De Falco M, Mansueto G, De Rosa G, Pollio F, Staibano S (2005) Preoperative administration of GnRH-a plus tibolone to premenopausal women with uterine fibroids: evaluation of the clinical response, the immunohistochemical expression of PDGF, bFGF and VEGF and the vascular pattern. Steroids 70:95–102

45. Ferrari MM, Berlanda N, Mezzopane R, Ragusa G, Cavallao M, Pardi G (2000) Identifying the indications for laparoscopically assisted vaginal hysterectomy: a prospective, randomised comparison with abdominal hysterectomy in patients with symptomatic uterine fibroids. Br J Obstet Gynaecol 107:620–625

46. Levens ED, Wesley R, Prekumar A, Blocker W, Nieman LK (2009) Magnetic resonance imaging and transvaginal ultrasound for determining fibroid burden: implications for research and clinical care. Am J Obstet Gynecol 200:537e1–537.e7

47. Lim SS, Sockalingam JK, Tan PC (2008) Goserelin versus leuprolide before hysterectomy for uterine fibroids. Int J Gynecol Obstet 101:178–183

48. Litta P, Fantinato S, Calonaci F, Cosmi E, Filippeschi M, Zerbetto I et al (2010) A randomized controlled study comparing harmonic versus electrosurgery in laparoscopic myomectomy. Fertil Steril 94(5):1882–1886

49. Mais V, Ajossa S, Guerriero S, Mascia M, Solla E, Melis GB (1996) Laparoscopic versus abdominal myomectomy: a prospective, randomized trial to evaluate benefits in early outcome. Am J Obstet Gynecol 174:654–658

50. Marana R, Busacca M, Zupi E, Garcea N, Paparella P, Catalano GF (1999) Laparoscopically assisted vaginal hysterectomy versus total abdominal hysterectomy: a prospective, randomized, multicenter study. Am J Obstet Gynecol 180:270–275

51. Miskry T, Magos A (2003) Randomized, prospective, double-blind comparison of abdominal and vaginal hysterectomy in women without uterovaginal prolapse. Acta Obstet Gynecol Scand 82:351–358

52. Palomba S, Orio F Jr, Russo T, Falbo A, Tolino A, Lombardi G et al (2005) Antiproliferative and proapoptotic effects of raloxifene on uterine leiomyomas in postmenopausal women. Fertil Steril 84:154–161

53. Palomba S, Orio F Jr, Russo T, Falbo A, Marconi D, Tolino A et al (2007) A multicenter randomized, controlled study comparing laparoscopic versus minilaparotomic myomectomy: short-term outcomes. Fertil Steril 88:942–951

54. Rein MS, Friedman AJ, Stuart JM, MacLaughlin DT (1990) Fibroid and myometrial steroid receptors in women treated with gonadotropin-releasing hormone agonist leuprolide acetate. Fertil Steril 53(6):1018–1023

55. Rutgers JL, Spong CY, Sinow R, Heiner J (1995) Leuprolide acetate treatment and myoma arterial Size. Obstet Gynecol 86:386–388

56. Sayyah-Melli M, Tehrani-Gadim S, Dastranj-Tabrizi A, Gatrehsamani F, Morteza G, Ouladesahebmadarek E et al (2009) Comparison of the effect of gonadotropin-releasing hormone agonist and dopamine receptor agonist on uterine myoma

growth. Histologic, sonographic, and intra-operative changes. Saudi Med J 30(8):1024–1033

57. Schutz K, Possover M, Merker A, Michels W, Schneider A (2002) Prospective randomized comparison of laparoscopic-assisted vaginal hysterectomy (LAVH) with abdominal hysterectomy (AH) for the treatment of the uterus weighing >200 g. Surg Endosc 16:121–125

58. Seracchioli R, Venturoli S, Vianello F, Govoni F, Cantarelli M, Gualerzi B et al (2002) Total laparoscopic hysterectomy compared with abdominal hysterectomy in the presence of a large uterus. J Am Assoc Gynecol Laparosc 9(3):333–338

59. Shergill SK, Shergill HK, Gupta M, Kaur S (2002) Clinicopathological study of hysterectomies. J Indian Med Assoc 100(4):238–239

60. Tan J, Sun Y, Zhong B, Dai H, Wang D (2009) A randomized, controlled study comparing minilaparotomy versus isobaric gasless laparoscopic assisted minilaparotomy myomectomy for removal of large uterine myomas: short-term outcomes. Eur J Obstet Gynecol Reprod Biol 145:104–108

61. Tan J, Sun Y, Dai H, Zhong B, Wang D (2008) A randomized trial of laparoscopic versus laparoscopic-assisted minilaparotomy myomectomy for removal of large uterine myoma: short-term outcomes. J Minim Invasive Gynecol 15:402–409

62. Van Dongen H, Emanuel MH, Wolterbeek R, Trimbos JB, Jansen FW (2008) Hysteroscopic morcellator for removal of intrauterine polyps and myomas: a randomized controlled pilot study among residents in training. J Minim Invasive Gynecol 15:466–471

63. Williams A, Critchley H, Osei J, Ingamells S, Cameron IT, Han C et al (2007) The effects of the selective progesterone receptor modulator asoprisnil on the morphology of the uterine tissues after 3 months treatment in patients with symptomatic uterine leiomyomata. Hum Reprod 22(6):1696–1704

64. Yen YK, Liu WM, Yuan CC, Ng HT (2002) Comparison of two procedures for laparoscopic-assisted vaginal hysterectomy of large myomatous uteri. J Am Assoc Gynecol Laparosc 9(1):63–69

65. Ylikorkala O, Tiitinen A, Hulkko S, Kivinen S, Nummi S (1995) Decrease in symptoms, blood loss and uterine size with nafarelin acetate before abdominal hysterectomy: a placebo-controlled, double-blind study. Hum Reprod 10(6):1470–1474

66. Zhu L, Lang JH, Liu CY, SHI HH, Zun ZJ, Fan R (2009) Clinical assessment for three routes of hysterectomy. Chin Med J 122(4): 377–380

67. Zullo F, Palomba S, Corea D, Pellicano M, Russo T, Fablo A et al (2004) Bupivacaine plus epinephrine for laparoscopic myomectomy: a randomized placebo-controlled trial. Obstet Gynecol 104: 243–249

68. Adelusola KA, Ogunniyi SO (2001) Hysterectomies in Nigerians: histopathological analysis of cases seen in Ile-Ife. Niger Postgrad Med J 8(1):37–40

69. Angle HS, Cohen SM, Hidlebaugh D (1995) The initial Worcester experience with laparoscopic hysterectomy. J Am Assoc Gynecol Laparosc 2(2):155–161

70. Banaczek Z, Sikora K, Lewandowska-Andruszuk I (2004) The occurrence of leiomyoma cellulare in the surgical material in the department of obstetrics and gynecology in the district specialized hospital in Radom. Ginekol Pol 75(11):858–862

71. Betjes HE, Hanstede M, Emanuel M, Stewart EA (2009) Hysteroscopic myomectomy and case volume hysteroscopic myomectomy performed by high- and low-volume surgeons. J Reprod Med 54:425–428

72. Bushaqer NJ, Dayoub N (2014) The effect of uterine leiomyomas size on presenting symptoms and accurate sonography assessment. Bahrain Med Bull 36(2):74–77

73. Butt JL, Jeffery ST, Van der Spuy ZM (2012) An audit of indications and complications associated with elective hysterectomy at a

74. Colgan TJ, Pendergast S, LeBlanc M (1993) The histopathology of uterine leiomyomas following treatment with gonadotropin-releasing hormone analogues. Hum Pathol 24(10):1073–1077

75. Corson SL, Brooks PG (1991) Resectoscopic myomectomy. Fertil Steril 55:1041–1044

76. Deligdisch L, Hirschmann S, Altchek A (1997) Pathologic changes in gonadotropin releasing hormone agonist analogue treated uterine leiomyomata. Fertil Steril 67:837–841

77. Dundr P, Mara M, Maskova J, Fucikova Z, Povysil C, Tvrdik D (2006) Pathological findings of uterine leiomyomas and adenomyosis following uterine artery embolization. Pathol Res Pract 202:721–729

78. El-Mowafi D, Madkour FW, Facharzt, Lall CL, Wenger JM (2004) Laparoscopic supracervical hysterectomy versus laparoscopic-assisted vaginal hysterectomy. J Am Assoc Gynecol Laparosc 11(2):175–180

79. Emanuel MH, Wamsteker K, Hart A, Metz G, Lammes FB (1999) Long-term results of hysteroscopic myomectomy for abnormal uterine bleeding. Obstet Gynecol 93:743–748

80. Emanuel M, Wamsteker K (2005) The intra uterine morcellator: a new hysteroscopic operating technique to remove intrauterine polyps and myomas. J Minim Invasive Gynecol 12:62–66

81. Fukuda M, Shimizu T, Fukuda K, Yomura W, Shimizu S (1993) Transvaginal hysterosonography for differential diagnosis between submucous and intramural myoma. Gynecol Obstet Investig 35:236–239

82. Gavai M, Hupuczi P, Papp Z (2006) Abdominalis myomectomia, mint a hysterectomia alternativaja: 504 eset analizise. Orv Hetil 147:971–8

83. Gaym A (2004) Leiomyoma uteri in Ethiopian women: a clinical study. Ethiop Med J 42:199–204

84. Goldrath MH (1990) Vaginal removal of the pedunculated submucous myoma. Am J Reprod Med 35(10):921–924

85. Gowri M, Mala G, Murthy S, Nayak V (2013) Clinicopathological study of uterine leiomyomas in hysterectomy specimens. J Evol Med Dent Sci 46(2):9002–9009

86. Grigoriadis C, Papaconstantinou E, Mellou A, Hassiakos D, Liapis A, Kondi-Pafiti A (2012) Clinicopathological changes of the uterine leiomyomas after GnRH agonist therapy. Clin Exp Obstet Gynecol 39(2):191–194

87. Gurung G, Pradhan N, Rawal S, Rana A, Ghimire S, Baral J (2009) Myomectomy: TU teaching hospital experiences. NJOG 4(1):15–18

88. Hallez J (1995) Single-stage total hysteroscopic myomectomies: indications, techniques, and results. Fertil Steril 63(4):703–708

89. Hanafi M (2005) Predictors of leiomyoma recurrence after myomectomy. Obstet Gynecol 105:877–881

90. Hanafi M (2013) Ultrasound diagnosis of adenomyosis, leiomyoma, or combined with histopathological correlation. J Hum Reprod Sci 6(3):189–193

91. Harmanli OH, Bevilacqua SA, Dandolu V, Chatwani AJ, Hernandez E (2005) Adenomyosis interferes with accurate ultrasonographic detection of uterine leiomyomas. Arch Gynecol Obstet 273:146–149

92. Hasson HM, Rotman C, Rana N, Sistos F, Dmowski WP (1992) Laparoscopic myomectomy. Obstet Gynecol 80(5):884–888

93. Hasson HM, Rotman C, Rana N, Asakura H (1993) Experience with laparoscopic hysterectomy. J Am Assoc Gynecol Laparosc 1(1):1–11

94. Huang JQ, Lathi RB, Lemyre M, Rodriguez HE, Nezhat CH, Nezhat C (2010) Coexistence of endometriosis in women with symptomatic leiomyomas. Fertil Steril 94:720–723

95. Jha R, Pant AD, Jha A, Sayami G (2006) Histopathological analysis of hysterectomy specimens. J Nep Med Assoc 45:283–290

public service hospital in South Africa. Int J Gynecol Obstet 116: 112–116

96. Johns D, Diamond MP (1994) Laparoscopically assisted vaginal hysterectomy. J Reprod Med 39:424–428

97. Kafy S, Huang JYJ, Al-Sunaidi M, Wiener D, Tulandi T (2006) Audit of morbidity and mortality rates of 1792 hysterectomies. J Minim Invasive Gynecol 13:55–59

98. Kamikabeya TS, Etchebehere RM, Nomelini RS, Murta EF (2010) Gynecological malignant neoplasias diagnosed after hysterectomy performed for leiomyoma in a university hospital. Eur J Gynaecol Oncol 31(6):651–653

99. Klimentova DV, Braila AD, Simionescu C, Ilie I, Braila MB (2012) Clinical and paraclinical study regarding the macro- and microscopic diagnosis of various anatomo-clinical forms of operated uterine fibromyoma. Romanian J Morphol Embryol 53(2):369–373

100. Leibsohn S, d'Ablaing G, Mishell DR, Schlaerth JB (1990) Leiomyosarcoma in a series of hysterectomies performed for presumed uterine leiomyomas. Am J Obstet Gynecol 162:968–976

101. Leung F, Terzibachian J, Gay C, Chung Fat B, Aouar Z, Lassabe C et al (2009) Hysterectomies performed for presumed leiomyomas: should the fear of leiomyosarcoma make us apprehend non laparotomic surgical routes? Gynecol Obstet Fertil 37:109–114

102. Lyons TL, Adolph AJ, Winer WK (2004) Laparoscopic supracervical hysterectomy for the larger uterus. J Am Assoc Gynecol Laparosc 11(2):170–174

103. MacKenzie IZ, Naish C, Rees M, Manek S (2004) 1170 consecutive hysterectomies: indications and pathology. J Br Menopause Soc 10(3):108–112

104. Mansour FW, Kives S, Urbach DR, Lefebvre G (2012) Robotically assisted laparoscopic myomectomy: a Canadian experience. J Obstet Gynaecol Can 34(4):353–358

105. Mecke H, Wallas F, Brocker A, Gertz HP (1995) Pelviskopische myomenukleation: technik, grenzen, komplikationen. Geburtsh Franuenheilk 55:374–379

106. Mettler L, Alvarez-Rodas E, Semm K (1995) Hormonal treatment and pelviscopic myomectomy. Diagn Ther Endosc 1:217–221

107. Moghadam R, Lathi RB, Shahmohamady B, Saberi NS, Nexhat CH, Nezhat F et al (2006) Predictive value of magnetic resonance imaging in differentiating between leiomyoma and adenomyosis. JSLS 10:216–219

108. Muhammad Z, Ibrahaim SA, Agu OC (2009) Total abdominal hysterectomy for benign gynaecological tumours in Jos University teaching hospital, Jos Plateau State. BoMJ 6(2):2–19

109. Munoz JL, Jimenez JS, Hernandez C, Vaquero G, Sagaseta P, Noguero R et al (2003) Hysteroscopic myomectomy: our experience and review. JSLS 7:39–48

110. Nezhat F, Nezhat CH, Admon D, Gordon S, Nezhat C (1995) Complications and results of 361 hysterectomies performed at laparoscopy. J Am Coll Surg 180:307–316

111. O'Hanlan KA, Dibble SL, Garnier A, Reuland ML (2007) Total laparoscopic hysterectomy: technique and complications of 830 cases. JSLS 11(1):45–53

112. Okezie O, Ezegwui HU (2006) Management of uterine fibroids in Enugu. Niger J Obstet Gynaecol 26(4):363–365

113. Ouldamer L, Rossard L, Arbion F, Marret H, Body G (2014) Risk of incidental finding of endometrial cancer at the time of hysterectomy for benign condition. J Minim Invasive Gynecol 21:131–145

114. Parker WH, Fu YS, Berek JS (1994) Uterine sarcoma in patients operated on for presumed leiomyoma and rapidly growing leiomyoma. Obstet Gynecol 83:414–418

115. Paul GP, Sejal A, Madhu KN, Thomas T (2010) Complications of laparoscopic myomectomy: a single surgeon's series of 1001 cases. Aust N Z J Obstet Gynaecol 50:385–390

116. Perveen S, Tayyab S (2008) A clinicopathological review of elective abdominal hysterectomy. JSP 13(1):26–29

117. Polena V, Mergui J, Perrot N, Poncelet C, Barranger E, Uzan S (2007) Long-term results of hysteroscopic myomectomy in 235 patients. Eur J Obstet Gynecol Reprod Biol 130:232–237

118. Radosa MP, Owsianowski Z, Mothes A, Weisheit J, Vorwergk J, Asskaryar FA et al (2014) Long-term risk of fibroid recurrence after laparoscopic myomectomy. Eur J Obstet Gynecol Reprod Biol 2-14(180):35–39

119. Reiter RC, Wagner PL, Gambone JC (1992) Routine hysterectomy for large asymptomatic uterine leiomyomata: a reappraisal. Obstet Gynecol 79(4):481–484

120. Rosenblatt P, Makai G, DiSciullo A (2010) Laparoscopic supracervical hysterectomy with transcervical morcellation: initial experience. J Minim Invasive Gynecol 17:331–336

121. Rovio PH, Helin R, Heinonen PK (2009) Long-term outcome of hysteroscopic endometrial resection with or without myomectomy in patients with menorrhagia. Gynecol Obstet 279:159–163

122. Sahagun Quevedo JA, Perez Ruiz JC, Cherem B, Efren PG (1994) Analysis of 1,000 hysterectomies. Technical simplifications and reflections. Ginecol Obstet Mex 62:35–39

123. Samaila M, Adesiyun AG, Agunbiade OS, Mohammed-Duro A (2009) Clinico-pathological assessment of hysterectomies in Zaria. Eur J Gen Med 6(3):150–153

124. Seidman MA, Oduyebo T, Muto MG, Crum CP, Nucci MR, Quade BJ (2012) Peritoneal dissemination complicating morcellation of uterine mesenchymal neoplasms. PLoS ONE 7(11):1–8

125. Seki K, Hoshihara T, Nagata I (1992) Leiomyosarcoma of the uterus: ultrasonography and serum lactate dehydrogenase level. Gynecol Obstet Investig 33:114–118

126. Shen C, Wu M, Kung F, Huang FJ, Hsieh CH, Lan KC et al (2003) Major complications associated with laparoscopic-assisted vaginal hysterectomy: ten-year experience. J Am Assoc Gynecol Laparosc 10(2):147–153

127. Sikora-Szczesniak DL, Sikora W, Szczesniak G (2013) Leimyoma cellular in postoperative material: clinical cases. Studia Medyczne 29(2):144–151

128. Takamizawa S, Minakami H, Usui R, Noguchi S, Ohwada M, Suzuki M et al (1999) Risk of complications and uterine malignancies in women undergoing hysterectomy for presumed benign leiomyomas. Gynecol Obstet Investig 48:193–196

129. Theben JU, Schellong A, Altgassen C, Kelling K, Schneider S, Grobe-Drieling D (2013) Unexpected malignancies after laparoscopic-assisted supracervical hysterectiomes (LASH): an analysis of 1,584 cases. Arch Gynecol Obstet 287:455–462

130. Uccella S, Cromi A, Serati M, Casarin J, Sturla D, Ghezzi F (2014) Laparoscopic hysterectomy in case of uteri weighing >1 kilogram: a series of 71 cases and review of the literature. J Minim Invasive Gynecol 21:460–465

131. Ueki M, Okamoto Y, Tsurunaga T, Seiki Y, Ueda M, Sugimoto O (1995) Endocrinological and histological changes after treatment of uterine leiomyomas with danazol or buserelin. J Obstet Gynaecol 21(1):1–7

132. Walid MS, Heaton RL (2010) Laparoscopic myomectomy: an intent-to-treat study. Arch Gynecol Obstet 281:645–649

133. West S, Ruiz R, Parker WH (2006) Abdominal myomectomy in women with very large uterine size. Fertil Steril 85:36–39

134. Wortman M, Daggert A (1995) Hysteroscopic myomectomy. J Am Assoc Gynecol Laparosc 3(1):39–46

135. Yoo EH, Lee PI, Huh CY, Kim DH, Lee BS, Lee JK et al (2007) Predictors of leiomyoma recurrence after laparoscopic myomectomy. J Minim Invasive Gynecol 14:690–697

136. Yoon HJ, Kyung MS, Jung US, Choi JS (2007) Laparoscopic myomectomy for large myomas. J Korean Med Sci 22:706–712

137. Harbour R, Miller J (2001) A new system for grading recommendations in evidence based guidelines. BMJ 323:334–336

138. Bradburn MJ, Deeks JJ, Berlin JA, Russell Localio A (2007) Much ado about nothing: a comparison of the performance of meta-analytical methods with rare events. Stat Med 26:53–77

139. Altman DG, Deeks JJ (2002) Meta-analysis, Simpson's paradox, and the number needed to treat. BMC Med Res Methodol 2:3

140. Kulinskaya E, Morgenthaler S, Staudte RG (2008) Meta Analysis: a guide to calibrating and combining statistical evidence, Chapter 2. Wiley, Chichester

141. Higgins J, Thompson SG, Spiegelhalter DJ (2009) A re-evaluation of random effects meta-analysis. J R Stat Soc Ser A Stat Soc 172: 137–159

142. Sutton AJ, Cooper NJ, Lambert PC, Jones DR, Abrams KR, Sweeting MJ (2002) Meta-analysis of rare and adverse event data. Expert Rev Pharmacoecon Outcomes Res 2:367–379

143. Menon GR, Sundram KR, Pandey RM, Prasad K, Handa BR, Singh P (2006) Application of hierarchical Bayesian linear model in meta-analysis. Int J Stat Sci 5:85–108

144. Rowland M, Lesnock J, Edwards R et al (2012) Occult uterine cancer in patients undergoing laparoscopic hysterectomy with morcellation. Gynecol Oncol S29

145. Leung F, Terzibackian JJ (2012) Re "The impact of morcellation during surgery on the prognosis of patients with apparently early uterine leiomyosacroma". Gynecol Oncol 124(1):172–173

16

Cross-linked xenogenic collagen implantation in the sheep model for vaginal surgery

Masayuki Endo · Iva Urbankova · Jaromir Vlacil · Siddarth Sengupta · Thomas Deprest · Bernd Klosterhalfen · Andrew Feola · Jan Deprest

Abstract The properties of meshes used in reconstructive surgery affect the host response and biomechanical characteristics of the grafted tissue. Whereas durable synthetics induce a chronic inflammation, biological grafts are usually considered as more biocompatible. The location of implantation is another determinant of the host response: the vagina is a different environment with specific function and anatomy. Herein, we evaluated a cross-linked acellular collagen matrix (ACM), pretreated by the anti-calcification procedure ADAPT® in a sheep model for vaginal surgery. Ten sheep were implanted with a cross-linked ACM, and six controls were implanted with a polypropylene (PP; 56 g/m²) control. One implant was inserted in the lower rectovaginal septum, and one was used for abdominal wall defect reconstruction. Grafts were removed after 180 days; all graft-related complications were recorded, and explants underwent bi-axial tensiometry and contractility testing. Half of ACM-implanted animals had palpable induration in the vaginal implantation area, two of these also on the abdominal implant. One animal had a vaginal exposure. Vaginal ACMs were 63 % less stiff compared to abdominal ACM explants ($p=0.01$) but comparable to vaginal PP explants. Seven anterior vaginal ACM explants showed areas of graft degradation on histology. There was no overall difference in vaginal contractility. Considering histologic degradation in the anterior vaginal implant as representative for the host, posterior ACM explants of animals with degradation had a 60 % reduced contractility as compared to PP ($p=0.048$). Three abdominal implants showed histologic degradation; those were more compliant than non-degraded implants. Vaginal implantation with ACM was associated with graft-related complications (GRCs) and biomechanical properties comparable to PP. Partially degraded ACM had a decreased vaginal contractility.

Keywords Graft-related complication · Biological graft · Prolapse · Biomechanics · Contractility

M. Endo · I. Urbankova · J. Vlacil · A. Feola · J. Deprest
Centre for Surgical Technologies, Faculty of Medicine, KU Leuven, Herestraat 49, 3000 Leuven, Belgium

M. Endo · I. Urbankova · J. Vlacil · S. Sengupta · T. Deprest · A. Feola · J. Deprest (✉)
Department of Development and Regeneration, Organ Systems Cluster, Faculty of Medicine, KU Leuven, Herestraat 49, 3000 Leuven, Belgium
e-mail: Jan.Deprest@uzleuven.be

M. Endo · J. Deprest
Pelvic Floor Unit, University Hospitals KU Leuven, Leuven, Belgium

I. Urbankova · J. Vlacil
Institute for Care of Mother and Child, Prague, Czech Republic

B. Klosterhalfen
Institute for Pathology, Düren Hospital, Düren, Germany

Introduction

Pelvic organ prolapse (POP) develops in half of parous women over 50 years, half of them being symptomatic with only 20 % of them seeking medical help [1, 2]. Lifetime risk of POP surgery is 19 % [3], and up to 25 % require later re-operation [4]. It was suggested that this may be reduced by using synthetic or biological implants [4, 5]. Although durable synthetic meshes are known to achieve good anatomical and functional results for cystocele repair, they may cause graft-related complications (GRCs) in over 10 % of women [4]. Alternative grafts that may reduce the number of GRC yet still provide durable results could be contemplated [6–10].

Biological grafts are derived from either human (autograft or allografts) or animal material (xenografts). Autografts, such as fascia lata, inherently have donor site-related morbidity and also have unpredictable durability [11, 12]. Allografts are retrieved from cadaveric tissue, and although fastidious steps are taken in preparation, concerns regarding transmission of possible prion disease or viruses remained. Xenografts are acellular collagen matrices (ACMs) that are either derived from the dermis, pericardium or small intestinal submucosa of animals that are purposely bred in strictly controlled conditions. Most ACMs are of bovine or porcine origin, which, during their production, undergo various chemical procedures (cross-linking, sterilization). After implantation, ACMs are remodelled and/or replaced by connective tissue within variable time periods. The latter can be modified using, e.g. cross-linking agents which leads to the formation of excessive intramolecular and intermolecular chemical bonds preventing decomposition by endogenous collagenases [13]. This alters the properties of the ACM either physically or chemically. A commonly used cross-linking agent is glutaraldehyde (GAD) [13] resulting in durable grafts that are slowly integrated and remodelled. However, residual GAD is cytotoxic and may cause calcification. To prevent this, Neethling et al. developed a multi-step anti-mineralization process called ADAPT® [14]. This enhances crosslink stability, removes residual GAD and modifies the non-bifunctionally reacted GAD residues. The process reduces lipid content and restores tissue elasticity [14]. ADAPT®-treated bovine pericardial patches have been successfully used in surgery of congenital heart defects without demonstrable calcification in a 36-month follow-up period [15]. These promising results demonstrating long-term stability in challenging circumstances are worthwhile considering for translation in pelvic floor surgery. Herein, we used ADAPT®-treated xenografts in a sheep model for transvaginal surgery, studying both the occurrence of GRCs and active and passive biomechanical properties of the vaginal wall. As a reference, we compared outcomes to repairs with light weight polypropylene (PP) implants.

Materials and methods

Implants and surgery

This study compares outcomes following vaginal and abdominal mesh insertion of either a xenogenic or synthetic implant in a sheep model. The xenogenic graft was a non-perforated acellular collagen matrix (ACM) derived from bovine pericardium which was cross-linked with an ultra-low concentration (0.05 %) of monomeric GAD. Further preimplantation processing included the so-called ADAPT® anti-calcification procedure and sterilization with propylene oxide [14, 16] (material donated by Prof WML Neethling, Fremantle, Australia). As a control, we used a commercially available monofilament polypropylene (PP) mesh

used for vaginal prolapse repair (PP) (Avaulta Solo; 56 g/m^2, Bard Medical, Covington, GA, USA). The latter was purchased and delivered sterile via the hospital pharmacy. Observations of these animals were earlier reported on elsewhere [17].

The anaesthetic, surgical technique and methodology used for outcome evaluation have been described in detail previously [18, 19]. Briefly, 16 parous Texel sheep (mean weight 68± 3.5 kg) were obtained from the Zootechnical Centre of the KU Leuven. They underwent simultaneous vaginal and abdominal implantation with either ACM (N=10) or PP (N=6). Surgery was conducted in sterile conditions under general anaesthesia with prophylactic antibiotics at induction and 3 days of postoperative analgesia. Following aqua dissection, a single incision was made in the recto-vaginal septum that was then dissected to create a suitable space for a 35×35 mm suture fixed prosthesis (posterior implant) (Fig. 1). Additionally, a 10×20 mm graft was inserted in the anterior vaginal wall (anterior implant). Finally, a 50 mm longitudinal paramedian cutaneous incision was made in the anterior abdominal wall, and a 40-mm primarily suture repaired full-thickness fascial incision was overlaid with the same graft as used vaginally (Fig. 1). All implants were fixed with interrupted PP 4/0 prolene sutures (Ethicon). Postoperatively, animals were allowed to move, drink and eat ad libitum and were clinically followed by a veterinarian.

Outcome measures

On average, 180 days later, animals were euthanized, and during necropsy graft-related complications (GRCs) or the presence of herniation was noted at each of the three implantation sites. Thereafter, the original implant together with the adjacent and ingrown tissue (further referred to as explant) was removed "en bloc" and its dimensions and thickness were determined as an average of three random measurements with a digital micrometer (Mitutoyo, Kawasaki, Japan; accuracy 0.01 mm). Contraction of the explant was defined as the explant area over initial graft area (1225 mm^2 for vaginal, 2500 mm^2 for abdominal implant, respectively). Explants were then divided to obtain specimens for histology and biomechanical testing as shown in Fig. 1. For vaginal explants, the anterior specimens were used for histology while the posterior explants were used for active and passive biomechanical testing. The larger abdominal explants were divided for both histology and passive biomechanics.

Histology quantified the inflammatory response and connective tissue formation on 5-µm-thick sections, stained with hematoxylin and eosin (H & E) and Movat pentachrome, using an ordinal scoring system [20, 21]. Two operators blinded to the initial treatment counted foreign body giant cell (FBGC), polymorphonuclear (PMN) cells, newly formed vessels and collagen organization, composition and amount in five randomly chosen areas at the implant–host

Fig. 1 Schematic drawing of abdominal (**a**) and vaginal (**b**) implantation in the sheep model. Specimens explanted (**c**) from the abdomen and anterior (*ant*) and posterior (*post*) vaginal wall were divided according with their respective testing method. The *arrow* is pointing cranially in the direction to the uterine cervix (illustration by Myrthe Boymans)

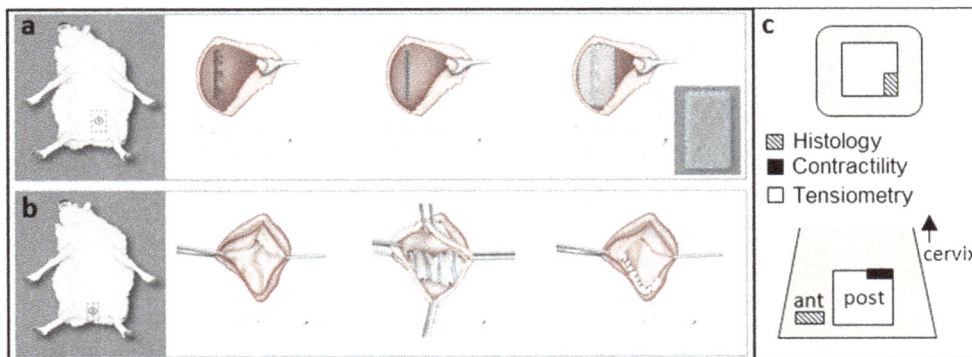

tissue interface at a magnification×400 (Zeiss Axioplan 400, Oberkochen, Germany). Infection was classified as either low grade ($\geq$15 PMN per HPF and no clinical evidence of infection) or high grade (presence of micro-abscesses, dense inflammatory infiltrate, fibrin exudation, bleeding and necrosis as well as clinical signs of infection, if any) [22]. All histological scores (FBGCs, PMN, vessel and collagen scores) were at least done in duplicate and averaged.

Passive biomechanics were tested using bi-axial tensiometry by a plunger test on a 500-N Zwick tensiometer with a 200-N cell load (Zwick GmbH & Co. KG, Ulm, Germany) using a protocol defined earlier [18]. A spherical 11.5 mm plunger was passed through an aperture $\varnothing$20 mm that exposing the explant compressed in $\varnothing$30-mm rings. All explants were placed with the graft facing upward. Records of the force–elongation relationship allowed to define the stiffness (N/mm) of the tested material, which we measured in the low-stress area also called as the "comfort" zone, the average slope of the force–elongation curve and the length of the former zone. These values were determined by TestXpert II software (Zwick GmbH & Co). Active biomechanics of a circumferential-oriented posterior vaginal explant as well as control strip (10×8 mm) were assessed by a contractility assay (Fig. 1) [23]. This is an ex vivo assessment quantifying the ability of the smooth muscles present in vaginal tissue strips to contract by immersing them in an organ bath at 80 mM KCl concentration (mN/mm^3), suggested as a proxy for vaginal function.

Statistical analysis and ethics committee approval

Data are reported as mean and standard deviation or as median and interquartile range depending on the distribution. Either a Student's t test or a Mann–Whitney U test was performed to compare PP and ACM. Chi-square was used for categorical data. Pairs of abdominal and vaginal explants from the same animal were also tested using a paired t test or Wilcoxon signed-rank test. All analyses were performed with Prism 5 (GraphPad Software, Inc., La Jolla, CA, USA), and the significance level was set up to $p<0.05$. Animals were housed in controlled conditions and treated in accordance with current

national guidelines on animal welfare. The experiment was approved by the Ethics Committee for Animal Experimentation of the Faculty of Medicine of the KU Leuven.

Results

Vaginal versus abdominal implantation of ACM

Five out of ten sheep implanted with ACM developed GRCs at the vaginal implantation site (50 %; Table 1). There was one exposure, two implants showed clinically obvious folding (Fig. 2), and two showed remarkable induration. The total GRC rate for xenogenic implants in the abdominal wall was 30 %. Animals that had induration in their vaginal implants also showed induration of their abdominal implants.

In one vaginal explant, there was macroscopically no visible implant in between the fixation sutures any more. Vaginal and abdominal explants were of comparable thickness, though the contraction rate was almost three times higher in vaginal explants ($p=0.0008$). There were significant differences between implantation sites for passive biomechanics: vaginal explants were 63 % less stiff than their abdominal counterparts ($p=0.01$), though the length of the comfort zone was comparable (Fig. 3a). Explants were also categorized by histologic signs of degradation. In the presence of histologic loss of implant integrity, degraded abdominal implants were more compliant than those without degradation (0.44 vs. 0.79 N/mm). Because of the low number, no statistics were done. For vaginal implants, the histology was taken from the anterior side. Of those animals with histologic signs of degradation, their corresponding posterior implants were compared to those without degradation. The compliance of posterior implants of animals with degradation in the anterior implant was lower than in those without (0.33 vs. 0.15 N/mm). Again, no statistics were done.

Histology of vaginal explants was scored on smaller anterior vaginal implants (Table 2). One must remember that this is a different location than the rectovaginal area described above. ACM abdominal explants had higher scores for FBGC ($p=0.0078$) yet similar amounts of PMN and vascularization

Table 1 Paired comparison of outcomes of vaginally and abdominally implanted ACMs

	ACM		Paired comparison
	Abdomen	Posterior vagina	
Graft-related complication	3/10 (30 %)	5/10 (50 %)	ns
Exposure	0/10 (0 %)	1/10 (10 %)	
Folding	0/10 (0 %)	2/10 (20 %)	
Induration	3/10 (30 %)	2/10 (20 %)	
Other gross anatomical findings			
Thickness (mm)	8.22±3.90	6.78±2.27	ns
Material not identifiable	0/10 (0 %)	1/10 (10 %)	ns
Contraction of identifiable mesh	−20.28 %±18.24	−61.18 %±17.25	0.0008
Biomechanics			
All ewes			
Comfort zone stiffness (N/mm)	0.68±0.2	0.41±0.46	ns
Comfort zone length (mm)	7.18±2.00	8.52±3.22	ns
Exclusion of outlier (n=9)			
Comfort zone stiffness (N/mm) (n=9)	0.73±0.29	0.27±0.19	0.0101
Comfort zone length (mm) (n=9)	7.30±2.00	8.90±3.17	ns

Biomechanical findings are displayed for all animals as well as results without the outlier, and contraction is displayed without those with unidentifiable or extruded material.

as vaginal ACM explants. Scores for collagen organization and composition were similar for both sites, but the amount of collagen was higher in the abdominal ACM explants ($p=0.0201$). All the above scores were averages. At closer look, explants fall apart in two categories. In 70 % of the anterior vaginal and 30 % of the abdominal explants, we could not trace the typically dense structure of the ACM on histology (Fig. 2d, e). In these cases, there was no measurable inflammation but limited areas of organized and mature connective tissue. Isolated pockets of inflammation were visible only when a suture was accidentally caught in the section. In the other cases, the ACM could be identified. In that case, there was an abundance of inflammatory cells, both FBGC and PMN, as evidenced by their score, as well as connective tissue deposition. In five ACM sections, we observed a precipitated material compatible with calcification (Fig. 2c). Four were abdominal explants; three of them were macroscopically categorized as indurated. In one of these ewes, also the anterior and posterior vaginal explants were indurated. The anterior explant showed calcification on histology, which coincided with histologic signs of infection).

Vaginal contractility and comparison to PP vaginal implants

Figure 3 displays the vaginal contractility findings. Posterior ACM explants where no graft was recognizable on histology ($n=7$) and the corresponding anterior vaginal implant had a 68 % lower contractility than those with recognizable material ($n=3$; Fig. 3b). Again, in view of the very low numbers, no statistics were attempted.

We compared the vaginal contractility and other findings to observations made earlier when using a PP vaginal implant (Table 3). In the PP group, there was one case of GRC

(folding), yet this apparently lower number was not significant. However, the 17 % contraction rate of PP explants was significantly less than for ACM ($p=0.0009$). Passive biomechanics of all vaginal ACM were comparable to observations in the PP explants. Compliance of degraded ACM (0.33 N/mm) was within the range of what was measured in PP (0.29 N/mm) explants. Active biomechanical findings were also comparable. However, the values of three animals with recognizable ACM were in the range of the PP-implanted animals. Conversely, the forces generated by the seven animals without degradation in the anterior ACM were 60 % lower than those of PP explants ($p=0.048$) (Fig. 3b).

The histology of vaginal explants with PP differed completely from those with recognizable ACM (Fig. 2f). PP induced a mild inflammation, with few cells, nearly all macrophages or FBGC, and less collagen deposition. These specimens showed no histologic signs of infection.

Discussion

In this study, we used the ovine model to document outcomes following insertion of a cross-linked ACM in the rectovaginal septum and, for histology, insertion of a smaller piece into the anterior vaginal wall. We used an investigational product that was treated with the ADAPT® procedure to prevent calcification, reduce lipid content and restore tissue flexibility. We used a double control, i.e. an internal control by implantation of the same material at a control site (the abdominal wall) and an external control by implantation of a durable PP implant at the same (vaginal) site.

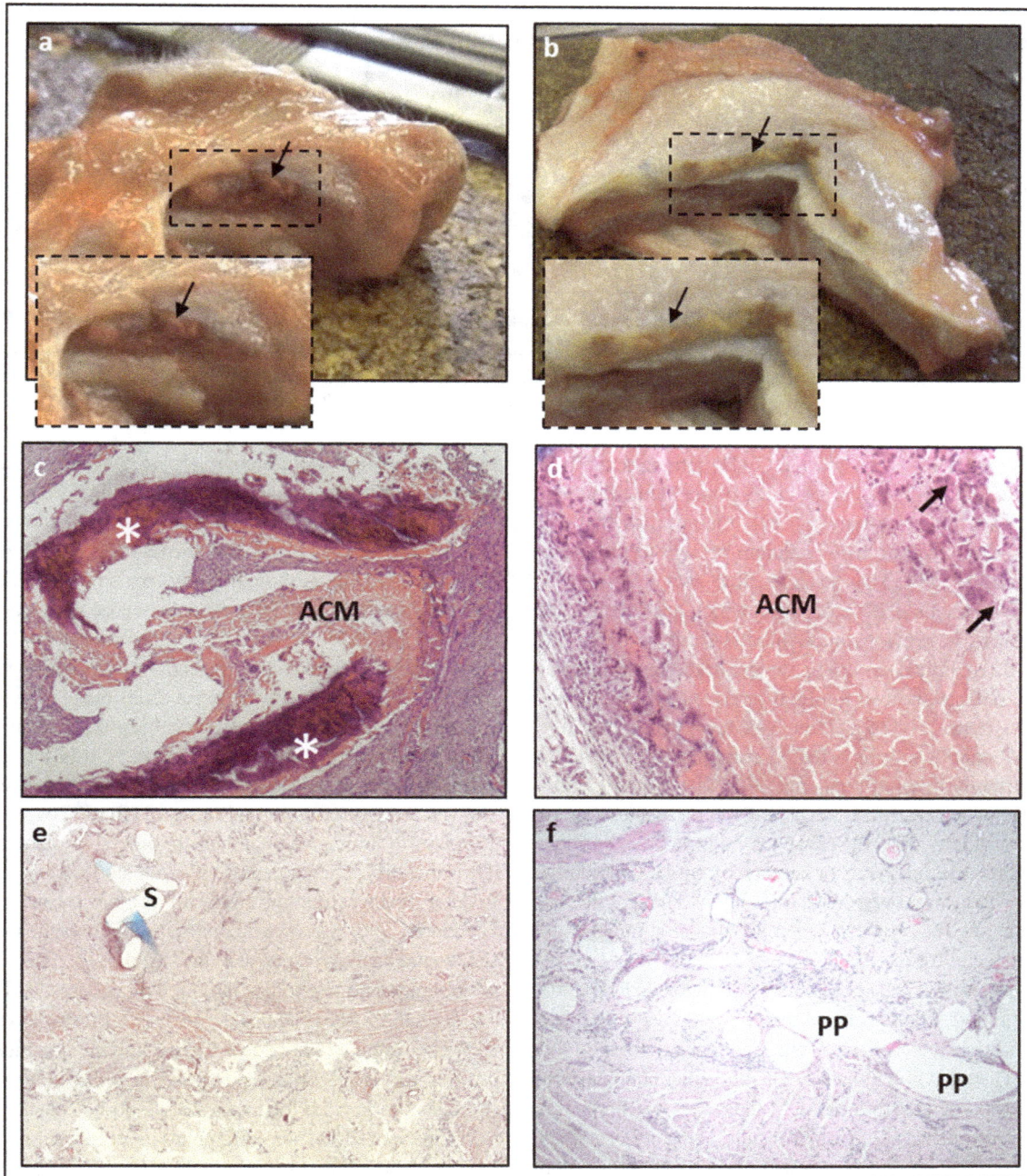

Fig. 2 Gross anatomy. Explants from the posterior vaginal wall (**a**) and the abdomen (**b**) with induration and folding visible in the below placed selections. The *dark area* (*arrows*) below the vaginal epithelium and above the abdominal muscles is the location of the implant, which looks complete. In these cases, the material was hard on palpation and surrounded with excessive amount of connective tissue. Histology showed variable host response (**c–e**), gradual degradation of ACM with mineral precipitation or calcification (*asterisk*; **c**) and FBGC (*arrow*) on the graft–tissue interface (**d**), or complete ACM degradation where just sutures (*S*) were identifiable (**e**). Polypropylene implant (*PP*) showed uniform response (**f**). (H & E, ×40, ×200, ×25, ×100, respectively)

Conceptually, ACM is the ideal matrix for gradual integration into the host. In order to avoid adverse reactions, ACMs are made free of allergens, DNA and other pathogens. Cross-linking should make them resistant to endogenous collagenase activity. However, several experimental and clinical studies report unfavourable outcomes with the use of a variety of ACM. Clinically, both GRC and failure were reported [24–27]. Also, our experiment revealed a number of GRC. The first striking observation was the presence of calcification on histology. This happened at both anatomical locations and not in the control group. Calcification of GA cross-linked grafts has been tied to residual non-viable cells and cellular

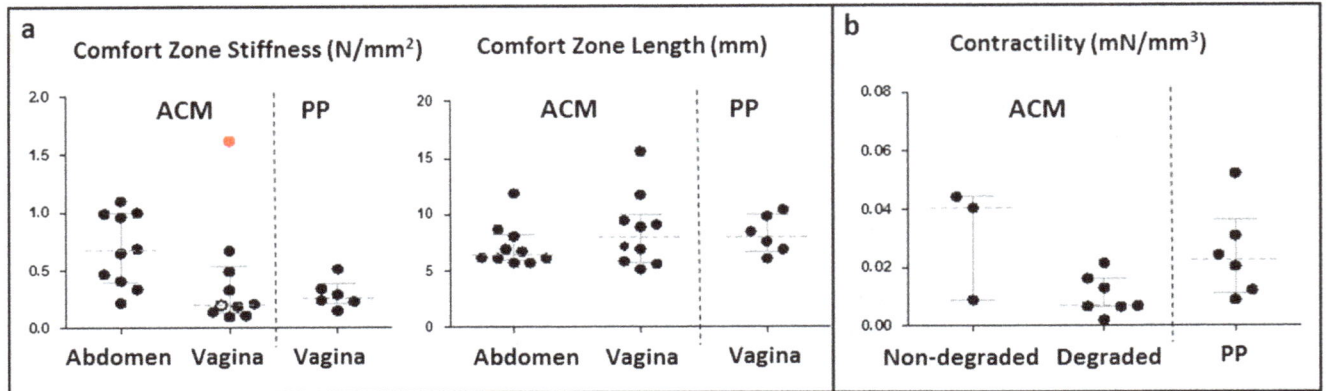

Fig. 3 Box plots and individual data of passive (**a**) and active (**b**) biomechanical tests. Individual data are plotted (*black circle*) with median and interquartile range marked with *gray lines*. The not identifiable implant is marked with an *empty circle* and outlier *red circle*

debris that were not removed during GAD pretreatment. They serve as nucleation sites for calcium phosphate minerals. GAD modifies phosphorous-rich cell membranes that are capable of mineralization using calcium present in the extracellular fluid [28, 29]. This adverse effect was meant to be prevented by the ADAPT® procedure, which has been earlier shown to work in previous experimental studies in rats and sheep [30–32]. Clinical studies on the use of the same material for cardiac defects showed minimal or no mineral precipitation in the matrices [15]. This was reassuring because pathological calcification is a feared complication in cardiac surgery, certainly in young patients [33, 34]. Another identified risk factor for calcification of grafts is the occurrence of infection or folding [35, 36]. These may add to other surgical factors, such as haemorrhage, or damage by surgical handling. To our knowledge, no previous studies have looked at the use of this material for surgical repair of the abdominal wall or a vaginal environment.

The most common local observation was palpable induration at the implant site. Histologically, this did not always coincide with calcification but may also with contraction, folding and wrinkling. There are no published data on contraction rates following insertion of cross-linked ACM in the vagina. Studies on abdominal insertion showed various results. Ozog et al. reported minimal or unchanged dimensions in 180 days with Pelvicol in rats, however, without visible deformation [37]. Conversely, Jenkins et al. reported a 50 % area reduction and wrinkling for abdominal wall reconstruction after 3 months in mini pigs using Collamend (another cross-linked porcine dermis; Bard, Davol, RI) [38]. They explained the process by the presence of encapsulation, though we observed that process also in non-contracted ACM [37]. Contraction is, however, not the privilege of ACM, as significant contraction rates have been reported following PP implantation both in the vagina (45 %) and abdomen (10 %) 90 days after surgery [18].

We also observed various stages of graft degradation in 30 % of abdominal and 70 % of vaginal explants. The occurrence of degradation of cross-linked ACM has been reported

by several groups in different models [39–42]. Claerhout et al. documented degradation in rabbit abdominal Pelvicol (Bard, Haasrode, Belgium) implants from 180 days onwards [40], and Pierce documented the same for vaginal Pelvisoft implants [41]. In a clinical study, we saw the same when Pelvicol was used for laparoscopic sacrocolpopexy, leading to recurrence [24]. Graft degradation coincided in 8 out of 9 cases with an abundance of foreign body (giant) cells on biopsy [43]. Description of the exact time course of degradation is currently impossible since clinical, as experimental studies usually involve only one time point. Interestingly, degradation does not occur in the same way at both locations. Pierce et al. showed more degradation of Pelvisoft (Bard, Covington, GA) 270 days following vaginal than abdominal implantation [44]. The same difference was present in our study. It is not possible to determine whether this is a faster or more vigorous process. However, Abramov et al. showed differences between the wound healing response in the vagina and in the abdomen, which may lead to another remodelling process [45].

Vaginal ACM explants were around 2.7 times less stiff than their abdominal counterparts. To our knowledge, there are no studies on biomechanics following simultaneous ACM implantation in both locations, so we do not have references to compare to. However, differences in biomechanics for these two environments were studied following insertion of PP (Gynemesh; Ethicon, Somerville, NJ) in a rabbit [44]. Vaginal explants were 1.5 less stiff than abdominal explants. Both observations follow a trend reported on biomechanics of cadaverous native tissue from the vagina and abdominal aponeurosis [46]. Gabriel et al. reported the vaginal wall being four times less stiff than abdominal aponeurosis. There are, to our knowledge, no published reference data on the biomechanics of native vaginal tissue and abdominal wall.

Graft degradation is another factor of relevance, as it interferes with the biomechanical properties. For that reason, we compared stiffness of those animals where no ACM was visible anymore versus those where the material was conserved. Effects seemed to be different according to the location of implantation. Yet,

Table 2 Histological scores of host response and connective tissue formation following insertion of ACM and PP in the vagina and abdominal wall

Histology	Abdomen ACM	Anterior vagina	Pair comparison	Anterior vagina PP	Unpaired comparison
	N= 10	N= 10		N=6	
FBGC	0.8 (0.88)	0.1 (0.53)	0.0078	0.40 (0.25)	
PMN	0.15 (0.38)	0.2 (0.67)		0.05 (0.23)	
Vascularity	1.0 (0.4)	1.15 (0.3)		2.05 (0.55)	0.0023
Collagen organization	1.5 (1.4)	1.4 (0.35)		1.3 (0.55)	
Collagen composition	1.8 (0.4)	2.1 (0.4)		2.3 (0.55)	
Collagen amount	2.7 (0.2)	2.5 (0.2)	0.0201	1.9 (0.35)	0.0061
Calcification	4/10	1/10		0/6	
Scores at the interface with identifiable material on histology	N= 7	N= 3		N= 6	
FBGC	1.1 (0.7)	0.8 (0.35)		0.40 (0.25)	
PMN	0.1 (0.45)	1.8 (0.85)		0.05 (0.23)	
Vascularity	0.7 (0.45)	1.5 (0.45)		2.05 (0.55)	
Collagen organization	1.4 (1.0)	0.8 (0.5)		1.3 (0.55)	
Collagen composition	1.8 (0.3)	2.4 (0.3)		2.3 (0.55)	
Collagen amount	2.8 (0.3)	2.8 (0.1)		1.9 (0.35)	

Scores are displayed for all explanted specimens and also for those with identifiable ACM. For later, statistics was not carried out due to a few specimens. Data for vaginal PP implants were previously published by Feola et al. 2014 [17]

FBGC foreign body giant cell, *PMN* polymorphonuclears

low numbers preclude actual statistical assessment, and more importantly, degradation was determined on the anterior implant, whereas biomechanics on the posterior implant. For those reasons, we prefer not to make any firm conclusions on this matter.

Smooth muscle contractility showed, at the first glance, no difference for the explants using different implant materials. Further analysis into two subgroups revealed a 68 % decline of forces in group without visible ACM. When there was still detectable ACM, findings were comparable to PP-implanted

tissues. In other words, the absence of material coincides with reduction in contractility. In line with other studies, we further demonstrated that ACM implants affect smooth muscle contractility [47]. This is somewhat counter-intuitive unless one assumes that earlier in time, the implant may have already compromised contractility, e.g. by a process of stress shielding, as described by others [47–49]. To elucidate that, one would, however, need a study with several time points and appropriate native tissue controls, and the mechanisms remain therefore unexplained.

Table 3 Outcomes and test results of vaginally implanted ACM and PP and their unpaired comparison (significance level $p<0.05$)

	ACM Posterior vagina N=10	PP Posterior vagina N=6	Unpaired comparison
Graft-related complication	5/10 (50 %)	1/6 (16.6 %)	0.0367
Exposure	1/10 (10 %)	0/6 (0 %)	
Folding	2/10 (20 %)	1/6 (16.6 %)	
Induration	2/10 (20 %)	0/6 (0 %)	
Contraction of identifiable mesh	−53.82 %±10.20 (n=7)	−23.06 %±16.63	0.0009
Biomechanics			
Comfort zone stiffness (N/mm)	0.27±0.19 (n=9)	0.29±0.12	ns
Comfort zone length (mm)	8.89±3.17 (n=9)	8.18±1.67	ns
Contractility (mN/mm³)	0.017±0.015 (n=10)	0.025±0.016	ns
Degraded (n=7)	0.010±0.007	0.025±0.016	0.0481
Non-degraded (n=3)	0.031±0.019	–	–

Our study has several limitations. Again, we only studied one time point, precluding insight into the time course of the host response; hence, it cannot learn on the processes driving the adverse events neither. Another is the use of a semiquantitative histological scoring system and limited staining methods. Though they are descriptive, it would be much more informative to also have biochemical and molecular read outs to document details on the nature of the immune response, neovascularization, collagen metabolism and nerve ingrowth [50]. This might be difficult to do, as those tools are not readily available in sheep and also add significantly to the cost. Further, we had to resort to use a second vaginal location for implantation so that we could obtain sufficient tissue for histology, without compromising the availability of tissue for biomechanical testing. Further, there are the limitations of the model; even though sheep can be used as a model for vaginal surgery as well as prolapse [18], it remains mostly an asymptomatic quadruped, with clinically different anatomical and pelvic floor loads, hence not an ideal disease model. It has however several advantages: apparently, sheep may clinically develop obvious pelvic floor relaxation and some degree of prolapse after delivery; further, this is a widely available, affordable alternative to the primate, which would be the closest model that we could think off.

In conclusion, we demonstrated that despite treatment with ADAPT®, ACM insertion into the rectovaginal septum was associated with a number of local adverse effects. Apart from that, the passive biomechanical properties were not better than what was obtained when a PP mesh was used. Following degradation of the ACM, there was a decrease in smooth muscle contractility. The ideal implant material has apparently not yet been identified.

Acknowledgment We thank to Ivan Laermans, Rosita Kinart, Ann Lissens (Centre for Surgical Technologies, KU Leuven, Leuven, Belgium), Godelieve Verbist (Dept. of Development and Regeneration, KU Leuven, Leuven, Belgium) for their technical support during the experiment. We thank Leen Mortier for help with data and manuscript management.

Conflict of interest Masayuki Endo and Andrew Feola are recipients of a Marie Curie Industry-Academia Partnership Programme grant of the European Commission. They, as well as Iva Urbankova, Jaromir Vlacil, Siddarth Sengupta and Thomas Deprest, declare that they have no conflict of interest.

Bernd Klosterhalfen is a consultant for FEG Textiltechnik, Aachen, and a plaintiff's expert witness in the litigation case Cisson vs. Bard.

Jan Deprest is a fundamental clinical researcher of the Fonds Wetenschappelijk Onderzoek Vlaanderen (1801207). The experiment was partly supported by an unconditional grant from Blasingame, Burch, Garrard and Ashley (Atlanta, GA, USA) and the University of Western Australia. Agreements are handled via the Leuven Research and Development transfer office. Sponsors did not interfere with the planning, execution or reporting of this experiment neither are they the owner of the results.

Contribution to the authorship ME contributed to protocol development, experimental surgery, data collection and data analysis. IU contributed to histological analysis, data collection and data analysis. IU and JD were responsible for initial manuscript writing. JV and AF contributed to protocol development, experimental surgery, data collection and analysis. JV, SS, TD and BK contributed to histological analysis and data collection. All authors contributed to manuscript editing.

References

1. Barber MD, Maher C (2013) Epidemiology and outcome assessment of pelvic organ prolapse. Int Urogynecol J 24:1783–90. doi:10.1007/s00192-013-2169-9
2. Milsom I, Altman D, Lapitan MC, et al. (2009) Epidemiology of urinary (UI) and faecal (FI) incontinence and pelvic organ prolapse (POP). 35–112.
3. Wu JM, Matthews CA, Conover MM et al (2014) Lifetime risk of stress urinary incontinence or pelvic organ prolapse surgery. Obstet Gynecol 123:1201–6. doi:10.1097/AOG.0000000000000286
4. Maher CM, Feiner B, Baessler K, Glazener CMA (2011) Surgical management of pelvic organ prolapse in women: the updated summary version Cochrane review. Int Urogynecol J 22:1445–57. doi:10.1007/s00192-011-1542-9
5. Keys T, Campeau L, Badlani G (2012) Synthetic mesh in the surgical repair of pelvic organ prolapse: current status and future directions. Urology 80:237–43. doi:10.1016/j.urology.2012.04.008
6. Mangera A, Bullock A, Chapple CR, MacNeil S (2012) Are biomechanical properties predictive of the success of prostheses used in stress urinary incontinence and pelvic organ prolapse? A systematic review. Neurourol Urodyn 21:13–21. doi:10.1002/nau
7. Salomon LJ, Detchev R, Barranger E et al (2004) Treatment of anterior vaginal wall prolapse with porcine skin collagen implant by the transobturator route: preliminary results. Eur Urol 45:219–225. doi:10.1016/j.eururo.2003.09.005
8. Meschia M, Pifarotti P, Bernasconi F et al (2007) Porcine skin collagen implants to prevent anterior vaginal wall prolapse recurrence: a multicenter, randomized study. J Urol 177:192–5. doi:10.1016/j.juro.2006.08.100
9. Botros SM, Sand PK, Beaumont JL et al (2009) Arcus-anchored acellular dermal graft compared to anterior colporrhaphy for stage II cystoceles and beyond. Int Urogynecol J Pelvic Floor Dysfunct 20:1265–71. doi:10.1007/s00192-009-0933-7
10. Mangera A, Bullock AJ, Roman S et al (2013) Comparison of candidate scaffolds for tissue engineering for stress urinary incontinence and pelvic organ prolapse repair. BJU Int 112:674–85. doi:10.1111/bju.12186
11. Trabuco EC, Klingele CJ, Weaver AL et al (2009) Medium-term comparison of continence rates after rectus fascia or midurethral sling

placement. Am J Obstet Gynecol 200:300.e1–6. doi:10.1016/j.ajog. 2008.10.017

12. Jeon M-J, Jung H-J, Chung S-M et al (2008) Comparison of the treatment outcome of pubovaginal sling, tension-free vaginal tape, and transobturator tape for stress urinary incontinence with intrinsic sphincter deficiency. Am J Obstet Gynecol 199:76.e1–4. doi:10. 1016/j.ajog.2007.11.060

13. Dunn RM (2012) Cross-linking in biomaterials: a primer for clinicians. Plast Reconstr Surg 130:18S–26S. doi:10.1097/PRS. 0b013e31825efea6

14. Neethling WML, Glancy R, Hodge AJ (2004) ADAPT-treated porcine valve tissue (cusp and wall) versus Medtronic Freestyle and Prima Plus: crosslink stability and calcification behavior in the subcutaneous rat model. J Heart Valve Dis 13:689–96

15. Neethling WML, Strange G, Firth L, Smit FE (2013) Evaluation of a tissue-engineered bovine pericardial patch in paediatric patients with congenital cardiac anomalies: initial experience with the ADAPT-treated CardioCel(R) patch. Interact Cardiovasc Thorac Surg 17: 698–702. doi:10.1093/icvts/ivt268

16. Neethling WML, Hodge AJ, Clode P, Glancy R (2006) A multi-step approach in anti-calcification of glutaraldehyde-preserved bovine pericardium. J Cardiovasc Surg (Torino) 47:711–8

17. Feola A, Endo M, Urbankova I et al (2014) Host reaction to vaginally inserted collagen containing polypropylene implants in sheep. Am J Obstet Gynecol. doi:10.1016/j.ajog.2014.11.008

18. Manodoro S, Endo M, Uvin P et al (2013) Graft-related complications and biaxial tensiometry following experimental vaginal implantation of flat mesh of variable dimensions. BJOG 120:244–50. doi: 10.1111/1471-0528.12081

19. De Tayrac R, Alves A, Thérin M (2007) Collagen-coated vs noncoated low-weight polypropylene meshes in a sheep model for vaginal surgery. A pilot study. Int Urogynecol J Pelvic Floor Dysfunct 18:513–20. doi:10.1007/s00192-006-0176-9

20. Badylak S, Kokini K, Tullius B et al (2002) Morphologic study of small intestinal submucosa as a body wall repair device. J Surg Res 103:190–202. doi:10.1006/jsre.2001.6349

21. Zheng F, Lin Y, Verbeken E et al (2004) Host response after reconstruction of abdominal wall defects with porcine dermal collagen in a rat model. Am J Obstet Gynecol 191:1961–70. doi:10.1016/j.ajog. 2004.01.091

22. Morawietz L, Tiddens O, Mueller M et al (2009) Twenty-three neutrophil granulocytes in 10 high-power fields is the best histopathological threshold to differentiate between aseptic and septic endoprosthesis loosening. Histopathology 54:847–53. doi:10.1111/ j.1365-2559.2009.03313.x

23. Feola A, Moalli P, Alperin M et al (2011) Impact of pregnancy and vaginal delivery on the passive and active mechanics of the rat vagina. Ann Biomed Eng 39:549–58. doi:10.1007/s10439-010-0153-9

24. Claerhout F, De Ridder D, Roovers JP et al (2009) Medium-term anatomic and functional results of laparoscopic sacrocolpopexy beyond the learning curve. Eur Urol 55:1459–67. doi:10.1016/j.eururo. 2008.12.008

25. Deprest J, De Ridder D, Roovers J-P et al (2009) Medium term outcome of laparoscopic sacrocolpopexy with xenografts compared to synthetic grafts. J Urol 182:2362–8. doi:10.1016/j.juro.2009.07.043

26. Quiroz LH, Gutman RE, Shippey S et al (2008) Abdominal sacrocolpopexy: anatomic outcomes and complications with Pelvicol, autologous and synthetic graft materials. Am J Obstet Gynecol 198:557.e1–5. doi:10.1016/j.ajog.2008.01.050

27. Hviid U, Hviid TVF, Rudnicki M (2010) Porcine skin collagen implants for anterior vaginal wall prolapse: a randomised prospective controlled study. Int Urogynecol J 21:529–34. doi:10.1007/s00192-009-1018-3

28. Jorge-Herrero E, Garcia Paez JM, Del Castillo-Olivares Ramos JL (2005) Tissue heart valve mineralization: review of calcification mechanisms and strategies for prevention. J Appl Biomater Biomech 3:67–82

29. Schoen FJ, Levy RJ (2005) Calcification of tissue heart valve substitutes: progress toward understanding and prevention. Ann Thorac Surg 79:1072–80. doi:10.1016/j.athoracsur.2004.06.033

30. Van den Heever JJ, Neethling WML, Smit FE et al (2013) The effect of different treatment modalities on the calcification potential and cross-linking stability of bovine pericardium. Cell Tissue Bank 14: 53–63. doi:10.1007/s10561-012-9299-z

31. Neethling WML, Glancy R, Hodge AJ (2010) Mitigation of calcification and cytotoxicity of a glutaraldehyde-preserved bovine pericardial matrix: improved biocompatibility after extended implantation in the subcutaneous rat model. J Heart Valve Dis 19:778–85

32. Neethling WML, Yadav S, Hodge AJ, Glancy R (2008) Enhanced biostability and biocompatibility of decellularized bovine pericardium, crosslinked with an ultra-low concentration monomeric aldehyde and treated with ADAPT. J Heart Valve Dis 17:456–63

33. Schoen FJ, Hobson CE (1985) Anatomic analysis of removed prosthetic heart valves: causes of failure of 33 mechanical valves and 58 bioprostheses, 1980 to 1983. Hum Pathol 16:549–59

34. Butany J, Leong SW, Cunningham KS et al (2007) A 10-year comparison of explanted Hancock-II and Carpentier-Edwards supraannular bioprostheses. Cardiovasc Pathol 16:4–13. doi:10. 1016/j.carpath.2006.06.003

35. Schoen FJ (1987) Biomaterial-associated infection, neoplasia, and calcification: clinicopathologic features and pathophysiologic concepts. ASAIO Trans 33:8–18

36. Cunanan C, Cabiling C, Dinh T (2001) Tissue characterization and calcification potential of commercial bioprosthetic heart valves. Ann Thorac Surg 417–421

37. Ozog Y, Konstantinovic M, Zheng F et al (2009) Porous acellular porcine dermal collagen implants to repair fascial defects in a rat model: biomechanical evaluation up to 180 days. Gynecol Obstet Invest 68:205–12. doi:10.1159/000235852

38. Jenkins ED, Melman L, Deeken CR et al (2011) Biomechanical and histologic evaluation of fenestrated and nonfenestrated biologic mesh in a porcine model of ventral hernia repair. J Am Coll Surg 212:327–39. doi:10.1016/j.jamcollsurg.2010.12.006

39. Deeken CR, Melman L, Jenkins ED et al (2011) Histologic and biomechanical evaluation of crosslinked and non-crosslinked biologic meshes in a porcine model of ventral incisional hernia repair. J Am Coll Surg 212:880–8. doi:10.1016/j.jamcollsurg.2011.01.006

40. Claerhout F, Verbist G, Verbeken E et al (2008) Fate of collagen-based implants used in pelvic floor surgery: a 2-year follow-up study in a rabbit model. Am J Obstet Gynecol 198:94.e1–94.e6

41. Pierce LM, Rao A, Baumann SS et al (2009) Long-term histologic response to synthetic and biologic graft materials implanted in the vagina and abdomen of a rabbit model. Am J Obstet Gynecol 200: 546.e1–8. doi:10.1016/j.ajog.2008.12.040

42. Melman L, Jenkins ED, Hamilton NA et al (2011) Early biocompatibility of crosslinked and non-crosslinked biologic meshes in a porcine model of ventral hernia repair. Hernia 15:157–64. doi:10.1007/ s10029-010-0770-0

43. Deprest J, Klosterhalfen B, Schreurs A et al (2010) Clinicopathological study of patients requiring reintervention after sacrocolpopexy with xenogenic acellular collagen grafts. J Urol 183: 2249–55. doi:10.1016/j.juro.2010.02.008

44. Pierce LM, Grunlan MA, Hou Y et al (2009) Biomechanical properties of synthetic and biologic graft materials following long-term implantation in the rabbit abdomen and vagina. Am J Obstet Gynecol 200:549.e1–8. doi:10.1016/j.ajog.2008.12.041

45. Abramov Y, Golden B, Sullivan M et al (2007) Histologic characterization of vaginal vs. abdominal surgical wound healing in a rabbit model. Wound Repair Regen 15:80–6. doi:10.1111/j.1524-475X. 2006.00188.x

46. Gabriel B, Rubod C, Brieu M (2011) Vagina, abdominal skin, and aponeurosis: do they have similar biomechanical properties? Int Urogynecol J 22:23–27. doi:10.1007/s00192-010-1237-7

47. Feola A, Abramowitch S, Jallah Z et al (2013) Deterioration in biomechanical properties of the vagina following implantation of a high-stiffness prolapse mesh. BJOG 120:224–32. doi:10.1111/1471-0528. 12077

48. Majima T, Yasuda K, Tsuchida T et al (2003) Stress shielding of patellar tendon: effect on small-diameter collagen fibrils in a rabbit model. J Orthop Sci 8:836–41. doi:10.1007/s00776-003-0707-x

49. Lo IKY, Marchuk L, Majima T et al (2003) Medial collateral ligament and partial anterior cruciate ligament transection: mRNA changes in uninjured ligaments of the sheep knee. J Orthop Sci 8:707–13. doi: 10.1007/s00776-003-0695-x

50. Liang R, Zong W, Palcsey S et al (2014) Impact of prolapse meshes on the metabolism of vaginal extracellular matrix in rhesus macaque. Am J Obstet Gynecol. doi:10.1016/j.ajog.2014.08.008

17

Adnexectomy by poor man's transvaginal NOTES

Anneleen Reynders[1] · Jan Baekelandt[1]

Abstract The purpose of this study was to demonstrate the feasibility and safety of adnexectomy by transvaginal natural orifice transluminal endoscopic surgery (vNOTES) for benign adnexal masses. Conventional, reusable laparoscopic instruments were used, inserted through aninexpensive, self-constructed single port device. Between November 2013 and November 2014, 20 adnexectomies by vNOTES were performed by a single surgeon (BJ). Only conventional, reusable laparoscopic instruments were used. The self-constructed single port device was made by assembling a surgical glove, a wound protector, one reusable 10-mm trocar, and four reusable 5-mm trocars. The adnexectomy was performed according to the technique for standard laparoscopic surgery, and the specimen was removed through the colpotomy incision. Patient and perioperative data were analysed. Twenty patients underwent adnexectomy by vNOTES, and no conversion to standard laparoscopy or laparotomy was necessary. Mean operation time was 32 min (20–50 min); mean drop in hemoglobin level was 0.9 g/dl (0–2.1 g/dl). There were no operative complications. Post-operative pain scores were very low. The mean size of the removed adnexal mass was 51.8 mm (35–110 mm). Adnexectomy by vNOTES is feasible even for masses up to 110 mm and even when performed with reusable, conventional laparoscopic instruments. The main advantages of vNOTES are better cosmetics, low postoperative pain scores and easy removal of the specimen without spillage. This frugally innovative technique also enables surgeons to perform adnexectomies by vNOTES in low resource settings.

Keywords Minimally invasive surgery · Natural orifice endoscopic surgery · Transvaginal · Adnexectomy · Frugal innovation · vNOTES · gloveport

Introduction

Driven by the desire to minimalise surgical morbidity, the evolution from laparotomy to laparoscopy has now extended to the era of even less invasive surgery such as robotics, minilaparoscopy, single incision laparoscopic surgery (SILS) and natural orifice transluminal endoscopy (NOTES). Minimally invasive surgery not only improves cosmetic outcome, it also reduces the surgical injury, which in turn decreases the inflammatory and neuroendocrine response resulting in less post-operative pain and quicker recovery [1, 2].

NOTES attempts to reach the abdominal cavity through an invisible scar, i.e. numerous surgical procedures are performed via a natural body orifice. It has gained popularity amongst general surgeons, urologists and gastroenterologist over the past few years, and its feasibility and safety have been approved [3].

NOTES can be performed through a variety of approaches including the stomach, oesophagus, bladder and rectum, but the vast majority of NOTES procedures have been performed transvaginally, as the vagina provides direct access [4]. Culdotomy has been used widely for several surgical procedures (by gynaecologists but also by general surgeons for extraction of large specimens), and it has been approved as safe and easy to close [5, 6].

✉ Jan Baekelandt
  jan.baekelandt@imelda.be

[1] Department of Obstetrics and Gynaecology, Imelda Hospital Bonheiden, Imeldalaan 9, 2820 Bonheiden, Belgium

In *hybrid* NOTES, the surgical procedure is performed through a natural body orifice with transabdominal assistance, whereas the term *pure* NOTES refers to procedures that involve only transluminal access.

Given its potential benefits, including no visible scars, fewer port-related complications and less painful and faster postoperative recovery, we introduced transvaginal pure NOTES (vNOTES) for benign adnexal masses in our surgical practice since November 2013. We describe here our initial clinical experience in poor man's tNOTES. We evaluate the feasibility and surgical outcome of vNOTES adnexectomy when performed with only conventional, reusable laparoscopic instruments, and an inexpensive, self-constructed single port device that can be quickly and easily assembled. We aimed to demonstrate that there is no need for expensive, commercially available disposable SILS-ports, other disposable instruments, or sealing devices, to perform a safe and equally time efficient adnexectomy by vNOTES.

Materials and methods

Patients

Between November 2013 and November 2014, a single surgeon (BJ) performed 20 adnexectomies by vNOTES. All patients were selected for adnexectomy for benign gynaecological disease. We selected each patient based on the following criteria: no contraindication for general anaesthesia, pneumoperitoneum or Trendelenburg position; no fixed uterus, strong pelvic adhesions or nodularity in the Pouch of Douglas on clinical examination; no history of pelvic inflammatory disease or moderate to severe endometriosis and mass not suspicious for malignancy. In our first 20 cases, we did not include patients with large fibroid uteri as these may impair visualisation. Virginity and pregnancy were considered as exclusion criteria whereas obesity (BMI =/> 30) and absence of vaginal delivery were not.

The following patient and perioperative data were collected and retrospectively analysed: patient age, body mass index (BMI), parity, history of vaginal delivery, previous pelvic surgery, type of surgery, total operating time, serum haemoglobin (Hb) drop (change between the preoperative Hb and postoperative Hb 1 day after surgery), (peri-) operative complications, post-operative pain score and size of the adnexal mass.

The duration of surgery was defined as the time from the start of colpotomy to the end of vaginal closure. Bowel, bladder, ureteral or vascular injuries, as well as blood loss >300 ml, were considered as intraoperative complications. Short-term post-operative complications were classified as urinary tract infection, post-operative ileus, vaginal vault bleeding or infection or hematuria.

Post-operative pain was assessed using the visual analog pain scale (VAS) (scoring from 0 = no pain to 10 = worst imaginable pain). The VAS score was evaluated at 6 and 24 h post-operatively. All patients received the same intraoperative analgesia: intravenous paracetamol 1000 mg and ketorolac trometamol 20 mg. Post-operative pain was managed by paracetamol 1000 mg, and ketorolac trometamol was administered on patient's demand.

No bowel preparation was done prior to surgery. A Foley catheter was placed just before surgery and removed the morning after surgery (range 12–22 h). Prophylactic intravenous antibiotic therapy, cefazoline 2 g and metronidazol 500 mg, was administrated during surgery.

As this was a new technique, the first patients were closely monitored post-operatively.

No vaginal intercourse was allowed for 6 weeks after the procedure. Each patient was re-assessed at the post-operative consultation 6 weeks after surgery.

Surgical technique

The patient was placed in lithotomy position under general anaesthesia. A rectovaginal examination was performed to exclude pelvic adhesions or obliteration of the Pouch of Douglas.

The operation field was disinfected and draped. A Foley catheter was placed. A 2.5-cm single incision was made in the posterior vaginal fornix. The Pouch of Douglas was opened to insert the self-constructed NOTES port (Fig. 1). The device was constructed before surgery, using an Alexis Wound Protector/Retractor (Applied Medical, Rancho Santa Margarita, CA, USA) attached to a size 8 surgical glove. One finger of the surgical glove was incised to place a 10-mm reusable trocar for CO2 insufflation and laparoscope insertion. Four 5-mm reusable trocars were placed through the remaining fingers for insertion of the reusable laparoscopic instruments.

Assembling five trocars into the gloveport before starting the procedure gives the option of leaving instruments inserted through the trocars throughout surgery; thus, alternating between instruments becomes less time consuming. We used a

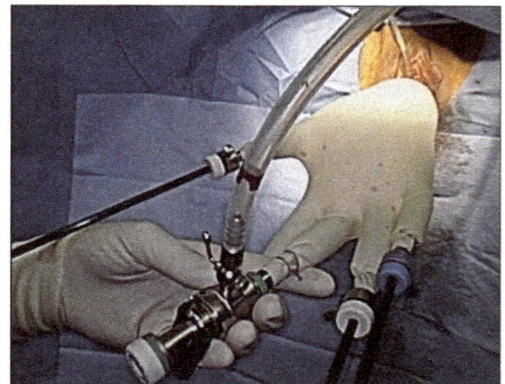

Fig. 1 Low cost self-constructed single port device

standard rigid zero-degree 10-mm laparoscope. The reusable conventional laparoscopic instruments were a bipolar forceps, a pair of cold scissors, an atraumatic forceps, and a suction-irrigation cannula.

After placing the patient in Trendelenburg position, carbon dioxide was insufflated to maintain an adequate pneumoperitoneum.

Adnexectomy was performed (Video 1) by dissection of the infundibulopelvic and ovarian ligament, and fallopian tube, using the bipolar forceps and cold scissors. No sealing or ligature device was used.

After complete resection, the specimen was extracted through the wound protector into the glove part of the self-constructed port. If the adnexal mass was too large, an endoscopic bag (Memobag 1200 ml; Teleflex) was used.The pursestring of the endobag was pulled through the colpotomy and was released outside of the vagina. Before removing the bag, the mass was first punctured to aspirate its content and reduce its volume. All adnexae were resected in toto, and no spilling into the abdominal cavity or vagina occurred.

After hemostasis and rinsing of the peritoneal cavity, the pneumoperitoneum was deflated and the port device removed with the specimen inside it. The colpotomy was closed using a Vicryl-1 (Ethicon, Piscataway, NJ, USA) running suture.

Results

Between November 2013 and November 2014, twenty adnexectomies were successfully performed by poor man's vNOTES using conventional, reusable laparoscopic instruments. No conversion to standard multi-incision laparoscopy or laparotomy was necessary. Fourteen patients underwent a unilateral adnexectomy. In six patients, a bilateral salpingo-oophorectomy was performed.

Table 1 presents an overview of patient and perioperative data. Individual patient details are presented in Table 2. Mean operation time was 32 min. Five patients had had previous pelvic surgery. There were no intraoperative complications, and only one patient had a post-operative cystitis for which

Table 1 Overview of patient and perioperative characteristics

Data	Mean	Range
Age (years)	51	31–75
BMI (kg/m^2)	24.0	17.2–28.7
Total operating time (min)	32	20–50
Serum hemoglobine drop (g/dl)	0.9	0–2.1
Postoperative pain score		
6 h	2.0	0–4
24 h	1.3	0–2
Size of adnexal mass (mm)	51.8	35–110

oral antibiotic therapy was administered. The mean drop in haemoglobin level was 0.9 g/dl. Most patients scored a low post-operative pain score (range 0–2) 24 h after surgery. Mean size of the removed adnexal mass was 51.8 mm with the largest cyst measuring 110 mm.

Each patient was examined 6 weeks after surgery. There was no vaginal wound infection nor dehiscence, and no patient complained of pain during pelvic examination. All patients were in good health and were all extremely satisfied with the result. One patient even mentioned playing tennis on day 1 post-surgery (against our medical advice).

Discussion

In this study, vNOTES for benign adnexal masses was successfully performed in 20 patients, using only conventional, reusable laparoscopic instruments and a self-constructed single incision port. The procedures were completed within a reasonable operation time and without complications. No conversion to laparotomy or standard laparoscopy was necessary.

An inexpensive, self-constructed single port device, which can quickly and easily be made by any surgeon, was used. Combining this self-constructed port device with easily available, conventional and reusable laparoscopic instruments, this study shows that adnexectomy via vNOTES is feasible without increasing the cost of laparoscopic surgery. This frugally innovative technique can potentially be performed in a low resource setting. It has been described as an approach for adhaesiolysis [7].

To the best of our knowledge, this is the first report of pure vNOTES for adnexectomy using this combination of a low cost port device with only reusable laparoscopic instruments.

A self-constructed port using a surgical glove has advantages when compared to commercial ports. It is less costly, it has flexible material that enables greater manipulation of instruments and a greater number and size of instruments can be passed through the incision.

Conventional transvaginal surgery has significant advantages compared to laparoscopic surgery such as the absence of abdominal scarring, reduced spillage by removing the specimen through the colpotomy and faster recovery from surgery [8]. By performing vNOTES, technical drawbacks of transvaginal surgery such as limited visualisation to attempt good hemostasis and the difficulty to perform adnexectomy in case of adhesions between the adnexa and the uterus can be overcome. Additionally, vNOTES abandons the risk of trocar related complications and induces less post-operative pain [9]. We did not encounter any difficulties in inserting the instruments using our poor man's vNOTES technique.

To perform vNOTES, various technical difficulties, comparable to those for transumbilical SILS, need to be overcome. The surgeon has to deal with problems due to instrument

Table 2 Patient and perioperative characteristics of consecutive patients

Patient no.	Age (years)	BMI (kg/m^2)	Parity	History of vaginal delivery	Previous pelvic surgery	Type of surgery	Total operating time (min)	Serum hemo-globine drop (g/dl)	(Peri-) operative complications	Post-operative pain score		Size of adnexal mass (largest diameter, mm)
										6 h	24 h	
1	54	24.1	P4	Yes	LS	BSO	40	0.4	-	2	2	70
2	44	17.2	P1	Yes	-	USO R	35	0.8	-	2	2	62
3	56	21.5	P2	Yes	LS	BSO	35	0.5	Cystitis	2	2	35
4	47	27.1	P2	Yes	-	USO R	30	0	-	2	1	50
5	58	26.0	P0	No	-	BSO	35	0.6	-	4	1	40
6	52	28.3	P0	No	-	USO R	35	0.6	-	1	1	36
7	66	22.9	P2	Yes	-	BSO	40	0.7	-	2	1	45
8	46	20.8	P0	No	-	USO R	22	1.4	-	2	1	35
9	51	25.4	P2	Yes	-	USO L	22	0.5	-	2	1	35
10	56	24.2	P1	Yes	-	USO R	25	1.2	-	2	1	42
11	63	26.7	P2	Yes	-	BSO	30	2.0	-	3	0	40
12	56	25.0	P2	Yes	-	USO R	22	0.5	-	1	1	39
13	75	23.2	P1	Yes	-	USO R	20	0.6	-	2	2	38
14	31	21.5	P2	Yes	-	USO R	35	1.8	-	2	2	60
15	45	28.7	P1	Yes	-	USO R	20	0	-	2	2	40
16	43	24.4	P2	No	CS	USO R	50	0.9	-	2	2	100
17	45	23.7	P2	Yes	CE	USO R	45	0.7	-	0	0	110
18	36	22.8	P2	Yes	CS	USO R	40	1.7	-	2	1	39
19	55	23.4	P1	Yes	-	BSO	35	1.2	-	2	1	70
20	38	22.5	P2	Yes	-	USO L	32	2.1	-	2	2	49

CE cystectomy, *CS* caesarean section, *LS* laparoscopic sterilisation, *USO* unilateral salpingo-oophorectomy, *BSO* bilateral salpingo-oophorectomy, *R* right, *L* left

collision, limited triangulation and reduced traction of tissue [10, 11]. Due to the colpotomy providing a more flexible entry compared to the infraumbilical fascia opening, we find these difficulties to be less restricting when compared with SILS.

As the camera is inserted through the Pouch of Douglas, the view through a vNOTES port is opposite to the standard laparoscopic view, i.e. caudal to cranial as opposed to cranial to caudal. Rotating the axis of the surgical field for vNOTES required a brief adaptation period.

For the poor man's vNOTES technique, a standard rigid 0° endoscope was used and provided good visualisation. Experience gained from performing vNOTES adnexectomies in a non poor man's setting, showed that a 30° 5-mm chip on tip endoscope provides even better visualisation and maneuverability.

One could argue the possibility of pelvic infection after vaginal surgery; however, none of our patients presented with this complication after the vNOTES procedure. Previous studies have also shown that post-operative pelvic infection is unlikely to happen especially when prophylactic antibiotics are administered [12, 13]. Further concern when performing transvaginal surgery is the development of post-operative dyspareunia. No difference between conventional compared to laparoscopic transvaginal surgery is to be expected, and

different studies show the absence of dyspareunia at a mid- and long-term follow-up [12–14]. As was the case for our study protocol, sexual abstinence should be recommended for 6 to 8 weeks as is the recommendation for conventional transvaginal surgery [14].

Some contra-indications should be considered before performing vNOTES. In patients with a massive hemoperitoneum, the endoscopic view will get disturbed [15]. If Pouch of Douglas adhesions can be expected, a thorough pelvic examination should be performed prior to surgery, and in case of unexpected Pouch of Douglas obliteration, conversion to transabdominal laparoscopy should be considered. Virginity is another contra-indication for vNOTES. On the other hand, nulliparity nor absence of history of vaginal delivery should be a reason not to perform vNOTES. In our case series, the highest BMI was 28.7. We did not, however, consider obesity (BMI =/> 30) a contra-indication. If a good Trendelenburg position can be achieved, the bowel and mesentary can be lifted out of the pelvis and will not impair visualisation.

Lee et al. [15] suggested that vNOTES should be avoided in patients with an adnexal mass larger than 80 mm due to technical difficulties. We, however, successfully managed to perform adnexectomy by vNOTES in two patients with an adnexal mass larger than 80 mm (110 and 100 mm, respectively) without significantly increasing the duration of surgery. All adnexae were resected in toto. In case of a large mass, an endoscopic bag was used. The pursestring of the endobag was pulled through the colpotomy and released outside the vagina. Before removing the bag, the mass was first punctured to aspirate its content and reduce its volume. All adnexae were resected in toto, and no spilling into the abdominal cavity or vagina occurred.

As previously mentioned by Lee et al. [15], the major limitation of vNOTES is the inability to overview the pelvicarea, in particular the vesico-uterine pouch, and thus lesions such as bladder endometriosis or anterior uterine wall myomas can be missed. Innovation of endoscopes is desirable to overcome this limitation and to have the ability with vNOTES to explore the entire abdominal cavity.

Further concern is the possibility of performing repeated vNOTES procedures. To date, only one group of surgeons has reported on repeated vNOTES, performed in two patients 6 and 8 months after previous vNOTES [16].

Conclusion

In this study, poor man's vNOTES for benign adnexal masses was successfully and safely completed in correctly selected patients. We showed this frugally innovative technique to be feasible with only reusable standard laparoscopic instruments and a low cost self-constructed single port device. This technique may potentially be applied in a low resource setting. Adnexal masses up to 110 mm could be easily and safely removed without spillage of contents into the abdomen. Less post-operative pain and a quicker recovery are recorded as other advantages of vNOTES. Additionally, it avoids abdominal wall wounds and trocar-related complications. The major limitation of vNOTES with the currently available instruments and endoscopes appears to be the inability to explore the vesico-uterine pouch. Innovations in instruments and endoscopes together with additional studies with larger cohorts and longer follow-up should lead to vNOTES being used to safely perform more complex gynaecological procedures in most patients suitable for laparoscopic surgery.

Contributions Anneleen Reynders collected the data, performed the literature review and wrote the article. She was first assistant during most of the procedures.

Jan Baekelandt recruited and operated all the patients. He supervised the data collection, reviewed and submitted the article and made the video.

References

1. Burpee SE, Kurian M, Murakame Y, Benevides S, Gagner M (2002) The metabolic and immune response to laparoscopic versusopen liver resection. Surg Endosc 16(6):899–904

2. Grande M, Tucci GF, Adorisio O et al (2002) Systemic acute-phaseresponse after laparoscopic and open cholecystectomy. Surg Endosc 16(2):313–316

3. Rattner D, Kalloo A (2006) ASGE/SAGES working group on natural Orifice translumenal endoscopic surgery. October 2005. Surg Endosc 20:329–333

4. Santos BF, Hungness ES (2011) Natural orifice translumenal endoscopic surgery:progress in humans since white paper. World J Gastroenterol 17:1655–1665

5. Tolcher MC, Kalogera E, Hopkins MR, Weaver AL, Bingener J, Dowdy SC (2012) Safety of culdotomy as a surgical approach: implications for natural orifice transluminal. JSLS 16:413–420

6. Uccella S, Cromi A, Bogani G, Casarin J, Serati M, Ghezzi F (2013) Transvaginal specimen extraction at laparoscopy without concomitant hysterectomy: our experience and systematic review of the literature. J Minim Invasive Gynecol 20:583–590

7. Baekelandt J (2014) Poor Man's NOTES: can it be a good approach for adhesiolysis? a first case report with video demonstration. J Minim Invasive Gynecol 4650(14):01530–01531. doi:10.1016/j.jmig.2014.11.001

8. Ferrari MM, Mezzopane R, Bulfoni A et al (2003) Surgical treatmentof ovarian dermoid cysts: a comparison between laparoscopicand vaginal removal. Eur J Obstet Gynecol Reprod Biol 109:88–91

9. Hackethal A, Sucke J, Oehmke F et al (2010) Establishing transvaginalNOTES for gynecological and surgical indications: benefits, limits, and patient experience. Endoscopy 42:875–878

10. Peak J, Kim SW, Lee SH et al (2011) Learning curve and surgical outcome for single-port access total laparoscopic hysterectomy in 100 consuctive cases. Gynecol Obstet Investig 72:227–233

11. Phongnarisorn C, Chinthakanan O (2011) Transumbilical single-incision laparoscopic hysterectomy with conventional laparosopic instruments in patients with symptomatic leimyoma and/or adenomysosis. Arch Gynecol Obstet 284:893–900

12. Zornig C, Mofid H, Siemssen L et al (2009) Transvaginal NOTES hybrid cholecystectomy:feasibility results in 68 cases with mid-term follow-up. Endoscopy 41:391–394

13. Lee CL, Wu KY, Su H, Wu PJ, Han CM, Yen CF (2014) Hysterectomy byTransvaginal Natural Orifice Transluminal Endoscopic Surgery (NOTES): a series of 137 patients. JMIG 21(5):818–824

14. Tanaka M, Sagawa T, Yamazaki R, Myojo S, Dohi S, Inoue M (2013) Evaluation of transvaginal peritoneal surgery in young femalepatients. Surg Endosc 27:2619–2624

15. Lee CL, Wu KY, Su H, Ueng SH, Yen CH (2012) Transvaginal Natural-Orifice Transluminal Endoscopic Surgery(NOTES) in Adnexal Procedures. JMIG 19:509–513

16. Perretta S, Vix M, Dallemagne B, Nassif J, Donatelli G, Marescauw J (2012) Repeated transvaginal notes: is it possible? Surg Endosc 26:565

18

Suggested spontaneous resolution of possible paediatric hydrosalpinx: a case report with discussion

Zainab Kazmi[1,2] · Sujata Gupta[2] · Michael Dobson[3]

Abstract Hydrosalpinx is a rare cause of abdominal pain in paediatric patients, though cases are documented in the literature. Its aetiology differs considerably from traditional hydrosalpinx due to ascending sexually transmitted infection. Hydrosalpinx can resent mimicking an acute abdomen or can be asymptomatic. Management of paediatric hydrosalpinx varies but often involves surgical removal of the affected tube. A 12-year-old girl presented with left-sided acute abdominal pain setting within 24 h. Initial ultrasound scan suggested presence of hydrosalpinx. Post-discharge follow-up appointment with a consultant paediatric gynaecologist demonstrated no symptomology, but repeated scan by another sonographer showed continued presence of possible hydrosalpinx, which had since grown. Later, MRI was performed to confirm site of the lesion. However, MRI revealed no tubal masses, suggesting spontaneously resolved hydrosalpinx. Consultant-administered ultrasound scan confirm no tubal abnormalities. Our case suggests spontaneous resolution in possible paediatric hydrosalpinx. Our recommendation is for conservative management of asymptomatic paediatric and adolescent hydrosalpinges, with emergency surgery offered if symptoms indicative of tubal or adnexal torsion.

✉ Zainab Kazmi
  Zainab.Kazmi@student.manchester.ac.uk

[1] University of Manchester School of Medicine, Stopford Building, Oxford Road, Manchester M13 9PT, UK

[2] Women's Health Directorate, Royal Preston Hospital, Sharoe Green Lane North, Preston, Lancashire PR2 9HT, UK

[3] Department of Radiology, Royal Preston Hospital, Sharoe Green Lane North, Preston, Lancashire PR2 9HT, UK

Keywords Paediatric hydrosalpinx · Abdominal tenderness · Gynaecological sonographer

Case report

A 12-year-old nulliparous girl presented to paediatric admissions unit with acute onset abdominal pain centralized to the left iliac fossa over the past 12 h, leading to one episode of sudden collapse. She reported no associated bowel or urinary symptoms. The patient had reached menarche aged 12 and had regular menstrual cycles. She denied any prior sexual activity, and her last menstrual period has occurred 1 week prior. She had no prior surgical or medical history of note. Social and family history was unremarkable.

On examination, abdominal tenderness was noted with no associated guarding or peritonism. Midstream urine and beta-hCG levels were tested and recorded, with normal findings. The patient was admitted for observation. However, the pain resolved within 24 h and no further symptoms were reported following resolution. Admission notes suggested initial working diagnosis was of an ovarian cyst. The patient was discharged and scheduled for a follow-up review and ultrasound scan in 2 weeks.

On the initial follow-up 2 weeks after discharge, an outpatient ultrasound scan was performed by an experienced gynaecological sonographer (Fig. 1). The sonographer reported an elongated fluid-filled structure within the left adnexa adjacent to the uterus measuring 5×1.3 cm 'consistent with hydrosalpinx'. There were no other adnexal pathology noted, and there was no evidence of free fluid.

Due to missed appointments, the next follow-up scan was performed 6.5 months later by a different experienced gynaecological sonographer (Fig. 2). This sonographer reported the presence of an $8.2 \times 3 \times 5.6$ cm fluid-filled

Fig. 1 Initial ultrasound image
(shows pathology)

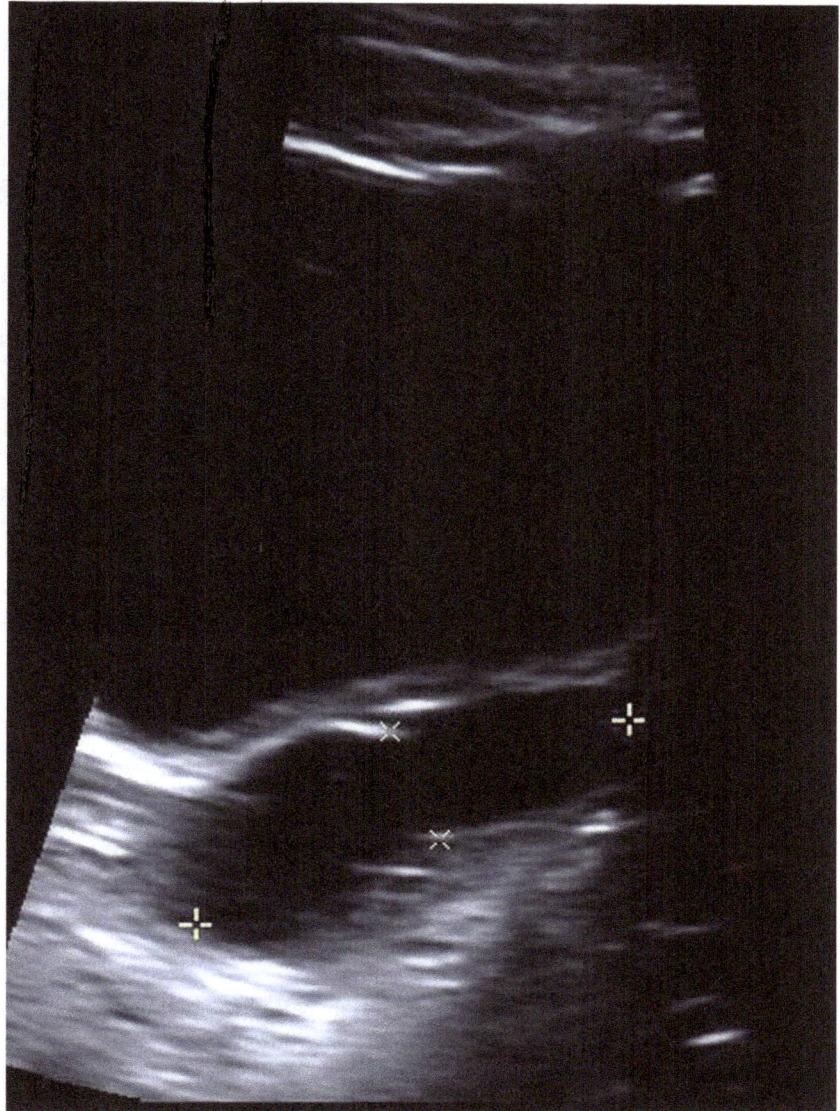

tubular structure in the left adnexa. She remarked also that the ultrasound appearances of an elongated cyst are suggestive of hydrosalpinx. No other adnexal pathology was seen, with no evidence of free fluid in the pelvis.

With the continued presence of what appeared to be a possible hydrosalpinx, a laparoscopy and salpingectomy were scheduled. Prior to the operation, a consultant radiologist-administered MRI of the pelvis was performed with the aim of confirming the site of the hydrosalpinx (Fig. 3). However, this MRI demonstrated no evidence of hydrosalpinx or any pelvic visceral abnormalities.

Due to these new imaging findings, a decision was made to review the patient using the original imaging modality: ultrasound. A pelvic ultrasound, using a trans-abdominal approach and performed by a consultant radiologist, demonstrated no evidence of a pelvic cyst or mass or any free fluid.

As there were no further troubling symptoms and no abnormalities reported on two separate imaging modalities, no treatment was indicated. The patient was reviewed one final time in follow-up clinic. The patient was discharged from gynaecology outpatient follow-up clinic. There has been no recurrence in symptomology reported as of time of writing.

Discussion

Aetiology

Adult hydrosalpinx is traditionally associated with pelvic inflammatory disease due to an ascending sexually transmitted infection such as *Chlamydia trachomatis* [1]. However, the aetiology in paediatrics differs considerably. In paediatric patients, resultant peritubal adhesions from past inflammation or

Fig. 2 Follow-up ultrasound
image (shows pathology)

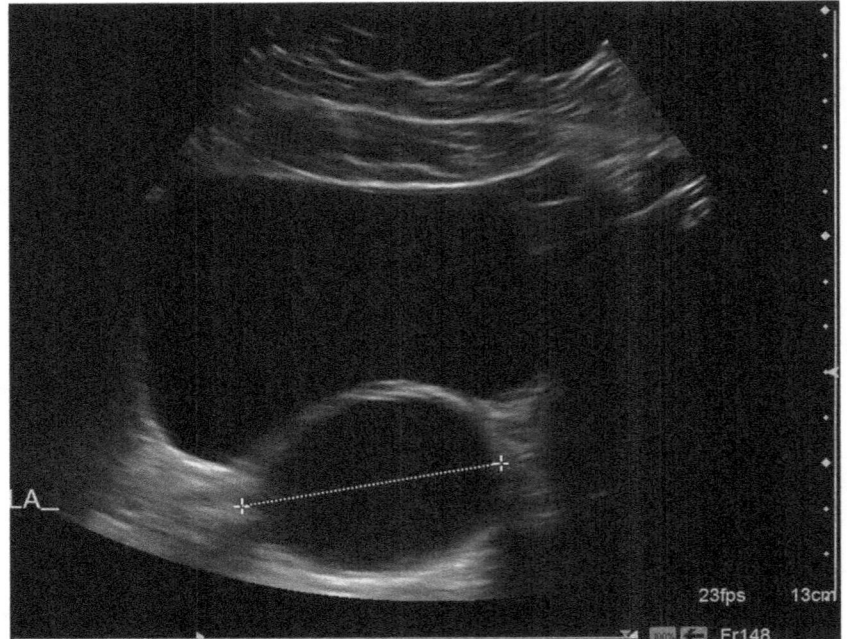

surgery can lead to pelvic venous congestion, which contribute to distal tubal occlusion disclosure [2]. Pelvic venous congestion may be caused by adnexal masses, usually either inflammatory or functional, like the corpus luteum [2]. Neoplastic adnexal masses, however, are very rare in this age range [2]. Overall, the pathogenesis of hydrosalpinx remains poorly defined in children [3]. In this case, there was no positive history for any of the above causes. Furthermore, the patient became and remained asymptomatic after admission.

Without clear pre-existing tubal or ovarian pathology, paediatric hydrosalpinx is likely due to increased fallopian tube mobility on the ligamentum latum [1]. As well, the perimenarcheal (early puberty) phase can be associated with higher follicle-stimulating hormone (FSH) levels due to the stimulated hypothalamic-pituitary-gonadal axis, which leads to new activation and increased mobility of ovarian and tubal function [1, 2]. This can cause a previously asymptomatic hydrosalpinx to become newly symptomatic [1].

New onset symptomology of previously asymptomatic hydrosalpinx can also be due to abnormal tubal peristalsis activity or inherent congenital tubal abnormalities [2]. These anatomical abnormalities include abnormal mesosalpinx length, spiral course of the salpinx and distal occlusion [2].

Fig. 3 MRI image (no
pathology)

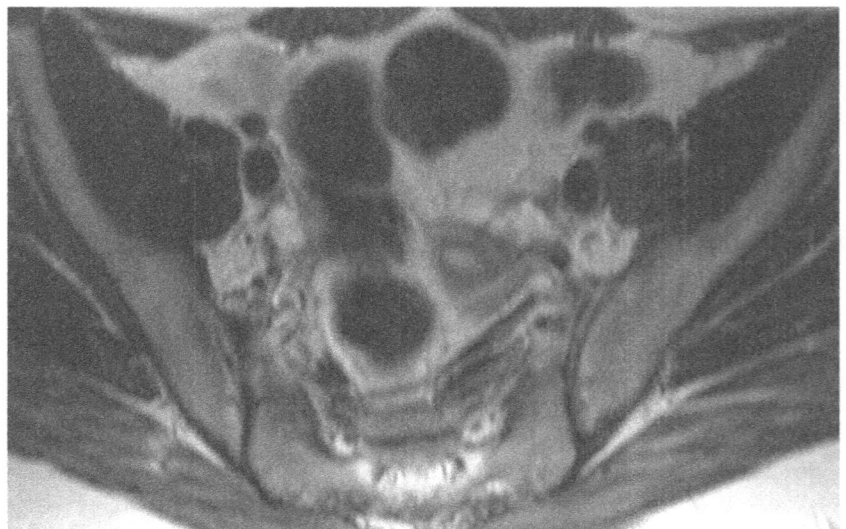

Presentation

Amongst paediatric patients, hydrosalpinx appears to be most common in the perimenarcheal phase [2], possibly due to the factors listed above.

Clinical onset of fallopian tube disease is highly variable. There is often associated pain, but occasionally, no pain may be noted [2]. Where the hydrosalpinx is symptomatic, it is often associated with nonspecific signs of infection [3]. Unfortunately, the nonspecific symptomology can contribute to difficulty making a diagnosis. Moreover, often, ongoing symptomology is only present in cases of continuing infection [4].

Investigations

Imaging is paramount in diagnosing hydrosalpinx. In children with acute or subacute-onset pelvic pain, trans-abdominal ultrasound is the preferred initial imaging modality [5]. Ultrasonography is cost-effective and very safe to use [5]. It can also give instantaneous answers and is useful as an initial imaging modality [6].

Ultrasonography of hydrosalpinx can easily demonstrate dilatation at the ampulla [2] or an elongated cystic pathology in the fallopian tubes [6] that is separated from and leading to the ovary [2]. Colour Doppler ultrasonography can provide evidence of hydrosalpinx by demonstrating increased vascularity and decreased resistance index (RI) when the cause is neoplastic or infective [1].

Magnetic resonance imaging is also useful to differentiate hydrosalpinx from other similar presentations [2, 5]. Fluid contents become apparent on MRI with low T1 and high T2 signals [2]. A different appearance is seen in haematosalpinx and pyosalpinx, based on the density of cystic content [2].

Imaging is also useful in allowing us to determine whether dilatation is acute or chronic. More acute conditions are demonstrated by the 'cogwheel sign', which shows subtle, linear projections protruding into the lumen [2]. Chronic conditions are shown as 'beads on a string', with small mural foci and flattened mucosal folds [2].

Furthermore, we can review potential complications using imaging. On both ultrasonography and MRI, a characteristic whirlpool sign is classically noted where tubal torsion is present [2]. This is critical as the earlier torsion is diagnosed and treated, the much higher the probability that the fallopian tube can be salvaged [1].

However, it is not possible to make a definite diagnosis without diagnostic surgery, thought this is obviously invasive. The benefits of surgical investigation, like laparoscopy, include possibility of simultaneous treatment if an abnormality is detected [6].

Future advances in imaging

There remain some drawbacks of using ultrasonography [7], including the possibility that ultrasonography alone is not always accurate. 3D ultrasound is a promising new imaging modality that avoids the common misdiagnosis of hydrosalpinx that often occurs with 2D sonography [8]. Presently, diagnostic surgery may be the most accurate imaging modality. A retrospective surgical study revealed that, for hydrosalpinx, there is a 100 % association between laparoscopic and final histological findings [9]. However, invasive approaches should be avoided wherever possible. Advances in imaging may pave the way for a more thorough preoperative assessment [10].

Complications

Hydrosalpinx is a known cause of fallopian tubal torsion, which can have an adverse impact on fertility due to possible tubal and ovarian necrosis. Moreover, torsion itself can result in acute abdominal pain, nausea and vomiting. Torsion is three times more frequent on the right tube than left, likely due to the cushioning effect of the sigmoid colon on the left tube [11]. Isolated tubal torsion is rare, with its incidence being reported as one in 1.5 million women [11]. Torsion of a normal tube has been previously reported, though incidence is dramatically higher where there is pre-existing tubal or ovarian pathology [4].

Hydrosalpinx itself can be painful with the enlargement of a mass in the abdomen. This can change with the waxing and waning of hydrosalpinx with reabsorption of hydrosalpinx and subsequent re-accumulation [12].

Management

Fallopian tube pathologies, including both ovarian cysts and hydrosalpinx, indicate surgical intervention when presenting as an acute abdomen [2]. A low threshold is required for surgical intervention as the associated symptomology for torsion is nonspecific [13].

The types of surgeries offered vary. Salpingectomy refers to the surgical removal of a Fallopian tube, and is often preferred over other surgeries where the tube and ovary are preserved, as those operations have a higher risk of future ectopic pregnancies. While salpingectomy is most often indicated for ectopic pregnancies, it is also used to manage tubal damage, as in hydrosalpinx.

Historically, salpingectomies were completed using a laparotomy approach. With technological advances, a laparoscopic approach is increasingly favoured as it avoids the larger laparotomy incision, leading to less post-operative pain and quicker discharge [5].

Bilateral salpingectomy is a cause of female sterility and should be avoided. Hydrosalpinx resection has previously been recommended where there is no functional ipsilateral ovary [5].

Other surgical procedures which may be considered include salpingostomy, salpingopexy and detorsion. Salpingostomy is a tubal corrective surgery and eliminates the need for tubal loss. However, it is also associated with a significantly increased rate of ectopic pregnancy post-operatively [14]. Salpingopexy refers to the fixation of the tube via suturing to the posterior broad ligament of the uterus or to the lateral pelvic wall with the intent of preventing future tubal or adnexal torsion [15]. However, this runs the risk of changing the normal anatomy of the pelvic organs [16]. Detorsion is relevant where the hydrosalpinx has caused the adnexa or the fallopian tube to tort. The untwisting of the tube can reduce the risk of ischaemic damage as it allows the potential for revascularization [17]. Another more conservative measure that may be implemented in the future is the aspiration of the hydrosalpinx, guided by ultrasound, through the abdominal wall [11]. This procedure can avoid an incision altogether.

In paediatrics, all cases requiring surgery must be considered carefully, with the decision to operate being weighed against the use of an invasive management approach in asymptomatic minors. Furthermore, often, paediatric operations can be inherently more challenging, with variable anatomy and aetiologies. The decision to operate in paediatric hydrosalpinx presents its own unique set of challenges. In managing paediatric hydrosalpinx, there is a fine line between under-treatment and over-treatment. In under-treatment, there is a risk of tubal or ovarian torsion, recurrence, tubal pregnancy and infertility [2]. With over-treatment, one runs the risk of subjecting a child to unnecessary surgery [2].

Prognosis

Hydrosalpinx often adversely affects future fertility. The presence of this structure can cause inflammation of the fallopian tubes, and free uterine fluid can impact implantation [18]. The presence of this structure can also block movement of the ovum into the uterine cavity [19].

There are reports of resolution of hydrosalpinx in adult patients in the literature. The findings from this case presentation are quite novel because a spontaneous resolution of this condition in paediatrics has never been clearly reported in the literature. However, in all cases of paediatric hydrosalpinx, a decision to operate is made quickly after presentation and diagnosis. Perhaps, in prior cases, due to the speed in operating, there was insufficient time for a spontaneous resolution.

Recommendations

Given that this case report suggests potential for spontaneous resolution, our proposed management for conservative management is as follows:

(1) Utilize a watch-and-wait approach for asymptomatic hydrosalpinx. Ensure that patients and parents/guardians are educated on the condition and all potential risks.
(2) Routine ultrasound scanning to assess changes in hydrosalpinx size/shape/location.
(3) If the hydrosalpinx is symptomatic and suggestive of possible tubal/ovarian torsion, emergency surgery should be offered, with detorsion or salpingectomy depending on potential for revascularization.

Conclusion

We have presented this case report of a 12-year-old girl with what appears to be spontaneous resolution of possible hydrosalpinx not requiring any medical or surgical management. Paediatric hydrosalpinx is often treated with surgery, particularly salpingectomy, in order to prevent future risk of ovarian torsion and thus to preserve fertility. However, salpingectomy can be associated with reduced fertility as well. We hope to propose a case for a watch-and-wait approach without any intervention for asymptomatic possible hydrosalpinx in order to minimize any unnecessary treatment in a paediatric patient.

Contribution to authorship   ZK was responsible for the project development, data collection, data analysis and manuscript writing. SG was responsible for the project development, data management and manuscript editing. MD was responsible for the data collection and data analysis.

Funding   No funding was provided for this research.

Informed consent   Informed consent was obtained from all individual participants included in the study.

References

1. Pampal A, Atac GK, Nazli ZS, Ozen IO, Sipahi T (2012) A rare cause of acute abdominal pain in adolescence: hydrosalpinx leading to isolated torsion of fallopian tube. J Pediatr Surg 47(12):e31–e34

2. Lucchetti MC, Orazi C, Silveri M, Marchetti P (2014) Fallopian tube diseases as a cause of pelvic pain in perimenarcheal girls: diagnostic tools and treatment pitfalls. 13th European Conference of Paediatric and Adolescent Gynaecology; 17–20 September 2014. British Society of Paediatric and Adolescent Gynaecology, London

3. Zhapa E, Rigamonti W, Castagnetti M (2010) Hydrosalpinx in a patient with complex genitourinary malformation. J Pediatr Surg 45(11):2265–2268

4. Ullal A, Kollipara PJ (1999) Torsion of a hydrosalpinx in an 18-year-old virgin. J Obstet Gynaecol 19(3):331

5. Monga J, Dwarakanath L, Chandran H (2007) Laparoscopic salpingectomy for hydrosalpinx in adolescent females—a report of two cases. Gynecol Surg 4(4):309–311

6. Ben-Rafael Z, editor. Hydrosalpinx in paediatric age—case report. 17th World Congress on Controversies in Obstetrics, Gynecology & Infertility (COGI); November 8–11, 2012; Lisbon, Portugal: Monduzzi Editoriale; 2013

7. Mesogitis S (2004) Ultrasound-guided procedures for the treatment of benign ovarian cysts. Ultrasound Rev Obstet Gynecol 4(4):257

8. Baba K (2011) Fetal and gynecological 3D ultrasound in daily practice. Donald Sch J Ultrasound Obstet Gynecol 5(1):1–6

9. Liberis V, Tsikouras P, Zografos C, Ammari A, Dislian V, Iatrou C et al (2009) The contribution of laparoscopy to the diagnosis of adnexal masses in young and premenopausal women. Eur J Gynaecol Oncol 30(4):402–407

10. Adnexal masses: characterization and imaging strategies. Seminars in Ultrasound, CT and MRI: Elsevier; 2010.

11. Dadhwal V, Gupta N, Gupta B, Deka D, Mittal S (2009) Laparoscopic management of isolated fallopian tube torsion in a premenarchal 13-year-old adolescent girl. Arch Gynecol Obstet 279(6):909–910

12. Garrett LA, Vargas SO, Drapkin R, Laufer MR (2008) Does the fimbria have an embryologic origin distinct from that of the rest of the fallopian tube. Fertil Steril 90(5)

13. Dunnihoo DR, Wolff J (1984) Bilateral torsion of the adnexa: a case report and a review of the world literature. Obstet Gynecol 64(3): 55S–59S

14. Taylor RC, Berkowitz J, McComb PF (2001) Role of laparoscopic salpingostomy in the treatment of hydrosalpinx. Fertil Steril 75(3): 594–600

15. Verlaenen H, Camus M, Amy J, Devroey P (1995) Laparoscopic treatment of adnexal torsion: a report of three cases and a review of the literature. J Gynecol Surg 11(4): 251–255

16. Visnjic S, Kralj R, Zupancic B (2014) Isolated fallopian tube torsion with partial hydrosalpinx in a premenarcheal girl: a case report. J Med Case Rep 8:197

17. Barisic D, Bagovic D (1999) Bilateral tubal torsion treated by laparoscopy: a case report. Eur J Obstet Gynecol Reprod Biol 86(1): 99–100

18. Strandell A (2012) Management of hydrosalpinx. Textbook of assisted reproductive techniques fourth edition: volume 2: clinical. Perspectives 2:308

19. Boukaidi SA, Delotte J, Steyaert H, Valla JS, Sattonet C, Bouaziz J et al (2011) Thirteen cases of isolated tubal torsions associated with hydrosalpinx in children and adolescents, proposal for conservative management: retrospective review and literature survey. J Pediatr Surg 46(7):1425–1431

19

Long-term clinical outcomes of repeat hysteroscopic endometrial ablation after failed hysteroscopic endometrial ablation

Grace W. Yeung[1] · George A. Vilos[1,4] · Angelos G. Vilos[1] · Ayman Oraif[1,2] · Hanin Abduljabar[1] · Basim Abu-Rafea[3]

Abstract The study aims to describe patient characteristics, uterine cavity shape and histopathology, complications, and long-term clinical outcomes of women who failed hysteroscopic rollerball or loop endometrial ablation (HEA) and subsequently consented to repeat hysteroscopic endometrial ablation (RHEA), and is a retrospective cohort study (Canadian Task Force classification II-2). The study was conducted in the university-affiliated teaching hospital. Patients included women who failed primary hysteroscopic endometrial ablation (PHEA, $n=183$) and subsequently underwent RHEA by the senior author (GAV) from 1993 through 2007 with a minimum follow-up of 5 years. RHEA was performed under general anesthesia using 26 F (~9 mm) resectoscope, monopolar loop electrode in 136 (74.3 %), 3–5 mm rollerball in 41 (22.4 %) or combination in 6 (3.3 %) women. Patient characteristics, uterine cavity, and clinical outcomes of women who failed PHEA and subsequently consented to RHEA were evaluated by retrospective chart review and patient follow-up including office visits and/or telephone interview. The corresponding median age (range) for PHEA and RHEA was 40 (26–70) and 43 (29–76) years. Indications for PHEA included abnormal uterine bleeding (AUB, 52.7 %), AUB and dysmenorrhea (25.8 %), dysmenorrhea (18.8 %), and others (2.7 %). Indications for RHEA included persistent AUB (53 %), AUB and uterine/pelvic pain (26.2 %), uterine/pelvic pain only (19.1 %), postmenopausal bleeding (1.1 %), and thickened endometrium (0.5 %). Complications of RHEA ($n=7$, 3.8 %) included false passage (3), uterine perforation (2), and bleeding (2). One patient with excessive bleeding required immediate hysterectomy. At a median follow-up of 9 years (5–19), 69 % of women avoided hysterectomy. Repeat hysteroscopic endometrial ablation is a feasible, safe, and long-term effective alternative to hysterectomy for abnormal uterine bleeding from benign causes when performed by experienced surgeons.

Keywords Abnormal uterine bleeding · Heavy menstrual bleeding · Menorrhagia · Hysteroscopic endometrial ablation · Repeat endometrial ablation

✉ George A. Vilos
george.vilos@lhsc.on.ca

[1] Division of Reproductive Endocrinology and Infertility, Department of Obstetrics and Gynecology, Western University, London, Ontario, Canada

[2] King Abdul Aziz University, Jeddah, Saudi Arabia

[3] Dalhousie University, Halifax, Nova Scotia, Canada

[4] The Fertility Clinic, Room E-3620A, London Health Science Centre, 800 Commissioners Road East, London, ON N6A 4G5, Canada

Introduction

First-generation endometrial ablation techniques performed by hysteroscopic endometrial ablation (HEA) were introduced in the 1980s as an alternative to hysterectomy to treat women with abnormal uterine bleeding (AUB) from benign causes. These included endometrial laser ablation and radiofrequency rollerball/bar or transcervical resection of the endometrium (TCRE) [1, 2]. Second-generation endometrial ablation technologies, also referred to as global endometrial ablation (GEA) or nonhysteroscopic endometrial ablation, were introduced in the 1990s as "automated," easier, and safer alternatives to hysteroscopic endometrial ablation requiring less skill and could be performed in the office [3, 4].

Following endometrial ablation by any technique and technology, including hysteroscopic endometrial ablation (HEA), long-term outcomes (within 10 years) indicate that 15 to 30 %

of women require additional surgery such as hysterectomy for persistent AUB, uterine/pelvic pain, or both [5–7]. The subsequent 30 % hysterectomy rate after endometrial ablation together with a high satisfaction rate of women who chose hysterectomy as primary treatment of their AUB [7] has raised some serious issues, questions, and concerns regarding the cost-effectiveness, ongoing utilization, and indeed the future of both hysteroscopic and nonhysteroscopic endometrial ablation for the treatment of AUB.

Consequently, many gynecologists resort to hysterectomy for both as primary treatment of AUB and as the next logical step in women who fail primary endometrial ablation. However, in spite of major technological advances in minimally invasive gynecological surgery, hysterectomy remains a major surgical procedure associated with significant morbidity, mortality, and health care costs and resources [7–11].

To minimize the post-ablation hysterectomy rate, a few gynecological surgeons have reported their experience with repeat hysteroscopic endometrial ablation (RHEA) using the resectoscope with [12] or without concomitant utilization of ultrasonic guidance [13–16]. Based on these reports, RHEA appears to be more challenging to perform and may be associated with a higher complication rate [16].

For the above reasons, in our center, we have developed a relatively easy and safe technique and we routinely offer RHEA as an alternative to hysterectomy when primary HEA [17] and non-HEA [18] fail and patients continue to complain of persistent AUB, uterine/pelvic pain, or both.

In the present study, we describe our technique and experience, as well as patient characteristics, indications, and long-term outcomes in women who failed hysteroscopic rollerball or loop endometrial ablation and subsequently consented to RHEA.

Materials and methods

From 1990 through December of 2007, the senior author (GAV) performed 3768 primary HEA using 3–5-mm rollerball electrodes, 8-mm cutting loop electrodes, or a combination of the two to treat women with AUB. In addition, 183 women who had failed primary HEA underwent RHEA by the same surgeon from January 1991 through December 2007. We are aware that some of our patients who failed primary HEA received various treatments, including repeat ablation and/or hysterectomy, by other gynecologists in the area. Therefore, 183 of 3768 cases represent a minimal rate of approximately 5 % repeat ablations among our initial population.

All women who presented with persistent AUB and/or uterine/pelvic pain after primary HEA had complete assessment including pelvic examination and imaging using abdominal and transvaginal ultrasound and/or MRI when indicated.

Endometrial biopsy was attempted in all women with uterine bleeding but, in the majority of cases, we were unable to access the uterine cavity or obtain an adequate/satisfactory sample in the clinic. For this reason, women with postmenopausal bleeding were also included if the endometrial cavity and endometrium could not be assessed in the office. Consequently, we performed endometrial resection in the majority of cases or D&C and we always obtained an endometrial sample in the operating room during RHEA.

Patients were offered several treatment options including medical therapy in the presence of adequate and normal endometrial histopathology especially if they were nearing menopause, RHEA, or hysterectomy. When RHEA was chosen, patients were counseled appropriately and informed consent was obtained. None of the patients undergoing RHEA was pretreated to thin the endometrium.

After general anesthesia, with the patient in appropriate stirrups and horizontal dorsolithotomy position, a bimanual pelvic examination was performed to assess the size, shape, mobility, and, most importantly, the position of the uterus. None of the RHEA was performed under ultrasonic or laparoscopic guidance although 30 (17 %) women underwent concomitant laparoscopy for a variety of additional indications including pelvic pain and/or pelvic mass.

Technique of repeat hysteroscopic endometrial ablation
Following bimanual pelvic examination, the anterior lip of the cervix was grasped with a double-toothed tenaculum and the cervical canal was gradually dilated up to the level of the internal os (approximately 4 cm) using Hagar dilators. Occasionally, a single-toothed tenaculum was applied to the posterior lip of the cervix to redistribute the tension between the anterior and posterior lip of the cervix to minimize the risk of cervical tears and maintain the cervical canal straight. If resistance was encountered with any of the dilators, a 5-mm hysteroscope was used to visualize the cervical canal and internal os. Bearing in mind the length and direction of the cervical canal and the position of the uterus, the cervical canal was subsequently dilated to 10 mm.

The resectoscope was introduced, and the endocervical canal was superficially resected to facilitate inflow and outflow of the distending/irrigant solution and visualize better the utero-isthmic junction and any residual uterine cavity. Up to the year 2000, if a uterine cavity was present, we used mostly a 3-mm rollerball electrode to ablate any visible endometrium and or endometrial pockets. In the absence of a recognizable uterine cavity or in the presence of narrow distorted cavities, the endometrial/endouterine cavity was resected taking small cuts with the loop electrode by alternating sides following any residual endometrial canal until the entire cavity was recreated and all visible endometrial remnants were resected (Fig. 1).

After we analyzed the results of using rollerball ablation versus loop resection for RHEA, we noticed that the rate of

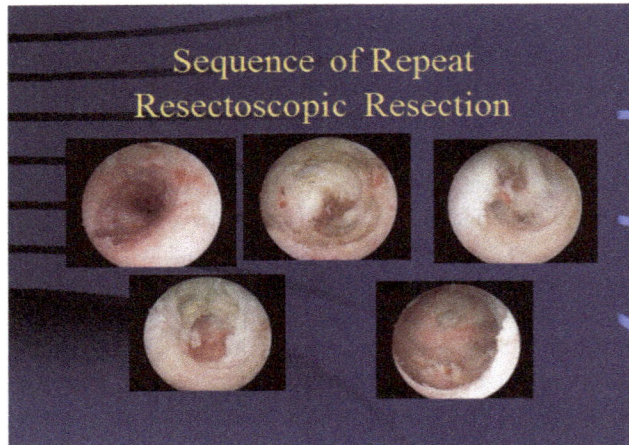

Fig. 1 Clockwise sequence of repeat hysteroscopic endometrial resection with the loop electrode

failed RHEA that underwent hysterectomy was 36.6 % for rollerball compared with 23.2 % for resection. In addition, we found that it was easier and safer to resect rather than rollerball the residual endometrial cavity. For this reason, around the year 2000, we started doing more RHEA using resection with the loop electrode rather than ablate with the rollerball (Fig. 2).

In the majority of RHEA, the uterus was distended using 1.5 % glycine solution via an automated fluid management system (Endomat; Karl Storz GmbH & Co., Tuttlingen, Germany) set at an infusion rate of 300 mL/min, pump pressure of 80 mmHg, and suction at 0.2 bar. Prior to the availability of this system, from the year 1990 to 2000, a gravity system was used, at 100 cmH_2O (~75 mmHg) infusion pressure with 80–100 mmHg wall suction, to evacuate smoke bubbles, clots, and debris from the uterus. We used a 26 F (9 mm diameter) monopolar resectoscope (Karl Storz GmbH & Co., Tuttlingen, Germany) with an 8-mm monopolar loop electrode at 120 W

of low voltage continuous (cut) waveform in 136 women (74.3 %), rollerball with high voltage interrupted (coag) waveform in 41 women (22.4 %), and a combination of the two in 6 women (3.3 %). Rollerball ablation was allowed if an endometrial cavity was reasonably well preserved. Time required to perform a RHEA is not different than that of primary HEA; approximately 15 min.

After the university ethics board approval (HSRB 13849E), we retrospectively identified and reviewed the medical records of these women and follow-up was conducted through office visits and/or telephone interviews. Exclusion criteria included patients who did not have a minimum follow-up of 5 years since their RHEA or did not wish to participate in the study.

Data collected included patient characteristics such as age, body mass index (BMI), parity, and obstetrical history (i.e., cesarean section, vaginal deliveries) at the time of primary HEA, type of primary ablation (i.e., rollerball, resection, or both) and indications for primary and RHEA. In addition, we recorded uterine cavity findings and appearance, laparoscopic findings and procedures performed at time of RHEA for women who underwent concomitant laparoscopy, and any complications encountered during all procedures.

Follow-up data included outcome of RHEA (i.e., requirement for additional treatment such as any medical therapy, third repeat ablation, or hysterectomy), patient satisfaction, and avoidance of hysterectomy. In those women who required no further treatment after RHEA, their menstrual blood loss was classified as amenorrhea, spotting, hypomenorrhea, and persistent AUB, taking into account their age and menopausal status.

Medical records were reviewed, and telephone interviews were conducted to determine if hysterectomy was performed by a different surgeon than the surgeon who performed the RHEA. If hysterectomy was performed, efforts were made to collect data including date, indication, and histopathology of the hysterectomy specimen.

Fig. 2 Type of repeat hysteroscopic endometrial ablation versus calendar year

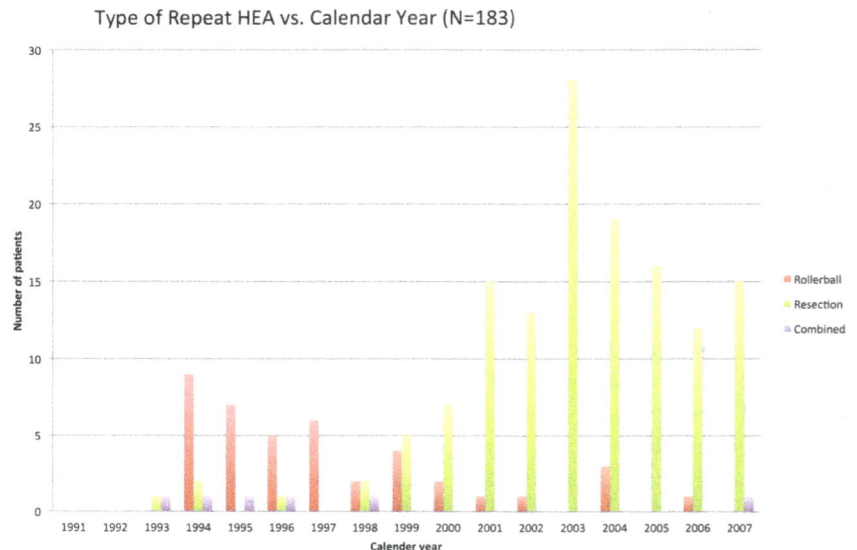

Type of Repeat HEA vs. Calendar Year (N=183)

Data were analyzed using SAS software (SAS Institute, Inc., Cary, NC). The median and range are used to describe non-normal data, and the mean (SD) and 95 % confidence interval are used to describe normal distribution variables. A p value <0.05 was considered statistically significant.

Results

An algorithmic summary of the 183 women who underwent repeat HEA is provided in Fig. 3. Twenty-five (13.6 %) women were lost to follow-up. Of the remaining 158 (86.3 %) women with a median follow-up of 9 years (range 5–19), 102 (64.6 %) required no further treatment. Two women (1.3 %) were deceased from etiologies unrelated to RHEA, one from cervical cancer and the other from disseminated breast cancer.

The patient with cervical cancer had RHEA 6 months after HEA. Following 5 years of amenorrhea, she developed irregular vaginal bleeding and cervical biopsy indicated invasive squamous cell carcinoma, moderately differentiated (stage II b). She died of her disease 1 year after radical surgery.

The patient with breast cancer had RHEA 2 years after HEA. Ten years later, she was diagnosed with breast cancer and died of her disease 6 years after therapy.

Fifty-six women (35.4 %) required further treatment including hysterectomy (n=49, 31.0 %), third HEA (n=3, 1.9 %), or short-term medical therapy (n=4, 2.5 %).

The interval from primary to repeat HEA is shown in Fig. 4 indicating that the majority (72.1 %) of RHEA were performed within the first 3 years of the primary HEA.

The demographics and characteristics of the women who received RHEA including body mass index (BMI), parity, and mode of delivery are shown in Table 1 while the indications for both are shown in Table 2. Persistent bleeding was the most common indication for both primary and RHEA.

Uterine cavity appearance and findings at RHEA The cavity appearance was described as contracted (n=56, 35.4 %), containing endometrial pockets (n=25, 15.8 %), and septum-like

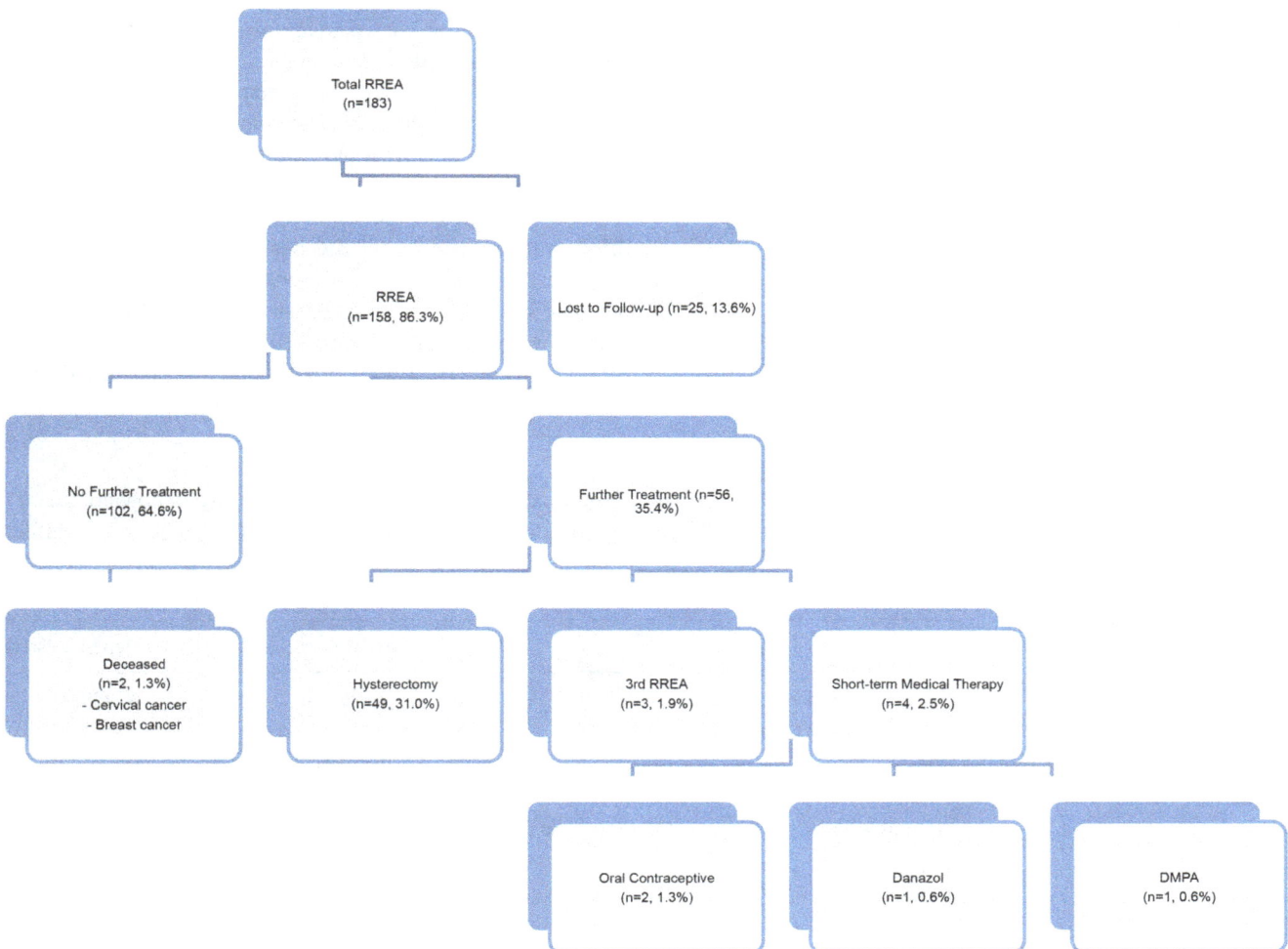

Fig. 3 Algorithmic summary of all patients who had repeat hysteroscopic endometrial ablation (HEA)

Fig. 4 Interval in years to repeat
hysteroscopic endometrial
ablation

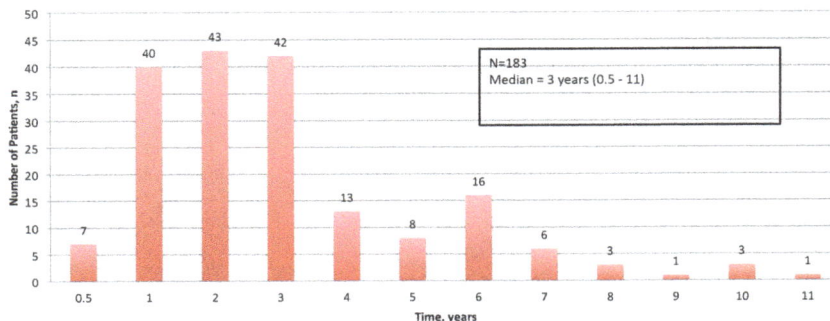

(n=4, 2.5 %). The cavity was described as normal in six cases
(3.8 %) and absent in seven cases (4.4 %). The cavity was not
described in 60 cases (38.0 %). Findings included leiomyoma
(n=17, 10.7 %), hematometra (n=14, 8.9 %), and polyp (n=1,
0.6 %). No specific lesions were described in 126 cases (80.0 %).

From 1991 through 1999, repeat HEA (n=49) was performed by rollerball (n=33, 67.3 %), resection (n=11,
22.4 %), and combined (n=5, 10.2 %). From the year 2000
and thereafter, RHEA (n=134) was performed by resection
(n=125, 93.3 %), rollerball (n=8, 6.0 %), or combination of
the two (n=1, 0.7 %) (Fig. 2).

Findings and procedures at concomitant laparoscopy At
RHEA, 30 women had concomitant laparoscopy for pain and/
or pelvic mass. Laparoscopic findings included endometriosis
in 24, adhesions in 10, and hematosalpinx in 3 women. Laparoscopic procedures included excision of endometriosis and
adhesiolysis, and bilateral salpingectomy in 15, salpingo-
oophorectomy in 6, and appendectomy in 1 woman. Of these
30 women, 13 (43.3 %) underwent hysterectomy at a later
date for pain (n=9), pain and bleeding (n=3), and
hematometra (n=1). Hysterectomy was performed vaginally
in 6, LAVH in 3, and abdominally in 4 women.

Perioperative complications of RHEA Among the 183
RHEA, complications were encountered in 7 women
(3.8 %) including uterine perforation (n=2), creation of false
passage (n=3), and excessive bleeding (n=2).

Uterine perforation with the resectoscope was encountered in two cases. One case resulted in incomplete resection
and laparoscopy identified no intra-abdominal injury. This
patient subsequently underwent vaginal hysterectomy for
pain. Histopathology of the uterine specimen identified
leiomyoma. The second case of uterine perforation did have
a complete endometrial resection; however, the patient
underwent abdominal hysterectomy in a peripheral hospital
within a week of the RHEA for infection. There was no
intra-abdominal injury noted. Histopathology of the uterine
specimen was not available.

Sub-endometrial false passage was created in three cases
all of which had complete resections. One patient was lost to
follow-up while the other two subsequently had vaginal hysterectomy and abdominal hysterectomy for pain. Histopathology demonstrated normal tissue in the first and adenomyosis
in the second case.

Two cases of RHEA resulted in excessive intraoperative
bleeding. In one case, the bleeding was resolved by
tamponade with a Foley catheter balloon. The second case
resulted in emergency vaginal hysterectomy and adenomyosis
and leiomyoma were found on histopathology.

Incomplete RHEA was performed in one patient who was
morbidly obese and was lost to follow-up.

Outcomes after RHEA Of the 158 women who were followed for a minimum of 5 years, 102 (64.6 %) required no further
treatment while 49 (31.0 %) had hysterectomy, 3 (1.9 %)

Table 1 Demographics and type
of endometrial ablation of 183
women who underwent RHEA
(%)

		Primary ablation	Repeat ablation
Age (years), median (range)		40 (26–70)	43 (29–76)
Body mass index (kg/m^2), median (range)		25.1 (17.7–61.2)	
Parity	Nulliparous	19 (10.4)	
	Parous	164 (89.6)	
Mode of delivery	Cesarean section	34 (18.6)	
	Vaginal delivery	130 (71.0)	
Type of ablation	Rollerball	87 (47.5)	41 (22.4)
	Resection	62 (33.9)	136 (74.3)
	Combined	34 (18.6)	6 (3.3)

Table 2 Indications for primary and repeat hysteroscopic endometrial ablation (N=183)

Indication	Primary	Repeat
AUB (1 with simple hyperplasia)	159 (86.9 %)	97 (53.0 %)
AUB+dysmenorrhea/pain	19 (10.4 %)	48 (26.2 %)
Dysmenorrhea/pain	2 (1.1 %)	35 (19.1 %)
PMB (undiagnosed)	3 (1.6 %)	2 (1.1 %)
Thickened endometrium	-	1 (0.5 %)
Total	183 (100 %)	183 (100 %)

underwent third HEA, and 4 (2.5 %) were administered short-term medical therapy including oral contraceptives (n=2, 1.3 %), danazol (n=1, 0.6 %, Sanofi-Aventis Canada Inc., Laval, QC, Canada), and depo-medroxyprogesterone acetate (DMPA, n=1, 0.6 %) (Fig. 3).

Indications for hysterectomy The most common indication for hysterectomy after RHEA was pelvic pain (n=22, 44.9 %) followed by pelvic pain and bleeding (n=17, 34.7 %), and bleeding alone (n=4, 8.2 %). Six women (12.2 %) had hysterectomy with or without salpingo-oophorectomy for other indications including uterine prolapse (n=1, 2.0 %), leiomyoma (n=3, 6.1 %), breast cancer (n=1, 2.0 %), and uterine perforation and sepsis (n=1, 2.0 %).

Type of hysterectomy The most common type of hysterectomy performed was vaginal (n=24, 49 %), followed by total abdominal (n=18, 36.7 %) and laparoscopic-assisted vaginal hysterectomy (LAVH, n=6, 12.2 %). One (2.0 %) hysterectomy was not performed by the senior author (GAV), and thus, the type of hysterectomy and histopathology was unknown as hospital records were not accessible.

Histopathology of hysterectomy specimens The most common histopathology of hysterectomy specimens after RHEA was adenomyosis (n=18, 37.0 %) followed by no specific pathology (n=14, 28.6 %), and leiomyoma (n=12, 24.5 %). Two specimens (4.1 %) included endometriosis and one specimen included simple endometrial hyperplasia without atypia (2.0 %). Four (8.2 %) histopathology results are unknown.

Discussion

Review of the available literature on long-term clinical outcomes of endometrial ablation for the treatment of AUB raises several observations, questions, and concerns.

One observation is that both HEA and non-HEA, by any technique or technology, appear to be of diminishing effectiveness with time [5–7]. As presented in the "Introduction," it is becoming more evident that within the first 10 years of endometrial ablation, up to 30 % of women end up with a hysterectomy for a variety of reasons mostly related to the original problem of AUB and/or pain.

Since the median age of women undergoing endometrial ablation is in their early 40s and 30 % of them require hysterectomy within the next 10 years to resolve their original problem of AUB/dysmenorrhea, it stands to reason that at least an additional 10 % of women will require hysterectomy for other indications including uterine neoplasia, pain, prolapse, etc., during their lifetime. If one accepts this reasoning with a hysterectomy rate exceeding 30 % after endometrial ablation, then endometrial ablation may no longer be cost-effective [19]..

For these reasons, if one is to preserve endometrial ablation in everyday clinical practice, strategies must be developed to improve its feasibility and increase its safety and long-term efficacy.

One strategy to maintain utilization of endometrial ablation and minimize hysterectomy may be a wider utilization of repeat endometrial ablation. As stated in the "Introduction," several authors have reported their experience with RHEA after failed HEA [12–16] and non-HEA [18, 20]. However, since the literature on repeat ablations is very scanty, it is reasonable to assume that this is not a very appealing and widely practiced option. This lack of appeal may be related to a number of reasons including the lack of surgical experience and expertise, increased complications, the absence of evidence-based long-term efficacy, and the ease of solving the problem definitively with a simple hysterectomy.

As stated above, from 1991 through 1999, RHEA in our center was performed mostly by rollerball (67 %) while from around the year 2000 to the present, RHEA is performed mostly by resection (93 %). We have found that the use of the loop electrode under direct vision is safer and more efficacious than the rollerball as shown by reduced rates of complications and hysterectomy in the present study and that of Istre and Langebrekke [14] using a similar technique to ours. On the other hand, Wortman and Daggett [12, 20] advocate the use of concomitant ultrasonic guidance during RHEA. This additional feature however, although conferring an element of safety, requires additional utilization of ultrasound equipment and personnel in the operating room.

We have previously reported higher complications associated with RHEA (OR 4.01, 95 % CI 1.63–9.87) than primary HEA. However, those numbers may reflect lack of experience at that time and the different technique we used prior to the year 2000. In our previous study, the overall complication rate for RHEA was 9.30 % (7 cases out of 75) versus 2.05 % (20 cases out of 800) for RHEA (p=0.006) [16].

In the present study, the overall complication rate with RHEA was 3.8 %. The present complications are similar to those reported by others, with one study reporting two uterine and one cervical perforations (4.5 %). The three women with perforation were operated by less-experienced endoscopic surgeons [15]. The three other studies reported no complications [12–14]. This indicates that RHEA may be a relatively safe procedure when performed by experienced surgeons.

Although RHEA has been reported to be feasible and relatively safe, feasibility is not an indication unless it is shown to be effective. In our study, following RHEA, 69 % of women avoided hysterectomy including 17/158 (10.8 %) women who had undergone concomitant laparoscopy This rate is within the range of 54 to 100 % within 5 years of follow-up reported by others [12–15]. Whether this rate is significant enough to justify repeat ablation as an alternative to hysterectomy or bypass it all together and go directly to a vaginal or laparoscopic hysterectomy cannot be answered at this time.

In the present study, indications for repeat ablation were persistent AUB (53 %), uterine/pelvic pain (19 %), or both AUB and pain (26 %) while the most common indication for hysterectomy after RHEA was pelvic pain (45 %) followed by pelvic pain and bleeding (35 %). Similar results have been reported by others reporting 33 (28 %) of RHEA receiving hysterectomy for pain (48 %), persistent bleeding (27 %), and pain and bleeding (10 %) [14]. It is of interest to note that all authors report that hysterectomy was performed at a median of approximately 3 years after RHEA [12, 14, 15].

Pelvic pain after endometrial ablation has been attributed to several conditions including adenomyosis, hematometra, post-ablation tubal sterilization syndrome (PATSS), endometriosis, and others [21–23]. Indeed, in our study, the most common histopathology of hysterectomy specimens after RHEA was adenomyosis (37 %). Adenomyosis in hysterectomy specimen was reported from 58 to 61 % in three other studies [12, 14, 15].

The low rate of hematometra ($n=14$, 8.9 %) and PATSS ($n=3$) may be related to our technique of meticulous electrocoagulation or complete resection of the tubal cornua as described previously [24]. Sterilization by tubal occlusion has been identified as a predictor of pain after endometrial ablation [23, 25, 26]. It is thought that some of these patients experience pain caused by medial tubal accumulation of blood originating from residual cornual endometrium [23].

In our study, 79 % of women reported amenorrhea, 8 % spotting, and 15 % hypomenorrhea. Of these, 96 % were satisfied and 99 % felt that it was worthwhile to have undergone RHEA. Gimpleson and Kaigh reported that RHEA resulted in amenorrhea in 10 women (63 %), staining in 3 (19 %), and light flow in 3 (19 %) [13], while Wortman and Daggett reported that 88.5 % achieved satisfactory results and avoided hysterectomy [12].

We did not use any pretreatment to thin the endometrium prior to RHEA believing that identification of residual endometrium may be more difficult. In fact, Hansen et al. reported that pretreatment increased the risk of subsequent hysterectomy (81 vs 30 %, $p>0.01$) possibly due to difficulties in identifying endometrial mucosa, in these scarred and distorted uterine cavities, when pretreatment is used [15].

Additional strategies to increase efficacy of primary endometrial ablation have included better patient [27] selection and/or endometrial ablation technology [28]. However, the long-term clinical outcomes (up to 10 years) are similar among all endometrial ablation technologies [6] and no significant differences in effectiveness or safety have been found between first- and second-generation endometrial ablation techniques [29, 30].

A final strategy may be to combine endometrial ablation with adjunct therapy.

Indeed, preliminary studies indicate that the combination of both HEA and non-HEA with DMPA [31, 32] or the levonorgestrel intrauterine system (LNG-IUS) [33–36] significantly improve short-term clinical outcomes in women with AUB as determined by amenorrhea, satisfaction, and reintervention rates.

This study is of clinical significance since it highlights several issues including feasibility, safety, and long-term effectiveness of repeat endometrial ablation. Strengths of the study include the largest number of patients treated by both primary and RHEA and the longest follow-up reported to date while weaknesses include the retrospective nature and reflection of only one surgeon's experience.

In summary, we have shown that RHEA is a feasible, relatively safe, and a long-term effective alternative to hysterectomy for AUB from benign causes when performed by experienced surgeons. However, two observations must be pointed out regarding RHEA.

The first observation is that all authors have reported on using the resectoscope to perform repeat ablations rather than any of the nonhysteroscopic technologies. This, together with the fact that the majority of endometrial cavities after primary ablation by all methods is significantly distorted [37, 38], indicates that repeat ablation may not be feasible and possibly dangerous, when attempted/performed by any technique other than the hysteroscopic approach.

The second observation is that RHEA has been reported mostly by some of the pioneers and expert surgeons on the use of resectoscopic surgery including HEA [12–16]. However, since presently, HEA has been mostly substituted by non-HEA techniques [39, 40], the art of HEA may be on its way to extinction. Consequently, the more technically difficult and skill-demanding RHEA will remain in the domain of a handful of surgeons and not an option provided by the majority of gynecologists.

Precis Repeat hysteroscopic endometrial ablation is a feasible, safe, and long-term effective alternative to hysterectomy for benign abnormal uterine bleeding when performed by experienced surgeons.

References

1. Papadopoulos NP, Magos A (2007) First-generation endometrial ablation: roller-ball vs loop vs laser. Best Pract Res Clin Obstet Gynaecol 21:915–929
2. (2007) ACOG Practice Bulletin No. 81, May 2007: endometrial ablation. Obstet Gynecol 109(5):1233-48
3. Garry R, for the Endometrial Ablation Group (2002) Evidence and techniques in endometrial ablation: consensus. 2002. Gynecol Endosc 11(1):5–17
4. Madhu CK, Nattey J, Naeem T (2009) Second generation endometrial ablation techniques: an audit of clinical practice. Arch Gynecol Obstet 280:599–602
5. Munro MG (2006) Endometrial ablation. Where have we been? Where are we going? Clin Obstet Gynecol 49(4):736–766
6. Longinotti MK, Jacobson GF, Hung YY, Learman LA (2008) Probability of hysterectomy after endometrial ablation. Obstet Gynecol 112(6):1214–1220
7. Bhattacharya S, Middleton LJ, Tsourapas A et al (2011) Hysterectomy, endometrial ablation and Mirena® for heavy menstrual bleeding: a systematic review of clinical effectiveness and cost-effectiveness analysis. Health Technol Assess 15(19):iii–xvi, **1-252**
8. Wright JD, Devine P, Shah M et al (2010) Morbidity and mortality of peripartum hysterectomy. Obstet Gynecol 115:1187–1193
9. Boyd LR, Novesky AP, Curtin JP (2010) Effect of surgical volume on route of hysterectomy and short-term morbidity. Obstet Gynecol 116:909–915
10. Roberts TE, Tsourapas A, Middleton LJ et al (2011) Hysterectomy, endometrial ablation, and levonorgestrel releasing intrauterine system (Mirena) for treatment of heavy menstrual bleeding: cost effectiveness analysis. BMJ 342:d2202. doi:10.1136/bmj.d2202
11. Clark-Pearson DL, Geller EL (2013) Complications of hysterectomy. Clin Exp Ser Obstet Gynecol 121:654–673
12. Wortman M, Daggett A (2001) Reoperative hysteroscopic surgery in the management of patients who fail endometrial ablation and resection. J Am Assoc Gynecol Laparosc 8(2):272–277
13. Gimpelson RJ, Kaigh J (1992) Endometrial ablation repeat procedures. Case studies. J Reprod Med 37(7):629–635
14. Istre O, Langebrekke A (2003) Repeat hysteroscopic surgery reduces the hysterectomy rate after endometrial and myoma resection. J Am Assoc Gynecol Laparosc 10(2):247–251
15. Hansen BB, Dreisler E, Stampe SS (2008) Outcome of repeated hysteroscopic resection of the endometrium. J Minim Invasive Gynecol 15(6):704–706
16. MacLean-Fraser E, Penava D, Vilos GA (2002) Perioperative complication rates of primary and repeat hysteroscopic endometrial ablations. J Am Assoc Gynecol Laparosc 9(2):175–177
17. Yeung GW, Vilos GA, Garcia-Erdeljan M, Marks JL, Vilos AG, Abu-Rafea B (2012) Repeat resectoscopic endometrial resection after failed primary resectoscopic ablation: Is it worth the risk? J Minim Invasive Gynecol 19(6):S22
18. Garcia-Erdeljan M, Vilos GA (2012) Repeat hysteroscopic endometrial resection after failed thermal balloon endometrial ablation: is it worth the risk? J Minim Invasive Gynecol 17:S25
19. Laberge P, Leyland N, Murji A, Fortin C, Martyn P, Vilos GA (2015) Endometrial ablation in the management of abnormal uterine bleeding. J Obstet Gynaecol Can 37(4):362–376
20. Wortman M (2013) Sonographically guided reoperative hysteroscopy (SGRH) for the management of global endometrial ablation (GEA) failures: a review of 50 cases. J Minim Invasive Gynecol 20:S53
21. Thomassee MS, Curlin H, Yunker A, Anderson TL (2013) Predicting pelvic pain after endometrial ablation: which preoperative patient characteristics are associated? J Minim Invasive Gynecol 20:642–647
22. Sharp TH (2012) Endometrial ablation: postoperative complications. Am J Obstet Gynecol 207(4):243–247
23. McCausland AM, McCausland VM (2010) Long-term complications of minimally invasive endometrial ablation devices. J Gynecol Surg 26(2):133–149. doi:10.1089/gyn.2009.0016
24. Vilos GA, Oraif A, Vilos AG, Ettler E, Edris F, Abu-Rafea B (2015) Long-term clinical outcomes following resectoscopic endometrial ablation of non-atypical endometrial hyperplasia in women with abnormal uterine bleeding. J Minim Invasive Gynecol 22:66–77. doi:10.1016/j.jmig.2014.07.009
25. El-Nashar SA, Hopkins MR, Creedon DJ, St Sauver JL, Weaver AL, McGree ME et al (2009) Prediction of treatment outcomes after global endometrial ablation. Obstet Gynecol 113:97–106
26. Peeters JA, Penninx JP, Mol BW, Bongers MY (2013) Prognostic factors for the success of endometrial ablation in the treatment of menorrhagia with special reference to previous cesarean section. Eur J Obstet Gynecol Reprod Biol 167:100–103
27. Wishall KM, Price J, Pereira N, Butts SM, Della Badia CR (2014) Postablation risk factors for pain and subsequent hysterectomy. Obstet Gynecol 124:904–910. doi:10.1097/AOG.0000000000000459
28. Daniels JP, Middleton LJ, Champaneria R, Khan KS, Cooper K, Mol BW et al (2012) Second generation endometrial ablation techniques for heavy menstrual bleeding: network metaanalysis. BMJ 344:e2564
29. Lethaby A, Hickey M, Garry R (2005) Endometrial destruction techniques for heavy menstrual bleeding. Cochrane Database Syst Rev 4. Wiley. [DOI: 10.1002/14651858]
30. Fernandez H (2011) Update on the management of menometrorrhagia: new surgical approaches. Gynaecol Endocrinol 1:1131–1136
31. Townsend DE, Richart RM, Paskowitz RA, Woolfork RE (1990) "Rollerball" coagulation of the endometrium. Am J Obstet Gynecol 76:310–313
32. Goldrath MH (1995) Hysteroscopic endometrial ablation. Obstet Gynecol Clin NA 22:559–572
33. Al-Shukri M, Burnett M (2009) Combined intervention with endometrial ablation plus LGN-IUS versus ablation alone for the treatment of menorrhagia. J Obstet Gynecol Can 31(5):S25
34. El-Nashar SA (2010) Combined bipolar radiofrequency endometrial ablation with levonorgestrel intrauterine system: a novel approach for challenging cases. J Minim Invasive Gynecol 17:S37
35. Vaughan D, Byrne P (2012) An evaluation of the simultaneous use of the levonorgestrel-releasing intrauterine device (LNG-IUS, Mirena ®) combined with endometrial ablation in the management of menorrhagia. J Obstet Gynaecol 32:372–374. doi:10.3109/01443615.2012.666581
36. Sohn B, Vilos GA, Vilos AG, Ternamian A, Abu-Rafea B, Oraif A (2013) Resectoscopic rollerball endometrial ablation and concomitant levonorgestrel-releasing intrauterine system in women with abnormal uterine bleeding: is the combination better? J Minim Invasive Gynecol 20:S22
37. Magos AM, Baumann R, Lockwood GM, Turnbull AC (1991) Experience with the first 250 endometrial resections for menorrhagia. Lancet 337:1074–1080
38. Taskin O, Onoglu A, Inal M et al (2002) Long-term histopathologic and morphologic changes after thermal endometrial ablation. J Am Assoc Gynecol Laparosc 9(2):186–190
39. Reid PC (2007) Endometrial ablation in England—coming of age? An examination of hospital episode statistics 1989/1990 to 2004/2005. Eur J Obstet Gynecol Reprod Biol 135:191–194
40. Fergusson RJ, Lethaby A, Shepperd S, Farquhar C (2013) Endometrial resection and ablation versus hysterectomy for heavy menstrual bleeding. Cochrane Database Syst Rev 11. Art. No.: CD000329. DOI:10.1002/14651858.CD000329.pub2

20

Intraoperative transvaginal sonography: a novel approach for localization of deeper myomas during laparoscopic myomectomy

P.G Paul[1] · Dimple K. Ahluwalia[1] · Dhivya Narasimhan[1] · Gaurav Chopade[1] · Saurabh Patil[1] · Varsha Rengaraj[1] · Tanuka Das[1]

Abstract The aim of this study is to assess the use of intraoperative transvaginal ultrasonography (TVS) to locate deep myomas that were not identified on laparoscopic view. The design of this study is a prospective observational study. This study was conducted in private Advanced Endoscopy and Infertility Treatment Centre, Kerala, India. The study comprised of 84 patients who underwent laparoscopic myomectomy from January 2011 to December 2013 in whom intraoperative TVS was used as an intervention. The number of additional deeper myomas removed was calculated, and recurrence at 1 year was calculated. The total number of myomas enucleated was 390, and the additional myomas enucleated after intraoperative TVS were 94. The recurrence of myomas at 1-year follow-up was 7.1 %. Intraoperative TVS was helpful to the surgeon for identifying deeper myomas making the surgery more effective.

Keywords Myomas · Intraoperative TVS · Laparoscopic myomectomy

Introduction

Laparoscopic myomectomy was described for the first time in the late 1970s for subserous myomas [1]. In the early 1990s, the technique was developed to include removal of intramural myomas [2]. As endoscopic surgeons gained experience, they started performing laparoscopic myomectomy for multiple and larger myomas, irrespective of size, number, or location of myoma [3].

One of the difficulties of laparoscopic myomectomy is locating the deeper and smaller myomas especially those closer to the endometrium (type 3) according to the International Federation of Gynecology and Obstetrics (FIGO) classification [4]. Laparoscopic myomectomy carries increased risk of residual myomas because unlike laparotomy, the uterus cannot be palpated to locate very small myomas. Postoperative recurrence may be either due to enlarged residual myomas or newly formed myomas. There are studies that show increased risk of recurrence (16.7–51.4 %) after 5 years of laparoscopic myomectomy [5, 6]. This increases the chance of reoperation and decreases the chances of symptom relief after the surgery. Several studies have shown that large myomas are associated with significant reduction in pregnancy rate after IVF [7, 8]. Khalaf et al. showed that smaller myomas (≤5 cm) not encroaching endometrial cavity were found to significantly reduce ongoing pregnancy rate at each cycle of IVF by 40 %; similarly, Stovall et al. concluded that implantation and pregnancy rates were one half that of matched controls [9, 10].

Technical problems in identifying deeper myomas lead to misplaced incision causing more blood loss, myometrial integrity, and increased operating time. Good preoperative myoma mapping is helpful, but it is difficult to locate deeper and smaller intramural myomas intraoperatively [11]. Intraoperative location of myomas with laparoscopic contact ultrasound probes can be done [12]. But it is costly and not available as standard ultrasound probes. To overcome this, we attempted to use intraoperative transvaginal ultrasonography (TVS) with

✉ P.G Paul
  drpaulpg@gmail.com

[1] Centre for Advanced Endoscopy and Infertility, Paul's Hospital, Vattekkattu Road, Kaloor, Kochi, Kerala 682 017, India

a simultaneous laparoscopic view to locate deep-seated and smaller myomas and to enucleate additional residual myomas.

The primary aim of the study was to assess the effectiveness of intraoperative transvaginal ultrasonography to locate deeper and smaller myomas, which were not identified on laparoscopic view.

Material and methods

This was a prospective observational study of women who underwent laparoscopic myomectomy for uterine leiomyomas from January 2011 to December 2013 when intraoperative TVS was done to identify the additional myomas.

For all patients, preoperative TVS and transabdominal scans were performed, and inclusion criteria were:

1) Patients with four or more myomas.
2) Patients with type 3 myoma, irrespective of the number of myomas (myoma that contacts the endometrium and is 100 % intramural) according to the FIGO classification [4].

Exclusion criteria were:

1) Patients with other coexisting diseases like endometriosis and severe pelvic adhesion.
2) Patients with submucous myomas type 0, 1, and 2 according to FIGO classification.
3) Postmenopausal women.

Laparoscopic myomectomy was not limited by factors such as location (anterior/posterior wall) and depth (subserosal/intramural). Data was collected on demographic characteristics, and the chief indication and symptoms were analyzed. The study was approved by the ethical committee of Paul's Hospital for the intervention.

Preoperatively GnRH agonists were not used before surgery because we found that degeneration of the myoma made the surgical dissection difficult. Postoperative patients were followed up with TVS by the first author for recurrence of myomas at 1 year, and any myoma of more than 2 cm was considered as recurrence (Fig. 1).

Fig. 1 Flow chart of patients from selection to 1 year after myomectomy

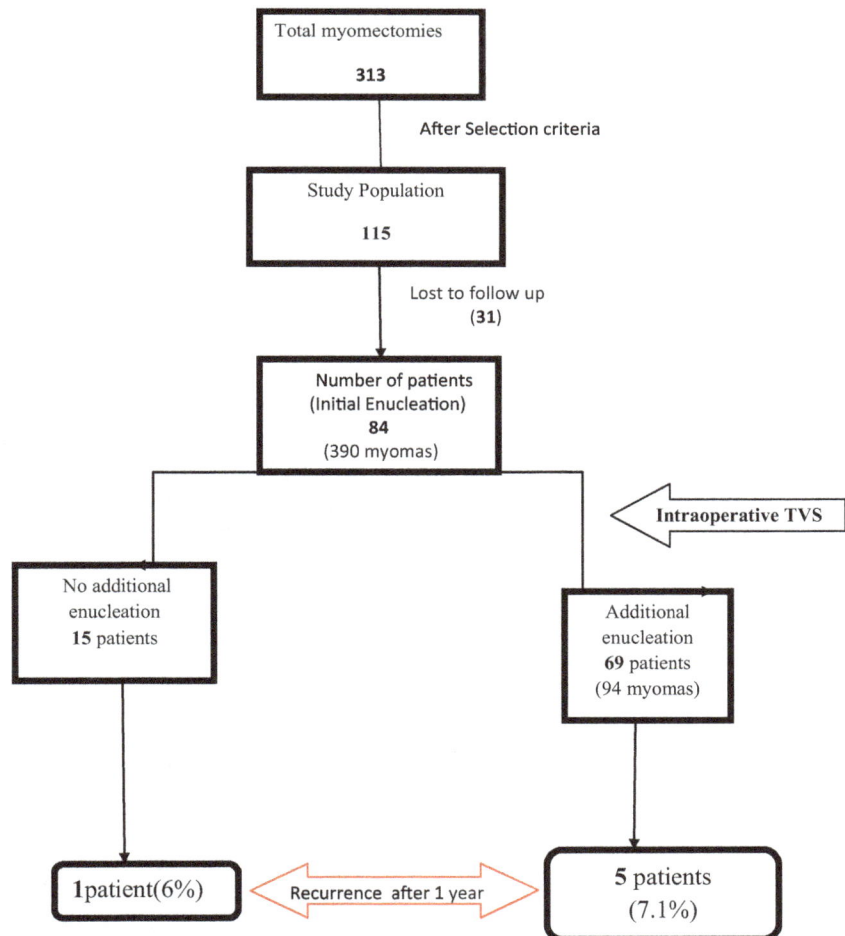

Fig. 2 Deep intramural myoma mapped preoperatively

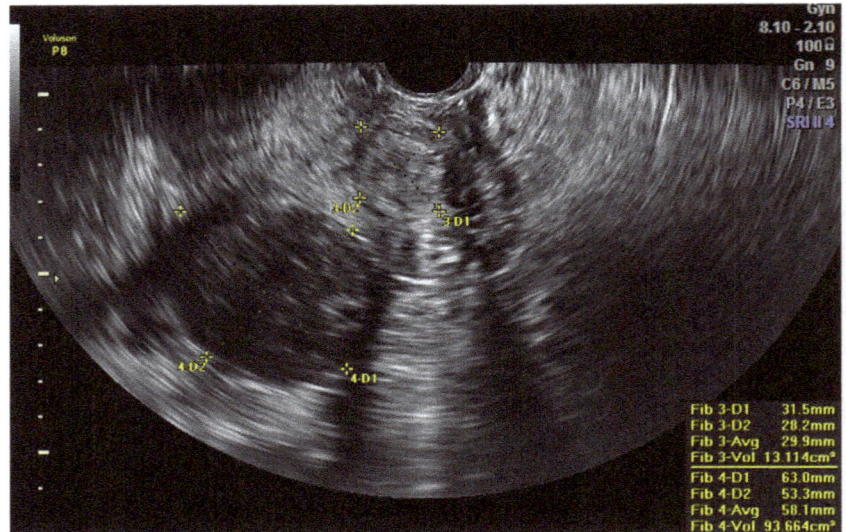

Surgical technique

All procedures were performed by the first author using similar technique under general anesthesia, as described in our previous publications [13, 14]. Hysteroscopy was performed to look for distortion of the endometrial cavity and to exclude any undiagnosed submucous myoma on ultrasonography. Entry into the abdominal cavity through an umbilical incision or a higher one in the case of larger uteri was accomplished using a 10-mm trocar. In patients with a previous history of an open surgery or in cases where intra-abdominal adhesions were suspected, entry under direct vision using a Ternamian Endotip (Karl Storz, Tuttlingen, Germany) was performed. Two ancillary 5-mm trocars lateral to the right and left epigastric vessels and a median supra-pubic trocar were inserted. Vasopressin 20 IU diluted in 60 ml of saline was infused into

the myometrium of the uterus to reduce the bleeding. A transverse or vertical incision was made over the myoma that was preoperatively mapped (Fig. 2) with Harmonic Ace (Ethicon Endosurgery, Cincinnati, Ohio).The myoma was kept under traction using myoma spiral and dissected with Harmonic Ace. The myomectomy site was sutured intracorporeally with polyglactin 910 (Vicryl, Ethicon, India) or 1-0 braided Lactomer (Polysorb, Tyco Healthcare) in single or double layers depending upon the depth of muscle defect. The myomas were removed with electromechanical morcellator (Karl Storz, Gynaecare, Tuttlingen, Germany). After enucleating all visible myomas, the intraoperative TVS was done, and additional myomas were identified.

Intraoperative TVS was done by either a second or third author and confirmed by an operating surgeon (first author). All preoperative TVS were done by the first author. We used

Fig. 3 Deep intramural myoma identified by intraoperative sonography

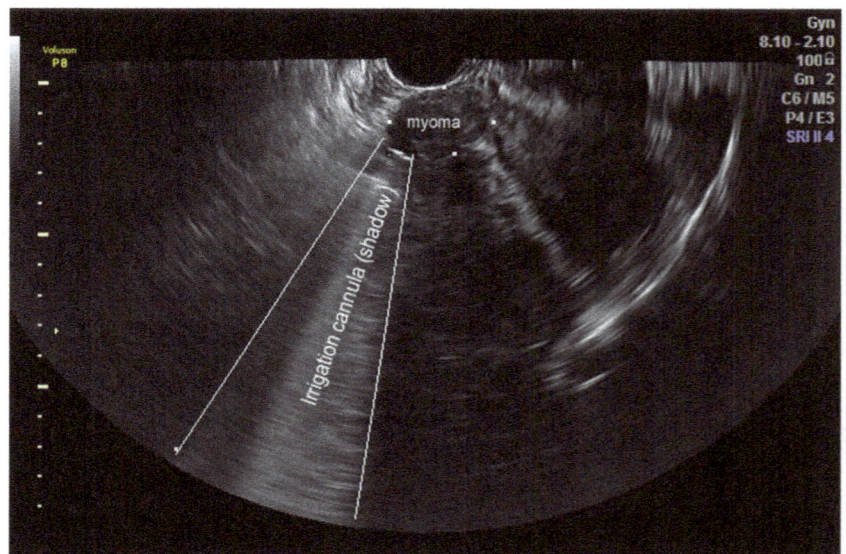

ultrasonic device Voluson E (GE Healthcare, Beethoven Street, 239 D m- 42,655, Solingen, Germany) with TVS probe RIC5-9W-RS/Gyn and detection frequency set at 8–14 MHz. The vaginal probe was covered with a sterile cover, and the whole uterus was scanned to identify any residual myoma. The laparoscopic surgeon (first author) filled the pouch of Douglas with normal saline to make an acoustic window for better ultrasonic visualization. The myoma identified on transvaginal ultrasound was located laparoscopically with a suction irrigation cannula by trial and error. The irrigating fluid from suction irrigation cannula seen as a comet shape on transvaginal ultrasound helps in the localization of the myoma (Fig. 3). The myoma thus identified was enucleated laparoscopically as described before (Fig. 4).

Table 1 Demographic characteristics/chief complaints

Demographic characteristics	
Age (years)	33.40 ± 5.13
BMI (mean)	32
Chief complaints	No. of patients
Abdominal pain	35 (41.7 %)
Primary infertility	22 (26.2 %)
Menorrhagia	14 (16.6 %)
Secondary infertility	4 (4.8 %)
Dysmenorrhea	5 (5.9 %)
Dysmenorrhea and menorrhagia	2 (2.4 %)
Irregular bleeding	2 (2.4 %)

Results

The total number of myomectomies performed from January 2011 to December 2013 was 313. One hundred fifteen patients met inclusion criteria, but 31 patients were lost to follow-up; of these, 84 patients who met the inclusion criteria were included in the study. The mean age of our patients was 33.40 ± 5.13 and mean BMI was 32. The proportion of parity was 52 %. The primary preoperative indications were abdominal pain in 35 patients (41.7 %) followed by primary infertility in 22 patients (13.1 %) and menorrhagia in 14 patients (16.7 %) and as shown in Table 1.

The size of the myomas enucleated is shown in Table 2. The average number of myomas enucleated per patient was 4.64. Sixty-three patients had four or more myomas. Twenty-one patients had less than four myomas, but these were all type 3.

The total number of myomas removed was 390. The mean size of the myomas removed was 3.28 cm.

The average blood loss in milliliter was 163.86 ± 18.92 in patients with intraoperative TVS, whereas 148.18 ± 21.44 without intraoperative TVS. The mean drop in hemoglobin concentration after surgery was 1 g%. The total time duration (induction to closure) was 134 ± 27.25 min in cases where intraoperative TVS was performed and 110 ± 21.02 min in cases without intraoperative TVS.

The additional myomas removed after performing intraoperative TVS were 94. These were visible during preoperative TVS also. Size (range) of the additional myomas removed was 2.5 (1.5–3.5 cm). Average number of additional myomas enucleated per patient was 1.1. Out of 94 additional myomas removed, 86 were FIGO type III and 8 were type IV. Recurrence of myoma at 1-year follow-up on ultrasound examination was 7.1 %.

Discussion

In patients with multiple myomas, an experienced laparoscopic surgeon can remove all visible myomas but identification of deeper and smaller myomas are difficult due to lack of tactile perception. The better way to overcome this limitation is the

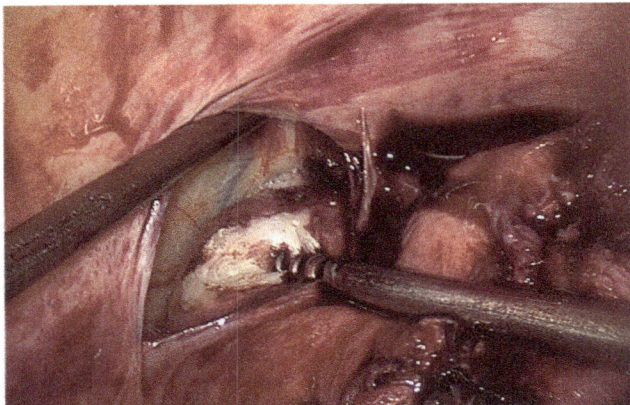

Fig. 4 Laparoscopic enucleation of deep intramural myoma

Table 2 Total number of myomas

Size (cm)	Number of myomas
<5	324 (83.08 %)
5–6	20 (5.13 %)
6–7	20 (5.13 %)
7–8	9 (2.31 %)
8	9 (2.31 %)
9	3 (0.77 %)
10	1 (0.26 %)
12	1 (0.26 %)
14	3 (0.77 %)
Mean size = 3.28 cm	Total—390 myomas

Table 3 Intraoperative findings

Intraoperative findings	With intraoperative TVS	Without intraoperative TVS
Total time duration (min)	134.63 ± 27.25	110 ± 21.02
Total blood loss (ml)	163.86 ± 18.92	148.18 ± 21.44
Number of additional myomas removed	1.1	

use of intraoperative ultrasonography. The aim of the study was to assess the effectiveness of intraoperative TVS to locate deeper and smaller myomas that were not identified on laparoscopic view. This is in contrast to a similar study where an intraoperative contact probe was used. However, this method is costly and not easily available [12]. To our knowledge, this is the first study where TVS is used intraoperatively to localize deep/hidden myomas.

In our study, mean size of myomas removed was 3.28 cm, which is not considered significant by Pritts et al. in his review article. Most of our patients were having a long duration of infertility and planning to go for IVF and that was the reason for removing smaller myomas. The size of the myomas removed is similar to other studies [9, 10, 15]. Additional myomas that were not visible laparoscopically were detected by intraoperative TVS in 69 of 84 patients. The mean size of the additional enucleated myomas was 2.5 (1.5 to 3.5 cm). In a similar study where intraoperative contact ultrasound probe was used, 25 additional myomas with a median diameter of 1.2 cm were enucleated in a group of 42 patients which is comparable to our study [12].

In our study, the operative time was more when intraoperative TVS was done due to the time taken for sonography and the surgical time for enucleating additional myomas. The blood loss was also more due to increased duration of the surgery. (Table 3) But blood loss was not clinically significant, and duration can be minimized with experience in intraoperative TVS.

Causes of postoperative recurrence are considered to be either enlargement of residual myomas or formation of new ones. Postoperative residual myomas greatly affect the recurrence rate. Some studies have reported that laparoscopic myomectomy is associated with a higher recurrence rate as compared with laparotomy recurrence rate [16, 17]. Doriot et al. and Hiroto Shimanuki et al. defined recurrence of a myoma >2 cm with transvaginal ultrasonography to be significant in their study after laparoscopic myomectomy [12]. In a study by Rossetti et al. which compares recurrence of myomas after 6 months in the abdominal and the laparoscopic group, there was a recurrence of 27 % in the laparoscopic group as compared to 23 % in the abdominal group [16]. In our study, recurrence at 1-year follow-up was 7.1 % that is lower than the above studies. In our study, recurrence was due to the formation of new ones as we had removed visible myomas.

The intraoperative ultrasound allowed precise localization of the myoma and determination of the best hysterotomy incision. A suboptimal incision would have caused greater trauma to the normal myometrium, as well as increased operating time for laparoscopic reconstruction of the uterus following the myomectomy. The other option would have been converting to an open procedure to enable palpation of the location of the known myomas and making an appropriate incision. Laparoscopic myomectomy is a well-accepted surgical approach for selected patients [16]. The intraoperative TVS allowed the surgeon to complete the myomectomy laparoscopically without tactile information.

Transvaginal sonography is a widely available imaging modality that every gynecologist is well versed with although there can be an interobserver variation. Its novel use intraoperatively to localize deep-seated myomas enables the surgeon to complete the myomectomy laparoscopically, despite the absence of tactile sensation. Limitation of the study was a lack of randomization and small sample size due to lost to follow-up (Fig. 1) and short follow-up time (1 year).

Conclusion

Intraoperative TVS is helpful to the surgeon for identifying deeper and smaller myomas, thus making the surgery more effective. Hence, intraoperative use of transvaginal sonography for patients with multiple and deep-seated myomas is advantageous.

Informed consent   All procedures followed were approved by the ethical standards of the responsible committee on human experimentation (institutional and national) and in accordance with the Helsinki Declaration of 1975, as revised in 2000(5). Informed consent was obtained from all patients for being included in the study.

Authors' contributions   Dr. P.G Paul was the operating surgeon responsible for the planning and conduct of research work. Dr. Dimple K. Ahluwalia and Dr. Dhivya Narasimhan were the assistant surgeons assigned in performing ultrasound during surgeries and conducting studies. Dr. Gaurav Chopade performed statistical analysis and also helped in conducting studies. Dr. Saurabh Patil took charge of the reporting and review of literature. Dr. Varsha Rengaraj and Dr. Tanuka Das were responsible for the preparation of the manuscript.

References

1. Semm K, Mettler L, et al (1980) Technical progress in pelvic surgery via operative laparoscopy. Am J Obstet Gynecol 138:121–127
2. Daniell JF, Gurley LD, et al (1991) Laparoscopic treatment of clinically significant symptomatic uterine myomas. J Gynecol. Surg 7: 37–39
3. Sinha R, Hegde A, Mahajan C, Dubey N, Sundaram M (2008) Laparoscopic myomectomy: do size, number, and location of the myomas form limiting factors for laparoscopic myomectomy? J Minim Invasive Gynecol 15:292–300
4. Munro MG et al (2011) FIGO Working Group on Menstrual Disorders: FIGO classification system (PALM-COEIN) for causes of abnormal uterine bleeding in nongravid women of reproductive age. Int J of Gynecol & Obstet. 113:3–13. doi:10.1016/j.ijgo.2010. 11.011
5. Doridot V, Dubisson J, Chapron C, et al (2001) Recurrence of leiomyomata after laparoscopic myomectomy. J Am Assoc Gynecol Laparosc 8:495–500
6. Nehzat FR, Roemisch M, Nezhat CH, et al (2001) Recurrence rate after laparoscopic myomectomy. J Am Assoc Gynecol Laparosc 8: 495–500
7. Benecke C, Kruger TF, Siebert TI, Van der Merwe JP, Steyn DW (2005) Effect of fibroids on fertility in patients undergoing assisted reproduction. A structured literature review. Gynecol Obstet Investig 59:225–230
8. Pritts EA, Parker WH, Olive DL (2009) Fibroids and infertility: an updated systematic review of the evidence. Fertil Steril 91:1215–1223
9. Khalaf Y, Ross C, El-Toukhy TH, Seed RP, Braude P, et al (2006) The effect of small intramural fibroids on the cumulative outcome of assisted conception. Hum Reprod 21:2640–2044
10. Stovall DW, Parrish SB, Van Voorhis BJ, et al (1998) Uterine leiomyomas reduce the efficacy of assisted reproduction cycles: results of a matched follow-up. Study; Hum Reprod vol.13(no.1): 192–197
11. Dubuisson JB, Fauconnier A (2007) Laparoscopic myomectomy. In: Atlas of operative laparoscopy and hysteroscopy. 3rd edn, Informa healthcare, U.K, p. 235
12. Shimanuki H et al (2006) Effectiveness of intraoperative ultrasound in reducing recurrent fibroids during laparoscopic myomectomy. J Reprod Med 51:683–688
13. Paul PG, Koshy A, Thomas T, et al (2006) Pregnancy outcomes following laparoscopic myomectomy and single layer myometrial closure. Hum Reprod 21:3278–3281
14. Paul PG, Koshy A, Thomas T, et al (2006) Laparoscopic myomectomy: feasibility and safety—a retrospective study of 762 cases. Gynecol Surg 3:97–102
15. Liselotte M, Thoralf Schollmeyer E, et al (2005) Update on laparoscopic myomectomy. Gynecol Surg 2:173–177
16. Rosette A, Sizzi O, et al (2001) Long-term results of laparoscopic myomectomy: recurrence rate in comparison with abdominal myomectomy. Hum Reprod 16:770–774
17. Miller CE et al (2000) Myomectomy. Comparison of open and laparoscopic techniques. Obstet Gynynecol Clin North Am 27: 407–420

21

The FAST-EU trial: 12-month clinical outcomes of women after intrauterine sonography-guided transcervical radiofrequency ablation of uterine fibroids

Hans Brölmann[1] · Marlies Bongers[2] · José Gerardo Garza-Leal[3] · Janesh Gupta[4] ·
Sebastiaan Veersema[5] · Rik Quartero[6] · David Toub[7,8]

Abstract The FAST-EU Trial was designed to establish the effectiveness and confirm the safety of transcervical intrauterine sonography-guided radiofrequency ablation with the VizAblate™ System in the treatment of symptomatic uterine fibroids. This was a multicenter, prospective, single-arm trial involving academic and community hospitals in the United Kingdom, the Netherlands, and Mexico. Women with qualifying uterine fibroids and heavy menstrual bleeding underwent intrauterine sonography-guided transcervical radiofrequency ablation (RFA) with the VizAblate System; anesthesia was individualized. Patients were required to have up to five fibroids from 1 to 5 cm in diameter. The primary trial endpoint was the percentage change in perfused fibroid volume, as assessed by contrast-enhanced MRI at 3 months by an independent core laboratory. Secondary endpoints, evaluated at 6 and 12 months, included safety, percentage reductions in the Menstrual Pictogram (MP) score, and the Symptom Severity Score (SSS) subscale of the Uterine Fibroid Symptom-Quality of Life (UFS-QOL) questionnaire, along with the rate of surgical reintervention for abnormal uterine bleeding and the mean number of days to return to normal activity. Additional assessments included the Health-Related Quality of Life (HRQOL) subscale of the UFS-QOL, nonsurgical reintervention for abnormal uterine bleeding, anesthesia regimen, patient satisfaction, and pain during the recovery period. An additional MRI study was performed at 12 months on a subgroup of patients. Fifty patients (89 fibroids) underwent transcervical radiofrequency ablation with the VizAblate System. At 3 and 12 months, perfused fibroid volumes were reduced from baseline by an average of 68.1 ± 28.6 and 67.4 ± 31.9 %, respectively, while total fibroid volumes were reduced from baseline by an average of 54.7 ± 37.4 and 66.6 ± 32.1 %, respectively (all $P<.001$ compared with baseline; Wilcoxon signed-rank test). At 12 months, mean MP score and SSS decreased by 53.8 ± 50.5 and 55.1 ± 41.0 %, respectively; the mean HRQOL score increased by 277 ± 483 %. There were four surgical reinterventions (8 %) within 12 months. This is the first report of the 12-month follow-up for patients in the FAST-EU Trial. In concert with previously reported 3- and 6-month endpoint data, the 12-month results of the FAST-EU Trial suggest that in addition to substantially reducing the perfused and total volume of targeted uterine fibroids, the VizAblate System is safe and effective through 12 months in providing relief of abnormal uterine bleeding associated with submucous, intramural, and transmural fibroids.

Keywords Fibroids · Radiofrequency ablation · VizAblate · Intrauterine sonography · Ultrasound

✉ David Toub
dtoub@mac.com

[1] Vrije Universiteit Medisch Centrum, Amsterdam, Netherlands

[2] Máxima Medisch Centrum, Veldhoven, Netherlands

[3] Universidad Autónoma de Nuevo León, Monterrey, Nuevo Leon, Mexico

[4] Birmingham Women's Hospital, Birmingham, UK

[5] Sint Antonius Ziekenhuis, Nieuwegein, Netherlands

[6] Medisch Spectrum Twente, Enschede, Netherlands

[7] Gynesonics, Inc., Redwood City, CA 94063, USA

[8] Albert Einstein Medical Center, 5501 Old York Road, Philadelphia, PA 19141, USA

Introduction

Uterine fibroids are highly prevalent and the primary indication for over 200,000 hysterectomies performed annually in the USA [1, 2]. While various fibroid treatments exist, they have limitations, such as being invasive, requiring general anesthesia, or being not optimally suited for treatment of both intramural and submucous myomata.

Radiofrequency ablation (RFA) involves the placement of one or more needle electrodes into a solid tumor in order to deliver thermal energy, resulting in thermal fixation and coagulative necrosis within the treated tissue [3, 4]. Recent studies have been performed using RFA in conjunction with simultaneous, real-time sonography to guide volumetric ablations, resulting in volume reduction and symptom improvement [3, 5, 6].

The VizAblate System (Gynesonics; Redwood City, CA) combines radiofrequency ablation with intrauterine sonography and is CE-marked and commercially available in the European Union. VizAblate permits real-time imaging and transcervical treatment of uterine fibroids, including those that are not amenable to hysteroscopic resection such as type 3, type 4, and types 2–5 (transmural) fibroids as well as large type 1 and type 2 myomata [7]. The Fibroid Ablation Study-EU (FAST-EU) was designed to examine the safety and effectiveness of transcervical radiofrequency ablation of uterine fibroids under intrauterine sonography guidance with the VizAblate System. The trial endpoints, reached at 3 and at 6 months, have previously been reported [8]. This paper presents the 12-month efficacy and safety results of women treated under the FAST-EU Trial.

Patients and methods

This was a prospective, single-arm, multicenter trial. The primary endpoint was the percentage change in target fibroid perfused volume as assessed by contrast-enhanced MRI by an independent core laboratory at baseline and at 3 months. Additional endpoints, reached at 6 months, included safety, percentage reductions in the Menstrual Pictogram (MP) score and the Symptom Severity Score (SSS) subscale of the Uterine Fibroid Symptom-Quality of Life (UFS-QOL) questionnaire, the rate of surgical reintervention for abnormal uterine bleeding, and the mean number of days to return to normal activity. The Health-Related Quality of Life (HRQOL) subscale of the UFS-QOL questionnaires, along with anesthesia regimen, patient satisfaction, and recovery pain, was also assessed.

Patients were enrolled across seven sites in three nations: Mexico (one site), the United Kingdom (two sites), and the Netherlands (four sites). The trial included women with one to five uterine fibroids of FIGO types 1, 2, 3, 4, and 2–5 (transmural) measuring between 1 and 5 cm in maximum diameter. Fibroids that did not contain an edge within the inner half of the myometrium were not counted in this total and were not targeted for ablation, as they were believed to be less likely to materially contribute to abnormal uterine bleeding

(AUB). At least one fibroid was required to indent the endometrial cavity.

Patients were 28 years of age or older and not pregnant, with regular, predictable menstrual cycles and heavy menstrual bleeding for at least 3 months. A Menstrual Pictogram score ≥ 120 was also required for inclusion along with a baseline UFS-QOL SSS ≥ 20. The Menstrual Pictogram was first described by Wyatt and colleagues and is a variant of the Pictorial Blood Loss Assessment Chart (PBAC) that patients complete to provide a visual assessment of menstrual blood loss during a single cycle [9, 10]. Unlike the original PBAC described by Higham and colleagues, the Menstrual Pictogram includes a greater range of icons representing different saturations of sanitary products, clots, and losses in a toilet and also distinguishes different absorbency levels of sanitary napkins and tampons [11].

Exclusions included a desire for future fertility, the presence of one or more type 0 fibroids, cervical dysplasia, endometrial hyperplasia, active pelvic infection, clinically significant adenomyosis (>10 % of the junctional zone measuring more than 10 mm in thickness as measured by MRI), and the presence of one or more treatable fibroids that were significantly calcified (defined as <75 % fibroid enhancement by volume on contrast-enhanced MRI). Screening included transvaginal sonography, as well as hysteroscopy or hysterosonography, contrast-enhanced MRI, endometrial biopsy, and a pregnancy test.

All records were de-identified and only the range of each patient's age was documented, as per clinical trial requirements in the Netherlands. Women were followed at 7–14 days, 30 days, 3 months, 6 months, and 12 months post-treatment. All MRI studies were forwarded to an independent core laboratory (MedQIA, Los Angeles, CA, USA) for quality control and interpretation to reduce variability in the measurements; the core laboratory also developed standardized imaging protocols for use at the individual trial sites, credentialed the sites, and trained MRI technologists at each trial site. Fibroid measurements consisted of the total voxel volume and perfused voxel volume via contrast-enhanced MRI at the specified time points.

Procedure

The VizAblate System, as well as its use, has previously been described in detail and includes a reusable intrauterine ultrasound (IUUS) probe and a single-use, articulating radiofrequency ablation handpiece that are combined into an integrated treatment device that is inserted transcervically (Fig. 1) [8]. A custom graphical interface provides the gynecologist with a real-time, image-guided treatment system that indicates the borders of the thermal ablation (Ablation Zone) as well as the border beyond which tissues are safe from ablation (Thermal Safety Border). Because the deployment path is

Fig. 1 The VizAblate treatment
device

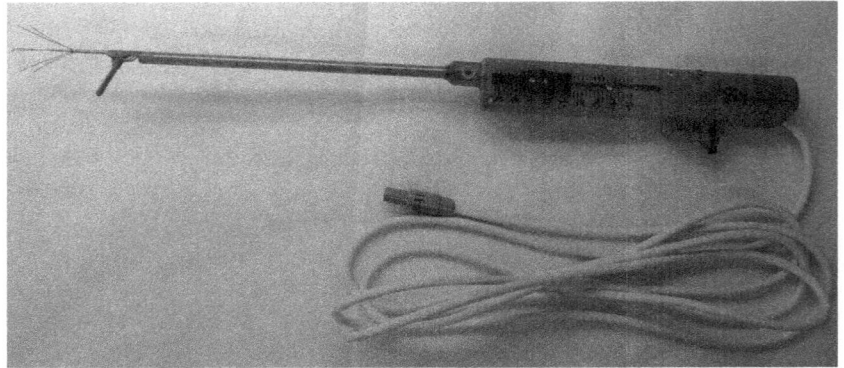

predictable relative to the ultrasound image, one can plan the ablation location and size before introducing any electrode elements into a fibroid. Additionally, the guidance software provides graphics that allow the gynecologist to maintain a safe margin from the ablation to the serosal margin and extra-uterine viscera. Mechanical stops provide definitive tactile limits, ensuring that the needle electrodes are deployed to the proper distance to achieve the ablation size as selected by the gynecologist. The radiofrequency generator modulates power (up to 150 W) to maintain a constant temperature of 105 °C at the needle electrode tips, and the ablation time is preset based on the ablation size. Depending on the width of the ablation, the distance from the Ablation Zone to the Thermal Safety Border will vary from 6.0 to 9.5 mm.

In this trial, the method of anesthesia was chosen by each investigator based on individual patient characteristics in consultation with an anesthesiologist. Treated fibroids received one or more ellipsoidal ablations under real-time intrauterine sonographic guidance, ranging from 1 to 4 cm in width and 2 to 5 cm in length. The number of ablations, along with their sizes, was at the discretion of the investigator and was chosen in order to maximize the ablation volume of the fibroid while maintaining the Thermal Safety Border within the uterine serosal margin.

Statistical analysis

The primary endpoint was the percentage change in target fibroid perfused volume at 3 months. The null hypothesis for the primary trial endpoint at 3 months was H_0: probability of success <50 % versus the alternative H_a: probability of success ≥50 %. A sample of 40 patients was sufficient to detect this difference of 22 % in probability of success with a power of 82 % using a one-group chi-square test with a 0.05 two-sided significance level. Allowing for an expected dropout rate of 20 % at the 12-month follow-up visit, the minimum recommended sample size for the initial trial protocol was 48. The primary trial endpoint success criterion was achievement of >30 % reduction in mean target fibroid perfused volume in at least 50 % of patients at 3 months.

The data in this report consist of the Full Analysis dataset. This includes all patients enrolled who provided a baseline fibroid volume assessment and received treatment with the VizAblate System. Patients who received a surgical reintervention were considered treatment failures, and their subsequent data was imputed using the last observation carried forward (LOCF) method. Missing data was not imputed for patients who conceived or who neglected to complete a questionnaire.

All statistical analyses were performed with SAS 9.3 (SAS, Cary, NC). Values were considered significant at the level of $\alpha=0.05$. The Wilcoxon signed-rank test was used to test if a change was significantly different from 0.

Ethics

The protocol was approved by the Ethics Committees of the respective institutions as well as by the Federal Commission for Protection against Health Risks (COFEPRIS) in Mexico. All enrolled patients provided written informed consent for treatment with the VizAblate System prior to enrollment. The trial overview was published on ClinicalTrials.gov (identifier: NCT01226290) and conducted in accordance with Standard ISO 14155 (Clinical investigation of medical devices for human subjects – Good clinical practice) of the International Organization for Standardization (ISO), the Helsinki Declaration of 1975, as revised in 2008, and the ethical standards of applicable national regulations and institutional research policies and procedures governing human experimentation.

Results

Patients

Fifty patients were treated in the FAST-EU trial at seven sites. Baseline characteristics for all treated patients are provided in Table 1. Anesthesia was provided as noted in Table 2.

Table 1 Baseline subject characteristics

Subjects treated	50
Most frequent age range	41–45 years of age[a]
Mean Menstrual Pictogram (MP) score	423±253 (range 119–1582)
Mean UFS-QOL SSS	61.7±16.9 (range 28.1–100.0)
Mean UFS-QOL HRQOL score	34.3±19.0 (range 0.0–73.3)
Total number of target fibroids identified on MRI	118
Mean number of target fibroids per patient	2.4±1.7 (range 1–7)[b]
Mean diameter of target fibroids	2.9±1.4 cm (range 1.0–6.9 cm)
Mean perfused fibroid volume	18.3±20.6 cm^3 (range 0.3–77.0 cm^3)
Mean total (perfused+nonperfused) fibroid volume	18.8±21.4 cm^3 (range 0.3–77.0 cm^3)

UFS-QOL Uterine Fibroid Symptom-Quality of Life Questionnaire, *SSS* Symptom Severity Score subscale, *HRQOL* Health-Related Quality of Life subscale

[a] Subject ages were specified as a range by each site to protect subject privacy

[b] Two small additional fibroids, beyond the upper limit of 5 target fibroids/patient, were identified on review of one MRI series after treatment

One patient (three fibroids) was excluded from analysis of the primary endpoint. This patient was deemed by the core MRI laboratory to have had unusable imaging for making precise baseline fibroid measurements, although eligibility based on fibroid diameter ≤5 cm and location was not in question. This patient was treated as she met the eligibility requirements and her treatment could contribute to patient-reported and safety data for the trial. Consequently, while 92 fibroids were ablated, accurate baseline volume measurements could only be performed for 89. One patient reported a pregnancy at the time of her 6-month follow-up visit and was thus excluded from the 6- and 12-month analyses. While all patients provided baseline MP data, one patient each at 3, 6, and 12 months declined to submit a Menstrual Pictogram. One patient did not turn in her baseline HRQOL portion of the UFS-QOL; her HRQOL data was not included in the analysis. A flow diagram depicting sample sizes for MRI and patient-reported outcomes at baseline and 3-, 6-, and 12 months is provided in Fig. 2.

The protocol required a baseline and 3-month MR study for the primary endpoint analysis (reduction in perfused fibroid volume). Approximately 14 months after the first patient was

Table 2 Anesthesia provided to FAST-EU subjects

Anesthesia option	No. of subjects
General anesthesia alone	15 (30.0 %)
Conscious sedation alone	15 (30.0 %)
Spinal anesthesia alone	8 (16.0 %)
Conscious sedation+epidural anesthesia	8 (16.0 %)
Epidural anesthesia alone	2 (4.0 %)
Paracervical blockade alone	1 (2.0 %)
General anesthesia+epidural anesthesia	1 (2.0 %)

treated, the protocol was amended to add an MR evaluation at 12 months in order to provide longer-term information about the effects of transcervical RFA. Twenty-eight patients (58.3 %) provided their informed consent to undergo another MR examination with contrast enhancement at 12 months post-ablation and underwent such imaging.

Effects on fibroid volume

Characteristics of fibroids that were ablated are shown in Table 3, and results of fibroid ablation on total and perfused volume at 3 and 12 months are provided in Table 4. Fibroids are classified in Table 3 as per the FIGO classification system [12]. Radiofrequency ablation with the VizAblate System was associated with statistically significant reductions (68.1 and 54.7 %, respectively) in both total and perfused fibroid volumes at 3 and 12 months. Seventy-nine of 89 treated fibroids (88.8 %) in all 49 patients with measurable MRI data met the primary trial endpoint success criterion at 3 months (achievement of >30 % reduction in mean target fibroid perfused volume at 3 months in at least 50 % of patients). By 12 months post-ablation (n=28 patients; 43 fibroids), treated fibroids experienced a mean reduction in total fibroid volume of 66.6± 32.1 % ($P<.001$). Thirty-seven fibroids (86.0 %) in 100 % of the 28 patients imaged at 12 months demonstrated >30 % reduction in perfused fibroid volume at 12 months.

Patient-reported outcomes

Patient-reported secondary endpoint data through 12 months are provided in Table 5. The mean MP score declined through 12 months, with mean and median reductions of 53.8 and 72.3 % at 12 months, respectively (all $P<.001$). By 3 months post-ablation, 44 of 49 patients (89.8 %) experienced a reduction in menstrual blood loss as reflected by their Menstrual

Fig. 2 Patient flow diagram

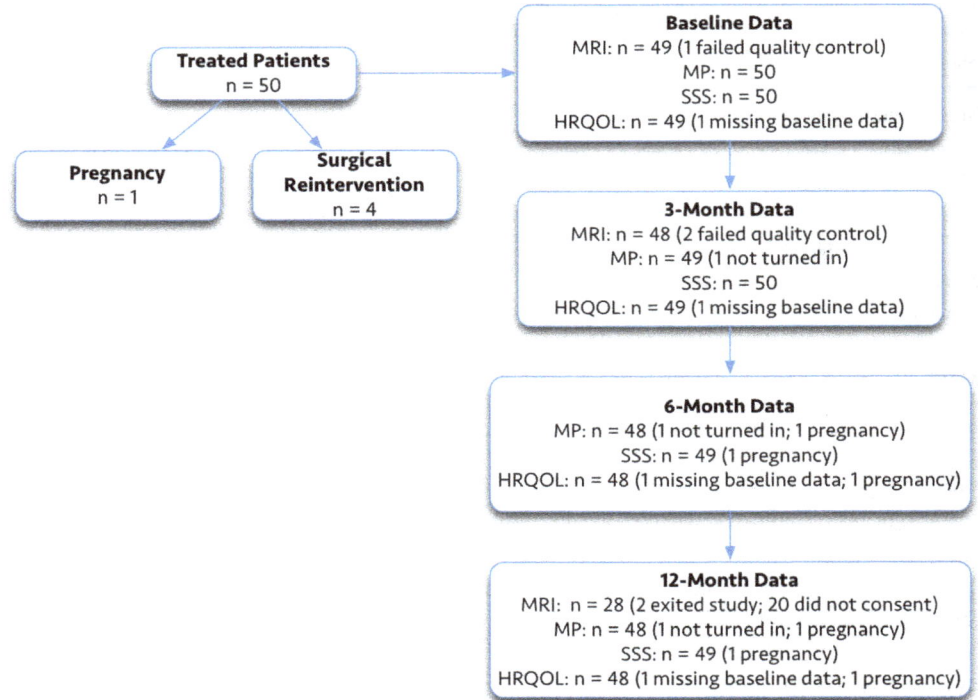

Pictogram scores. Of these 49 patients at 3 months, 28 (57.1 %) had >50 % reduction in MP scores; this proportion increased to 35 of 48 patients (72.9 %) at 6 months and was realized by 31 of 48 patients (64.6 %) at 12 months. The proportion of patients achieving >50 % bleeding reduction at 6 months was not significantly different from the proportion at 12 months (P=.095).

Lukes and colleagues reported that a 22 % or greater reduction in menstrual blood loss was meaningful to the majority of women [13]. In the FAST-EU Trial, 37 of 49 (75.5 %) patients had achieved such clinically meaningful reductions in menstrual bleeding by 3 months. This increased to 41 of 48 patients (85.4 %) at 6 months and 38 of 48 patients (79.2 %) at month 12, which was not significantly different from 6 months (P=.175).

As shown in Table 5, the reductions in the transformed SSS subscale of the UFS-QOL questionnaire at 3, 6, and 12 months were statistically significant, as were the increases in the transformed HRQOL subscale. Patients experienced a 55.1 % reduction in SSS at 12 months, corresponding to a mean reduction in transformed SSS of 35.3 points from baseline. At all post-ablation time points studied, the majority of patients experienced at least a clinically significant 10-point reduction in SSS (82 % of patients at 3 months, 86 % at 6 months, 78 % at 12 months).

Adverse events

There were 34 adverse events deemed possibly, probably, or definitely related to the VizAblate System or overall

Table 3 Characteristics of ablated fibroids

Total number of ablated target fibroids[a]	92
Mean number of ablated target fibroids per subject	1.8±1.1 (range 1–5)
Total number of type 0 ablated fibroids	0
Total number of type 1 ablated fibroids	14
Total number of type 2 ablated fibroids	42
Total number of type 3 ablated fibroids	3
Total number of type 4 ablated fibroids	25
Total number of type 2–5 (transmural) ablated fibroids	8
Mean diameter of ablated fibroids	3.2±1.4 cm (range 1.1–6.9 cm)

[a] Includes three fibroids that were ablated in a subject whose MRI data was not evaluable with regard to precise fibroid measurements

Table 4 Reduction in mean perfused and total fibroid volumes through 12 months

	Baseline	3 months	% Reduction from baseline	P value[a]	12 months[b]	% Reduction from baseline	P value[a]
No. of ablated fibroids	89	89			43		
No. of subjects	49	49			28		
Perfused fibroid volume (cm^3)	18.3±20.6 9.5 (0.3–77.0)	5.8±9.6 1.6 (0.0–45.7)	68.1±28.6 % 76.9 % (−33.3 to 100 %)	<.001	6.6±11.3 1.0 (0.0–56.1)	67.4±31.9 % 73.3 % (−32.7 to 100 %)	<.001
Total fibroid volume (cm^3)	18.8±21.4 9.5 (0.3–77.0)	8.0±12.0 1.9 (0.0–56.3)	54.7±37.4 % 62.5 % (−85.7 to 100 %)	<.001	6.8±11.4 1.2 (0.0–56.1)	66.6±32.1 % 73.3 % (-32.7–100 %)	<.001

Data are mean±standard deviation; median (range)

[a] Wilcoxon signed-rank test, null hypothesis of no change

[b] A 12-month MRI study was added through a protocol amendment after several patients had been treated, and 28 patients provided informed consent to undergo this additional imaging study

procedure over a 12-month period. These included seven women with dysmenorrhea, six with abnormal uterine bleeding above baseline, four with pelvic pain and/or cramping, two urinary tract infections (both within 30 days of treatment), and one fibroid expulsion that had no significant consequences. There were two readmissions within 30 days of the procedure. One patient was admitted overnight on post-procedure day #9 to receive parenteral antibiotics for lower abdominal pain believed secondary to cystitis (one of the two instances of urinary tract infection previously noted) and was discharged on the following day. Another patient developed bradycardia down to 38 bpm shortly after the procedure and was kept overnight in the hospital for successful treatment with atropine and observation.

Surgical reintervention

Four patients (8 %) underwent surgical reintervention, all after 6 months post-ablation. One patient underwent hysteroscopy and nonresectoscopic endometrial ablation (ThermaChoice®; Ethicon, Somerville, NJ) at 10 months. At the time of her endometrial ablation, hysteroscopy confirmed the presence of a normal endometrial cavity; no residual fibroid tissue was noted. Two patients, both treated by the same investigator, underwent hysteroscopic myomectomy at 6.5 and 7 months post-ablation, respectively, due to AUB felt secondary to fibroid sloughing. In both cases, the ablated fibroids had a 70–85 % reduction in perfused volume at 3 months. A fourth patient underwent total abdominal hysterectomy at 11 months secondary to abnormal uterine bleeding above baseline. The patient was noted post-operatively to have had an abnormal bleeding duration at baseline that had not been reported in her menstrual history, constituting a protocol violation. The patient may have had a component of anovulation contributing to her abnormal uterine bleeding.

Pregnancy

There was a single pregnancy reported within the first 6 months after ablation with the VizAblate System. The patient presented with 12 weeks of amenorrhea at her 6-month trial visit, had a positive pregnancy test at that time, and delivered a live-born male infant at term via elective repeat Cesarean section [14].

Return to normal activity, patient satisfaction, and pain during recovery

Forty-eight patients provided results of a 10-point visual analogue scale (VAS) regarding their pain during the recovery period (up to 14 days post-treatment). On average, they reported a mean VAS score of 3.0±1.7 (median 3.0, range 0–9). Forty-seven patients completed a recovery diary relating to how long it took them to return to their normal activities of daily life. On average, return to normal activity took 4.4± 3.1 days (median 4.0 days, range 1–14 days). There was an overall satisfaction rate of 87.8 % (43/49 patients) at 12 months; 69.4 % were "very satisfied," 10.2 % were "satisfied," and 8.2 % were "somewhat satisfied," with their treatment. At 12 months, 49 patients provided a mean scoring of 8.8±2.4 out of 10 in terms of how likely they would be to recommend the treatment to a friend or relative.

Discussion

It is of particular importance to determine how well patients fared beyond the previously reported 3- and 6-month endpoints from the FAST-EU Trial. The results outlined in this report confirm and extend the results of the 3- and 6-month endpoints and demonstrate that intrauterine sonography-

Table 5 Improvement in patient-reported outcomes through 12months

	Baseline	3months	Change from baseline	% Change from baseline	P value^a	6months	Change from baseline	% Change from baseline	P value^a	12 months	Change from baseline	% Change from baseline	P value*
MP	50 423±253 361 (119–1582)	49 202±202 170 (0–1011)	49 221±290 191 (−700, 1265)	49 45.2±57.9% 56.9% (−225–100%)	<.001	48 181±209 107 (0–1011)	48 244±302 191 (−700, 1307)	48 51.9±59.8% 68.6% (−225–100%)	<.001	48 173±200 85 (0–786)	48 243±296 217 (−343, 1543)	48 53.8±50.5% 72.3% (−103–100%)	<.001
SSS	50 61.7±16.9 60.9% (28.1–100%)	50 31.7±20.1 31.3% (0.0–93.8%)	50 30.0±22.2 31.3 (−18.8–84.4)	49 46.7%±32.8% 52.5% (−33.3–100%)	<.001	49 25.1±19.3 18.8 (0.0–78.1)	49 36.7±22.6 37.5 (−6.3, 75.0)	49 57.6±31.4% 66.7% (−22.2–100%)	<.001	49 26.6±24.0 21.9 (0.0–78.1)	49 35.3±26.9 37.5 (−18.8, 93.8)	49 55.1±41.0% 62.5% (−66.7–100%)	<.001
HRQOL	49 34.3±19.0 30.2 (0.0–73.3)	49 76.4±22.2 83.6 (5.2–100)	49 42.1±25.6 40.5 (−7.8, 95.7)	49 336±846% 123% (−11.1–5550%)	<.001	48 79.5±22.7 85.3 (0.9–100)	48 44.5±26.7 45.3 (−5.2, 96.6)	48 266±475% 118% (−28.6–2800%)	<.001	48 80.7±24.7 91.4 (0.9–100)	48 45.7±30.5 45.7 (−33.6, 96.6)	48 277±483% 127% (−54.2–2800%)	<.001

Data are number of subjects; mean±standard deviation; median (range)

MP Menstrual Pictogram, SSS Symptom Severity Score, HRQOL Health-Related Quality of Life

^a Wilcoxon Signed-Rank Test, null hypothesis of no change

guided transcervical radiofrequency ablation of fibroids provides significant reductions in fibroid volume and bleeding symptoms through 12 months.

Transcervical radiofrequency ablation avoids many of the potential complications associated with a laparoscopic or open procedure for the treatment of fibroids. There are no incisions, eliminating the potential for wound infection, seroma, and hematoma. The peritoneal cavity is not entered nor is the serosa penetrated or coagulated, so that intraperitoneal adhesiogenesis is unlikely. There is no overt risk of ureteral injury, unlike hysterectomy. In contrast to operative hysteroscopy, only a small quantity of hypotonic fluid is used for acoustic coupling, no large venous sinuses are exposed, and intrauterine pressure is not raised to levels above mean arterial pressure, avoiding the risk of significant fluid intravasation. The integral intrauterine sonography probe permits real-time visualization of the myometrium and serosa, providing a perspective of the myometrium and intramyometrial pathology that are not achievable with a hysteroscope and enabling treatment of intramural and transmural fibroids as well as larger submucous myomata.

The trial success criterion was >30 % reduction in mean target fibroid perfused volume at 3 months in at least 50 % of patients. This success criterion stems from the MR-guided focused ultrasound data of Stewart and colleagues, which found that sustained relief of fibroid symptoms up to 24 months is associated with nonperfused volume ratios >20 % after hyperthermic ablation [15]. Initially, it was not known if total fibroid volume would be significantly reduced at that early time point, which was the rationale for using reduction in perfused fibroid volume (measured via contrast-enhanced MRI) as the primary endpoint as opposed to reduction in total fibroid volume. In the FAST-EU Trial, contrast-enhanced MRI demonstrated significant mean reductions at 3 months in both the volume of perfused fibroid tissue as well as in total fibroid volume at 3 months (68.1 and 54.7 %, respectively). At 12 months, patients demonstrated significant reductions (67.4 and 66.6 %, respectively) in mean perfused and total fibroid volumes. It has been previously demonstrated that hyperthermic ablation of >20 % of a fibroid may provide sustained relief from fibroid symptoms [15].

There were statistically significant reductions in menstrual blood loss, as evidenced by 45.2, 51.9, and 53.8 % reductions in the menstrual pictogram at 3, 6, and 12 months, respectfully, as well as significant improvements in both subscales of the UFS-QOL questionnaire. The majority of patients (57.1–72.9 %, depending on time point) realized more than a 50 % reduction in their menstrual pictogram scores, with 75.5 % of patients achieving a clinically meaningful reduction in menstrual bleeding as early as 3 months after treatment. Similarly, 78–86 % patients realized at least a 10-point reduction in SSS (depending on time point), with a mean reduction from baseline of 35.3 points at 12 months; a 10-point reduction in SSS represents a moderate effect size and was required by the US Food and Drug Administration for the approval of MRgFUS [16].

Patients typically experienced mild or no pain through the first post-ablation visit. Return to normal activity was just over 4 days and patient satisfaction was high (87.8 %). Two patients (4 %) were hospitalized overnight, one for abdominal pain secondary to apparent cystitis and the other for observation after bradycardia that responded to atropine. Neither event was deemed to have been related to the VizAblate System upon review by an independent medical advisory board.

This trial has several noteworthy attributes. Care was taken to exclude women with abnormal uterine bleeding secondary to anovulation through strict adherence to the inclusion criterion regarding the menstrual history. Additionally, at least one fibroid was required to have indented the endometrial cavity, making it more likely that a patient's bleeding symptoms are largely or exclusively secondary to fibroids rather than another etiology. A core MRI facility was used to reduce variability and bias in MRI imaging quality, interpretation, and measurements relative to the primary trial endpoint. In addition, the use of multiple clinical sites included academic medical centers as well as community hospitals to provide a more realistic assessment of the use of the VizAblate System in different treatment locations.

As a nonrandomized single-arm trial that does not directly compare against another fibroid treatment, this trial cannot be used to compare treatment with VizAblate to standard fibroid therapy. Only a subset of patients (28/48 eligible; 58.3 %) underwent MRI at 12 months. Finally, follow-up was limited to 12 months; longer surveillance and greater numbers of patients will be required to establish definitive efficacy and safety data. Toward that end, a larger clinical trial is underway.

Conclusions

These results from the FAST-EU Trial demonstrate that the initial endpoint results reported at 3 and 6 months were sustained in the treated population through 12 months. Patients realized significant reductions in perfused and total fibroid volume, menstrual bleeding, overall symptoms, and improvements in quality of life. The data demonstrate the potential of intrauterine sonography-guided, transcervical radiofrequency ablation with the VizAblate System as a promising uterus-preserving technology for the treatment of submucous, intramural, and transmural fibroids without incisions or the need for general anesthesia.

Acknowledgments The authors would like to acknowledge Mark Holdbrook, PhD, for expert guidance with statistical analysis.

Adherence to ethical standards All procedures followed were in accordance with the ethical standards of the responsible committee on human experimentation (institutional and national) and with the Helsinki Declaration of 1975, as revised in 2000.

Informed consent Informed consent was obtained from all patients included in the trial.

Contributions of the Authors Doctors Bongers, Brölmann, Gupta, Veersema, Quartero, and Garza-Leal were responsible for the conception and design of the study, data collection, patient recruitment, and preparation of the manuscript and were the responsible surgeons. Dr. Toub was responsible for the conception and design of the study, data collection, data analysis and interpretation, statistical analysis, and preparation of the manuscript.

References

1. Baird DD, Dunson DB, Hill MC et al (2003) High cumulative incidence of uterine leiomyoma in black and white women: ultrasound evidence. Am J Obstet Gynecol 188(1):100–7
2. Dembek CJ, Pelletier EM, Isaacson KB et al (2007) Payer costs in patients undergoing uterine artery embolization, hysterectomy, or myomectomy for treatment of uterine fibroids. J Vasc Interv Radiol 18(10):1207–13
3. Ghezzi F, Cromi A, Bergamini V et al (2007) Midterm outcome of radiofrequency thermal ablation for symptomatic uterine myomas. Surg Endosc 21(11):2081–5
4. Luo X, Shen Y, Song WX et al (2007) Pathologic evaluation of uterine leiomyoma treated with radiofrequency ablation. Int J Gynaecol Obstet 99(1):9–13
5. Cho HH, Kim JH, Kim MR (2008) Transvaginal radiofrequency thermal ablation: a day-care approach to symptomatic uterine myomas. Aust N Z J Obstet Gynaecol 48(3):296–301
6. Iversen H, Lenz S (2008) Percutaneous ultrasound guided radiofrequency thermal ablation for uterine fibroids : A new gynecological approach. Ultrasound Obstet Gynecol 32(3):325
7. Garza-Leal JG, Toub D, León IH et al (2011) Transcervical, intrauterine ultrasound-guided radiofrequency ablation of uterine fibroids with the VizAblate System: safety, tolerability, and ablation results in a closed abdomen setting. Gynecol Surg 8(3):327–334
8. Bongers M, Brolmann H, Gupta J et al (2015) Transcervical, intrauterine ultrasound-guided radiofrequency ablation of uterine fibroids with the VizAblate(R) System: three- and six-month endpoint results from the FAST-EU study. Gynecol Surg 12(1):61–70
9. Wyatt KM, Dimmock PW, Walker TJ et al (2001) Determination of total menstrual blood loss. Fertil Steril 76(1):125–31
10. Higham JM, O'Brien PM, Shaw RW (1990) Assessment of menstrual blood loss using a pictorial chart. Br J Obstet Gynaecol 97(8):734–9

11. Warrilow G, Kirkham C, Ismail KMK et al (2004) Quantification of menstrual blood loss. Obstetrician & Gynaecologist 6(2):88–92

12. Munro MG, Critchley HO, Broder MS et al (2011) FIGO classification system (PALM-COEIN) for causes of abnormal uterine bleeding in nongravid women of reproductive age. Int J Gynaecol Obstetrics 113(1):3–13

13. Lukes AS, Muse K, Richter HE et al (2010) Estimating a meaningful reduction in menstrual blood loss for women with heavy menstrual bleeding. Curr Med Res Opin 26(11):2673–8

14. Garza-Leal JG, León IH, Toub D (2014) Pregnancy after transcervical radiofrequency ablation guided by intrauterine sonography: case report. Gynecol Surg 11(2):145–149

15. Stewart EA, Gostout B, Rabinovici J et al (2007) Sustained relief of leiomyoma symptoms by using focused ultrasound surgery. Obstet Gynecol 110(2 Pt 1):279–87

16. Stewart EA, Rabinovici J, Tempany CM et al (2006) Clinical outcomes of focused ultrasound surgery for the treatment of uterine fibroids. Fertil Steril 85(1):22–9

22

First-generation endometrial ablation revisited: retrospective outcome study—a series of 218 patients with premenopausal dysfunctional bleeding

S. Knaepen[1,3] · S. Van Calenbergh[2]

Abstract Premenopausal dysfunctional bleeding (PDB) is a common medical problem. Surgery is typically performed after the failure of a medical approach. Surgical options include endometrial ablation techniques or a hysterectomy. The aims of our study are to measure the outcome parameters of first-generation endometrial ablations (fgEA) and to identify patient-related prognostic factors. We included all fgEAs performed between September 2001 and December 2011 at the General Hospital of Turnhout, Belgium (n=218). The outcome was defined by the need for a postoperative therapy (group 1—no therapy; group 2—therapy, but no hysterectomy; group 3—hysterectomy). We also rated postoperative amenorrhea and patient satisfaction. The prognostic factors examined were associated dysmenorrhea, a history of cesarean section, preoperative duration of blood loss, age, parity, and a history of tubal ligation sterilization. We used Excel 2011, Version 14.0.0, and Statplus Mac LE 2009 for our statistical analysis. The hysterectomy rate post-fgEA was 10 % (22/218). The rate of amenorrhea (defined as cessation of bleeding from 3 months postprocedure until the moment the patient was interviewed) was 76 % (165/218). Ninety-two percent (202/218) of patients were either satisfied or very satisfied with the procedure and outcome. The only significant prognostic factor was the age of the patient at the time of the fgEA (p=0.0004 for mean age at time of fgEA and p=0.0433 for comparison pre- versus perimenopausal age). The outcome of this fgEA technique is often underestimated and can still result in a high amenorrhea and satisfaction rate and low postoperative hysterectomy rate.

Keywords Premenopausal dysfunctional bleeding · Treatment · First-generation endometrial ablation · Hysterectomy rate · Amenorrhea rate · Patient satisfaction · Prognostic factors

Background

Premenopausal dysfunctional bleeding (PDB) is a very common reason for women to consult a general practitioner or gynecologist. Approximately one third of women will be affected by heavy or abnormal uterine bleeding at some point in their lives. While PDB significantly diminishes the quality of life, serious complications are rare [1].

Causes can be anatomical (uterine fibroids, adenomyosis, endometrial polyps, endometrial carcinoma, uterine vascular malformations, myometrial hypertrophy), systemic (coagulation disorders, hypothyroidism, chronic liver failure, systemic lupus erythematosus), functional (dysfunctional uterine bleeding), or involve a combination of these factors. We can distinguish between a medical and a surgical approach to dealing with PDB [2].

Medical solutions include the use of levonorgestrel intrauterine systems (LNGIUS), non-steroidal anti-inflammatory drugs (NSAID), antifibrinolytic drugs (tranexamic acid), progesterones, oral contraceptives, and danazol.

✉ S. Knaepen
 knaepensenne@gmail.com

1 Department of Obstetrics and Gynecology, General Hospital Hasselt, Hasselt, Belgium

2 Department of Obstetrics and Gynecology, General Hospital Turnhout, Turnhout, Belgium

3 Rummenweg 57, 3800 Sint-Truiden, Belgium

Surgical approaches involve either a hysterectomy or less invasive endometrial resection/ablation procedures. With regard to the latter, two generations of techniques can be differentiated [3, 4]. First-generation techniques, the gold standard, involve hysteroscopy-dependent endometrial resection/ablation with resectoscopic electrosurgical instruments (rollerball, wire loop, vaporizing electrode) or with laser. Second-generation, non-resectoscopic endometrial ablation is performed with a disposable device, inserted into the uterine cavity, delivering energy to uniformly destroy the endometrial lining. This includes bipolar radiofrequency, hot liquid-filled balloon, cryotherapy, circulating hot water, and microwave techniques. These techniques demand less expertise and can sometimes be performed in an office setting, lowering the price of the procedure.

In general, in the first year after the procedure, surgery reduces menstrual bleeding to a greater extent than medical treatments, but LNGIUS appears to be equally beneficial to improving the quality of life and may control bleeding as effectively as conservative surgery over the long term. Oral medication only suits a minority of patients for a longer period [2].

When comparing different endometrial ablation generations/techniques, the 2013 Cochrane review of Lethaby et al. concludes that the existing evidence suggests comparable rates of success, satisfaction, and complications [5]. First-generation techniques have the disadvantage of higher risk of complications, such as perforation, water intoxication, and injury of the urogenital tract [6–8]. Second-generation techniques try to compensate for these weaknesses and have the advantages of being more rapid, safe, and easy to apply [3, 9–11].

Although these less invasive techniques have proven effective compared to a hysterectomy, there are still a proportion of patients for whom persisting symptoms necessitate a repeat ablation procedure or hysterectomy after a first ablation [12–14]. The 2013 Cochrane review of Fergusson and Lethaby states that both procedures are effective and that satisfaction rates are high. The advantage of a hysterectomy is the guarantee of permanent relief from bleeding. Endometrial resection/ablation is cheaper, but total costs are higher in the case of recurrence [15].

The aim of this retrospective study is to provide an overview of the outcome of first-generation endometrial ablation (fgEA) procedures performed on patients at the General Hospital of Turnhout, Belgium. We also assess possible prognostic patient-related factors, predicting the outcome of the ablation. El-Nashar et al. carried out a comparable study for second-generation endometrial ablation techniques. For a series of 816 patients, they noted an amenorrhea rate of 23 % (defined as cessation of bleeding immediately after ablation until at least 12 months after the procedure). Predictors of amenorrhea were age >45 years, uterine length <9 cm, endometrial thickness <4 mm, and use of radiofrequency ablation instead of thermal balloon ablation [16].

Methods

The study population consisted of patients undergoing an fgEA between September 2001 and December 2011 at the General Hospital of Turnhout, Belgium.

1. Satisfaction regarding the fgEA and the stay at daycare unit ?

Absolutely not satisfied	Not satisfied	Neutral opinion	Satisfied	Very satisfied
Score 1	Score 2	Score 3	Score 4	Score 5

2. Would you recommend the fgEA to friends/relatives with the same problem ?

Absolutely not	No	Neutral opinion	Yes	Absolutely
Score 1	Score 2	Score 3	Score 4	Score 5

3. Amenorrhea 3 months post-fgEA until now ?

No	Yes
Score 1	Score 2

4. What was the interval between the first bleeding symptoms and the fgEA ?

> 12 months	6 – 12 months	< 6 months
Score 1	Score 2	Score 3

5. Was any kind of therapy needed because of relapse AFTER the fgEA ? If so, please indicate the kind of therapy and the interval between the fgEA and the start of this new therapy (expressed in years).

Yes/No ? If yes: How many years after the procedure ? What kind of therapy ?
1) Hormonal medication combined estrogen-progesterone or progesterone only
2) Tranexamic acid
3) NSAID
4) LNGIUS
5) Hysterectomy
6) D and C
7) Another hysteroscopic ablation
8) Subdermal contraceptive implant

6. Was any kind of therapy applied BEFORE the fgEA ? If so, please indicate the kind of therapy and the interval between the start of this previous therapy and the fgEA (expressed in years).

Yes/No ? If yes: How many years before the procedure ? What kind of therapy ?
1) Hormonal medication combined estrogen-progesterone or progesterone only
2) Tranexamic acid
3) NSAID
4) LNGIUS
5) D and C
6) Subdermal contraceptive implant
7) Another hysteroscopic ablation

7. What kind of contraception was used since the procedure?

1) Copper-containing IUS
2) Condom
3) Sexual withdrawal peri-ovulatory
4) None
5) Patient had a sterilisation
6) Patient's partner had a sterilisation

8. The following questions apply to the moment the procedure was performed:

1) How many children did you have?
2) Did you have any twins or triplets ?
3) Can you tell me for every childbirth whether the way of delivery was vaginally or by caesarean section ?
4) Did you ever have a provocated abortion ?
5) Did you ever have a miscarriage ?

Fig. 1 Questionnaire

Until 2009, a unipolar loop technique was applied. After that, a bipolar loop mode was used. The procedures in our center were performed by two gynecologists, using the exact analogue method of transcervical resection of the endometrium. A radical resection of the endometrial lining over the total area of the cavity was applied. This was achieved using a technique developed and perfected over many years with resection up to the level of the myometrium over the anterior and posterior wall as well as the fundus, including the area of the ostia and the central part, up to the endocervical canal. Significant bleeding points were also coagulated. The minimum follow-up period was almost 2 years, as data collection started at the end of 2013.

A first inclusion criterion was a preoperative indication of PDB. All postoperative anatomopathological examinations were reviewed and cases of malignancies, myomas, polyps, and atypical hyperplasia were excluded. Postmenopausal patients were excluded as well. The preoperative bleeding patterns were menorrhagia or metrorrhagia, while intermenstrual blood loss was excluded. Patients who used hormonal contraception after the fgEA were excluded, as this could have been a confounding factor for the outcome.

By reviewing the patients' case notes and by contacting all patients by phone, we completed a questionnaire consisting of eight questions (Fig. 1). The first two questions emphasized on patient satisfaction. The third question estimated the amenorrhea rate. The fourth question determined how long the patient had suffered from PDB, before the procedure was applied. The next question concerned postoperative recurrence of the bleeding disorder. In the case of recurrence, we determined the timing of the associated intervention applied. Question six dealt with the therapeutic options used before the resection procedure and their timing related to the fgEA, while question seven investigated contraceptive methods used since the operation. The last question assessed the obstetric history of the patient. The remaining data was obtained by reviewing the patients' case notes.

Therapeutic options for PDB were defined as hormonal medication (combined estrogen-progesterone or progesterone only, applied in an oral or transdermal way or using ring application), LNGIUS, subdermal contraceptive implant, tranexamic acid, NSAID, hysterectomy, dilatation/curettage, and hysteroscopic ablation. Danazol was not included as it is no longer available in Belgium. Hormonal pretreatment before the fgEA is not a standard practice in our hospital.

Three categories of outcome were determined based on whether patients required additional therapy or not and on the type of intervention needed in case of failure. Group 1 involved patients who did not require therapy after the operation. Group 2 involved patients who required some kind of therapy after the operation, but not a hysterectomy. Group 3 involved patients who required a hysterectomy after primary ablation therapy.

We investigated the following prognostic parameters: dysmenorrhea versus no dysmenorrhea associated with the problem of PDB, a history of cesarean section, the duration of preoperative blood loss, age, and a parous compared to a nulliparous obstetric history. We also compared the outcome between premenopausal and perimenopausal women. Perimenopause was defined based on a minimum age of 47 years [17]. Finally, we emphasized on the influence of a history of tubal ligation sterilization.

Dysmenorrhea was examined because it can be a negative prognostic factor for patients still experiencing pain rather than problematic bleeding after the fgEA, thus necessitating further therapy. Parity could influence the volume of the uterus and, hence, also the operative technique and outcome. Also, in a uterus with a cesarean section scar, radical resection at the level of the anterior uterine isthmus could be limited due to risks of perforation.

Table 1 Patient characteristics

Age (mean) at the time of fgEA in years	43.81 ± 5.1
Parity (mean) at the time of fgEA	2.12 ± 0.98
History of cesarean section at the time of fgEA	41 (19 %)
Preoperative bleeding pattern	
Menorrhagia	202 (93 %)
Metrorrhagia	16 (7 %)
Dysmenorrhea associated with the problem of PDB	39 (18 %)
Duration of blood loss before the fgEA in months	
>12	160 (73 %)
6–12	45 (21 %)
<6	13 (6 %)
Therapy before the fgEA	119 (55 %)
Hormonal medication	85 (39 %)
Tranexamic acid	17 (8 %)
NSAID	7 (3 %)
LNGIUS	35 (16 %)
Dilation/curettage	20 (9 %)
Subdermal contraceptive implant	2 (1 %)
Another hysteroscopic ablation	1 (<1 %)
Therapy after the fgEA	36 (17 %)
Hormonal medication	9 (4 %)
Tranexamic acid	2 (1 %)
NSAID	0 (0 %)
LNGIUS	4 (2 %)
Hysterectomy	**22 (10 %)**
Dilation/curettage	2 (1 %)
Another hysteroscopic ablation	1 (<1 %)
Subdermal contraceptive implant	1 (<1 %)
Interval (mean) between previous therapy and the fhEA in years	2.94 ± 3.75
Interval (mean) between the fhEA therapy after in years	1.38 ± 1.42

Mean (±standard deviation) or fraction (a total of 218 patients)

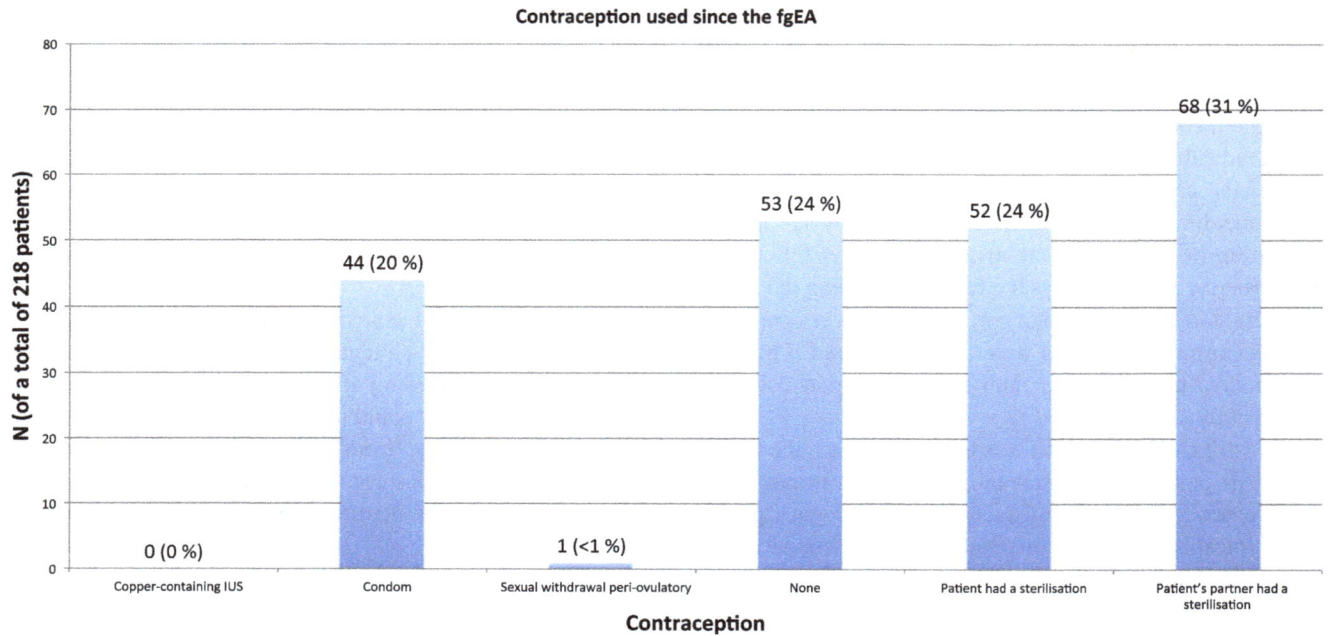

Fig. 2 Contraception used since the fgEA

Amenorrhea was defined as cessation of blood loss from 3 months post-fgEA until the moment the patient was contacted to complete the study questionnaire.

We used Excel 2011, Version 14.0.0, and Statplus Mac LE 2009, analysis of variance, and chi-square analysis for our statistical investigations. For all statistical analyses, a p value cutoff of <0.05 was considered significant.

Findings

A total of 363 patients were retained in the first phase, and eventually, 218 patients were included in our study. Patients were excluded if they did not fit the inclusion criteria (e.g., postoperative malignant pathological analysis, postmenopausal state, intermenstrual bleeding pattern).

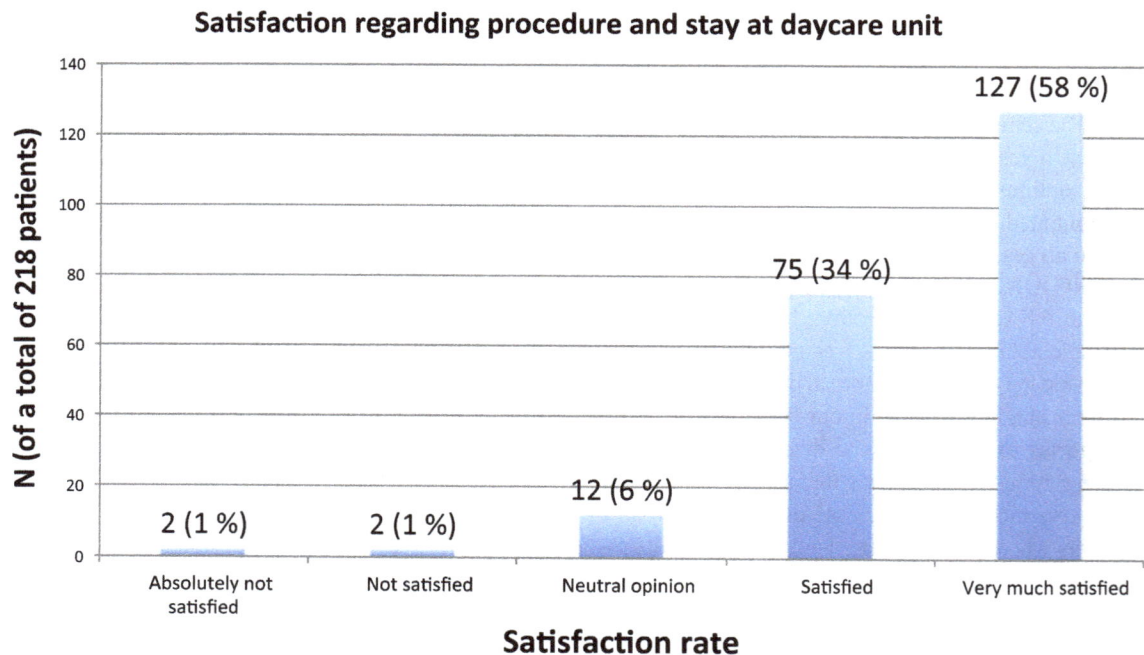

Fig. 3 Satisfaction regarding procedure and stay at daycare unit

Would you recommend the procedure to friends or relatives?

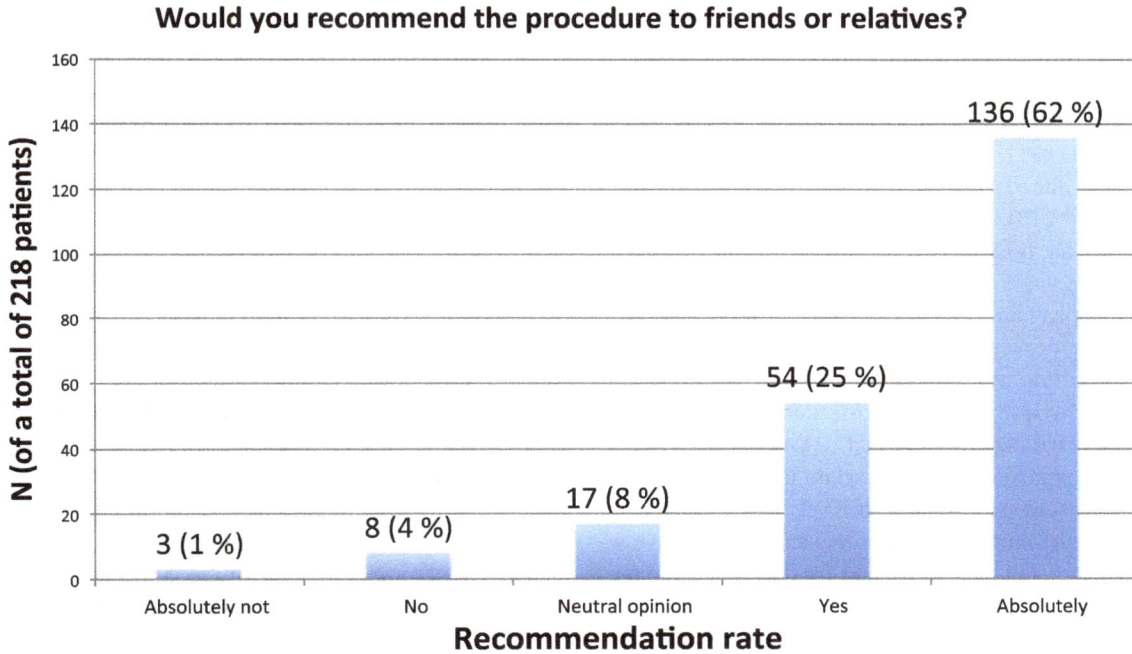

Fig. 4 Would you recommend the procedure to friends or relatives?

Table 1 gives an overview of patient characteristics. All percentages are calculated using the same denominator: 218, which is the total number of patients included. The age of included patients at the time of the fgEA ranged from 25 to 55 years. Parity ranged from 0 to 5. Since some people received multiple therapeutic options before the procedure, the absolute sum of pre-fgEA therapeutic approaches is higher than 119. The same applies to post-fgEA therapy. To calculate

Table 2 Statistical analysis on prognostic factors

Therapy after fgEA?	None Group 1	Yes, but no hysterectomy Group 2	Yes, but hysterectomy Group 3	p value	Statistical test
Dysmenorrhea associated?					
No (179 patients)	154 (71 %)	10 (5 %)	15 (7 %)	0.0921	Chi-square
Yes (39 patients)	28 (13 %)	4 (2 %)	7 (3 %)		
History of caesarian section					
No (177 patients)	148 (68 %)	11 (5 %)	18 (8 %)	0.9654	Chi-square
Yes (41 patients)	34 (16 %)	3 (1 %)	4 (2 %)		
Duration of preoperative blood loss					
>12 months (160 patients)	133 (46 %)	10 (3 %)	17 (6 %)	0.9935	Chi-square
6–12 months (45 patients)	38 (13 %)	3 (1 %)	4 (1 %)		
<6 months (13 patients)	11 (4 %)	1 (<1 %)	1 (1 %)		
Mean age at time of EA in years	42±4.88	43.64±5.98	39.77±5.28	0.0004	Analysis of variance
Pre-versus perimenopausal age at time of fgEA					
Premenopausal	121 (56 %)	8 (4 %)	20 (9 %)	0.0433	Chi-square
Perimenopausal	61 (28 %)	9 (3 %)	2 (1 %)		
Nulliparous versus parous					
Nullipara (13 patients)	10 (5 %)	1 (<1 %)	2 (1 %)	0.7828	Chi-square
Para (205 patients)	172 (79 %)	13 (6 %)	20 (9 %)		
History of sterilization?					
No (166 patients)	139 (64 %)	10 (5 %)	17 (8 %)	0.9084	Chi-square
Yes (52 patients)	43 (20 %)	4 (2 %)	5 (2 %)		

Mean (±standard deviation) or fraction (a total of 218 patients)

the mean interval between the fgEA and therapy (before or after), we noted all therapy intervals, divided by the total number of applied therapeutic options. The percentage of women who did not receive any kind of therapy after the fgEA (group 1) was 83 % (182/218). The proportion of women who needed therapy due to recurrence, but no hysterectomy (group 2), was 6 % (14/218). It turns out that the hysterectomy rate (group 3) after the fgEA was 10 % (22/218) of all cases. The amenorrhea rate was 76 % (165/218).

Figure 2 depicts an overview of contraception used after the fgEA. None of these options affect blood loss, since hormonal contraception was excluded.

Figures 3 and 4 describe patient satisfaction. For both question 1 (satisfaction regarding procedure and stay at daycare unit) and question 2 (recommendation of procedure to friends/relatives), the majority of women responded positively or very positively. For question 1, the proportion of positive and very positive responses was 92 % (34 %+58 %), and for question 2, the proportion was 87 % (25 %+62 %).

Table 2 is a synthesis of our findings on prognostic factors for the outcome of the fgEA. It turns out that only one of these is statistically significant: age at time of the fgEA ($p=0.0004$ for mean age at time of fgEA and $p=0.0433$ for comparison pre- versus perimenopausal age). No significant difference was seen for associated dysmenorrhea ($p=0.0921$), history of cesarean section ($p=0.9654$), or duration of preoperative blood loss ($p=0.9935$). Neither did there appear to be a significant difference in outcome when comparing parous versus nulliparous women ($p=0.7828$) or comparing patients with or without a history of tubal ligation sterilization ($p=0.9084$).

Conclusions

Table 1 shows that hormonal oral medication is still the first approach to the problem of PDB, followed by LNGIUS and dilatation/curettage. In the case of recurrence after fgEA, the most commonly chosen option is hysterectomy (partly explained by the fact that in most cases, the majority of conservative approaches have already been tried), followed by hormonal medication and LNGIUS. A consequence of radical ablation is impaired fertility or even total infertility. This explains why the procedure is only performed in those patients who do not plan to have (more) children in the future. Therefore, the mean age at fgEA is 43.81±5.15 years.

The most common methods of contraception after the fgEA (Fig. 2) were a vasectomy, tubal ligation sterilization, and the use of condoms. A significant proportion of patients no longer used contraception, typically those of an advanced age, because they assumed no longer to be fertile. Others were not sexually active.

We defined amenorrhea as cessation of blood loss starting from 3 months postprocedure instead of immediately after the fgEA. The reason for this is that in the first postoperative period, the healing reaction itself typically causes blood loss. There is also the possible expulsion of some retained resected tissue that could not be removed during the operation. We tried to quantify the amount of blood loss pre- versus postprocedure. However, since the operation had been performed at least 2 years before the time of our interviews, we found that patients were unable to recall exact details. This is why we used the simple approach of a postoperative amenorrhea versus no amenorrhea rate.

Figure 3 shows a very high satisfaction rate with respect to the procedure itself. Patients were highly motivated to recommend the procedure to others (Fig. 4).

The statistical analysis of prognostic factors in Table 2 shows that associated dysmenorrhea has a tendency to be a negative prognostic factor for the outcome. We notice a higher likelihood of a patient requiring extra therapy after the fgEA and a higher rate of post-fgEA hysterectomies. The same is true for a younger age at the time of the fgEA. It could be that the associated dysmenorrhea itself, regardless of the PDB, is sometimes the real indication for therapy afterwards. Concerning the differences based on age, one would expect that older patients would have a better long-term outcome, since some of them reach menopause in the first years after the fgEA.

A limitation of this study is its retrospective nature, restricting the possibility of examining additional possible prognostic factors, such as body mass index and hemoglobin. Another shortcoming of the retrospective approach is the difficulty some patients experience in recalling the details relevant to answering our questionnaire. This is why a quantification of pre- versus postoperative blood loss was impossible. This could be an interesting prognostic factor to examine in prospective studies.

We conclude that the fgEA technique is very effective in the treatment of PDB, particularly for perimenopausal patients. The results show a high satisfaction rate, a high percentage of postoperative amenorrhea, and a low number of hysterectomies required afterwards. Given these findings, the added value of less invasive (first-generation) endometrial ablation techniques should be reconsidered.

Authors' contributions Project development was accomplished by S. Van Calenbergh. Data collection and manuscript writing was performed by S. Knaepen.

Informed consent Informed consent was obtained from all individual participants included in the study. We received a signed approval from the local ethics committee as well.

Statement of responsibility I, Senne Knaepen, the corresponding author, declare that (a) every author allowed me to serve as the primary contact person, (b) I received consent for publication from every author, and (c) every author contributed sufficiently to the development of this manuscript.

References

1. Bonafede MM, Miller JD, Laughlin-Tommaso SK et al (2014) Retrospective database analysis of clinical outcomes and costs for treatment of abnormal uterine bleeding among women enrolled in US Medicaid programs. Clinicoecon Outcomes Res 6:423–429
2. Marjoribanks J, Lethaby A, Farquhar C (2003) Surgery versus medical therapy for heavy menstrual bleeding. Cochrane Database Syst Rev 2:CD003855
3. Lethaby A, Hickey M, Garry R et al (2009) Endometrial resection/ablation techniques for heavy menstrual bleeding. Cochrane Database Syst Rev 4:CD001501
4. Woods S, Taylor B (2013) Global ablation techniques. Obstet Gynecol Clin North Am 40(4):687–695
5. Lethaby A, Penninx J, Hickey M et al (2013) Endometrial resection and ablation techniques for heavy menstrual bleeding. Cochrane Database Syst Rev 8:CD001501
6. Pinion SB, Parkin DE, Abramovich DR et al (1994) Randomised trial of hysterectomy, endometrial laser ablation, and transcervical endometrial resection for dysfunctional uterine bleeding. BMJ 309(6960):979–983
7. Sinha A (1999) A randomised trial of endometrial ablation versus hysterectomy for the treatment of dysfunctional uterine bleeding: outcome at four years. Br J Obstet Gynaecol 106(9):1002
8. Vilos GA, Brown S, Graham G et al (2000) Genital tract electrical burns during hysteroscopic endometrial ablation: report of 13 cases in the United States and Canada. J Am Assoc Gynecol Laparosc 7(1):141–147
9. Madhu CK, Nattey J, Naeem T (2009) Second generation endometrial ablation techniques: an audit of clinical practice. Arch Gynecol Obstet 280(4):599–602
10. Kroft J, Liu G (2013) First- versus second-generation endometrial ablation devices for treatment of menorrhagia: a systematic review, meta-analysis and appraisal of economic evaluations. J Obstet Gynaecol Can 35(11):1010–1019
11. Daniels JP, Middleton LJ, Champaneria R (2012) Second generation endometrial ablation techniques for heavy menstrual bleeding: network meta-analysis. BMJ 23 344:E2564
12. Bansi-Matharu L, Gurol-Urganci I, Mahmood TA et al (2013) Rates of subsequent surgery following endometrial ablation among English women with menorrhagia: population-based cohort study. BJOG 120(12):1500–1507
13. Shavell VI, Diamond MP, Senter JP et al (2012) Hysterectomy subsequent to endometrial ablation. J Minim Invasive Gynecol 19(4):459–464
14. Longinotti MK, Jacobson GF, Hung YY et al (2008) Probability of hysterectomy after endometrial ablation. Obstet Gynecol 112(6):1214–1220
15. Fergusson RJ, Lethaby A, Shepperd S (2013) Endometrial resection and ablation versus hysterectomy for heavy menstrual bleeding. Cochrane Database Syst Rev 29 11:CD000329
16. El-Nashar SA, Hopkins MR, Creedon DJ et al (2009) Prediction of treatment outcomes after global endometrial ablation. Obstet Gynecol 113(1):97–106
17. McKinlay SM, Brambilla DJ, Posner JG (2008) The normal menopause transition. Maturitas 61(1-2):4–16

23

Office Hysteroscopy. An operative gold standard technique and an important contribution to Patient Safety

J. Mairos [1] · P. Di Martino [1]

Abstract According to World Health Organization (WHO), about 1 out of 10 hospitalized patients suffers an adverse event, in developed countries, being an adverse event an injury related to medical management, in contrast to complications of disease. These events cause both unnecessary suffering and huge cost to health systems. This issue is so important that WHO has defined it as a global health problem and in 2004 launched the World Alliance for Patient Safety, with the aim to coordinate, disseminate and accelerate improvements in Patient Safety. Office Hysteroscopy (OH), as an independent technique of the hospital circuit, has the ideal conditions to be qualified as the gold standard technique for the surgical treatment of intracavitary uterine pathology. It does not require the use of an operating room, hospital admission and general or locoregional anaesthesia. The appropriate surgical techniques, allied to pain control, allow OH to resolve much more than 90 % of the surgical needs of the intracavitary uterine pathology, thus being an important contribution for Patient Safety.

Keywords Office Hysteroscopy · Patient Safety · Health Quality

Background

The problem of adverse events in health care is known since 1950s. The subject remained largely neglected until early 1990s, when the results of the Harvard Medical Practice Study in 1991 [1, 2] warned of the dimension of the problem in a new economic and social context. Subsequent research in Australia [3], the United Kingdom of Great Britain and Northern Ireland [4] and the USA and in particular the 1999 publication *To err is human: building a safer health system by the Institute of Medicine* [5] provided further data and brought the subject to the top of the policy agenda and the forefront of public debate worldwide. Today, this is a well-known problem and the World Health Organization launched in 2004 the World Alliance for Patient Safety. Some facts mentioned in this Forward Programme in 2004 (http://www.who.int/patientsafety/worldalliance/en/) illustrate the problem:

Estimates show that in developed countries as many as 1 in 10 patients is harmed while receiving hospital care. The harm can be caused by a range of errors or adverse events (http://www.who.int/patientsafety/worldalliance/en/).

Hospital infections affect 14 out of every 100 patients admitted (http://www.who.int/patientsafety/worldalliance/en/).

Surgical care is associated with a considerable risk of complications. Surgical care errors contribute to a significant burden of disease despite the fact that 50 % of complications associated with surgical care are avoidable (http://www.who.int/patientsafety/worldalliance/en/).

Safety studies show that additional hospitalization, litigation costs, infections acquired in hospitals, disability, lost productivity and medical expenses cost some countries as much as US$ 19 billion annually. The economic benefits of improving Patient Safety are therefore compelling (http://www.who.int/patientsafety/worldalliance/en/).

Industries with a perceived higher risk such as the aviation and nuclear industries have a much better safety record than health care. There is 1 in 1,000,000 chances of a traveler being harmed while in an aircraft. In comparison, there is 1 in 300

✉ J. Mairos
joaomairos@sapo.pt

[1] Department of Gynecology and Obstetrics, Hospital das Forças Armadas - Pólo de Lisboa, Azinhaga dos Ulmeiros, 1649-020 Lisbon, Portugal

chances of a patient being harmed during health care (http://www.who.int/patientsafety/worldalliance/en/).

There is now growing recognition that Patient Safety and Quality are a critical dimension of universal health coverage.

A research carried out in three public hospitals in great Lisbon area in 2011 based on a sample of 1669 hospitalized patients and a total of 47,783 hospital admissions showed an Adverse Event's (AE) incidence of 11.1%, and the most critical places were the room or nursery (49.7 % of the AE) and the operating room (23.9 % of the AE) [6].

Regarding office practice in gynaecological and obstetrics procedures, a task force was convened in 2008 by the American College of Obstetricians and Gynaecologists (ACOG). The primary impetus to creating this task force was the steady migration of surgical procedures to the office that had solely been performed in the hospital or ambulatory surgical center, and this transition began with hysteroscopy in the 1980s [7].

In 2004, Bettochi et al. [8] reported on 4863 operative hysteroscopic procedures performed using a 5.0-mm diameter operative hysteroscope and 5F instruments. The procedures included the removal of cervical and endometrial polyps along with adhesiolysis and repair of "anatomic impediments", by using a vaginoscopic technique "without analgesics or anaesthesia", and noted that patients reported little discomfort, although those undergoing removal of endometrial polyps were more likely to experience "moderate" discomfort [9].

So, why would Office Hysteroscopy be such an important contribution for the Patient Safety?

Because, firstly, it is a procedure independent from the hospital circuit, thus avoiding risk of adverse events associated to hospitalization. Secondly, OH has clear advantages before operating room (OR) hysteroscopy, eliminating complications of general or locoregional anaesthesia, being limited only by its surgical ability and pain control.

Methods

All our OH have been performed by *see and treat* hysteroscopy and by vaginoscopic approach at the Department of Gynaecology and Obstetrics of the Hospital das Forças Armadas in Lisbon.

Preceding all hysteroscopies, patients were evaluated regarding need to treat vaginal pathological discharge, need for local or systemic hormonal treatment and use of misoprostol.

All patients were submitted to pelvic transvaginal ultrasound prior to procedure.

In the day of the hysteroscopy, rectal 10 mg butylscopolamine with 800 mg paracetamol and oral 5 mg diazepam were administered to all patients before the procedure.

Hysteroscopies were performed using rigid 5Fr Bettocchi® hysteroscopes with 30° optic. The distension medium used was saline solution at 37 °C, and the electrodes were Twizzle type bipolar from Versapoint®, apart from mechanical instruments. Hysteroscopic anaesthesia (HA), a method of local anaesthesia using an endoscopic needle, was given when requested by the patients, using a Williams Cystoscopic Injection Needle, 22 ga (length 35 cm, point 8 mm) [10]. This method was first described in 2009 by Skensved [11] and allows administration of focal local uterosacral, endocervical or even intracavitary anaesthesia (1 % lidocaine), under hysteroscopic visualization, with no need to interrupt the procedure or use of speculum [10]. When HA was decided, according to specific locations, 1 % lidocaine was injected through the hysteroscope: around 1 cm^3 per location in the endocervical region, near the internal os or intracavitarily, or 2 cm^3 at both uterosacral ligaments, if necessary, to a limit of 10 cm^3 maximum per hysteroscopy.

Procedures were performed by both experienced hysteroscopists and trainees, recorded on DVD, photographed and registered in our database during the global period of February 2012 to April 2014, accordingly to Table 1.

We questioned the patients about pain felt during procedures, by an anonymous survey using a 0–10 pain scale, in which 0 corresponded to no pain and 10 to maximum pain experienced before.

We rely on three retrospective studies conducted in our department: one between April 2011 and April 2014 (330 procedures) that assessed the number of patients sent to the OR, another between May 2010 and March 2012 (207 procedures) that evaluated effectiveness of HA and another between January 2010 and December 2012 (230 procedures) that evaluated the dimensions of the excised masses in OH.

Findings

In our study that assessed the efficacy of Office Hysteroscopy, 45 % of women were in premenopause and 55 % of them were in postmenopause. Regarding parity, 28 % were nulliparous or never had a vaginal delivery and 72 % had at least one vaginal delivery. Procedures were performed by both experienced hysteroscopists and trainees and were chirurgical in 239 cases,

Table 1 Characterization of hysteroscopies according to the degree of professional experience

Office Hysteroscopy		Hysteroscopic time (average—min)			Sent to OR
		Total	Experts	Trainees	
Diagnostic	24.7 %	24.6	21.7	24.6	5.7 %
Operative	75.3 %				

mainly polypectomies (191), followed by myomectomies (29), tubal ligation by Essure® (24) and adhesion lysis (3). We performed 87 diagnostic hysteroscopies.

Of the total 330 hysteroscopies, only 23 % had HA. Fifty-six per cent of those patients who received HA referred good tolerance to the procedure, 37 % had a level of pain between 7 and 10, on a 0–10 scale, and in 7 %, the procedure was not concluded.

In this study, we concluded that OH was successful in about 92–95 % of the cases [9], without resorting to the OR. The procedures were generally well tolerated. In 330 cases by "see and treat" OH, 97.85 % [12] of the cases were successfully concluded and only 2.15% [9] of the patients were sent to the OR.

In the study that evaluated effectiveness of HA, patients had ages between 14 and 91 years (average 54); 95 of them were in premenopause and 112 in post menopause [12]. Regarding parity, 49 were nulliparous or never had a vaginal delivery and 158 had at least one vaginal delivery [12]. Procedures were performed by both experienced hysteroscopists and trainees and were chirurgical in 148 cases, mainly polypectomies (119), followed by myomectomies (15), tubal ligation by Essure® (15) and adhesion lysis (1) [12]. Only 59 hysteroscopies were diagnostic [12].

We concluded the procedure in 85 % [12] of patients, with mild to moderate pain referred. When HA was administered, in 54 cases [12], the intensity of pain was clearly inferior, allowing procedure closure in 93 % [12] of these patients, which otherwise would be sent to OR. Therefore, it proved to be effective and more comfortable to the patient, since there is no need for the use of speculum or procedure interruption.

In the study that evaluated the dimensions of the excised masses, patients had ages between 14 and 91 years (average 57), 40 % of them were in premenopause and 60 % in post-menopause [13]. Regarding parity, 26 % were nulliparous or never had a vaginal delivery and 74 % had at least one vaginal delivery [13]. Procedures were performed by both experienced hysteroscopists and trainees and were all chirurgical, mainly polypectomy, followed by myomectomy [13]. The biggest polyp removed was 72 mm long, and the biggest myoma was 58 mm long [13].

Population was divided in three groups, considering removed masses size: group 1, masses measuring less than 2 cm (158 procedures); group 2, masses of 2 cm or larger and inferior to 5 cm (55 procedures); and group 3, masses of 5 cm or larger (17 procedures) [13].

Most patients reported only slight pain or discomfort during the procedure [13]. The pain level was ≤5 in 73.1 % [13] of patients. Only 17 % [13] requested HA and 10 % [13] expressed willingness for general anaesthesia, but only 7.4 % were sent to OR, 52 % of those belonging to group 1 [13].On univariate analysis, size or number of masses was not related to the intensity of pain felt, or with the willingness for general anaesthesia [13].

We concluded that the probability of more than one procedure per mass was higher with larger masses, being 20 % of patients submitted to more than one hysteroscopy. Masses smaller than 2 cm did not need more than two procedures, and one patient with a mass larger than 5 cm needed four procedures [13].

In this study, we were able to excise 17 masses larger than 5 cm [13], thus concluding that the removal of masses larger than 5 cm is practicable in OH.

In 92.6 % [13] of patients, we were able to avoid the risks associated with general or locoregional anaesthesia as well as the adverse effects and costs associated to hospitalization.

Conclusions

Office Hysteroscopy is a safe and effective technique, independent of the hospital circuit, not requiring the use of OR, hospital admission and general or locoregional anaesthesia, being therefore an important contribution for Patient Safety and Health Quality in gynaecology. Actually, OH has the ideal conditions to be qualified as the gold standard technique for the surgical treatment of intracavitary uterine pathology.

HA guaranties more comfort to the patient because it is speculum free and needs no hysteroscopy interruption. The use of HA, only when solicited, reduces costs and risks, effectively reducing pain, which allows closure of the procedure. Its focal characteristic also enhance HO capability, especially in myomectomies, where it can be administrated intracavitarily, preventing posterior OR procedure.

The removal of masses larger than 5 cm is controversial, but is possible, although it might imply more procedures per mass. That factor does not limit OH capability since the intensity of pain felt, or the willingness for general anaesthesia, is not directly related to the number of procedures.

It is therefore feasible to remove these masses, although it is technically challenging for the experienced hysteroscopist, because it implies balancing the tolerability of the patient and the control of the uterine cavity.

References

1. Brennan TA, Leape LL, Laird N, et al. (1991) Incidence of adverse events and negligence in hospitalised patients: results of the Harvard Medical Practice Study. N Engl J Med 324(6):370–377

2. Leape LL, Brennan TA, Laird N, et al. (1991) The nature of adverse events in hospitalized patients. Results of the Harvard Medical Practice Study II. N Engl J Med 324(6):377–384

3. Wilson RM, Runciman WB, Gibberd RW, et al. (1995) The Quality in Australian Health Care Study. Med J Aust 163:458–471

4. Vincent C, Neale G, Woloshynowych M (2001) Adverse events in British hospitals: preliminary retrospective record review. Br Med J 322:517–519

5. Kohn LT, Corrigan JM, Donaldson MS Eds. 1999 To err is human: building a safer health system. Institute of Medicine, National Academy Press

6. Sousa P, Uva AS, Serranheira F, et al. (2011) Eventos adversos em hospitais portugueses: estudo piloto de incidência, impacte e evitabilidade. Escola Nacional de Saúde Pública, Lisboa

7. Keats JP (2013) –12-01 Patient Safety in the obstetrics and gynecologic office setting. Obstet Gynecol Clin 40(Issue 4):611–623

8. Bettochi S, Ceci O, Nappi L, et al. (2004) Operative hysteroscopy without anesthesia: analysis of 4863 cases performed with mechanical instruments. J Am Assoc Gynecol 11:59–61

9. Wortman M, Daggett A, Ball C (2013) 01-01 Operative hysteroscopy in an office-based surgical setting: review of Patient Safety and satisfaction in 414 cases. J Minim Invasive Gynecol 20(Issue 1):56–63

10. Vinagre C, Mairos J, Di Martino P (2013) Hysteroscopic anesthesia: a new method of anesthesia in ambulatory hysteroscopy. Acta Obstet Ginecol Port 7(4):274–277

11. Skensved H. 2009 Treatment of symptomatic submucous fibroids in a true office setting: enucleation of fibroids in focal anaesthesia—a report on 401 cases. ESGE Congr 28–30 October

12. Mairos J, Di Martino P 2014 An operative gold standard technique and an important contribution to Patient Safety. ESGE Congr 24–27 September

13. Rodrigues M, Di Martino P, Mairos J (2014) Excision of intracavitary masses in Office Hysteroscopy—what are the limits? Acta Obstet Ginecol Port 8(3):252–256

24

Intravesical mini-laparoscopic repair of vesicovaginal fistulas

Antoni Llueca [1,2] (ID) · Jose Luis Herraiz [1,2] · Miguel Rodrigo [1,2] · Yasmin Mazzouzi [1,2] ·
Dolores Piquer [1,2] · Miriam Guijarro [1,2] · Arhoa Cañete [1,2] · Javier Escrig [1,2]

Abstract Vesicovaginal fistulas (VVF) constitute the most common type of genitourinary fistulas. In developed countries, VVF are almost always iatrogenic and frequently a secondary result of gynecological surgery. Some minimally invasive techniques have been introduced to decrease the morbidity related to standard open procedures for the treatment of VVF. One such procedure is the intravesical mini-laparoscopic approach. The aim of this study was to present our initial clinical experience using this technique for transvesical VVF repair. In 2013 and 2014, we carried out mini-laparoscopic repair of VVF in two women who did not respond to conservative treatment with a Foley catheter. The procedure was performed transvesically with a 3-mm instrument and a 5-mm, 30° scope. The fistulous tract was dissected and partially excised. The bladder and vaginal wall defects were closed in two layers with two separated continuous barbed, resorbable 3-0 sutures (V-Loc 90 Absorbable Wound Closure Device; Covidien, Norwalk, CT, USA). The median operative time for the two patients was approximately 100 min, and the blood loss was not clinically significant. The patients were released from the hospital 24 h after surgery. A Foley catheter was left in place for 14 days. Imaging examinations performed 6 weeks postoperatively revealed no VVF. In patients with simple fistulas, this technique provides a minimally invasive, easily reproducible approach with few associated complications. Nevertheless, further experience and observations are necessary.

Keywords Vesicovaginal fistula · Minimally invasive surgery · Mini-laparoscopy

Introduction

Vesicovaginal fistulas (VVF) constitute the most common type of genitourinary fistulas. In developed countries, VVF are almost always iatrogenic and frequently a secondary result of gynecological surgery. In underdeveloped countries, obstetric treatment is the primary cause of VVF [1]. The incidence of VVF in developed countries such as Great Britain is 1 in 788 hysterectomies [2].

Laparoscopic surgery has undergone exponential development during the last 2 decades because of its intraoperative and postoperative advantages over conventional surgery. It is now applied in many surgical procedures. One of the described applications of laparoscopic surgery in recent years is the treatment of VVF by means of minimally invasive surgery [3, 4].

Fistulas can be treated by a vaginal or abdominal approach depending on their location. For supratrigonal fistulas in a posterior position with difficult vaginal approach, one of the most used techniques is that described by O'Connor [5], in which the fistula is addressed transvesically, carrying out anterior cystotomy to reach the posterior aspect for complete resection. The purpose of this study was to describe our initial experience with VVF repair by means of an intravesical mini-laparoscopic approach in two patients.

✉ Antoni Llueca
antonillueca@gmail.com

[1] Multidisciplinary Unit of Abdominal Pelvic Oncology Surgery (MUAPOS), University General Hospital of Castellon, Av Benicasim s/n, 12004 Castellón, Spain

[2] Department of Medicine, University Jaume I, Castellón de la Plana, Spain

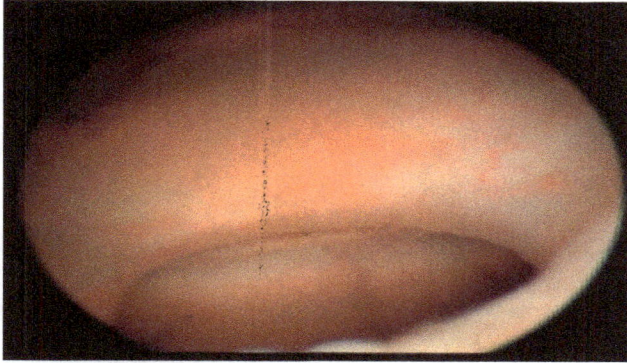

Fig. 1 Supratrigonal fistula on the dorsal vesical side

Clinical cases

A 45-year-old woman presented to our center in March 2013 for evaluation of urine leakage. She had undergone a laparoscopic hysterectomy for treatment of a uterine myoma in January 2013. Preliminary tests showed vaginal discharge of urine, and subsequent explorations showed a 3-cm supratrigonal fistula on the dorsal vesical side (Fig. 1).

Another woman, aged 72 years, presented to our center in January 2014 for evaluation of continual involuntary leaking of vaginal urine. The patient had undergone an abdominal laparotomic hysterectomy in October 2013 for treatment of pelvic endometriosis. Examination revealed a supratrigonal fistula. As the first therapeutic measure, permanent bladder catheterization was performed in both patients. Surgical treatment was performed after persistent demonstration of the VVF for 4 weeks. Informed consent was obtained from both patients before surgery.

Laparoscopic treatment was initially considered in both cases because of the location of the VVF. The same surgical technique was carried out for both patients. The patients were placed in the lithotomy position, and ureteral catheterization was performed. By means of cystoscopic visualization, two silk 0 sutures were introduced with a straight needle through the abdominal wall and into the interior of the bladder (Fig. 2). The needle was then extracted to the exterior through the urethra. The sutures were cut and tied together and then immediately reintroduced into the interior of the bladder.

Upon exerting exterior pressure on both sutures at the suprapubic level, the bladder remained immobile and fixed to the abdominal wall. After this procedure had been carried out, we introduced one 5-mm trocar for viewing and three 3-mm trocars for mini-laparoscopy (Karl Storz, Tuttlingen, Germany). A rigid 30° scope (Karl Storz) was introduced for an intravesical view. All instruments that were introduced through the trocars were 3 mm in diameter (scissors, clamps, needle holders, and bipolar coagulation forceps) (Karl Storz).

The mini-laparoscopic intravesical view was sufficient for recognition of the fistulous orifices and identification of the anatomical structures. The vesical mucosa was separated from the vaginal mucosa by means of dissection with scissors through the fistulous orifice (Fig. 3). In both patients, the mucosal vesical ring and affected vaginal area were cut out with scissors to create fresh surgical edges. The vaginal and vesical orifices were closed with two separated continuous barbed, resorbable 3-0 sutures (V-Loc 90 Absorbable Wound Closure Device; Covidien, Norwalk, CT, USA) (Figs. 4, 5, and 6).

The integrity of the bladder was checked by filling it with 300 ml of saline solution. The mean operative time for the two patients was approximately 100 min, and the blood loss was insignificant. The ureteral catheters were removed before finalizing the intervention, and a size 18-0 vesical Foley catheter was used for 2 weeks. Prophylactic antibiotics were used for 3 days. The patients were released from the hospital 24 h after surgery.

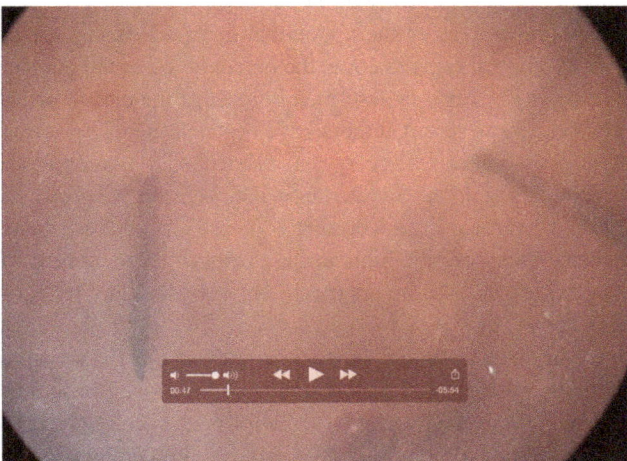

Fig. 2 Cystoscopic view from the bladder neck

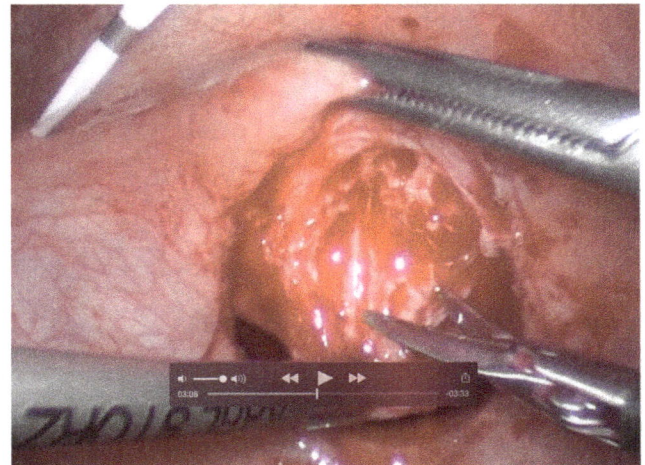

Fig. 3 Dissection of the bladder mucosa

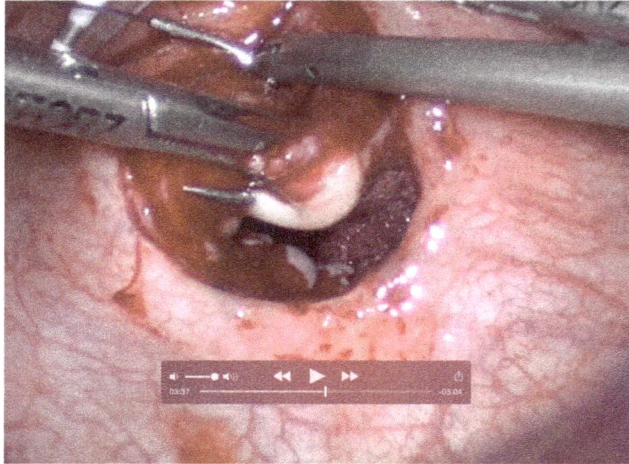

Fig. 4 Suturing of the bladder mucosa

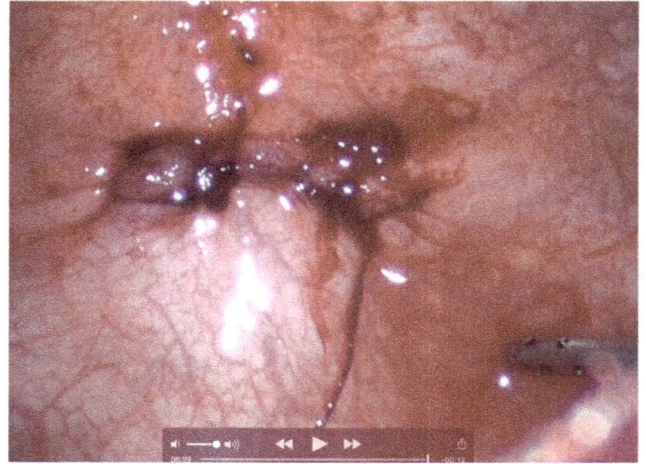

Fig. 6 Suturing of the bladder mucosa

Imaging examinations 6 weeks postoperatively revealed no VVF. The patients were asymptomatic at the time of this writing.

Discussion

Although some series report success between 5 and 25 % with permanent bladder catheterization in small VVF [6], in our cases, the urine vaginal leakage was present at the end of the 4-week period of bladder catheterization. We agree with the general opinion that the use of bladder catheter is useless in macroscopic fistulas.

No absolute consensus has yet been reached regarding the best approach for treating VVF. The vaginal approach is much less aggressive with less complications and a much faster recovery but requires proper training and familiarity in vaginal surgery. Supratrigonal fistulas are more challenging, but with an experienced vaginal surgeon, they can be repaired without

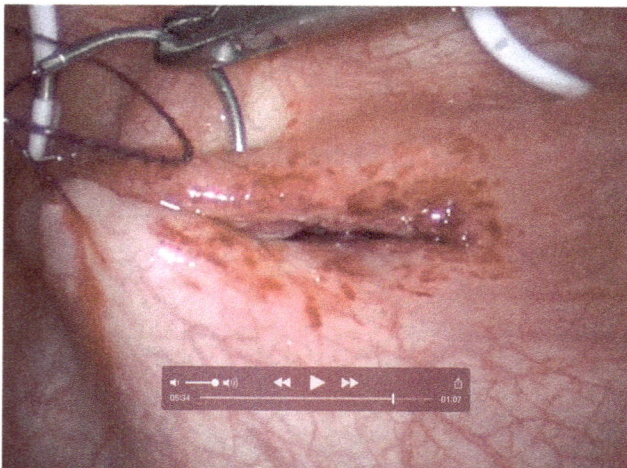

Fig. 5 Suturing of the vagina

any particular difficulty. There are some series with good results in transvaginal VVF repair [7].

The abdominal route allows the realization of other associated procedures (cystoplasty, ureteral reimplantation, etc.); it also provides access to high-location VVF in the cases of difficult vaginal approach (narrow vaginas, post irradiation, etc.). Nonetheless, some authors believe that the best approach for VVF is that which the surgeon best knows how to perform [1].

In recent years, laparoscopy has been frequently performed in place of laparotomy for treatment of VVF, and comparable results have been obtained [4, 8]. Almost all laparoscopic techniques are performed in an attempt to imitate the classic technique described by O'Connor [8]. Some authors have carried out minimally invasive transvesical approaches through only one aperture [9].

Our approach involves a minor skin incision, minor vesical trauma, and the ability to triangulate the working instruments. Following the directive of the most commonly used techniques for the treatment of VVF, adequate exposure of the damaged tissues and their previous exeresis before repair facilitates adequate scarring of the tissues.

And, advantage of the abdominal approach is the use of pedicle omental flaps to cover the defect between the bladder and the vagina, as it is described in most of the classic series [8]. Some more recent authors have describe the interposition of a fleece-bound sealing system (Thachosil®, Takeda Pharmaceuticals, Zurich, Switzerland) between the two lines of suture when repairing a recurrent VVF [10]. In contrast, some other authors describe high success rates in the treatment of VVF with laparoscopic approach without using any interposition flap [11].

In the present cases, the two orifices of the fistula were sutured separately with resorbable continuous barbed sutures (V-Loc); we were thus able to simplify the technique and reduce the time of surgery while avoiding implementation of intravesical knots.

One of the major problems when suturing the layers of the repaired VVF are the lines of suture of the vagina and the bladder and perhaps, the inflammation produced by the knots when tying the suture, is one of the most important factors in the relapse of the defect [12]. Some authors have described an intracorporeal suturing for the bladder and transvaginal suturing of the resultant vaginal defect without the observation of any recurrences within their series of extravesical repairs of VVF [11]. The suture employed in our patients does not have any knot, as it is integrated in the tissue; therefore, this could reduce the posterior inflammation of the tissues. However, we still need more cases over time to verify this affirmation.

This approach may not be the most adequate in patients with complicated or recurring fistulas or when another surgical treatment may be required to repair the fistula. However, in patients with simple fistulas, this minimally invasive approach is easily reproducible and associated with few complications.

Because of the limited number of patients treated, a larger number of cases are needed to establish the effectiveness of this technique in the long term.

Acknowledgments The authors would like to thank Michelle Fuerch and Marta Llueca for their editorial assistance in the preparation of the manuscript.

Authors' contributions A Llueca: Technique development, Manuscript writing
    JL Herraiz: Data collection
    M Rodrigo: Technique development
    Y Mazzouzi: Data collection
    D Piquer: Manuscript editing
    M Guijarro: Data management
    A Cañete: Data analysis
    J Escrig: Data analysis

Conflict of interest The authors report no conflicts of interest.
    A Llueca: declares that he has no conflict of interest
    JL Herraiz: declares that he has no conflict of interest
    M Rodrigo: declares that he has no conflict of interest
    Y Mazzouzi: declares that she has no conflict of interest
    D Piquer: declares that she has no conflict of interest
    M Guijarro: declares that she has no conflict of interest
    A Cañete: declares that she has no conflict of interest
    J Escrig: declares that he has no conflict of interest

Informed consent Informed consent was obtained from all individual participants included in the study.

References

1. Tenggardjaja CF, Goldman HB (2013) Advances in minimally invasive repair of vesicovaginal fistulas. Curr Urol Rep 14:253–261
2. Hilton P, Cromwell DA (2012) The risk of vesicovaginal and urethrovaginal fistula after hysterectomy performed in the english national health service–a retrospective cohort study examining patterns of care between 2000 and 2008. BJOG 119(12):1447–1454
3. Shah SJ (2009) Laparoscopic transabdominal transvesical vesicovaginal fistula repair. J Endourol 23:1135–1137
4. Guzen AS, Teber D, Canda AE, Rassweiller J (2009) Transperitoneal laparoscopic repair of iatrogenic vesicovaginal fistulas: Heil-Bronn experience and review of the literature. J Endourol 23:475–479
5. O'Connor JR (1980) Review of vesicovaginal fistula repair. J Urol 123:367–369
6. Lee RA, Symmonds RE, Williams TJ (1998) Current status of genitourinary fistula. Obstet Gynecol 72:313–319
7. Singh V, Sinha RJ, Sankhwar SN (2011) Transvaginal repair of complex and complicated vesicovaginal fistulae. Int J Gynaecol Obstet 114(1):51–55
8. Shah SJ (2009) Laparoscopic transabdominal transvesical vesicovaginal fistula repair. J Endourol 23:1135–1137
9. Roslan M, Markuszewski M, Bagińska J, Krajka K (2012) Suprapubic transvesical laparoendoscopic single-site surgery for vesicovaginal fistula repair: a case report. Video Surg Mini Invasive 7(4):307–310
10. Erdogru T, Sanli A, Celik O, Baykara M (2008) Laparoscopic transvesical repair of recurrent vesicovaginal fistula using with fleece-bound sealing system. Arch Gynecol Obstet 277(5):461–464
11. Lee JH, Choi JS, Lee KW (2010) Immediate laparoscopic nontransvesical repair without omental interposition for vesicovaginal fistula developing after total abdominal hysterectomy. JSLS 14(2):187–191
12. Greenberg JA (2010) The use of barbed sutures in obstetrics and gynecology. Rev Obstet Gynecol 3:82–91

25

A new approach to simplify surgical colpotomy in laparoscopic hysterectomy

L. van den Haak[1] · J. P. T. Rhemrev[2] · M. D. Blikkendaal[1] · A. C. M. Luteijn[1] ·
J. J. van den Dobbelsteen[3] · S. R. C. Driessen[1] · F. W. Jansen[1,3]

Abstract New surgical techniques and technology have simplified laparoscopic hysterectomy and have enhanced the safety of this procedure. However, the surgical colpotomy step has not been addressed. This study evaluates the surgical colpotomy step in laparoscopic hysterectomy with respect to difficulty and duration. Furthermore, it proposes an alternative route that may simplify this step in laparoscopic hysterectomy. A structured interview, a prospective cohort study, and a problem analysis were performed regarding experienced difficulty and duration of surgical colpotomy in laparoscopic hysterectomy. Sixteen experts in minimally invasive gynecologic surgery from 12 hospitals participated in the structured interview using a 5-point Likert scale. The colpotomy in LH received the highest scores for complexity (2.8 ± 1.2), compared to AH and VH. Colpotomy in LH was estimated as more difficult than in AH (2.8 vs 1.4, $p < .001$). In the cohort study, 107 patients undergoing LH were included. Sixteen percent of the total procedure time was spent on colpotomy (SD 7.8 %). BMI was positively correlated with colpotomy time, even after correcting for longer operation time. No relation was found between colpotomy time and blood loss or uterine weight. The surgical colpotomy step in laparoscopic hysterectomy should be simplified as this study demonstrates that it is time consuming and is considered to be more difficult than in other hysterectomy procedures. A vaginal approach to the colpotomy is proposed to achieve this simplification.

Keywords Laparoscopic hysterectomy · Colpotomy · New technology · Innovation of surgical technique

Introduction

New surgical techniques and technical equipment have attempted to facilitate laparoscopic hysterectomy (LH), after shortcomings of LH in comparison with vaginal hysterectomy (VH) and abdominal hysterectomy (AH) were demonstrated [1]. New alternatives for conventional suturing, such as bipolar coagulation, have improved hemostasis of the uterine and ovarian pedicles [1]. Furthermore, in a systematic review, the superiority of vessel-sealing devices with respect to blood loss and shorter operation time in some abdominal procedures was demonstrated compared to other electrothermical devices [2]. Finally, barbed sutures have been introduced for vaginal vault closing, and this technique appears to be equal compared to standard sutures with respect to time to cuff closing, cuff healing, and sexual function [3]. Although some of these effects are debatable, for instance due to possible contributing factors such as learning curve, they do demonstrate the efforts to facilitate the LH. Certainly, notwithstanding the well-known benefits of LH, VH remains the gold standard for the hysterectomy procedure [1, 4], even though in contrast with this statement, recent studies have shown that LH was associated with shorter hospital stay, less blood loss, and less postoperative pain compared to VH

✉ L. van den Haak
l.van_den_haak@lumc.nl

✉ F. W. Jansen
f.w.jansen@lumc.nl

[1] Department of Gynecology, Leiden University Medical Center, PO Box 9600, 2300 RC Leiden, The Netherlands

[2] Department of Obstetrics and Gynecology, Bronovo Hospital The Hague, The Hague, The Netherlands

[3] Department BioMechanical Engineering, Delft University of Technology, 2628 CD Delft, The Netherlands

[5, 6]. Yet, LH is still associated with a longer operating time [4, 7]. Furthermore, previous studies have demonstrated that LH is regarded as more difficult when compared to AH and VH [8]. Learning curve issues and implementation errors have contributed to these results. However, there still are technical opportunities to simplify the LH procedure. Our hypothesis is that the colpotomy should be addressed in this context. Colpotomy is part of the final surgical steps in the LH procedure, following the ligation of the uterine arteries, the skeletonizing of the cervix, and the dissection of the bladder from the cervix. These steps are relatively hazardous and time consuming in the procedure. It is in this anatomical area where most of the bleeding and ureter injuries occur [9, 10]. Moreover, the delicacy of laparoscopic surgery in this anatomical area was demonstrated by the initial higher incidence of ureter injuries during LH, which only decreased after a certain learning curve was passed [11]. In this light, an alternative route for colpotomy has been investigated: analysis of the current colpotomy procedure demonstrated that the main difficulties of this surgical step are the limited visibility during colpotomy (due to the anterior view of the endoscope combined with the location of the cervix deep in the pelvis), and the need for a 360° circular cutting motion during colpotomy. To overcome these difficulties, a vaginal approach to the colpotomy was suggested. The first test with a prototype of a vaginal colpotomy device on an in vitro vaginal model demonstrated a significant reduction of colpotomy time [12].

The aims of this study were to substantiate our hypothesis and to further evaluate the possibilities of a vaginal approach to colpotomy. The experienced difficulty, the duration of the surgical colpotomy step, and possible agents of change are evaluated. In addition, the idea of a vaginal approach to colpotomy is shaped into a new surgical instrument that may simplify colpotomy [13].

Materials and methods

Firstly, to investigate the difficulty of the colpotomy procedure, a structured interview was performed among experts in minimally invasive gynecologic surgery working at different hospitals throughout the Netherlands. The interview assessed the participants perception regarding the surgical step of the colpotomy. Furthermore, they were asked about their opinion regarding several features of the proposed facilitation of the colpotomy. (Figure 1) Participants were asked to answer using a 5-point Likert scale: 1 meaning "easy"/"not important", to 5 meaning "complex"/"important."

Next, a prospective cohort study was performed at two hospitals specialized in minimally invasive gynecologic surgery. From June 2010 to May 2014, LH procedures were timed to assess the duration of colpotomy. The total operating time (TOT) was defined as the time from the insertion of the Veress needle to the final stitches used for closing last trocar incision site. Colpotomy time (CT) was defined as the time from the first incision in the vaginal fornix (after ligating the uterine arteries and all uterine ligaments) until the complete separation of the cervix from the vaginal wall. An extrafascial technique was used to perform total laparoscopic hysterectomy. The vaginal wall was opened anteriorly at the vesicovaginal fold, after which the colpotomy was completed. All consecutive LH procedures were eligible for inclusion. This study was exempt from approval by the medical ethics committee. Procedures were performed by five gynecologists who perform LH on a regular basis and have experience in well over 100 TLH procedures. The number of participating gynecologists was chosen to enhance the external validity of the outcome. Inter-surgeon variability was minimized by using similar surgical procedure protocols. Furthermore, all surgeons received their training at the Leiden Residency Program. The Valtchev or Clermont Ferrand uterine manipulator was used. Bipolar and ultrasonic instruments were used for colpotomy. Basic patient characteristics

Fig. 1 Structured interview

1. What is your estimation of the total procedure time of a total hysterectomy and what is the estimated time required for the separation of the uterus from the vagina (absolute time and relative to the total procedure time)?
2. Can your estimate the complexity of separating the uterus from the vaginal wall for the different procedures?
3. How important is it to maintain the possibility to manipulate the possibility to manipulate the uterus with a manipulator while dissecting the uterus?
4. What is the importance of coagulation when separating the uterus from the vaginal wall with respect to the following items: Easy cutting, less bleeding, impaired wound healing, accurate dissection, less colla teral tissue damage.
5. How important is a visual position mark of the dissection device in a uterus extraction product such that the position of the instrument in the vagina can be seen through the laparoscopic endoscope?
6. What effort will it take to adapt the surgical procedure in your hospital and implement the use of this instrument?
7. All in all, do you think the envisioned instrument may provide a benefit enabling a faster and/or easier uterus extraction?

were gathered. The uterine weight and the total amount of blood loss were measured in the operating room. Patients were excluded in case of missing colpotomy time. Complications were classified according to the severity of the complications on the basis of the framework set by the Dutch Society for Obstetrics and Gynecology (NVOG) [14].

Statistical analysis

Baseline characteristics were summarized by means and standard deviations and, when applicable, by numbers and percentages. For the structured interview, an independent sample t test and a paired t test were used to compare experts versus residents and the type of hysterectomy, respectively. For the prospective study, t tests were used when applicable. A Pearson's correlation coefficient and analysis of variance (ANOVA) techniques were used to test any correlation between different variables and colpotomies. A generalized linear model was performed to assess the independent effect of certain parameters (such as uterine weight, body mass index (BMI)) on the duration of colpotomy. All tests were performed at the .05 level of significance. SPSS 20 was used to analyze all data.

Results

Structured interview

Sixteen experts from 12 hospitals were interviewed (Tables 1 and 2). On average, the experts performed 35 (SD 24) hysterectomy procedures annually, of which 59 % (SD 24) LH

Table 1 Participants opinion regarding colpotomy ($N = 16$ expert)

	Mean (SD)	p value
Number of hysterectomy procedures per year	35 (24)	
Amount of TLH (%)	59 (24)	
Amount of VH (%)	19 (21)	
Amount of AH (%)	22 (15)	
Estimated length of TLH procedure (minutes)	114 (24)	
Estimated colpotomy time TLH (minutes)	20 (10)	
Complexity of colpotomy TLH[a]	2.8 (1.2)	
Complexity of colpotomy VH[a]	2.0 (1.3)	
Complexity of colpotomy AH[a]	1,4 (.6)	
Estimated colpotomy vs total OR time (%)	18 (11)	
TLH vs VH	2.8 vs 2.0	.08
TLH vs AH	2.8 vs 1.4	< .001
VH vs AH	2.0 vs 1.4	.02

TLH total laparoscopic hysterectomy, *VH* vaginal hysterectomy, *AH* abdominal hysterectomy

Vaginal hysterectomy

[a] 1 easy–5 complex

Table 2 Preferred functions and adaptation of the new device ($N = 16$)

	Mean	SD
Importance of a uterine manipulator	4.5	1.4
The Importance of coagulation instead of cutting when separating the uterus from the vagina	2.3	1.6
-Collateral tissue damage	3.5	2.0
-Easy cutting	2.6	1.6
-Wound healing	2.6	1.6
-Accurate dissection	3.1	2.2
-Bleeding	4.2	1.1
Importance of markings so that a vaginal instrument is visible during laparoscopy	4.6	.7

Scale 1–5 = not–moderate–important

procedures, 19 % (SD 21) VH, and 22 % (SD 15) AH. The estimated TOT is 114 (SD 24) minutes, and they estimated this to spend 18 % (SD 11) on the colpotomy. The colpotomy in LH received the highest scores for difficulty (2.8 ± 1.2), compared to AH and VH. Colpotomy in LH was estimated as more difficult than in AH (2.8 vs 1.4, $p < .001$). The same trend is seen for the difficulty of colpotomy in LH versus VH (2.8 vs 2.0); however, this difference was not significant ($p = .08$). With respect to the vaginal approach to simplify colpotomy, the following functions of the envisaged instrument were regarded as moderately important to important by the participants: the ability to manipulate the uterus (4.5, SD 1.4), the presence of coagulation to stop bleeding during the colpotomy procedure (4.2, SD 1.1), and the existence of markings on the device to help visualize the device by the camera (4.6, SD .7).

Colpotomy analysis

Out of 164 consecutive patients, 107 patients undergoing LH were included. Fifty-seven (35 %) were excluded due to missing colpotomy time. Patient characteristics and procedure data are shown in Table 3. Most common indications for surgery were abnormal bleeding and/or uterine myoma. The mean total operating time was 116.4 min (SD 35.3 min), and the mean colpotomy time was 17.9 min (SD 7.8 min). On average, 16 % of the total procedure time was spent on colpotomy. BMI was positively correlated with colpotomy time (.320 and .311, both $p = .001$), and the generalized linear model confirmed the identified correlation and proved that it was independent from the other variables (Table 4). No statistically significant correlation was found between colpotomy time and uterine weight or blood loss.

Discussion

This study demonstrates that the surgical colpotomy is a time-consuming step in the LH procedure, that is preceded by the

Table 3 Patient characteristics and procedure data ($N=107$; 91 Leiden University Medical Center and 16 Bronovo hospital)

		Mean	SD	p value
Age (years)		49.4	10.6	
BMI (kg/m^2)		27.4	7.0	
Parity[a]		2	1.4	
		Number (%)		
Previous operations	None	66 (62)		
	One or more abdominal surgeries	41 (38)		
Indication for operation	Abnormal bleeding and / or uterine leiomyoma	68 (64)		
	(pre-)malignancy	37 (35)		
	Other[b]	2 (2)		
Total operating time (min)		116.4	35.3	
Colpotomy time (min)		17.9	7.8	
TOT minus CT (min)		98.5	31.5	
Uterine weight (g)		242.8	175.0	
Estimated blood loss (ml)		142.5	194.7	
Complications (total and %)	Peri-operative lesions[c]	1 (1 %)		
	Post-operative infection[d]	6 (6 %)		
	Other[e]	9 (9 %)		
Colpotomy-total OR time (%)		16	5	
Colpotomy time	No complications occurred ($N=91$)	18.0	8.1	
	A complication occurred ($N=15$)	17.9	6.0	1.0
Colpotomy time	No previous abdominal surgery	17.6	7.3	.6
	With previous abdominal surgery	18.4	8.6	

BMI body mass index

[a] Median

[b] 1 endometritis and salpingitis, 1 abdominal pain

[c] 1 bladder injury

[d] 5 urinary tract infections, 1 pneumonia

[e] 1 ileus, 1 urinary retention, 1 re-admittance for unexplained fever, 1 lost needle during surgery resulting in enlargement of the trocar incision, 1 patient with facial subcutaneous emphysema that required admittance at the intensive care unit, 1 infected hematoma, 1 vaginal cuff dehiscence occurring 4 weeks after surgery, 1 abdominal pain that led to additional surgery 10 days after TLH resulting in a partial oophorectomy, and 1 repeat laparoscopy on the same day regarding a loss of blood exceeding 300 ml

hazardous dissection of the uterine arteries, bladder, and cervix, risking blood loss and ureter injuries. Colpotomy time comprises 16 % of the total operation time, even reaching 45 %. Albeit an extreme value, it does demonstrate the difficulty that can be experienced when performing this task. This is substantiated by our structured interview. In accordance with a previous study [8], our structured interview revealed that experts find colpotomy in LH significantly more difficult than in AH, and that the same trend is seen for colpotomy in LH compared to VH (although not significant). It is also demonstrated that a rise in BMI proved to be associated with a longer colpotomy time. This effect of BMI on the duration of surgery is in line with other studies [15, 16]. However, in our study, the effect of BMI on the colpotomy time remained even after correcting for total operation time. Apparently, higher BMI apart from the additional procedure time, accounts for an additional complicating factor regarding the colpotomy step. These

women especially may benefit from the simplification of this procedure. Moreover, as the incidence of obesity is increasing, higher BMI will become part of everyday work in laparoscopic surgery [17]. No other factors, such as the amount of blood loss, previous abdominal surgery, or the presence of complications seemed to influence the duration of colpotomy. Surprisingly, also for uterine weight no correlation was found with colpotomy time. It is our opinion, that the colpotomy procedure can be regarded as independent from "uterine" factors, such as uterine weight. Indeed, when performing the colpotomy after all uterine ligaments and arteries have been dissected, the obtained additional mobility of the uterus will compensate for restrictions due to uterine weight. However, although uteri weighing up to 930 g were removed, the vast majority of uteri in our cohort weighed below 360 g. Therefore, we realize that, based on the results from our cohort, our statement may not fully apply to very large uteri. Yet,

Table 4 Pearson correlation and generalized linear model (*N* = 107; 91 LUMC and 16 Bronovo)

	Colpotomy time (min)		
	Pearson correlation	Sig.	N
BMI (kg/m²)	.329	.001	104
Age (years)	.278	.004	107
TOT minus CT (min)	.380	.000	105
Uterine weight (g)	.092	.349	105
Estimated blood loss (ml)	.082	.399	107
	Generalized linear model B[a]		
BMI (kg/m²)	.403	<.001	
Uterine weight (g)	−.002	.703	

BMI body mass index

[a] B unstandardized regression coefficient

support of our opinion can be found in literature, where the feasibility of LH in women with larger uteri has already been established [18, 19]. A limitation of our study is the high number of exclusions, especially given the prospective design of this study. However, the overall effect of the exclusions on the outcome of our study is limited. Missing data can be considered random and therefore effect cohort size rather than the results, although the introduction of bias cannot be fully excluded. Only one surgical protocol was used for our prospective study, and this raises the question of external validity regarding other surgical protocols. However the relative colpotomy time that resulted from our prospective study matches the estimated relative colpotomy time from our interview (16 % vs 18 %, respectively), in which gynecologists participated who use different protocols. This study did not focus on procedural steps of the LH other than colpotomy, which could be considered a flaw. For instance, dissection and sealing of the uterine artery would have been an interesting addition. On the other hand, this step has already been enhanced by new surgical techniques and technology. All other steps of the hysterectomy procedure are relatively straightforward and appear to be in no apparent need of improvement. Notwithstanding these shortcomings, our findings regarding colpotomy time are important. A recent study demonstrated that operative time was an independent predictor of postoperative morbidity and reoperation [20]. Furthermore, a cost analysis of different approaches to hysterectomy showed that patient operation room costs and total patient costs are higher for LH when compared to VH, and that longer operation time proved to be an important contributor to these higher costs [21]. In light of these studies, reducing CT and thereby the TOT may have beneficial effects on patient morbidity as well as on health care costs. This will become increasingly important, since there is an increase of laparoscopic hysterectomy procedures at the expense of the number of vaginal hysterectomies [22].

Vaginal approach for colpotomy

A prototype for a vaginal colptomizer device has been assembled [13]. Although several methods exist to perform the surgical colpotomy such as bipolar and harmonics, to our knowledge, the vaginal route to colpotomy has not yet been proposed. Figure 2 demonstrates our prototype. The intrauterine part of the manipulator has mobility in all planes (i.e., anterior-posterior, lateral, and rotation). After introducing the manipulator into the uterus, a cap is positioned over the cervix. This cervical cap, which rotates, has several functions: it presents the vaginal cuff and helps to push the uterus cranially. Furthermore, it houses the knife that enables the vaginal colpotomy. The knife is deployed and operated by moving the knife driver and the handle of the manipulator. The exact location where the knife is introduced into the vaginal wall (and hence in the abdominal cavity) is identified by a light source in the manipulator. Figures 3 and 4 demonstrate the knife during colpotomy in a human cadaver test and in detail, respectively. Finally, after colpotomy is completed, the entire surgical specimen and the manipulator are removed. Certain questions remain to be answered. For instance, our interview tried to assess the preference for a coagulation-based or "cold knife"-based cutting mechanism. Coagulation was preferred in case of bleeding and, to lesser extent, to facilitate the cutting action. However, some concerns were raised over the possible negative effects of coagulation with respect to wound healing. Several studies have reported a higher incidence of vaginal vault dehiscence after LH when compared to VH and AH [23–25]. It has been suggested that electrocoagulation may be the cause for this higher incidence, due to more extensive tissue damage and/or suboptimal tissue healing [26, 27]. However, in large series, no effect of electrocoagulation was demonstrated with respect to the occurrence of vaginal vault dehiscence [28]. Moreover, no effect of the power settings was observed [28]. It was concluded that the current available scientific evidence does not support one technique over the other, and it is expected that this topic will continue to be a main point of interest for gynecological societies. However, in light of the feasibility of the device, a cold knife cutting mechanism was designed. The structured interview also demonstrated the need for a manipulator function integrated in the

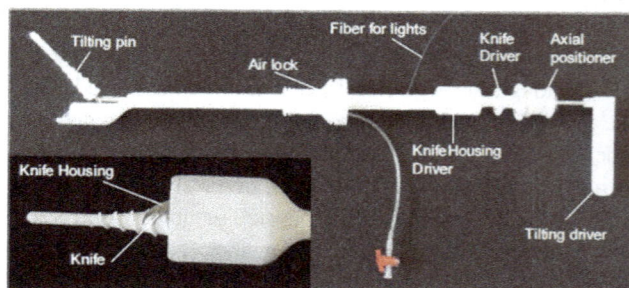

Fig. 2 MobiSep prototype

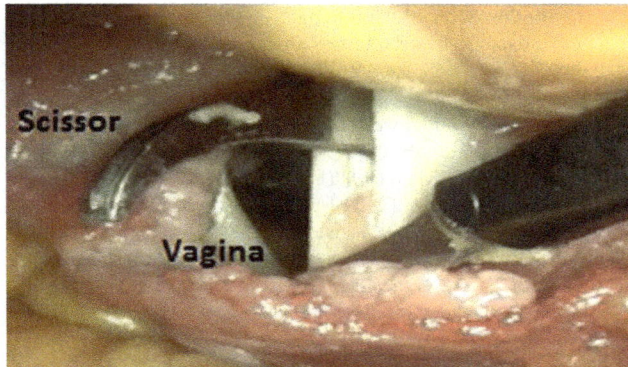

Fig. 3 Vaginal colpotomy with MobiSep prototype in human cadaver test

device. The importance of a uterine manipulator during LH has been demonstrated in literature. A manipulator is considered to increase the distance between the ureter and uterine arteries, thereby creating more space for the dissection of the uterine arteries [29]. Furthermore, in a recent Delphi study, full agreement was reached regarding the use of a uterine manipulator during LH to prevent ureter injuries during LH [30]. This resulted in the final design of the prototype: a uterine manipulator with an integrated vaginal colpotomizer.

In all, the significance of the present study is the clinically driven approach to the innovating the difficult surgical colpotomy step. Experiences in the past have shown the need for a careful introduction of new technology in daily practice [31, 32]. Consequently, innovation should start with a thorough analysis of the problem at hand. The eVALuate study has taught us that LH has certain disadvantages with respect to patient safety when compared to VH and AH [1]. Technical developments have already contributed to the enhanced safety of LH. However, further simplifying the LH is necessary, since our study demonstrates that the surgical colpotomy step takes place in an anatomical area which is at risk for complications, is regarded as difficult, and comprises a considerable amount of the total duration of the LH procedure. Therefore, much can be gained by simplifying this step.

Conclusions

Earlier studies have taught us that LH has certain disadvantages with respect to patient safety when compared to VH and AH. Technical developments have already contributed to the enhanced safety of LH. However, further simplifying the LH is necessary, since reducing the operation time of LH may reduce health care costs and complication rates [20, 21]. Our study demonstrates that the colpotomy step in LH should be simplified. Not only is this surgical step time consuming bu it is also regarded as significantly more difficult when compared to AH. A vaginal approach of the colpotomy step may solve these issues. A surgical instrument was designed as a uterine manipulator with an integrated vaginal colpotomizer. The device intends to address the shortcomings of the current colpotomy technique. Clinical studies will commence shortly to evaluate the efficacy and safety of the vaginal approach to colpotomy.

Authors' contribution L. van den Haak contributed the following: project development, data collection, data analysis, and manuscript writing. J.P.T. Rhemrev contributed the following: project development, data collection, data analysis, and manuscript writing. M.D. Blikkendaal contributed the following: data collection, data analysis, and manuscript writing. A.C.M. Luteijn contributed the following: data collection, and data analysis. J.J. van den Dobbelsteen contributed the following: project development and data analysis. S.R.C. Driessen contributed the following: data collection, data analysis, and manuscript writing. F.W. Jansen contributed the following: project development, data collection, data analysis, and manuscript writing.

Compliance with ethical standards A grant for this study was provided by the European Regional Development Fund.

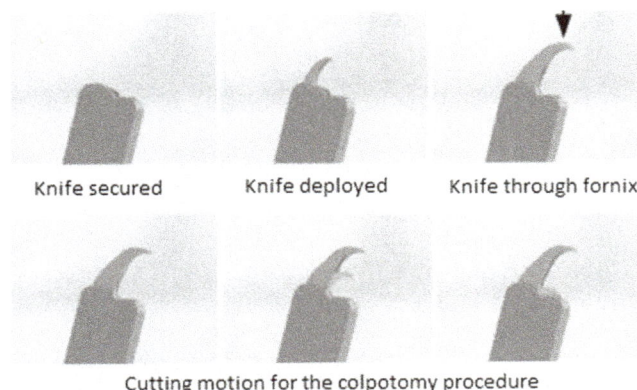

Knife secured   Knife deployed   Knife through fornix

Cutting motion for the colpotomy procedure

Fig. 4 Detail of the knife action of the vaginal colpotomizer in relation to safety cap

Informed consent This study was exempt from approval by the medical ethics committee. Only anonymous data from charts were analyzed. Patients were not subjected to experimental treatments, nor were they interviewed, nor were they in any way hindered during their treatment. Therefore, in agreement with Dutch regulations, informed consent was not obtained.

References

1. Garry R, Fountain J, Brown J et al (2004) EVALUATE hysterectomy trial: a multicentre randomised trial comparing abdominal, vaginal and laparoscopic methods of hysterectomy. Health Technol Assess 8:1–154

2. Janssen PF, Brolmann HA, Huirne JA (2012) Effectiveness of electrothermal bipolar vessel-sealing devices versus other electrothermal and ultrasonic devices for abdominal surgical hemostasis: a systematic review. Surg Endosc 26:2892–2901

3. Einarsson JI, Cohen SL, Gobern JM et al (2013) Barbed versus standard suture: a randomized trial for laparoscopic vaginal cuff closure. J Minim Invasive Gynecol 20:492–498

4. Nieboer TE, Johnson N, Lethaby A et al (2009) Surgical approach to hysterectomy for benign gynaecological disease. Cochrane Database Syst Rev 8:CD003677

5. Candiani M, Izzo S (2010) Laparoscopic versus vaginal hysterectomy for benign pathology. Curr Opin Obstet Gynecol 22:304–308

6. Candiani M, Izzo S, Bulfoni A et al (2009) Laparoscopic vs vaginal hysterectomy for benign pathology. Am J Obstet Gynecol 200:368–7

7. Johnson N, Barlow D, Lethaby A et al (2005) Methods of hysterectomy: systematic review and meta-analysis of randomised controlled trials. BMJ 330:1478

8. Nieboer TE, Spaanderman ME, Bongers MY et al (2010) Gynaecologists estimate and experience laparoscopic hysterectomy as more difficult compared with abdominal hysterectomy. Gynecol Surg 7:359–363

9. Janssen PF, Brolmann HA, Huirne JA (2013) Causes and prevention of laparoscopic ureter injuries: an analysis of 31 cases during laparoscopic hysterectomy in the Netherlands. Surg Endosc 27:946–956

10. Elliott SP, McAninch JW (2006) Ureteral injuries: external and iatrogenic. Urol Clin North Am 33(55-66):vi

11. Makinen J, Brummer T, Jalkanen J et al (2013) Ten years of progress—improved hysterectomy outcomes in Finland 1996-2006: a longitudinal observation study. BMJ Open 3:e003169

12. Gahler MM, van de Berg NN, Rhemrev J et al (2010) Vaginal approach for uterus separation during laparoscopic hysterectomy. J Med Devices 4:027514

13. Jansen FW, Rhemrev J (2013) MobiSep: a new approach to colpotomy in TLH. J Minim Invasive Gynecol 20:S51

14. Twijnstra AR, Zeeman GG, Jansen FW (2010) A novel approach to registration of adverse outcomes in obstetrics and gynaecology: a feasibility study. Qual Saf Health Care 19:132–137

15. Bardens D, Solomayer E, Baum S et al (2014) The impact of the body mass index (BMI) on laparoscopic hysterectomy for benign disease. Arch Gynecol Obstet 289:803–807

16. Osler M, Daugbjerg S, Frederiksen BL et al (2011) Body mass and risk of complications after hysterectomy on benign indications. Hum Reprod 26:1512–1518

17. Wang Y, Beydoun MA (2007) The obesity epidemic in the United States—gender, age, socioeconomic, racial/ethnic, and geographic characteristics: a systematic review and meta-regression analysis. Epidemiol Rev 29:6–28

18. O'Hanlan KA, McCutcheon SP, McCutcheon JG (2011) Laparoscopic hysterectomy: impact of uterine size. J Minim Invasive Gynecol 18:85–91

19. Uccella S, Cromi A, Serati M et al (2014) Laparoscopic hysterectomy in case of uteri weighing >/=1 kilogram: a series of 71 cases and review of the literature. J Minim Invasive Gynecol 21:460–465

20. Hanwright PJ, Mioton LM, Thomassee MS et al (2013) Risk profiles and outcomes of total laparoscopic hysterectomy compared with laparoscopically assisted vaginal hysterectomy. Obstet Gynecol 121:781–787

21. Wright KN, Jonsdottir GM, Jorgensen S et al (2012) Costs and outcomes of abdominal, vaginal, laparoscopic and robotic hysterectomies. JSLS 16:519–524

22. Driessen SRC, Baden NLM, van Zwet EW, Twijnstra ARH, Jansen FW. Trends in the implementation of advanced minimally invasive gynecologic surgical procedures in the Netherlands. J of Minim Invasive Gynecol. In press.

23. Kho RM, Akl MN, Cornella JL et al (2009) Incidence and characteristics of patients with vaginal cuff dehiscence after robotic procedures. Obstet Gynecol 114:231–235

24. Hur HC, Donnellan N, Mansuria S et al (2011) Vaginal cuff dehiscence after different modes of hysterectomy. Obstet Gynecol 118:794–801

25. Croak AJ, Gebhart JB, Klingele CJ et al (2004) Characteristics of patients with vaginal rupture and evisceration. Obstet Gynecol 103:572–576

26. Klauschie J, Wen Y, Chen B et al (2014) Histologic characteristics of vaginal cuff tissue from patients with vaginal cuff dehiscence. J Minim Invasive Gynecol 21:442–446

27. Sowa DE, Masterson BJ, Nealon N et al (1985) Effects of thermal knives on wound healing. Obstet Gynecol 66:436–439

28. Uccella S, Ceccaroni M, Cromi A et al (2012) Vaginal cuff dehiscence in a series of 12,398 hysterectomies: effect of different types of colpotomy and vaginal closure. Obstet Gynecol 120:516–523

29. Koh CH (1998) A new technique and system for simplifying total laparoscopic hysterectomy. J Am Assoc Gynecol Laparosc 5:187–192

30. Janssen PF, Brolmann HA, Huirne JA (2011) Recommendations to prevent urinary tract injuries during laparoscopic hysterectomy: a systematic Delphi procedure among experts. J Minim Invasive Gynecol 18:314–321

31. Stefanidis D, Fanelli RD, Price R et al (2014) SAGES guidelines for the introduction of new technology and techniques. Surg Endosc 28:2257–2271

32. Strasberg SM, Ludbrook PA (2003) Who oversees innovative practice? Is there a structure that meets the monitoring needs of new techniques? J Am Coll Surg 196:938–948

26

The Thessaloniki ESHRE/ESGE consensus on diagnosis of female genital anomalies

Grigoris F. Grimbizis [1,2] · Attilio Di Spiezio Sardo [1] · Sotirios H. Saravelos [1] ·
Stephan Gordts [1] · Caterina Exacoustos [1] · Dominique Van Schoubroeck [1] ·
Carmina Bermejo [1] · Nazar N. Amso [1] · Geeta Nargund [1] · Dirk Timmermann [1] ·
Apostolos Athanasiadis [1] · Sara Brucker [1] · Carlo De Angelis [1] · Marco Gergolet [1] ·
Tin Chiu Li [1] · Vasilios Tanos [1] · Basil Tarlatzis [1] · Roy Farquharson [1] ·
Luca Gianaroli [1] · Rudi Campo [1]

Abstract What is the recommended diagnostic work-up of female genital anomalies according to the European Society of Human Reproduction and Embryology (ESHRE)/ European Society for Gynaecological Endoscopy (ESGE) system? The ESHRE/ESGE consensus for the diagnosis of female genital anomalies is presented. Accurate diagnosis of congenital anomalies still remains a clinical challenge due to the drawbacks of the previous classification systems and the non-systematic use of diagnostic methods with varying accuracy, with some of them quite inaccurate. Currently, a wide range of non-invasive diagnostic procedures are available, enriching the opportunity to accurately detect the anatomical status of the female genital tract, as well as a new objective and comprehensive classification system with well-described classes and sub-classes. The ESHRE/ESGE Congenital Uterine Anomalies (CONUTA) Working Group established an initiative with the goal of developing a consensus for the diagnosis of female genital anomalies. The CONUTA working group and imaging experts in the field have been appointed to run the project. The consensus is developed based on (1) *evaluation of the currently available diagnostic*

methods and, more specifically, of *their characteristics* with the use of the experts panel consensus method and of *their diagnostic accuracy* performing a systematic review of evidence and (2) consensus for (a) the definition of where and how to measure uterine wall thickness and (b) the recommendations for the diagnostic work-up of female genital anomalies, based on the results of the previous evaluation procedure, with the use of the experts panel consensus method. Uterine wall thickness is defined as the distance between interostial line and external uterine profile at the midcoronal plane of the uterus; alternatively, if a coronal plane is not available, the mean anterior and posterior uterine wall thickness at the longitudinal plane could be used. Gynaecological examination and two-dimensional ultrasound (2D US) are recommended for the evaluation of asymptomatic women. Three-dimensional ultrasound (3D US) is recommended for the diagnosis of female genital anomalies in "symptomatic" patients belonging to high-risk groups for the presence of a female genital anomaly and in any asymptomatic woman suspected to have an anomaly from routine avaluation. Magnetic resonance imaging (MRI) and endoscopic evaluation are recommended for the sub-group of patients with suspected complex anomalies or in diagnostic dilemmas. Adolescents with symptoms suggestive for the presence of a female genital anomaly should be thoroughly evaluated with 2D US, 3D US, MRI and endoscopy. The various diagnostic methods should be used in a proper way and evaluated by experts to avoid mis-, over- and underdiagnosis. The role of a combined ultrasound examination and outpatient hysteroscopy should be prospectively evaluated. It is a challenge for further research, based on diagnosis, to objectively evaluate the clinical consequences related to various degrees of uterine deformity.

This manuscript is being published simultaneously in the journals of Human Reproduction and Gynaecological Surgery.

✉ Grigoris F. Grimbizis
grimbi@med.auth.gr; grigoris.grimbizis@gmail.com

[1] Congenital Uterine Malformations (CONUTA) Common ESHRE/ ESGE Working Group and Invited Experts, Leuven, Belgium

[2] 1st Department of Obstetrics and Gynecology, Aristotle University of Thessaloniki, Tsimiski 51 Street, 54623 Thessaloniki, Greece

Keywords Genital tract · Female genital anomalies ·
Mullerian anomalies · Uterine anomalies · ESHRE/ESGE
system · Diagnosis · Classification

Introduction

Female genital malformations are deviations from normal anatomy that could impair the reproductive potential of a woman or, in complex cases (e.g. obstructing anomalies), woman's health [8, 12, 20, 21, 24, 25, 32, 43, 52, 56, 59]. They arise embryologically from failure of Müllerian ducts' formation, canalization, fusion or absorption either as a single defect or in combination with different expression in the various parts of the female genital tract resulting in the so-called complex anomalies.

Accurate diagnosis of congenital anomalies still remains a clinical challenge with serious consequences in the management of those patients. This is the result of the following methodological bias: (1) absence of clear definitions and objective diagnostic criteria in the existing classification systems, mainly that of the American Fertility Society [1] for their diagnosis and differential diagnosis and (2) use of diagnostic methods with different accuracy, some of them quite inaccurate to make the correct diagnosis of the anomaly [54]. Thus, over the years, different investigators adopted their own subjective criteria, for the categorization of mainly uterine anomalies, that varied widely from one study to another, having as a result a poor selection and definition of the various patients' populations [54, 26, 16].

In view of these diagnostic methological and clinical drawbacks, the estimation of their exact prevalence in the general and selected populations was very difficult and the evaluation of the clinical consequences of each different types of anomaly inaccurate [54, 11]. Furthermore, comparisons between different studies and their grouping are hampered not only by the differences in study populations but also by differences in diagnostic methods and criteria used to differentiate between various types of uterine anomalies [59]. Moreover, the exact value of surgery is not known for patients' counselling and treatment underlying the urgent need to test available interventions in well-designed studies with properly defined groups [59].

In the recently published European Society of Human Reproduction and Embryology (ESHRE)/European Society for Gynaecological Endoscopy (ESGE) classification of female genital anomalies, a clear definition of all types of anomalies was provided and the anomalies were categorised in well-described classes and sub-classes [27, 28]. Thus, the previously mentioned diagnostic drawback of subjectivity in definitions is effectively answered enhancing their objective categorization [27, 28, 16]. It seems that with the use of the new system, all the existing, previously AFS poorly described and un-classified cases could be effectively described and classified with very rare exceptions offering a common "language"

of communication between the clinicians working in this field [16].

Currently, a wide range of non-invasive diagnostic procedures are available enriching the opportunity to detect the anatomical status of the female genital tract in an accurate way. However, the various existing methods have different characteristics, availability, invasiveness and diagnostic accuracy [5, 11, 54]. Thus, it is important to clarify their current role in the diagnostic work-up and objective documentation of female genital tract anomalies. Furthermore, standardised and systematic evaluation of asymptomatic women and of selected "high-risk" populations for the presence of female genital anomalies is fundamental for their management.

The aim of the Thessaloniki ESHRE/ESGE consensus is to provide the researchers with recommendations for the diagnostic work-up of female genital anomalies; the definitions of the ESHRE/ESGE classification were used as basis for their development. This is an initiative of the Congenital Uterine Anomalies (CONUTA) Working Group, which was started during the ESHRE Campus Workshop on Female Genital Anomalies in Thessaloniki.

Strategy for the consensus development

The development of the Thessaloniki ESHRE/ESGE consensus for the diagnosis of female genital anomalies by the CONUTA Working group was designed as follows:

1. *Evaluation of the currently available diagnostic methods,* including

   (1a) *The evaluation of the characteristics* of each different currently available diagnostic technique by the group of invited imaging experts and the members of the CONUTA group with the use of the *experts panel consensus method* [33]; a draft was circulated in two rounds for comments and a live meeting was arranged for the consensus

   (1b) *The evaluation of the diagnostic accuracy* of the different diagnostic methods performing a *systematic review of evidence* by SS, ADS and GG and

2. *Consensus development,* based on the results of the evaluation procedure, *including*

   (2a) *the definition of where and how to measure uterine wall thickness* by the invited imaging experts and the members of the CONUTA group with the use of the *experts panel consensus method*; a draft was circulated in two rounds for comments and a live meeting was arranged for the consensus

   (2b) *The recommendations* for the diagnostic work-up of female genital anomalies with the use of the *experts panel consensus method*, an initial proposal was circulated and the final document was prepared based on the comments.

The final document, including all the parts, was circulated again for final comments and approval from all the members of the consensus.

Evaluation of the currently available diagnostic methods

Diagnostic methods and their characteristics (consensus between experts)

Background Anatomy of the female genital tract is the basis of the ESHRE/ESGE classification system. More specifically, *uterine anatomy* is the basis for the *main classes and sub-classes.* Cervical and vaginal anomalies are classified independently in supplementary subcategories. Thus, diagnosis of uterine anomalies has to be based on diagnostic modalities that determine the anatomical status of the female genital tract in an objective way.

Each diagnostic method should ideally provide objective and measurable information on the anatomical status of: (i) the vagina, (ii) the cervix, (iii) the uterine cavity, (iv) the uterine wall, (v) the external contour of the uterus and (vi) the other intra-peritoneal structures.

Question What is the diagnostic potential, advantages, disadvantages and way of proper use of the available imaging techniques in the diagnosis of female genital tract congenital anomalies?

Gynaecological examination

Diagnostic potential inherent to the method

Some vaginal and some cervical malformations (aplasia, double cervices, longitudinal septa reaching to the external cervical os) can be diagnosed *objectively by inspection. Palpation* (through the vagina and/or the rectum in cases of vaginal aplasia) *cannot* provide *information* for the *uterine cavity and uterine wall* and could provide only some useful, but *highly subjective, information* for the uterine body (e.g. complete bicorporeal uterus). *Palpation* could provide information *in cases of dilatation secondary to obstruction of menstrual flow* (hematocolpos/hematometra/hemato-cavity in cases of non-communicating uterine horns).

Advantages

Gynaecological examination is always *the starting point and an essential part* of any woman's clinical evaluation. It is non-

invasive, simple, easy and low cost. It offers *unique information* in cases of some vaginal and cervical anomalies; it is also crucial that vaginal examination could elicit tenderness, which can aid diagnosis. It is included in the basic training of Obstetricians and Gynaecologists needing *no additional expertise.*

Disadvantages

It should not be used for the diagnosis of uterine anomalies due to its inherent inability to provide reliable information for uterine anatomy. It is not a primary approach in women who have never been sexually active.

Recommendations for its proper use

In cases of primary amenorrhea, careful inspection of the external genitalia for the presence of distal vaginal aplasia. Careful inspection of the vagina, to avoid mis-diagnosis in cases of longitudinal vaginal septa, by entering only in one of the two existing vaginal spaces. Careful inspection of the vaginal vault with a speculum to establish the presence of one or more cervical body(ies) or one cervical body with one or two external cervical opening(s). In cases of cyclic pelvic pain, with or without primary amenorrhea, careful palpation for palpable masses secondary to accumulation of menstrual blood (obstructed parts).

X-ray hysterosalpingography

Diagnostic potential inherent to the method

It *provides some reliable information* for the anatomy of the *uterine cavity* in the absence of cervical obstruction. It *could provide, also, information* for the anatomy of the *cervical canal* in the absence of cervical obstruction; the information on the anatomy of the cervical canal may be limited due to the instruments placed within and in the vicinity of the cervix. It *does not provide* any information for *the vagina* (exception: blind vagina with small opening), *the uterine wall and the external contour of the uterus.* It *does not provide any information* for rudimentary *non-communicating horns or cavities.*

Advantages

It is widely available and offers printable films that could be re-evaluated anytime. It offers additional useful information in cases of infertile women for potential intra-cavitary pathology (presence of defects/differential diagnosis between adhesions, polyps, myomas) and tubal morphology

Disadvantages

Its disadvantages include painful, risk of infection and irradiation of the patient. It is *more invasive than ultrasound,* not always easy and *needing radiological unit*. It *cannot be used for the differential diagnosis of uterine anomalies* due to its inherent inability to provide reliable information for uterine wall and the uterine outline anatomy; uterine anomalies represent the vast majority of malformations. Its diagnostic accuracy is restricted by false-positive and false-negative results; air bubbles might be mistaken for intra-cavity pathology; distension of the cavity due to fluid injection might distort the shape of the cavity to a degree that is related to whether there is a tubal ostia obstruction or not and, hence, limiting the value of assessing the interior contour. It *cannot be used for the diagnosis of obstructing anomalies*.

Recommendations for its proper use

The examiner has to be very cautious in order to be precise: *pulling the uterus is necessary* for the best imaging of the uterine cavity (otherwise small indentations could be missed). *Careful inspection of the vagina and the cervix* must be done to avoid mis-diagnosis in cases of double or septate cervix with or without longitudinal vaginal septa; *catheterization of both cervical* canals, if present, is necessary.

Two-dimensional ultrasound

Diagnostic potential inherent to the method

It could provide *reliable, objective and, most importantly, measurable information* for the anatomy of the *cervix, uterine cavity, uterine wall and external contour of the uterus*. It could provide *useful information of associated pelvic pathology*, e.g. ovarian pathology (e.g. benign and malignant tumours, endometriosis), hydrosalpinges, renal anomalies etc. It could provide, also, measurable information even for obstructing parts of the female genital tract. Transperineal 2D ultrasound may provide information on the vaginal cavity, especially in the presence of imperforate hemivagina.

Advantages

It is non-invasive, simple, low cost and available in almost every setting. *Gynaecologists are familiar* with the technique since training in ultrasound is included in the basic training in obstetrics and gynaecology; nowadays, *ultrasound examination is an essential part of women's routine evaluation*. Electronic storage of the diagnostic procedure is nowadays feasible for re-evaluation. It could provide the required planes in a flexible way since the examiner could change the position of ultrasound probes according to the needs of imaging. It offers additional valuable information in cases of infertile women for potential intra-cavitary (major adhesions might be suspected presented as "bridges" between the walls, polyps, myomas) and intramural pathology (myomas, adenomyosis).

Disadvantages

The *diagnostic accuracy of two-dimensional ultrasound (2D US)* being a dynamic examination, is highly dependent on the *experience of the examiner* and on the proper and *systematic way* of performing the procedure. It is not always feasible to have the required planes due to the patient's anatomical characteristics.

Recommendations for its proper use

The endometrial line should be well visible for precise imaging of the uterine cavity (late proliferative or secretory phase or intra-cavitary fluid enhancement/avoid early follicular phase). *Serial sagittal planes* from beyond the outer margin of one side of the uterus to the other including both cervix and uterine body if feasible *and transverse planes* from the cervix to beyond the uterine fundal level should be taken in a systematic way. In cases of vaginal obstruction or stenosis, if the woman consents, *transrectal ultrasound with vaginal probe or transperineal* could be performed to evaluate vaginal canal and uterus (not in children nor in adolescents). Abdominal palpation should be applied to improve the image by pushing away the bowel and to assess mobility of the pelvic organs; gynaecologists are better able to do this compared with sonographers.

Hysterosalpingo-contrast sonography

Diagnostic potential inherent to the method

It can provide *reliable, objective and, most importantly, measurable information* for the anatomy of the *cervix, uterine cavity, uterine wall, external contour of the uterus and* for other peritoneal structures (e.g. ovaries) with the exception of tubes. The *imaging of uterine cavity is better* due to the use of the contrast medium or saline enhancing the accuracy in identifying uterine cavity defects. Hysterosalpingo-contrast sonography could be used as a *tubal patency test* (infertile patients).

Advantages

It is minimally invasive, simple, low cost, potentially available in almost every setting (since only contrast medium is needed). *Gynaecologists could easily apply* the technique since training in ultrasound is included in the basic training in obstetrics and gynaecology, and insertion of an intra-uterine catheter could be done easily by them. *Electronic storage* of the diagnostic procedure is, nowadays, feasible for re-evaluation. It could provide *the required planes in a flexible way* since the examiner could change the position of ultrasound probes according to the needs of imaging. It offers *additional, more reliable information than that of 2D US* in cases of infertile women for *potential intra-cavitary* (adhesions presented as "bridges" between the walls, polyps, myomas) and *intramural pathology* (myomas, adenomyosis) but not necessarily for uterine malformations.

Disadvantages

The *diagnostic accuracy of hysterosalpingo-contrast sonography (HyCoSy)*, being a dynamic examination, is highly dependent on the *experience of the examiner* and on the proper and *systematic way* of performing. Distension of the uterine cavity could potentially modify internal uterine contour resulting *in false-negative imaging of the uterine cavity* especially in marginal uterine anomalies. It is not always feasible to have the required planes due to the patient's anatomical characteristics. It is rarely painful with difficulties in the insertion of the catheter.

Recommendations for its proper use

Early follicular phase is recommended as appropriate to avoid pregnancies and artefacts due to thick secretory endometrium. *Serial sagittal planes* from beyond the outer margin of one side of the uterus to the other including both cervix and uterine body if feasible *and transverse planes* from the cervix to beyond the uterine fundal level should be taken in a systematic way

Three-dimensional ultrasound

Diagnostic potential inherent to the method

It can provide *highly reliable, objective and, most importantly, measurable information* for the anatomy of the *cervix, uterine cavity, uterine wall, external contour of the uterus* and for associated pelvic pathology; the coronal plane of the uterus does provide a clear image of the cavity and *the external profile of the uterine fundus*. 3D volumes give *reliable and objective representation* of the *examined* organs *more independently of the examiner* overcoming the limitations of obtaining coronal images with 2D sonography. It can provide, also, measurable *information even for obstructed parts* of the female genital tract.

Advantages

It is non-invasive and easily applied to the patient (no difference from conventional ultrasound). *Reliable imaging of the uterus* since *uterine anatomy is presented* in the sagittal, transverse and coronal planes in an objective way independently of the examiner's ability. It provides *precise and objective measurements of the uterine dimensions* which is the absolute advantage in differential diagnosis between different classes. *Electronic storage* of the volume is, nowadays, routinely done for re-evaluation giving the opportunity for off-line analysis enabling the assessment of the uterus/uterine wall in different slices and to choose the plane of maximum interest in the coronal/sagittal or transverse sections for measurements. It offers *additional*

information, which is more reliable than that of 2D US, in cases of infertile women for potential intra-cavitary (adhesions presented as "bridges" between the walls, polyps, myomas) and intramural pathology (myomas, adenomyosis). *Transperineal three-dimensional ultrasound (3D US)* may offer the opportunity to view pelvic structures including the vagina and cervix.

Disadvantages

It is not so widely available as 2D US (up to now). It needs experienced sonographers with *special and adequate training* in 3-dimensional image acquisition and post-processing techniques. *Beware for artefacts* due to inappropriate volume acquisition and/or manipulation of the volume. It cannot provide very detailed and reliable data in very few cases of complex anomalies. 3D US without saline infusion or contrast medium cannot be used as a real time tubal patency test in cases of infertile patients.

Recommendations for its proper use

This method should be started with a 2D evaluation of the uterus. Use in midcycle or luteal phase is encouraged as this demonstrates the endometrial wall and the outline of the cavity at its best. Contrast medium could be used for the evaluation of the cavity and the tubes; in these cases, the examination has to be performed in the early follicular phase. Save a 3D volume for off-line analysis. The reconstructed coronal plane of the uterus might show the cavity and the external uterine profile as well as the tubal angle and the junctional zone, if possible along all the endometrium and cavity. Acquisition of an isolated cervical volume, without including the uterus: from a mid-sagittal plane, an axial plane of cervix can be obtained in 80 % and a coronal plane in 20 % of the cases; in cases of uterine malformations, the extent of the cervix and the limits of the cervical canal may be studied better. Diagnosis of associated vaginal anomalies can be done by transperineal acquisition of the pelvic floor volume after filling the vagina with gel or saline; an axial plane can be obtained from a mid-sagittal plane.

Magnetic resonance imaging

Diagnostic potential inherent to the method

It can provide *highly reliable and objective information* for the anatomical status of the vagina *cervix, uterine cavity, uterine wall, external contour of the uterus* and for other peritoneal structures with the exception of tubes. It provides, also, *reliable information even for dilated (obstructed) parts* of the female genital tract.

Advantages

It is non-invasive and it has no radiation. It gives *a reliable and objective representation* of the examining organs *in the sagittal, transverse and coronal plane* (three dimensions). It can be used for *diagnosis in cases of complex and obstructing anomalies*. *Electronic storage* of the diagnostic procedure is, nowadays, routinely done for re-evaluation

Disadvantages

It is more expensive and less available than ultrasound and not appropriate for patients with claustrophobia and morbid obesity. It needs *experience and training* in the assessment of the results. *The required planes are provided in a non-flexible way* since planes are pre-defined and independent of the examiner, a disadvantage that could potentially impair the diagnostic accuracy of the method in the absence of an experienced radiologist. It cannot be used as a tubal patency test in cases of infertile patients.

Recommendations for its proper use

Gynaecologists should be trained in magnetic resonance imaging (MRI) reading and work closely with radiologists to review the images as the clinical background knowledge of the former supplements the radiological interpretation of the images by the latter.

Hysteroscopy

Diagnostic potential inherent to the method

It provides *highly reliable information* for the anatomical status of the vagina (vaginoscopic approach), the *cervical canal and, mainly, the uterine cavity and the tubal ostia.*

Advantages

It is minimally invasive giving the additional *opportunity of treating T-shaped, septate and bicorporeal septate uterus. Its objective includes estimation of the cervical canal and endometrial cavity* (differential diagnosis of T-shaped and infantile uterus). It provides a minimal invasive *evaluation of the vagina and/or cervix in case of virgo.* *Electronic storage* of the procedure is, nowadays, routinely done for re-evaluation.

Disadvantages

It is more complex to organise but includes *no information for uterine wall thickness and uterine outline* and is unable to offer differential diagnosis between septate and bicorporeal uterus. It needs *experience and training*. Evaluation of the cavity is not feasible in cases of obstructed anomalies. It could not be used as a tubal patency test in cases of infertile patients.

Recommendations for its proper use

It complements ultrasound in the initial investigation of female genital tract malformations.

Endoscopy; laparoscopy and hysteroscopy

Diagnostic potential inherent to the method

It provides *highly reliable information* for the anatomical status of the vagina (vaginoscopic approach), *cervical canal, uterine cavity, tubal ostia, external contour of the uterus and the intraperitoneal structures.*

Advantages

It is a direct visualisation of the cervical canal, endometrial cavity and the *external contour* of the uterus representing until now the *"gold standard"* in the diagnosis and differential diagnosis. *Electronic storage* of the procedure is, nowadays, routinely done for re-evaluation. Endoscopic approach represents the minimally invasive route of choice in the *treatment of a wide variety of female genital anomalies.*

Disadvantages

It is invasive with no objective estimation of the uterine wall thickness. The diagnosis is mainly based on the subjective impression of the clinician performing them, and this is thought to be a limitation in the objective estimation of the anomaly. It needs *experience and training.*

Recommendations for its proper use

The invasiveness of the laparoscopic approach makes it not acceptable as a first-line screening procedure; it complements indirect imaging in the diagnosis of more complex anomalies in combination with possible surgical actions. It offers supplementary information about partial or total absence of Fallopian tubes and abnormal localization of ovaries.

Computerized tomography scanning (CTS)

Computerized tomography scanning (CTS) has no place any longer in the diagnosis of female genital anomalies due to radiation and poor depiction of the female genital structures and it was not included in the evaluation.

Diagnostic accuracy of the different methods (systematic review of evidence)

Question What is the diagnostic accuracy of the available imaging techniques in the diagnosis of female genital tract congenital anomalies as compared to the combined hysteroscopic and laparoscopic investigation (reference standard) based?

Limitations Prior to approaching this problem, the limitations have to be recognised and disclosed as follows. Firstly, the studies to date will not have based the assessment of different diagnostic accuracies on the current ESHRE/ESGE classification. Therefore, evidence will inevitably have to be drawn from the period following the initial Buttram and Gibbons classification [9], which was later revised into the American Fertility Society classification [1], the most widely accepted classification worldwide for the last 25 years.

Secondly, the gold standard method of comparison for diagnosis to date has been the combined hysteroscopy and laparoscopy investigation, which allows for the direct visualisation of the internal and external contour of the uterus but does not always allow accurate and objective uterine measurements. With the new ESHRE/ESGE classification and need to measure fundal, septal and lateral uterine wall thickness, it might be possible and necessary that the gold standard test may evolve to become another imaging modality in the future.

Methods Articles assessing the diagnostic accuracy of the most widely used imaging techniques were searched through MEDLINE, EMBASE and the Cochrane Library from 1988 to 2014. A combination of text words and Medical Subject Headings (MeSH) were used to generate the list of citations (Table 1); these were primarily designed for MEDLINE and were modified appropriately for EMBASE and the Cochrane Library. In addition to the electronic searches, relevant articles were hand searched from further citations. The study selection process is shown in Fig. 1.

The diagnostic accuracy was estimated by combining the values of sensitivity, specificity, positive predictive value (PPV) and negative predictive value (NPV) of each imaging technique according to the formula of Altman [14]; as reference standard was used the combined hysteroscopic and laparoscopic investigation. When studies did not report these values in text, 2×2 tables were manually constructed where

Table 1 Search terms used in the systematic review (either as MeSH terms or free text terms)

Uterus/abnormalities (MeSH)	Ultrasonography (MeSH)
Mullerian ducts/abnormalities (MeSH)	Hysterosalpingography (MeSH)
Female genital abnormalit[a]	Magnetic resonance imaging (MeSH)
Female genital anomal[a]	Hysteroscopy (MeSH)
	Laparoscopy (MeSH)

[a] Any character

possible, and these variables were individually estimated. Data were analysed on IBM SPSS version 21 for Windows (SPSS Inc., IL, USA). Means and 95 % confidence intervals (CI) for sensitivity, specificity, PPV and NPV and accuracy were calculated for each individual methodology.

Primary outcome of this systematic review was the accuracy of each diagnostic method in terms of identifying a congenital malformation.

Results Thirty-eight studies of high quality were included in the primary analysis. Several studies were excluded due to inadequate gold standard methodology used and incomplete/absent data regarding the diagnostic accuracy. There were no studies found reporting on the use of MRI as a screening tool (studies included patients with a previous diagnosis of congenital malformations undergoing further evaluation), and therefore the secondary outcome but not the primary outcome could be assessed for this methodology.

Pooled analysis of the included studies showed that the highest degrees of overall diagnostic accuracy were in decreasing order: 3D US (97.6 %), sonohysterography (SHG; 96.5 %), 2D US (86.6) and hysterosalpingography (HSG; 86.9 %). MRI was shown to be able to correctly subclassifiy 85.8 % of anomalies, which implies that the accuracy of identifying the presence of a malformation is well above 90 % (Tables 2, 3, 4, 5 and 6). Overall, it appears that 3D US may be more accurate than MRI in sub-classifying malformations, although it should be noted that sub-classification is hindered due to the subjective nature of the previous classifications adopted.

Consensus development

Measurement of the uterine wall thickness (consensus between experts)

Background Uterine wall thickness *is an important parameter and a reference point* for the definitions of dysmorphic T-shaped, septate and bicorporeal uteri according to the new classification system. The adoption of an objective criterion for the definition of uterine deformity is one of the advantages of the new classification system since according to AFS classification the detection of anomalies was based only on the subjective impression of the clinician performing the test. Although myometrial thickness at the various uterine regions cannot be easily assessed with endoscopic techniques, *it can be measured* with *ultrasound or MRI*.

However, the thickness of the uterine wall as the reference value for the estimation of the internal indentation at the mid-fundal level in cases of septate uterus, external indentation in cases of bicorporeal and lateral wall thickness in cases of T-shaped uterus might, indeed, vary in different regions of the

Fig. 1 The study selection process for the systematic review on the diagnostic accuracy of the different methods used to assess female genital anomalies

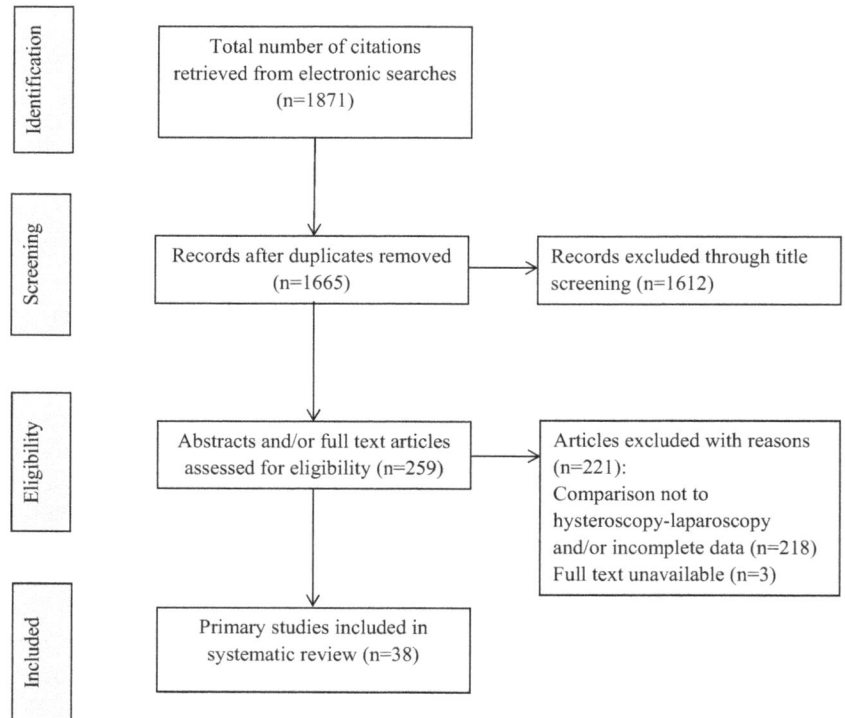

Identification

Total number of citations retrieved from electronic searches (n=1871)

Screening

Records after duplicates removed (n=1665) → Records excluded through title screening (n=1612)

Eligibility

Abstracts and/or full text articles assessed for eligibility (n=259) → Articles excluded with reasons (n=221): Comparison not to hysteroscopy-laparoscopy and/or incomplete data (n=218) Full text unavailable (n=3)

Included

Primary studies included in systematic review (n=38)

uterus. Thus, recommendations for the measurement of uterine dimensions and accurate description of uterine deformity are very important.

Question Where and how to measure the reference value of the uterine wall thickness?

Main option This include the distance between the interostial line and external uterine profile at the midcoronal plane of the uterus (fitted to 3D US, MRI and, at times, 2D US).

Definition of the reference value of the uterine wall thickness

This is the distance between the line connecting the tubal ostia and the external uterine profile *obtained with 3D US, MRI and, at times, with 2D US. Comments:* in cases of an external indentation (fusion defects), the distance between the two lines: one connecting the tubal ostia and the other the external outline of the two uterine bodies.

Why to use this as a reference parameter

Uterine anomalies are (fusion and/or absorption) defects at the uterine fundal midline and, therefore, measurements should be oriented there. Until now, imaging at that level has always been used until now to diagnose congenital uterine anomalies.

How to measure (Figs. 2, 3a-c and 4a-d):

Step 1   Imaging of the uterus in a midcoronal plane; a sectional plane or a rendered 3D ultrasound image of a coronal section of the uterus is now widely accepted as the most accurate plane for measurements.

Step 2   Draw the line connecting the two tubal ostia; in cases of an external indentation, draw a second line connecting the external profile of the two uterine bodies.

Step 3   In cases of patients with normal external uterine surface, the distance between the line connecting the tubal ostia and the external uterine outline is defined as the uterine wall thickness (reference value); in cases of patients with an existing external indentation, the distance between the two previously described lines is defined as the uterine wall thickness (reference value).

Step 4   Estimate the length of any existing internal indentation by measuring the distance between the interostial line and the indentation's edge at the cavity; septum is considered any indentation >50 % of the previously measured total fundal uterine wall thickness. Estimate of the lateral wall thickness by measuring at an angle of 90° to the lining of the myometrial-endometrial border.

Table 2 Diagnostic accuracy of HSG compared with hysteroscopy±laparoscopy in diagnosing female genital tract congenital anomalies

Study	Cases (n)	Sensitivity	Specificity	PPV	NPV	Accuracy
Bocca et al. [6]	125	50	94	71	87	76
Ludwin et al. [37]	83	77	100	100	35	78
De Felice et al. [14]	208	100	100	100	100	100
Momtaz et al. [44]	38	95	78	65	97	84
Guimaraes Filho et al. [30]	54	63	98	83	94	85
Valenzano et al. [58]	54	91	100	100	94	96
Traina et al. [57]	80	100	97	85	100	96
Alborzi et al. [3]	186	70	92	83	88	83
Preutthipan and Linasmita [48]	336	100	97	69	100	92
Brown et al. [7]	46	100	100	100	100	100
Soares et al. [55]	65	44	96	67	92	75
Alatas et al. [2]	62	100	100	100	100	100
Garglione 1997	70	100	100	100	100	100
Goldberg et al. [23]	32	100	100	100	100	100
Keltz et al. [34]	18	90	20	53	67	58
Raziel et al. [51]	60	74	59	62	72	67
Mean (95 % CI)		84.6 (74.4–94.9)	89.4 (80.0–100)	83.6 (74.6–92.6)	89.1 (79.7–98.5)	86.9 (79.8–94.0)

HSG hysterosalpingogram, *PPV* positive predictive value, *NPV* negative predictive value, *CI* confidence interval

Comments: 1. Tubal ostia should be considered as the ultrasound border between uterine cavity and the proximal intramural part of the tubes. 2. *External uterine contour should be delineated clearly* in ultrasound images to avoid under- or overestimation of the uterine wall thickness. A non-rendered image in the C plane may give a sharper outline compared with a (thin) sliced rendered image.

Drawbacks Drawback include the following: (1) When an anomaly is present, measurements in certain parts (fundus) could not be, sometimes, either feasible or representative, (2) external profile of the uterus at the fundal level is not always clearly assessable leading to an inaccurate evaluation and (3) in cases of bicorporeal uterus, sometimes the two uterine bodies are not very close to each other and this could create some diagnostic bias.

Alternative option This include the mean thickness of the anterior and posterior uterine wall (fitted to 2D US).

Definition of the reference value of the uterine wall thickness

This is the mean thickness of the anterior and posterior wall in 2D or 3D US longitudinal planes at the mid-point of the

Table 3 Diagnostic accuracy of 2D US compared with hysteroscopy±laparoscopy in diagnosing female genital tract congenital anomalies

Study	Cases (n)	Sensitivity (%)	Specificity (%)	PPV (%)	NPV (%)	Accuracy (%)
Ludwin et al. [38]	117	91	92	99	52	84
De Felice et al. [14]	104	100	99	86	100	96
Momtaz et al. [44]	38	55	95	84	83	79
Valenzano et al. [58]	54	86	100	100	91	94
Ragni et al. [50]	98	73	100	100	97	93
Traina et al. [57]	80	64	99	88	94	86
Soares et al. [55]	65	44	100	100	92	84
Alatas et al. [2]	62	50	100	100	97	87
Nicolini et al. [46]	89	43	98	94	68	76
Mean (95 % CI)		67.3 (51.0–83.7)	98.1 (96.0–100)	94.6 (89.4–99.8)	86.0 (73.7–98.3)	86.6 (81.3–91.8)

2D US two-dimensional ultrasound, *PPV* positive predictive value, *NPV* negative predictive value, *CI* confidence interval

Table 4 Diagnostic accuracy of HyCoSy compared with hysteroscopy±laparoscopy in diagnosing female genital tract congenital anomalies

Study	Cases (n)	Sensitivity (%)	Specificity (%)	PPV (%)	NPV (%)	Accuracy (%)
Ludwin et al. [38]	117	94	83	99	65	85
Ludwin et al. [37]	83	96	89	99	73	89
De Felice et al. [14]	104	100	100	100	100	100
Guimaraes Filho et al. [30]	55	100	94	73	100	92
Valenzano et al. [58]	54	100	100	100	100	100
Ragni et al. [50]	98	91	100	100	99	98
Alborzi et al. [3]	186	91	100	100	96	97
Dodero et al. [17]	52	100	100	100	100	100
Brown et al. [7]	46	100	100	100	100	100
Soares et al. [55]	65	73	100	100	97	93
Alatas et al. [2]	62	100	100	100	100	100
Goldberg et al. [23]	32	100	100	100	100	100
Keltz et al. [34]	18	100	100	100	100	100
Mean (95 % CI)		95.8 (91.1–100)	97.4 (94.1–100)	97.8 (93.3–100)	94.6 (87.6–100)	96.5 (93.4–99.5)

HyCoSy hysterosalpingo-contrast sonography, *PPV* positive predictive value, *NPV* negative predictive value, *CI* confidence interval

uterine corpus. *Comments:* in cases of septate or bicorporeal uteri with an internal indentation covering more than 50 % of the uterine cavity, the longitudinal plane at the mid-cavity level is affected by the indentation and it could not be used as a reference plane for measurements. In that case, a longitudinal plane of the lateral cavities could be used as the reference for measurements in the same described way.

Why to use this as a reference parameter:

This part of the uterine wall could be considered as representative for measurements since it is not affected in cases of

uterine anomalies and if it is affected alternatives could be provided.

How to measure:

Step 1   Imaging of the uterus in longitudinal plane,
Step 2   Estimation of mid-point between the fundal part of uterine cavity and the internal cervical os and
Step 3   Measurements of uterine wall thickness of the anterior and posterior wall at the mid-point level (estimated in step 2) taking the mean of those measurements as the reference point

Table 5 Diagnostic accuracy of 3D US compared with hysteroscopy±laparoscopy in diagnosing female genital tract congenital anomalies

Study	Cases (n)	Sensitivity (%)	Specificity (%)	PPV (%)	NPV (%)	Accuracy (%)
Imboden et al. [31]	10	100	100	100	100	100
Laganà et al. [35]	224	100	100	100	100	100
Ludwin et al. [38]	117	97	100	100	80	94
Moini et al. [42]	214	87	97	99	54	84
Bocca et al. [6][a]	125	100	100	100	100	100
Faivre et al. [18]	31	100	100	100	100	100
Ghi et al. [22]	284	100	100	100	100	100
Makris et al. [39]	248	100	100	100	100	100
Momtaz et al. [44]	38	97	96	92	99	96
Radoncic and Funduk-Kurjak [49]	267	100	100	100	100	100
Wu et al. [61]	40	100	100	100	100	100
Mean (95 % CI)		98.3 (95.6–100)	99.4 (98.4–100)	99.2 (97.6–100)	93.9 (84.2–100)	97.6 (94.3–100)

3D US three-dimensional ultrasound, *PPV* positive predictive value, *NPV* negative predictive value, *CI* confidence interval

[a] Performed in conjunction with saline infusion

Table 6 Diagnostic accuracy of MRI compared with hysteroscopy± laparoscopy in diagnosing female genital tract congenital anomalies

Study	Cases (*n*)	Correct sub-classification (*n*; %)
Imboden et al. [31]	13	7/13 (54 %)
Faivre et al. [18]	31	24/31 (77 %)
Santos et al. [53]	26	23/26 (89 %)
Mueller et al. [45]	105	83/105 (81 %)
Deutch et al. [15]	7	2/7 (29 %)
Marten et al. [40]	4	4/4 (100 %)
Console et al. [13]	22	21/22 (95 %)
Minto et al. [41]	9	7/9 (78 %)
Letterie et al. [36]	16	12/16 (75 %)
Pellerito et al. [47]	24	24/24 (100 %)
Carrington et al. [10]	29	29/29 (100 %)
Fedele et al. [19]	18	18/18 (100 %)
Weighted mean		254/296 (85.8 %)

MRI magnetic resonance imaging;

Sensitivity, specificity, PPV and NPV cannot be assessed for MRI as this was not used as a *screening* tool in the studies identified

Drawbacks

Drawbacks include the following: (1) Uterine wall thickness at the posterior, anterior and lateral uterine walls' level is, probably, different from that observed at the fundal level even in the absence of any pathology, (2) uterine wall thickness at that level (mean of the anterior and posterior walls' thickness on a longitudinal section) has never been used to define congenital uterine anomalies, (3) uterine wall thickness at the posterior and anterior level will be affected by a number of uterine conditions like fibromas and adenomyosis. Furthermore, with the vascular network placed laterally, the wall thickness might well be different and (4) uterine anomalies are (fusion and/or absorption) defects at the uterine fundal midline and, therefore, measurements should be oriented there.

Recommendations (consensus between CONUTA group members and invited experts)

Background Female genital anomalies are common benign entities with an estimating prevalence ranging from ~6 % in the general population up to ~15 % in selected population with recurrent pregnancy losses. Thus, women of reproductive age during their routine examination should be examined for the presence of a potential congenital anomaly. Certainly in symptomatic patients or, otherwise, in patients with higher risk for the presence of an anomaly, special attention should be paid during their diagnostic work-up.

The recommendations for the diagnostic work-up were based on the diagnostic potential of the different methods and their diagnostic accuracy. Additional parameters (e.g. accessibility, need for training and expertise, cost etc.) were also taken into account. The diagnostic methods should be used in a systematic way taking into consideration the comments for their proper use. The anatomical characteristics should be recorded and documented as described previously based on the anatomical varieties of the ESHRE/ESGE classification system.

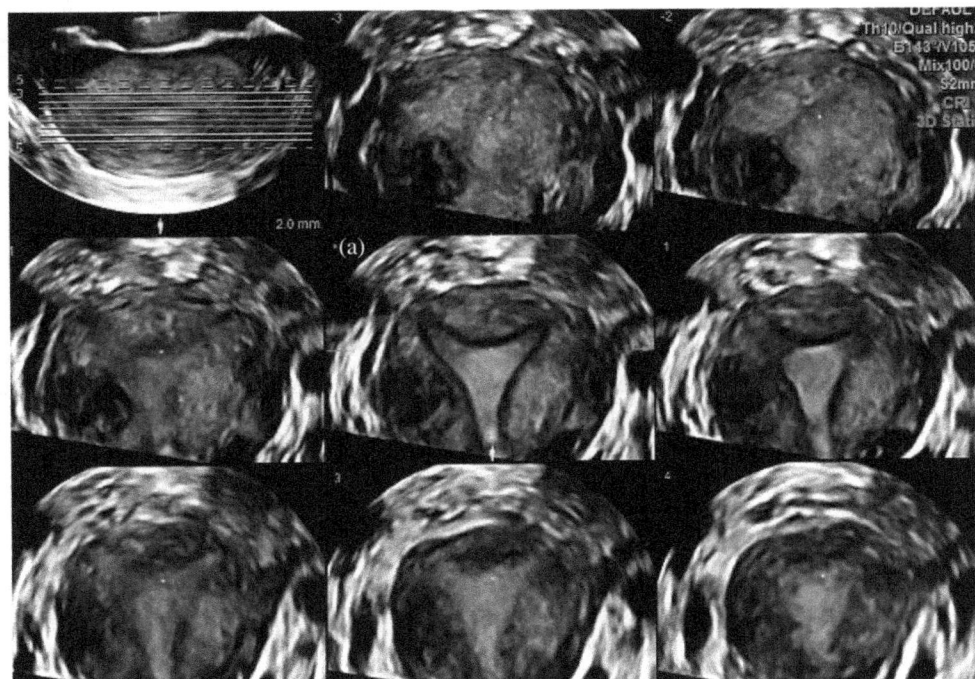

Fig. 2 How to obtain an optimal 3D US coronal plane: tomographic ultrasound imaging (TUI) is the representation by a series of parallel slices through the volume and the distance between the slices as well as their number can be configured; the plane is optimal only if the slices or cutting line is exactly on the endometrium and the junctional zone at the level of the tubal ostia and isthmus (a) at the central plane

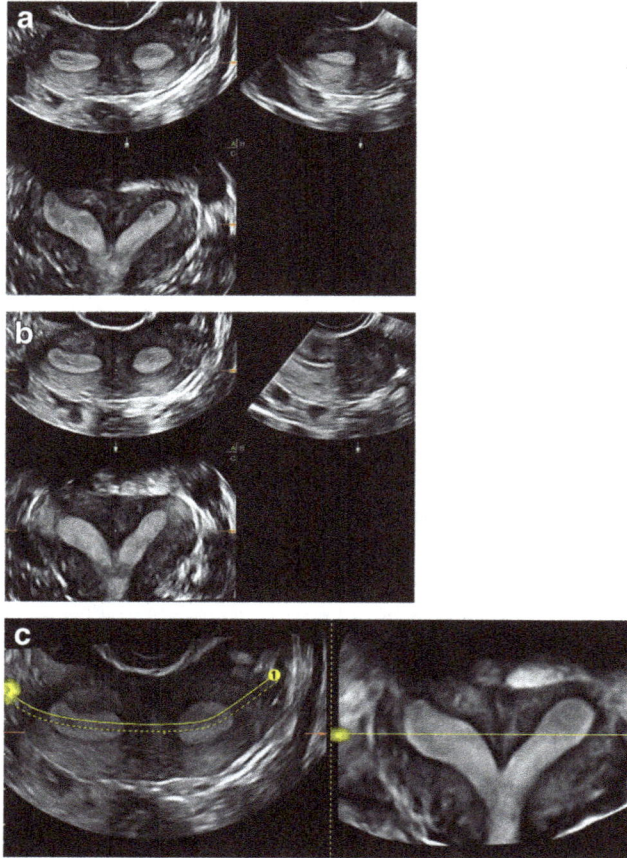

Fig. 3 a–c How to obtain an optimal 3D US coronal plane: cutting line is not perfect on the endometrium in (**a**) and (**b**); thus, if necessary, the *dotted line* can be curved to follow the endometrium and the tubal ostia like in plane (**c**)

Definitions

Asymptomatic patients	Patients consulting for routine gynaecological examination without complaints of chronic pelvic pain (i.e. dysmenorrhea, dyspareunia, cyclic low abdominal pain) and history of poor reproductive outcome having normal gynaecological findings at clinical examination.
Symptomatic or high risk patients	Groups of patients presenting with clinical problems that could be associated with the presence of female genital anomalies and expected to have higher prevalence than that of the general population. Thus, as symptomatic groups should be considered: (1) patients with *primary amenorrhea, inability of normal intercourse, chronic pelvic pain* (dysmenorhea, dyspareunia, cyclic

abdominal pain); (2) patients *with poor reproductive outcome*, including (a) patients with *two or more IVF failures*, (b) women with *two or more 1st trimester pregnancy losses* and/or one *2nd trimester loss* and (c) women with a history of *preterm delivery*; and (3) *adolescents with symptoms* suggestive for the presence of a female genital anomaly.

Recommended evaluation of asymptomatic women
Clinicians should, always, be attentive for the presence of a congenital anomaly in asymptomatic women of reproductive age during their routine examination, supplementing gynaecological examination with a 2D US as follows:

- Gynaecological examination: the anatomy of the external genitalia, the vagina and the cervix should be carefully evaluated.
- 2D US: it should be done in a pre-defined and systematic manner to increase its diagnostic accuracy. The shape and the dimensions of the uterine cavity, the uterine wall (anterior, posterior, lateral and fundal width) and external uterine contour should be recorded in a systematic way in longitudinal and transverse planes.
- The absence of findings suspicious for the presence of an anomaly should not be considered as definite and the presence of one could not be excluded.
- Positive findings should be used for documentation only and counselling of the patients for further investigation given that they are asymptomatic women.

Recommended diagnostic work-up of selected population
The following thorough, preferably non-invasive, high accuracy diagnostic work-up is recommended for (1) *all symptomatic patients* of reproductive age, sexually active, *belonging to "high risk" groups* for the presence of a female genital anomaly and (2) *any asymptomatic woman suspected* to have anomaly from routine evaluation and wishing to undergo a more thorough evaluation. Furthermore, although they could not be considered as symptomatic, careful inspection is recommended for infertile patients after a first trimester miscarriage where foetal heart beats and for those entering IVF and/or older than 35 years old.

- Gynaecological examination with carefull evaluation and recording of the external genitalia, vaginal and cervical anatomy.
- 2D US (vaginal) in a pre-defined and systematic manner (to increase its diagnostic accuracy), where the shape and the dimensions of the uterine cavity, the uterine wall (anterior, posterior, lateral and fundal width) and external

Fig. 4 (**a**) Coronal 3D US view of a normal uterus; uterine wall thickness: *distance between the line joining tubal ostia (interostial line) and a parallel line on the top of the fundus*. (**b**) Coronal 3D US view of a partial septate uterus; *1*, uterine wall thickness: distance between the line joining tubal ostia (interostial line) and a parallel line on the top of uterine fundus; *2*, internal midline indentation: distance between the interostial line and a parallel line on the top of midline indentation. (**c**) Coronal 3D US view of a complete septate uterus: *1*, uterine wall thickness: distance between the line joining tubal ostia (interostial line) and a parallel line on the top of uterine fundus; *2*, internal midline indentation: distance between the interostial line and a parallel line on the top of midline indentation (the line reaches the internal cervical os). (**d**) Coronal 3D US view of a bicorporeal septate uterus: uterine wall thickness: distance between the interostial line and a parallel line joining the external outline of the uterine horns

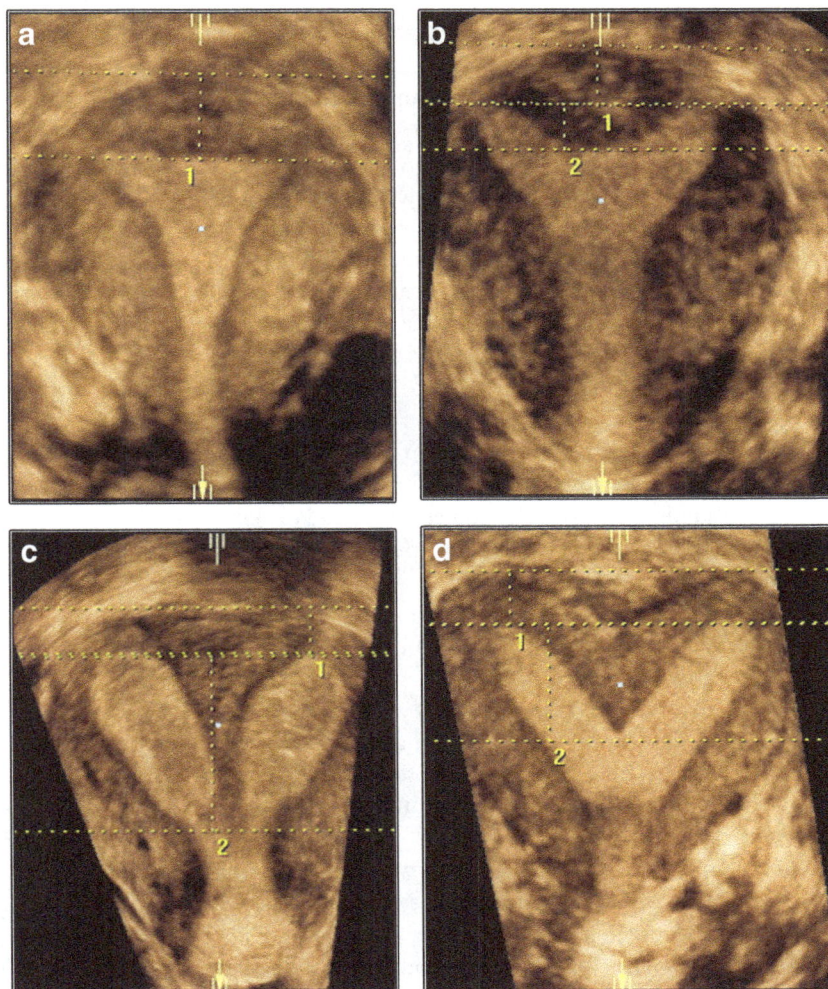

uterine contour should be recorded in a systematic way and pre-defined way in longitudinal and transverse planes. Measurements of 2D US examination should be used as a referendum for the evaluation of uterine anatomy deviations in 3D ultrasound.

- 3D US (vaginal) in a pre-defined and systematic manner where the shape and the deviations from normal cervical and uterine anatomy should be recorded and documented.

In subgroups of patients with *subfertility, recurrent IVF failures or recurrent pregnancy losses* additional examinations can be performed:

- HyCoSy or 2D or 3D SHG by an experienced sonographer when available.
- Hysteroscopy and, in cases of suspected adnexal pathology, hydrolaparoscopy or laparoscopy. Those techniques should be offered by clinicians, endoscopic reproductive surgeons, having also the ability to surgically treat any discovered pathology.

- X-ray HSG, nowadays, should not be considered anymore as a "first-line" diagnostic procedure and should be reserved only for settings where the pre-mentioned diagnostic methods are not available or for health systems where indicated for other reasons. Congenital uterine anomaly may be suspected from HSG performed in women with infertility to verify tubal patency".

Recommended diagnostic work-up for complex anomalies
Sub-groups of patients with suspected *complex anomalies* (defined as anomalies resulting from disturbances in more than one stage of normal embryological development and having as a result anatomical deviations in more than one organ of the female genital tract) and *those where the application of the previously mentioned methods could not be applied* (e.g. obstructing anomalies) should be evaluated as follows:

- Abdominal and/or transrectal 3D US in a pre-defined and systematic manner where the shape and the deviations from normal cervical and uterine anatomy should be recorded and documented.

- MRI: evaluation of the results is recommended to be done by an imaging expert in collaboration with an experienced gynaecologist.
- Hysteroscopy and laparoscopy: these techniques should be offered by clinicians (endoscopic reproductive) and surgeons with experience in the management of complex female genital anomalies in special centres after thorough non-invasive evaluation and, mainly, in the context of concomitant surgical treatment of any discovered pathology.

Recommended diagnostic work-up for adolescents
Adolescents with symptoms suggestive for the presence of a female genital anomaly (primary amenorrhea and/or pelvic masses or pathology and/or cyclic pelvic pain) should be evaluated as follows:

- Gynaecological examination with careful evaluation and recording of the external genitalia.
- Abdominal and/or transrectal 2D US where the presence, the shape and the dimensions of the uterus (cavity, wall and external contour) should be recorded in a systematic and pre-defined manner in longitudinal and transverse planes.
- Abdominal and/or transrectal 3D US where the shape and the deviations from normal cervical and uterine anatomy should be recorded and documented.
- MRI as a first-line diagnostic procedure. Evaluation of the results is recommended to be done by an imaging expert in collaboration with an experienced gynaecologist.
- Hysteroscopy and laparoscopy: those techniques should be offered in the context of concomitant surgical treatment of any discovered pathology and only by endoscopic reproductive surgeons with experience in the management of complex female genital anomalies in special centres after thorough non-invasive evaluation.

In patients with female genital anomalies, *investigation of the urinary tract* is also recommended as mandatory.

Conclusion The combination of gynaecological examination and 2D US could be recommended as the current standard for the evaluation of asymptomatic women; 3D US could be considered the standard for diagnosis of female genital anomalies supplemented by MRI, hysteroscopy and laparoscopy in complex ones or in diagnostic dilemmas.

Open issues for further research The role of a combined ultrasound examination together with outpatient hysteroscopy as a one-stop diagnostic evaluation of symptomatic "high-risk" patients should be prospectively evaluated. The ESHRE/ESGE classification should be considered as a guide for diagnosis offering a common terminology among the clinicians to convey the exact anatomical status of the female genital tract [29, 16]; based on that, it is a challenge for further research to objectively estimate the clinical consequences related to various degrees of uterine deformity, e.g. the length of the septum and the potential co-factors that are associated with poor reproductive outcome. Large prospective studies with correct classifications and accurate measurements of the length of midline indentations are needed to establish optimal indications of reconstructive surgery in patients with congenital uterine anomalies.

References

1. American Fertility Society (1988) The AFS classification of adnexal aghesions, distul tubal occlusion, tubal occlusion secondary to tubal ligation, tubal pregnancies, Mullerian anomalies and intrauterine adhesions. Fertil Steril 49:944–955
2. Alatas C, Aksoy E, Akarsu C, Yakin K, Aksoy S, Hayran M (1997) Evaluation of intrauterine abnormalities in infertile patients by sonohysterography. Hum Reprod 12:487–490
3. Alborzi S, Dehbashi S, Khodaee R (2003) Sonohysterosalpingographic screening for infertile patients. Int J Gynaecol Obstet 82:57–62
4. Altman DG (1991) Practical statistics for medical research. Chapman & Hall, London
5. Bermejo C, Ten Martínez P, Cantarero R, Diaz D, Pérez Pedregosa J, Barrón E, Labrador E, Ruiz López L (2010) Three-dimensional ultrasound in the diagnosis of Müllerian duct anomalies and concordance with magnetic resonance imaging. Ultrasound Obstet Gynecol 35(5):593–601
6. Bocca SM, Oehninger S, Stadtmauer L, Agard J, Duran EH, Sarhan A, Horton S, Abuhamad AZ (2012) A study of the cost, accuracy, and benefits of 3-dimensional sonography compared with hysterosalpingography in women with uterine abnormalities. J Ultrasound Med 31(1):81–85
7. Brown SE, Coddington CC, Schnorr J, Toner JP, Gibbons W, Oehninger S (2000) Evaluation of outpatient hysteroscopy, saline infusion hysterosonography, and hysterosalpingography in infertile women: a prospective, randomized study. Fertil Steril 74:1029–1034
8. Brucker SY, Rall K, Campo R, Oppelt P, Isaacson K (2011) Treatment of congenital malformations. Semin Reprod Med 29:101–112
9. Buttram VC, Gibbons WE (1979) Mullerian anomalies: a proposed classification (an analysis of 144 cases). Fertil Steril 32:40–46
10. Carrington BM, Hricak H, Nuruddin RN, Secaf E, Laros RK Jr, Hill EC (1990) Müllerian duct anomalies: MR imaging evaluation. Radiology 176:715–720

11. Chan YY, Jayaprakasan K, Zamora J, Thornton JG, Raine-Fenning N, Coomarasamy A (2011) The prevalence of congenital uterine anomalies in unselected and high-risk populations: a systematic review. Hum Reprod Update 17:761–771

12. Chan YY, Jayarpakasan K, Tan A, Thornton JG, Coomarasamy A, Raine-Fenning NJ (2011) Reproductive outcomes in women with congenital uterine anomalies: a systematic review. Ultrasound Obstet Gynecol 38:371–382

13. Console D, Tamburrini S, Barresi D, Notarangelo L, Bertucci B, Tamburrini O (2001) The value of the MR imaging in the evaluation of Müllerian duct anomalies. Radiol Med 102(4):226–232

14. De Felice C, Porfiri LM, Savelli S, Alfano G, Pace S, Manganaro L, Vestri AR, Drudi FM (2009) Infertility in women: combined sonohysterography and hysterosalpingography in the evaluation of the uterine cavity. Ultraschall Med 30(1):52–57

15. Deutch T, Bocca S, Oehninger S et al (2006) Magnetic resonance imaging versus three-dimensional transvaginal ultrasound for the diagnosis of Müllerian anomalies. Fertil Steril 86:S308

16. Di Spiezio Sardo A, Campo R, Gordts S, Spinelli M, Cosimato C, Tanos V, Brucker S, Li TC, Gergolet M, De Angelis C, Gianaroli L, Grimbizis G (2015) The comprehensiveness of the ESHRE/ESGE classification of female genital tract congenital anomalies: a systematic review of cases not classified by the AFS system. Hum Reprod 30(5):1046–1058

17. Dodero D, Corticelli A, Caporale E, Cardamone C, Francescangeli E (2001) Benign uterine pathology in premenopause and transvaginal sonohysterography: personal experience. Minerva Ginecol 53(6):383–387

18. Faivre E, Fernandez H, Deffieux X, Gervaise A, Frydman R, Levaillant JM (2012) Accuracy of three-dimensional ultrasonography in differential diagnosis of septate and bicornuate uterus compared with office hysteroscopy and pelvic magnetic resonance imaging. J Minim Invasive Gynecol 19(1):101–106

19. Fedele L, Dorta M, Brioschi D, Massari C, Candiani GB (1989) Magnetic resonance evaluation of double uteri. Obstet Gynecol 74(6):844–847

20. Fedele L, Bianchi S, Zanconato G, Berlanda N, Bergamini (2005) Laparoscopic removal of the cavitated noncommunicating rudimentary uterine horn: surgical aspects in 10 cases. Fertil Steril 83:432–436

21. Gergolet M, Rudi Campo R, Verdenik I, Kenda Suster N, Gordts S, Gianaroli L (2012) No clinical relevance of the height of fundal indentation in subseptate or arcuate uterus: a prospective study. Reprod Biomed Online 24:576–582

22. Ghi T, Casadio P, Kuleva M, Perrone AM, Savelli L, Giunchi S, Meriggiola MC, Gubbini G, Pilu G, Pelusi C, Pelusi G (2009) Accuracy of three-dimensional ultrasound in diagnosis and classification of congenital uterine anomalies. Fertil Steril 92(2):808–813

23. Goldberg JM, Falcone T, Attaran M (1997) Sonohysterographic evaluation of uterine abnormalities noted on hysterosalpingography. Hum Reprod 12(10):2151–2153

24. Grimbizis GF, Camus M, Tarlatzis BC, Bontis JN, Devroey P (2001) Clinical implications of uterine malformations and hysteroscopic treatment results. Hum Reprod Update 7:161–164

25. Grimbizis GF, Tsalikis T, Mikos T, Papadopoulos N, Tarlatzis BC, Bontis JN (2004) Successful end-to-end cervico-cervical anastomosis in a patient with congenital cervical fragmentation: case report. Hum Reprod 19:1204–1210

26. Grimbizis GF, Campo R (2010) Congenital malformations of the female genital tract: the need for a new classification system. Fertil Steril 94:401–407

27. Grimbizis GF, Gordts G, Di Spiezio SA, Brucker S, De Angelis C, Gergolet M, Li T-C, Tanos V, Brölmann H, Gianaroli L, Campo R (2013) The ESHRE/ESGE consensus on the classification of female genital tract congenital malformations. Hum Reprod 28:2032–2044

28. Grimbizis GF, Gordts G, Di Spiezio SA, Brucker S, De Angelis C, Gergolet M, Li T-C, Tanos V, Brölmann H, Gianaroli L, Campo R (2013) The ESHRE/ESGE consensus on the classification of female genital tract congenital malformations. Gynecol Surg 10:199–212

29. Grimbizis GF, Gordts G, Di Spiezio SA, Brucker S, De Angelis C, Gergolet M, Li T-C, Tanos V, Brölmann H, Gianaroli L, Campo R (2014) Reply: are the ESHRE/ESGE criteria of female genital anomalies for diagnosis of septate uterus appropriate? Hum Reprod 29:868–869

30. Guimaraes Filho HA, Mattar R, Pires CR, Araujo Junior E, Moron AF, Nardozza LM (2006) Comparison of hysterosalpingography, hysterosonography and hysteroscopy in evaluation of the uterine cavity in patients with recurrent pregnancy losses. Arch Gynecol Obstet 274:284–288

31. Imboden S, Müller M, Raio L, Mueller MD, Tutschek B (2014) Clinical significance of 3D ultrasound compared to MRI in uterine malformations. Ultraschall Med 35(5):440–444

32. Joki-Erkkilä MM, Heinonen PK (2003) Presenting and long-term clinical implications and fecundity in females with obstructing vaginal malformations. J Pediatr Adolesc Gynecol 16:307–312

33. Jones J, Hunter D (1995) Consensus methods for medical and health services research. BMJ 311:376–380

34. Keltz MD, Olive DL, Kim AH, Arici A (1997) Sonohysterography for screening in recurrent pregnancy loss. Fertil Steril 67:670–674

35. Laganà AS, Ciancimino L, Mancuso A, Chiofalo B, Rizzo P, Triolo O (2014) 3D sonohysterography vs hysteroscopy: a cross-sectional study for the evaluation of endouterine diseases. Arch Gynecol Obstet 290(6):1173–1178

36. Letterie GS, Haggerty M, Lindee G (1995) A comparison of pelvic ultrasound and magnetic resonance imaging as diagnostic studies for Müllerian tract abnormalities. Int J Fertil Menopausal Stud 40:34–38

37. Ludwin A, Ludwin I, Banas T, Knafel A, Miedzyblocki M, Basta A (2011) Diagnostic accuracy of sonohysterography, hysterosalpingography and diagnostic hysteroscopy in diagnosis of arcuate, septate and bicornuate uterus. J Obstet Gynaecol Res 37(3):178–186

38. Ludwin A, Pityński K, Ludwin I, Banas T, Knafel A (2013) Two- and three-dimensional ultrasonography and sonohysterography versus hysteroscopy with laparoscopy in the differential diagnosis of septate, bicornuate, and arcuate uteri. J Minim Invasive Gynecol 20(1):90–99

39. Makris N, Kalmantis K, Skartados N, Papadimitriou A, Mantzaris G, Antsaklis A (2007) Three-dimensional hysterosonography versus hysteroscopy for the detection of intracavitary uterine abnormalities. Int J Gynaecol Obstet 97:6–9

40. Marten K, Vosshenrich R, Funke M, Obenauer S, Baum F, Grabbe E (2003) MRI in the evaluation of Müllerian duct anomalies. Clin Imaging 27(5):346–350

41. Minto CL, Hollings N, Hall-Craggs M, Creighton S (2001) Magnetic resonance imaging in the assessment of complex Müllerian anomalies. BJOG 108(8):791–797

42. Moini A, Mohammadi S, Hosseini R, Eslami B, Ahmadi F (2013) Accuracy of 3-dimensional sonography for diagnosis and classification of congenital uterine anomalies. J Ultrasound Med 32(6):923–927

43. Mollo A, De Franciscis P, Colacurci N, Cobellis L, Perino A, Venezia R, Alviggi C, De Placido G (2009) Hysteroscopic resection of the septum improves the pregnancy rate of women with unexplained infertility: a prospective controlled trial. Fertil Steril 91:2628–2631

44. Momtaz MM, Ebrashy AN, Marzouk AA (2007) Three-dimensional ultrasonography in the evaluation of the uterine cavity. Middle East Fertil Soc J 12(1):41–46

45. Mueller GC, Hussain HK, Smith YR, Quint EH, Carlos RC, Johnson TD, DeLancey JO (2007) Müllerian duct anomalies:

comparison of MRI diagnosis and clinical diagnosis. AJR Am J Roentgenol 189(6):1294–1302

46. Nicolini U, Bellotti M, Bonazzi B, Zamberletti D, Candiani GB (1987) Can ultrasound be used to screen uterine malformations? Fertil Steril 47:89–93

47. Pellerito JS, McCarthy SM, Doyle MB, Glickman MG, DeCherney AH (1992) Diagnosis of uterine anomalies: relative accuracy of MR imaging, endovaginal ultrasound, and hysterosalpingography. Radiology 183:795–800

48. Preutthipan S, Linasmita V (2003) A prospective comparative study between hysterosalpingography and hysteroscopy in the detection of intrauterine pathology in patients with infertility. J Obstet Gynaecol Res 29(1):33–37

49. Radoncic E, Funduk-Kurjak B (2000) Three-dimensional ultrasound for routine check-up in in vitro fertilization patients. Croat Med J 41:262

50. Ragni G, Diaferia D, Vegetti W, Colombo M, Arnoldi M, Crosignani PG (2005) Effectiveness of sonohysterography in infertile patient work-up: a comparison with transvaginal ultrasonography and hysteroscopy. Gynecol Obstet Investig 59(4):184–188

51. Raziel A, Arieli S, Bukovsky I, Caspi E, Golan A (1994) Investigation of the uterine cavity in recurrent aborters. Fertil Steril 62:1080–1082

52. Rock JA, Roberts CP, Jones HW (2010) Congenital anomalies of the uterine cervix: lessons from 30 cases managed clinically by a common protocol. Fertil Steril 94:1858–1863

53. Santos XM, Krishnamurthy R, Bercaw-Pratt JL, Dietrich JE (2012) The utility of ultrasound and magnetic resonance imaging versus surgery for the characterization of Müllerian anomalies in the pediatric and adolescent population. J Pediatr Adolesc Gynecol 25(3): 181–184

54. Saravelos SH, Cocksedge KA, Li T-C (2008) Prevalence and diagnosis of congenital uterine anomalies in women with reproductive failure: a critical appraisal. Hum Reprod Update 14:415–419

55. Soares SR, Barbosa dos Reis MM, Camargos AF (2000) Diagnostic accuracy of sonohysterography, transvaginal sonography, and hysterosalpingography in patients with uterine cavity diseases. Fertil Steril 73:406–411

56. Strawbrigde LC, Crough NS, Cutner AS, Creighton SM (2007) Obstructive Mullerian anomalies and modern laparoscopic management. J Pediatr Adolesc Gynecol 20:195–200

57. Traina E, Mattar R, Moron AF, Neto LCA, Matheus EDE (2004) Diagnostic accuracy of hysterosalpingography and transvaginal sonography to evaluate uterine cavity diseases in patients with recurrent miscarriage. Rev Bras Ginecol Obstet 26:527–533

58. Valenzano MM, Mistrangelo E, Lijoi D, Fortunato T, Lantieri PB, Risoo D, Constantini S, Ragni N (2006) Transvaginal sonohysterographic evaluation of uterine malformations. Eur J Obstet Gynecol Reprod Biol 124:246–249

59. Venetis C, Papadopoulos S, Campo R, Gordts S, Tarlatzis BC, Grimbizis GF (2014) Clinical implications of congenital uterine anomalies: a meta-analysis of comparative studies. Reprod Biomed Online 29(6):665–683

60. Wu MH, Hsu CC, Huang KE (1997) Detection of congenital Müllerian duct anomalies using three-dimensional ultrasound. J Clin Ultrasound 25:487–492

Authors' Roles

Scientific coordinators: Grigoris Grimbizis and Rudi Campo

Coordination of recommendations development: Stephan Gordts

Systematic evaluation of diagnostic accuracy: Sotirios Saravelos, Attilio Di Spiezio Sardo and Grigoris Grimbizis

CONUTA scientific committee and faculty members: Sara Brucker, Rudi Campo, Carlo De Angelis, Attilio Di Spiezio Sardo, Roy Farquharson, Marco Gergolet, Luca Gianaroli, Stephan Gordts, Grigoris Grimbizis, Tin Chiu Li, Vasilios Tanos, Basil Tarlatzis

Invited experts: Nazar Amso, Apostolos Athanasiadis, Carmina Bermejo, Caterina Exacoustos, Geeta Nargund, Dirk Timmermann, Dominique Van Schoubroeck

27

Delivery and pregnancy outcome in women with bowel resection for deep endometriosis: a retrospective cohort study

Silvia Baggio[1] · Paola Pomini[1] · Alessandro Zecchin[1] · Simone Garzon[1] · Cecilia Bonin[1] · Lorenza Santi[2] · Anna Festi[1] · Massimo Piergiuseppe Franchi[1]

Abstract Endometriosis affects women in reproductive age and can involve bowel in 6–12 % of the patients. In case of bowel occlusion or deep pain, radical laparoscopic endometriosic surgery associated with bowel resection is recommended. The purpose of this study was to analyze the conception rate, the obstetric complications, and the pregnancy outcome. This is a retrospective study; we investigated 51 patients with deep endometriosis who underwent surgical treatment with bowel resection during the period between 2000 and 2007. Among the 30 patients who gave birth to at least one live child after surgery, we considered only the first pregnancy following bowel resection and we investigated the incidence of pregnancy disorders, the gestational age at delivery, the baby birth weight, and the complications related to the different ways of delivery. We compared the results with a control group of 93 patients with no previous abdominal surgery. The whole group of 51 patients tried to conceive after surgery, and 30 women had at least one pregnancy with the birth of an alive baby. Considering only the first pregnancies after surgery, 6 (20 %) experienced gestational hypertensive disorders, 3 (10 %) had placenta previa, 6 (20 %) had preterm birth (<37 weeks), and 1 patient (3.3 %) gestational diabetes. In this group, the average newborn weight was 3000±545 g. Compared with the control group, women with previous bowel resection for deep endometriosis had a higher risk of hypertensive disorders ($p<0.05$), placenta previa ($p<0.05$), and lower newborn weight ($p<0.05$), while the association with preterm birth and gestational diabetes was not statistically significant. These patients experience 12 vaginal deliveries (40 %) and 18 caesarean sections (60 %). Comparing with the caesarean rate in the control group (29.03 %), the incidence of caesarean section in the study population was substantially higher ($p<0.01$) with 33.3 % of the sections performed because of previous bowel surgery. No differences in severe complication rates were observed between vaginal and caesarean deliveries (ns). Complete removal of endometriosis with bowel segmental resection seems to improve the pregnancy rate, but in this group, there is an increased incidence of hypertensive disorders, placenta previa, and lower newborn weight. Despite the small number of patients, we do not observe more complications in the vaginal group than in the caesarean group, so we hypothesize the previous radical surgery should not influence the way of delivery.

Keywords Endometriosis · Bowel resection · Pregnancy

Introduction

Endometriosis is characterized by the presence of the endometrial glands and stroma outside the uterine cavity. It primarily affects women of fertile age and represents a relevant clinical issue as it causes severe abdominal pain [1, 2] and infertility [2, 3].

Endometriosis is classified depending on location, extent and depth of implants, presence and severity of adhesions, and presence and size of ovarian endometriomas.

The incidence of bowel implants among women with endometriosis is between 6 and 12 % [4–7]. The most affected sites are the rectum and recto-sigmoid junction, which account

✉ Silvia Baggio
silvia.baggio1@gmail.com

[1] Department of Obstetrics and Gynaecology, University of Verona, Piazzale L.A. Scuro 10, 37134 Verona, Italy

[2] Department of Endocrinology, University of Verona, Piazzale L.A. Scuro 10, 37134 Verona, Italy

for up to 93 % [8–10] of all intestinal endometriosis lesions. When this kind of lesion is associated with deep pain, stenosis, or massive bowel involvement, the recommended approach is the complete excision of deep endometriosis with bowel resection [11]. In these last years, many authors have reported different surgical procedures to remove endometriosis nodules from bowel like the shaving technique that consists in the excision of nodule after its complete resection from the rectum without resection [12]. Bowel endometriosis removal let the patient have a reliable and persistent relief of pain symptoms and improvement of quality of life [13–22] and leads to a better fertility and pregnancy rate [23].

Considering the young age of women who undergo this radical surgery, and the related fertility improvement, the aims of our study were to analyze the obstetric complications and the outcome of the pregnancies conceived after surgery and to evaluate if there is a recommended way of delivery conscious of short- and long-term complications related to a bowel segmental resection.

Methods

From July 1996 to February 2007, 329 infertile women with severe endometriosis underwent laparoscopic surgery treatment at the Gynecology and Obstetrics Department of the Ospedale Sacro Cuore (Negrar, Italy).

In our study, we analyze only the 77 patients who had a colorectal segmental resection. The indications for radical surgery with bowel resection were severe pelvic pain refractory to medical treatments and/or severe bowel stenosis caused by endometriosis implants.

In our Unit, in case of deep endometriosis with muscularis involvement, the treatment of choice is bowel segmental resection. The shaving technique is performed if the endometriotic nodule involves only the serosa.

In all cases, surgery was performed by laparoscopy. Each procedure was performed using a 10-mm laparoscope in the umbilical position and three 5-mm trocars. After an accurate check of the pelvic and abdominal organs, adnexal adhesions, when present, were sectioned with micro-scissors. Where endometriomas were present, steeping and temporary ovarian suspension was performed. Complete excision of all visible endometriosis lesions from healthy tissue was obtained using 5-mm bipolar scissors according to the technique described by Redwine [24]. Pre- and post-operative management has already been reported in previous studies [21, 25, 26]. The intestinal surgery was performed by a colorectal surgeon with a T–T colorectal anastomosis. All women were clinically evaluated at 1 month, 6 months 1 year up to 4 years after surgery, and all findings were recorded in a specific database.

In this retrospective study, data about history, surgery, complications, and follow-up were obtained from database and medical records, while data concerning obstetric outcomes were updated contacting the 77 patients between July and August 2013.

Only 51 of 77 patients who underwent bowel resection were considered in our study; 26 patients were not contactable. Among the patients who conceived after surgery, we retrieved data from medical records about conception, complications during pregnancy, gestational age at delivery, birth weight, way of delivery, indications (caesarean section), and possible complications. Previous caesarean delivery was considered an obstetric indication. We collected the same obstetric data from a population without endometriosis who delivered in January and February 2007 in our Unit (control group) to compare the incidence of obstetric complications and the way of delivery in the two groups. The control group included 92 women with good health, no previous caesarean section or bowel surgery, regular menstrual cycle, no dysmenorrhea, no dyspareunia, no dyschezia, and normal gynecological evaluation before the conception. Subjects with medical conditions, previous bowel surgery, or suspicion of endometriosis were excluded.

Statistics

All statistical analysis was carried out with a SPSS 21.0 software. Continuous variables were expressed as arithmetic mean+SD; in case of asymmetric quantitative variables, the indicators were associated with the median, maximum, and minimal values. Categorical variables were expressed as distributions of absolute or relative frequencies. The distribution of conceptions and deliveries during follow-up was studied with the Kaplan–Meier curves. The chi-square test and Fisher exact test were used to compare data obtained by cross tabs. Statistical significance was declared at $p<0.05$.

Results

Demographic data were similar in the case and control group population; none had previous caesarean section, and they did not differ in age and gestational age at delivery (Table 1).

Pregnancies

After surgery, all patients tried to conceive and 38 (70.37 %) obtained at least one pregnancy with a total of 68 pregnancies. Spontaneous miscarriage was observed in 19/68 (23.53 %) and ectopic pregnancy in 2/68 (2.94 %). The remaining 47/68 (73.53 %) had ongoing pregnancies with a live child delivery.

In summary, 30 patients had at least one ongoing pregnancy with delivery, in particular, 14/30 (46.6 %) had one

Table 1 Demographic characteristics of case and control patients

	Case	Control	p
Number of patients	51	93	
Age (years)	30.9±3.3	30.7±4.0	N.S.
Gestational age (w)	38.1±2.2	38.3±3.3	N.S.
Hypertension/preeclampsia	20 %	5.4 %	<0.05
Abnormal placentation	10 %	2.2 %	<0.05
Neonatal weight (g)	3000±545	3287±671	<0.05

NS no significative, *W* weeks

pregnancy, 15/30 (50 %) had two pregnancies, and one patient (3.3 %) had 3 ongoing pregnancies.

Before radical surgery with bowel resection, only 2/51 (3.9 %) patients had an ongoing pregnancy with a live child delivery, even if 32/51 (62.7 %) were trying to conceive for more than 1 year, while after surgery 30/51 (58.8 %). This difference is statistically significant ($p<0.001$).

Conception

Most of the ongoing pregnancies with delivery were obtained spontaneously (71 %), while 14/47 (29 %) were obtained with in vitro fertilization (IVF). The mean age at the first conception was 30.1 years (d.s. 3.2). Spontaneous pregnancies had a mean interval from surgery of 13.8 months (d.s. 14.1) and a median of 9 months, with a minimum interval of 0 month and a maximum of 53 months. Pregnancies obtained with IVF had a mean interval of 26.8 months (d.s. 21.4) and a median of 22 months, with a minimum interval of 6 and a maximum of 85 months.

Gestational age and fetal growth

We considered only the first pregnancy with the birth of a live child. The mean gestational age at delivery was 38.10 weeks (d.s. 2.25), with a median of 38 weeks, a minimum gestational age of 33 weeks, and a maximum of 42.

Six of thirty pregnancies (20 %) ended with a preterm delivery (before 37 weeks), with a mean gestational age of 34.62 weeks (d.s. 1.21). Among these pregnancies, 1 ended because of a preterm labor with consequent vaginal delivery during the 36th week without any complications, while 5 had caesarean delivery with a mean gestational age of 34.40 weeks (d.s. 1.14). The indications of these caesarean sections were different; 2 were performed at 35 and 36 weeks after the diagnosis of labor because of the previous bowel resection, to protect the anastomosis, 1 for breech presentation and premature rupture of membranes at 34 weeks, 1 for severe IUGR (<5 % percentile) and Doppler velocimetry alterations at 34 weeks, and 1 for twin pregnancy and preterm labor at 33 weeks of gestation. Excluding the twin newborns, the mean

weight at birth was 3000 g (d.s. 545) with a median of 3100 g, a minimum weight of 1900 g, and a maximum of 3880 g.

In the control group the mean gestational age at the delivery was 38.3 weeks (d.s. 3.3), with a median of 37.9 weeks, a minimum gestational age of 27 weeks and a maximum of 41.6 weeks.

Thirteen of 93 pregnancies (14 %) ended with a preterm delivery (before 37 weeks), with a mean gestational age of 33.2 weeks (d.s. 3.8). The newborn mean weight at birth was 3287 g (d.s. 671) with a median of 3365 g, a minimum weight of 540 g, and a maximum of 4300 g.

Pregnancy complications

In the case group, 6/30 pregnancies (20 %) were complicated by hypertensive disorders (gestational hypertension and pre-eclampsia, with one case of severe eclampsia). Only one pregnancy (3 %) was complicated by diabetes mellitus. The abnormal placentation complicated 3 pregnancies (10 %); in particular, 2 pregnancies presented placenta previa (all obtained with IVF) and one placental flow alterations.

In the control group, 5/93 pregnancies (5.4 %) were complicated by hypertensive disorders while 10/93 (10.8 %) were complicated by diabetes mellitus. Abnormal placentation complicated 2 pregnancies (2.2 %); in particular, 1 pregnancy presented placenta previa (1.1 %) and 1 (1.1 %) placental flow alterations.

Delivery

Among the 30 pregnancies in the case group, there were 12 vaginal deliveries (40 %) and 18 caesarean deliveries (60 %). No significant difference was observed in the two groups concerning the interval time between surgery and delivery ($p=0.9$). Dividing the 18 caesarean deliveries into two groups based on the indications, 10 (55.6 %) had an obstetric indication, while 8 (44.4 %) were performed to protect the colon-rectal anastomosis, to prevent bowel perforation in this minor resistance point, in particular during labor expulsive stage when there is the maximum increase of abdominal pressure.

In the study population, vaginal deliveries were mainly complicated by minor injuries: first or second degree perineal laceration (50 %), episiotomy (16.6 %), and manual removal of placenta (8.3 %). Only one vaginal delivery (8.3 %), 10 months after surgery, was severely complicated with a wide laceration of the cervix, vagina, and rectum at the level of the suture of the previous bowel resection. The patient had a reconstructive surgery, without long-term complications.

Regarding caesarean deliveries, only two were severely complicated (11.1 %). The first case, 33 months after the radical surgery, presented a severe adhesion syndrome and developed severe intra-operative uterine bleeding and was admitted to ICU. In the second case, 24 months after bowel surgery, the diffuse adhesions between the uterus and bladder determined a large full-thickness bladder incidental laceration with reconstructive urological surgery. The patient developed urine retention with intermittent self-catheterization.

In the control group, there were 27/93 (29.03 %) caesarean sections and 66/93 (70.07 %) vaginal deliveries. The complications during vaginal deliveries were first or second degree perineal laceration (45.4 %), episiotomy (18.2 %), and tracheloraffia (1.5 %). There were no urinary tract injuries during the caesarean sections in the control group, but 2 patients (7.4 %) had severe intra-operative bleeding with necessity of blood transfusion in one case (3.7 %).

Discussion

Many studies have demonstrated the close relationship between endometriosis and infertility and the improvement of the pregnancy rate and pelvic pain after radical surgery [16, 18, 19, 23, 27, 28]. In particular, among women with bowel endometriosis, articles in literature confirm that the postoperative fertility rate is improved if segmental bowel resection is performed (Table 2).

Stepniewska et al. [23] reported a cumulative pregnancy rate of 35 % after bowel surgery in infertile women; Darai [27] reported 5 pregnancies in 12 infertile patients (42 %), and Kavallaris [16] reported 8 pregnancies in 15 infertile women (47 %) with previous bowel surgery. Our study shows a statistical significant improvement of pregnancy rate in infertile woman, after bowel surgery for endometriosis with the highest pregnancy rate, 70.4 % after surgery versus 3.9 % before ($p<0.01$).

The cumulative pregnancy rate is 50 % at 9 months for spontaneous conceptions and at 16 months for conceptions obtained with artificial reproductive techniques (ART), which is comparable to the results obtained by other authors [29]. This confirms that the maximum fertility rate is immediately after surgery considering both spontaneous and ART pregnancies (Fig. 1).

Donnez et al. reported an important increase of pregnancy rate after shaving technique too (57 %) [12]. Whether one technique is better than the other or not in terms of pain relief, fertility, and short- and long-term complications is still controversial, and it often depends on the surgeon and its experience. The high pregnancy rate observed after surgery both with bowel resection and shaving approach suggests that the increase in fertility is more likely to be related to the removal of the endometriotic disease rather than a specific surgical technique.

Although fertility after bowel surgery has been wide studied, outcome and way of delivery of the pregnancies obtained after this surgery have only been considered in few papers.

In a study including more than 1.4 million singleton births, Stephansson et al. [30] observed that endometriosis was associated with preterm birth, preeclampsia, and placental complications.

In our study, the mean gestational age at delivery was 38.16 weeks and 20 % of deliveries were before 37 weeks. Considering that the rate of preterm delivery in the general population is 10 %, and in the control group 14 %, we observed a significant increase in the risk of preterm birth in the case population ($p=0.005$). Moreover, in women with previous bowel surgery, the newborn weight at birth was significantly lower than the control group ($p=0.04$).

Another important finding is the incidence of hypertensive disorders during pregnancy in our population (20 %) which, compared with the rate of hypertension/preeclampsia in the control group population (5.4 %), confirms that women operated for deep endometriosis had a higher risk to develop this disorder ($p=0.024$). This is in contrast with the results reported by Brosen et al. [31], who showed a decrease in risk of preeclampsia in women with endometriosis.

Vercellini et al. [32] in his study did not detect any particular findings with regard to the incidence of hypertension, preeclampsia, preterm birth, and abruption placenta, but he found an incidence of 3.7 % of placenta previa in women with endometriosis, more than 10 times the figure of 0.3 % reported in the general population.

Our study confirms this increased risk of placenta previa with an incidence of 6.6 % in the case population and only 1.1 % in the control group ($p=0.045$). This risk in women with endometriosis is probably related to abnormal endometrial receptivity and a subsequent alteration in placentation, but further data are needed.

No significant differences were observed in the incidence of diabetes ($p=0.19$) between the case and the control groups.

Besides the obstetric outcome, there is another fundamental point to analyze regarding women who undergo bowel resection for deep endometriosis, the way of delivery.

There are no studies in literature that focus on this issue, and there is no common consensus. In our study, 60 % of deliveries were caesarean sections and 33.3 % were performed because of previous bowel surgery. In control group, the caesarean rate was clearly lower, 29.3 %. Refusing to perform an intestinal resection in a symptomatic patient who desires a child, persuaded that pregnancy hormones would solve the situation, is not the way to avoid caesarean sections, and sometimes, it could be dangerous. There are studies in literature that show the existence of a specific entity of deep endometriosis reacting differently to the hormonal environment of a pregnancy and responsible of severe bowel complications during the third trimester of pregnancy, like perforations or intestinal occlusions [33]. To find if there is a safer way to deliver after bowel surgery, in this pilot study, we decided to compare complication incidence after vaginal and caesarean

Table 2 Studies regarding the fertility outcome after bowel resection for intestinal endometriosis, compared with the conducted study

Study	No. of patients	No. of infertile patients searching offspring	Obtained pregnancies	Length of follow-up after surgery	Surgical treatment	Other considerations	Note
Darai 2005	34 (colorectal endometriosis)	12	5 (PR=42 %)	24 months (mean FU), min 6 months	LPS segmental intestinal resection	PR in the whole group = 45% (10/22)	9 spontaneous pregnancies, 3 with IVF
Thomassin 2004	27 (colorectal endometriosis)	8	2	15 months (mean FU), range 3–22 months	Segmental intestinal resection: 25 LPS, 2 LPT	4 pregnancies in the whole group (4/27)	All spontaneous pregnancies
Fleisch 2005	23 (infiltrative endometriosis of bowel or bladder)	4	2	45±18 months	LPT, 22 segmental resections	4 pregnancies in the whole group (4/17)	Only a pregnancy obtained with IVF, other 3 were spontaneous
Kavallaris 2003	50 (rectal endometriosis)	17 searching offspring (38 infertile PZ)	8 (PR=47 %)	32 months	LPS, segmental intestinal resection	3 early abortion, non-EP	2 pregnancies after IVF, others were spontaneous
Possover 2000	34 (segmental intestinal resection)	15	8 (PR=53 %)	16 months (mean FU)	Via vaginal resection laparoscopically assisted	All patients with primary infertility	
Stepniewska 2009	60 (bowel endometriosis)	48	17 (PR=35 %)	26.9 months (mean FU)	LPS, segmental intestinal resection	PR compared with no resection surgery	PR improved by intestinal resection when there are lesions
Our study	54 (bowel endometriosis)	54	33 (PR=61 %)	Mean 113 months (d.s. 16), range 68–153, median 113	LPS, segmental intestinal resection	50 pregnancies with newborns	36 spontaneous (71.43 %), 14 with IVF e IUI (28.57 %)

delivery in the two groups. In the case population, vaginal deliveries were mainly complicated by minor injuries; only one vaginal delivery (8.3 %) was severely complicated with

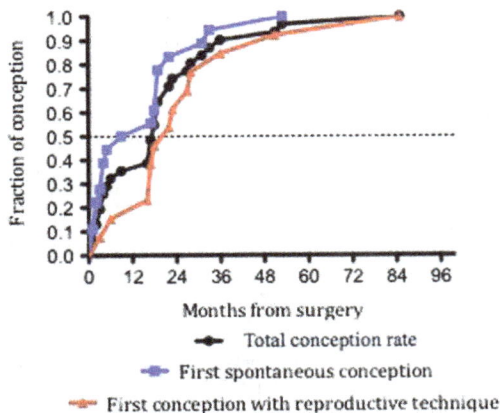

Fig. 1 Time distribution (months from surgery) of the first pregnancy conceptions (Kaplan–Meier). *Dashed line* shows the 50 % of conceptions after surgery. *Black*: total conceptions; *blue*: spontaneous conceptions; *red*: conceptions with reproductive technique

a laceration of the rectum at the level of the suture of the previous bowel resection. Among the patients who underwent caesarean section, two had severe complications (11.1 %). In conclusion, our results show no difference in complications in women with bowel endometriosis who had a vaginal birth or a caesarean section ($p=0.8$) and no differences in complications during caesarean or vaginal delivery comparing the case and control group ($p=0.09$). More studies with larger population are needed to confirm these preliminary results.

In literature, we found some studies that analyze the way of delivery in women who underwent ileal pouch-anal anastomosis (IPAA) for chronic ulcerative colitis. The condition of these populations and the case group is similar; they are young women looking for pregnancy, who undergo abdominal surgery and intestine resection, with consequent risk of massive adhesions and the presence of a rectal/anal point of minor resistance, dangerous with the increased abdominal pressure during delivery.

Many retrospective studies have documented that the pouch function in women with IPAA during labor and delivery is well preserved. Hanloser et al. [34] used the Mayo Clinic database to evaluate delivery outcomes in women after IPAA, and they found no increases in pouch complications or functional problems in those who had vaginal birth rather than caesarean section. Among the women who had vaginal delivery before and after IPAA, no differences were found concerning the duration of labor or labor complication rates pre-IPAA versus post-IPAA in the same women. Studies by Juhasz et al. [35] and Ravid et al. [36] echo the same findings.

A 2005 report from Cleveland Clinic [37] concluded that recommendation for vaginal delivery should be cautious because it found a major incidence of sphincter defects in women with an IPAA who had a vaginal delivery versus those who had a caesarean section. A 2007 review of literature confirmed that vaginal delivery places all women at risk of sphincter injury (in the general population, the incidence is 0.3 %) in particular if compared with caesarean section, but it underlined that there is no evidence to suggest that this risk is greater in women with an IPAA [38].

The review of literature regarding IPAA confirms the results of our study; there is no contraindication to vaginal delivery for women who undergo bowel resection for deep endometriosis as ACOG recommended [39]. In these women, the way of delivery should be chosen considering only obstetrical concerns. In fact, the Committee of Obstetric Practice believes that in the absence of maternal or fetal indications for caesarean delivery, a plan for vaginal delivery is safe and appropriate with a shorter maternal hospitalization, lower infection rates, fewer anesthetic complications, and lower risk of respiratory problems for the infant. Moreover, the presence of endometriosis increases the risk of surgery complications during caesarean section, in particular lower urinary tract injury, often related to bladder adhesions high up on the lower uterine segment. Previous caesarean section and severe endometriosis with bladder-uterine localizations are the major risk factors for bladder injury during caesarean section [40].

To reduce the incidence of the worst complications during labor and vaginal delivery in women with previous bowel resection, we think it would be interesting to study if there is a safe time interval between surgery and delivery. In our study, the rectum laceration during labor was in the patient with the smallest interval between surgery and delivery (10 months), maybe too short for a correct healing. On the other hand, it is well known that the best period to conceive is the closest to surgery, so waiting too much could be unfavorable.

Further studies may be necessary to evaluate if there is a safe interval of time to wait after bowel resection to conceive without an important reduction of the pregnancy rate.

Compliance with ethical standards All procedures followed were in accordance with the ethical standards of the responsible committee on human experimentation (institutional and national) and with the 1964 Helsinki Declaration and its later amendments or comparable ethical standards.

Informed consent Informed consent was obtained from all individual participants included in the study.

References

1. Koninckx PR, Meuleman C, Demeyere S, Lesaffre E, Cornillie FJ (1991) Suggestive evidence that pelvic endometriosis is a progressive disease, whereas deeply infiltrating endometriosis is associated with pelvic pain. Fertil Steril 55:759–65

2. Fauconnier A, Chapron C, Dubuisson JB, Vieira M, Dousset B, Bréart G (2002) Relation between pain symptoms and the anatomic location of deep infiltrating endometriosis. Fertil Steril 78:719–26

3. Pouly JL, Drolet J, Canis M, Boughazine S, Mage G, Bruhat MA et al (1996) Laparoscopic treatment of symptomatic endometriosis. Hum Reprod 11(Suppl 3):67–88

4. Macafee CH, Greer HL (1960) Intestinal endometriosis. A report of 29 cases and a survey of the literature. J Obstet Gynaecol Br Emp 67:539–55

5. Weed JC, Ray JE (1987) Endometriosis of the bowel. Obstet Gynecol 69:727–30

6. Jerby BL, Kessler H, Falcone T, Milsom JW (1999) Laparoscopic management of colorectal endometriosis. Surg Endosc 13:1125–8

7. Chapron C, Fauconnier A, Dubuisson JB, Barakat H, Vieira M, Bréart G (2003) Deep infiltrating endometriosis: relation between severity of dysmenorrhoea and extent of disease. Hum Reprod 18:760–6

8. Coronado C, Franklin RR, Lotze EC, Bailey HR, Valdés CT (1990) Surgical treatment of symptomatic colorectal endometriosis. Fertil Steril 53:411–6

9. Bailey HR, Ott MT, Hartendorp P (1994) Aggressive surgical management for advanced colorectal endometriosis. Dis Colon Rectum 37:747–53

10. Tran KT, Kuijpers HC, Willemsen WN, Bulten H (1996) Surgical treatment of symptomatic rectosigmoid endometriosis. Eur J Surg 162:139–41

11. Wattiez A, Puga M, Albornoz J, Faller E (2013) Surgical strategy in endometriosis. Best Pract Res Clin Obstet Gynaecol 27:381–92

12. Donnez J, Squifflet J (2010) Complications, pregnancy and recurrence in a prospective series of 500 patients operated on by the shaving technique for deep rectovaginal endometriotic nodules. Hum Reprod 25:1949–1958

13. Canis M, Botchorishvili R, Slim K, Pezet D, Pouly JL, Wattiez A et al (1996) [Bowel endometriosis. Eight cases of colorectal resection]. J Gynecol Obstet Biol Reprod (Paris) 25:699–709

14. Duepree HJ, Senagore AJ, Delaney CP, Marcello PW, Brady KM, Falcone T (2002) Laparoscopic resection of deep pelvic endometriosis with rectosigmoid involvement. J Am Coll Surg 195:754–8

15. Abbott JA, Hawe J, Clayton RD, Garry R (2003) The effects and effectiveness of laparoscopic excision of endometriosis: a prospective study with 2-5 year follow-up. Hum Reprod 18:1922–7

16. Kavallaris A, Köhler C, Kühne-Heid R, Schneider A (2003) Histopathological extent of rectal invasion by rectovaginal endometriosis. Hum Reprod 18:1323–7

17. Ford J, English J, Miles WA, Giannopoulos T (2004) Pain, quality of life and complications following the radical resection of rectovaginal endometriosis. BJOG 111:353–6

18. Thomassin I, Bazot M, Detchev R, Barranger E, Cortez A, Darai E (2004) Symptoms before and after surgical removal of colorectal endometriosis that are assessed by magnetic resonance imaging and rectal endoscopic sonography. Am J Obstet Gynecol 190:1264–71

19. Fleisch MC, Xafis D, De Bruyne F, Hucke J, Bender HG, Dall P (2005) Radical resection of invasive endometriosis with bowel or bladder involvement—long-term results. Eur J Obstet Gynecol Reprod Biol 123:224–9

20. Dubernard G, Piketty M, Rouzier R, Houry S, Bazot M, Darai E (2006) Quality of life after laparoscopic colorectal resection for endometriosis. Hum Reprod 21:1243–7

21. Landi S, Mereu L, Pontrelli G, Stepniewska A, Romano L, Tateo S et al (2008) The influence of adenomyosis in patients laparoscopically treated for deep endometriosis. J Minim Invasive Gynecol 15:566–70

22. Ferrero S, Anserini P, Abbamonte LH, Ragni N, Camerini G, Remorgida V (2009) Fertility after bowel resection for endometriosis. Fertil Steril 92:41–6

23. Stepniewska A, Pomini P, Bruni F, Mereu L, Ruffo G, Ceccaroni M et al (2009) Laparoscopic treatment of bowel endometriosis in infertile women. Hum Reprod 24:1619–25

24. Redwine DB (2004) Surgical management of endometriosis. Martin Dunitz, Taylor & Francis, New York, USA

25. Landi S, Ceccaroni M, Perutelli A, Allodi C, Barbieri F, Fiaccavento A et al (2006) Laparoscopic nerve-sparing complete excision of deep endometriosis: is it feasible? Hum Reprod 21:774–81

26. Mereu L, Ruffo G, Landi S, Barbieri F, Zaccoletti R, Fiaccavento A et al (2007) Laparoscopic treatment of deep endometriosis with segmental colorectal resection: short-term morbidity. J Minim Invasive Gynecol 14:463–9

27. Daraï E, Marpeau O, Thomassin I, Dubernard G, Barranger E, Bazot M (2005) Fertility after laparoscopic colorectal resection for endometriosis: preliminary results. Fertil Steril 84:945–50

28. Possover M, Diebolder H, Plaul K, Schneider A (2000) Laparascopically assisted vaginal resection of rectovaginal endometriosis. Obstet Gynecol 96:304–7

29. Chapron C, Fritel X, Dubuisson JB (1999) Fertility after laparoscopic management of deep endometriosis infiltrating the uterosacral ligaments. Hum Reprod 14:329–32

30. Stephansson O, Kieler H, Granath F, Falconer H (2009) Endometriosis, assisted reproduction technology, and risk of adverse pregnancy outcome. Hum Reprod 24:2341–7

31. Brosens I, Brosens JJ, Fusi L, Al-Sabbagh M, Kuroda K, Benagiano G (2012) Risks of adverse pregnancy outcome in endometriosis. Fertil Steril 98:30–5

32. Vercellini P, Parazzini F, Pietropaolo G, Cipriani S, Frattaruolo MP, Fedele L (2012) Pregnancy outcome in women with peritoneal, ovarian and rectovaginal endometriosis: a retrospective cohort study. BJOG 119:1538–43

33. Setubal A, Sidiropoulou Z, Torgal M, Casal E (2014) Bowel complications of deep endometriosis during pregnancy or in vitro fertilization. Fertil Steril 101(2):442–6

34. Hahnloser D, Pemberton JH, Wolff BG, Larson D, Harrington J, Farouk R et al (2004) Pregnancy and delivery before and after ileal pouch-anal anastomosis for inflammatory bowel disease: immediate and long-term consequences and outcomes. Dis Colon Rectum 47:1127–35

35. Juhasz ES, Fozard B, Dozois RR, Ilstrup DM, Nelson H (1995) Ileal pouch-anal anastomosis function following childbirth. An extended evaluation. Dis Colon Rectum 38:159–65

36. Ravid A, Richard CS, Spencer LM, O'Connor BI, Kennedy ED, MacRae HM et al (2002) Pregnancy, delivery, and pouch function after ileal pouch-anal anastomosis for ulcerative colitis. Dis Colon Rectum 45:1283–8

37. Remzi FH, Gorgun E, Bast J, Schroeder T, Hammel J, Philipson E et al (2005) Vaginal delivery after ileal pouch-anal anastomosis: a word of caution. Dis Colon Rectum 48:1691–9

38. Cornish J, Tan E, Teare J, Teoh TG, Rai R, Clark SK et al (2007) A meta-analysis on the influence of inflammatory bowel disease on pregnancy. Gut 56:830–7

39. American College of Obstetricians and Gynecologists (2013) ACOG committee opinion no. 559: cesarean delivery on maternal request. Obstet Gynecol 121:904–7

40. Phipps MG, Watabe B, Clemons JL, Weitzen S, Myers DL (2005) Risk factors for bladder injury during cesarean delivery. Obstet Gynecol 105:156–60

28

Laparoscopic versus robotic-assisted sacrocolpopexy for pelvic organ prolapse: a systematic review

Geertje Callewaert[1,2] · Jan Bosteels[3] · Susanne Housmans[2] · Jasper Verguts[2,4] ·
Ben Van Cleynenbreugel[1,5] · Frank Van der Aa[1,5] · Dirk De Ridder[1,5] ·
Ignace Vergote[2,6] · Jan Deprest[1,2]

Abstract The use of robot-assisted surgery (RAS) has gained popularity in the field of gynaecology, including pelvic floor surgery. To assess the benefits of RAS, we conducted a systematic review of randomized controlled trials comparing laparoscopic and robotic-assisted sacrocolpopexy. The Cochrane Library (1970–January 2015), MEDLINE (1966 to January 2015), and EMBASE (1974 to January 2015) were searched, as well as ClinicalTrials.gov and the International Clinical Trials Registry Platform. We identified two randomized trials ($n = 78$) comparing laparoscopic with robotic sacrocolpopexy. The Paraiso 2011 study showed that laparoscopic was faster than robotic sacrocolpopexy (199 ± 46 vs. 265 ± 50 min; $p < .001$), yet in the ACCESS trial, no difference was present (225 ± 62.3 vs. 246.5 ± 51.3 min; $p = .110$). Costs for using the robot were significantly higher in both studies, however, in the ACCESS trial, only when purchase and maintenance of the robot was included (LSC US\$11,573 $\pm$ 3191 vs. RASC US\$19,616 $\pm$ 3135; $p < .001$). In the Paraiso study, RASC was more expensive even without considering those costs (LSC US\$ 14,342 $\pm$ 2941 vs. RASC 16,278 $\pm$ 3326; $p = 0.008$). Pain was reportedly higher after RASC, although at different time points after the operation. There were no differences in anatomical outcomes, pelvic floor function, and quality of life. The experience with RASC was tenfold lower than that with LSC in both studies. The heterogeneity between the two studies precluded a meta-analysis. Based on small randomized studies, with surgeons less experienced in RAS than in laparoscopic surgery, robotic surgery significantly increases the cost of a laparoscopic sacrocolpopexy. RASC would be more sustainable if its costs would be lower. Though RASC may have other benefits, such as reduction of the learning curve and increased ergonomics or dexterity, these remain to be demonstrated.

Keywords Sacrocolpopexy · Laparoscopy · Pelvic organ prolapse · Vault prolapse · Robotics · Costs

Introduction

Robotic-assisted surgery

Robot-assisted surgery (RAS) has become popular in various surgical fields, including gynaecology and urology. Accordingly, the robot has been used for the surgical treatment of pelvic organ prolapse (POP). The most frequently quoted advantages of RAS are its 3D view, the elimination of surgeon tremor whilst permitting precise and intuitive movements. Further to this the use of wristed instruments improves

✉ Jan Deprest
jan.deprest@uzleuven.be

[1] Department of Development and Regeneration, Cluster Organ Systems, Faculty of Medicine, Group Biomedical Sciences, KU Leuven, 3000 Leuven, Belgium

[2] Department of Obstetrics and Gynaecology, University Hospitals Leuven, 3000 Leuven, Belgium

[3] Belgian Center for Evidence Based Medicine (CEBAM), Belgian Branch of the Cochrane Collaboration, 3000 Leuven, Belgium

[4] Department of Obstetrics and Gynaecology, Jessa Hospital, 3500 Hasselt, Belgium

[5] Department of Urology, University Hospitals Leuven, Leuven, Belgium

[6] Department of Gynaecologic Oncology, Leuven Cancer Institute, University Hospitals Leuven, KU Leuven, 3000 Leuven, Belgium

dexterity offering more favorable ergonomics. RAS combines these advantages with the minimally invasive approach, i.e., those already demonstrated for conventional or "straight stick" laparoscopy. Wide introduction of RAS is mainly limited by the high acquisition and maintenance cost (usually around 10 % of the purchase cost per year) and the repetitive costs of the consumables [1]. In Europe, the *initial cost* is typically depreciated over 7 or more years, which amounts to more than 1000 € per patient, when used for 300 or more procedures per year [2]. When used in fewer patients, this will result in higher per-case charges. The use of robotic instruments is limited to 10 cases, and the list charge price for three instruments is easily more than 1500 € [3]. Next to the high costs, other disadvantages are the lack of tactile feedback and instrument crowding, especially in a narrow operating field, such as the pelvis [2].

Minimally invasive pelvic floor surgery

Whereas most patients with symptomatic POP can be adequately managed by the vaginal route, correction of apical descent or multi-compartment prolapse with a so-called level I defect is better treated by the abdominal approach [4]. In sacrocolpopexy (SC), the vaginal vault and/or cervix is fixed by means of a graft to the anterior longitudinal ligament over the sacrum. Sacrocolpopexy by laparotomy further referred to as abdominal sacrocolpopexy (ASC) yields an over 90 % success rate, which improves on sacrospinous fixation. This is however at the expense of longer operation times, higher morbidity, and increased hospital cost [4]. These shortcomings are avoided by performing SC by minimal access, either by laparoscopy (LSC) or by its robotic-assisted equivalent (RASC). Despite the lower performance of spinofixation, single incision vaginal mesh prolapse repair seemed to be a reasonable alternative to LSC, as it was supposed to combine the durability and comprehensiveness of a mesh repair and the advantages of the vaginal route. In Maher's randomized clinical trial (RCT), LSC was associated with a shorter hospital stay, earlier return to daily activity, better 2-year anatomical outcomes, less graft related complications, and, as a consequence, less reinterventions as well as lower hospital costs, despite longer operation times [5, 6].

Only by 2012, level I evidence became available supporting the hypothesis that a laparoscopic SC yields as good anatomic (point C) and subjective (patient global impression score) outcomes as the same operation by laparotomy [7]. Moreover, LSC was associated with less blood loss, less pain, and a shorter hospital stay. Conversely, operation time, return to normal activities, or functional effects were similar for both modalities.

LSC unfortunately did not become widely implemented, because of its steep learning curve and long operation times,

adding to the generic disadvantages of a limited number of degrees of freedom and its two-dimensional vision [8]. These disadvantages could be circumvented by robotic assistance. The da Vinci Surgical System® (Intuitive Surgical Inc., Sunnyvale, CA, USA) is at present the only operational and commercially available surgical robot. Its increased magnification, three-dimensional vision, physiologic tremor filtering, and 7 degrees of freedom are believed to provide the surgeon with an enhanced ergonomic environment, simplifying complex laparoscopic tasks such as suturing and knot tying, which are essential techniques for SC. The implementation of robots was surprisingly quick into the clinical practice of gynaecologists in many Western countries. This may be by a combination of extensive marketing but certainly because RAS answers the needs of some robotic surgeons *not familiar with conventional laparoscopic surgery*. Subsequently, there has been a significant body of reassuring studies on RASCP demonstrating safety and efficacy, reviewed by Serati et al. [9]. Though there is to our knowledge no RCT comparing RASCP to ASCP, it seems that anatomical and functional outcomes are comparable, though with reduced morbidity, which logically would be the consequence of the minimal access route.

This experience has led to statements that RAS is "better than conventional surgery"—which is clearly stated on the manufacturer's website [10]. The latter is misleading at least, because today conventional sacrocolpopexy no longer is the synonym of ASC [10]. Given the level I evidence that LSC overall is better than ASC, the laparoscopic approach should theoretically be the standard and point of reference. Herein, we aimed to investigate whether there is at present any evidence that RASC would by any outcome measure be superior to LSC. Acceptable advantages would be respectively, a clinical benefit to the patient, a reduced health care cost, or improved surgeon's ergonomics. This question is timely: with the aging and increasing activity of the population, the demand for prolapse surgery is only expected to increase. Given the movement away from vaginal mesh use, minimal access sacrocolpopexy will become an increasingly popular procedure.

Methods

Literature search strategy

Relevant studies were identified from the Cochrane Library (1970–January 2015), MEDLINE (1966 to January 2015), and EMBASE (1974 to January 2015). Furthermore, ClinicalTrials.gov and the International Clinical Trials Registry Platform were searched for ongoing and completed clinical trials. Language restrictions were not applied. There was no systematic attempt to search the grey literature. Details of the search strategy can be found as an online resource. Essentially,

RCTs or controlled studies were included if they compared laparoscopic (LASC) with robotic-assisted sacrocolpopexy (RASC) as the primary surgical intervention with or without concomitant surgery.

Data collection and analysis

All titles and abstracts retrieved by electronic searching were independently assessed by two review authors (GC and JB). Studies that did not meet the inclusion criteria were excluded, and full-text copies of the potential eligible studies were obtained. The full-text articles were assessed for eligibility independently. Disagreements were resolved through discussion or arbitration by a third review author (JD).

For data extraction, a standard form available from the website of the Cochrane Library was used (data collection form for intervention reviews: RCTs only, version 3, April 2014). Two review authors (JB, GC) extracted data from eligible studies. When studies included data from multiple publications, the main trial report was used, supplemented by a previous published protocol if available. Differences were resolved through discussion or arbitration by a third review author (JD).

Primary outcomes were the use of resources and costs (including equipment/theatre costs, length of hospital stay in days, duration of operation in minutes, number of outpatient attendances, number of days off work, direct medical resource use, direct medical costs. Secondary outcomes were patient satisfaction parameters, measured by any validated questionnaire (e.g., PGI-I, PGIC, POP-specific quality of life (P-QoL)); objective measurement of cure rate (POP-Q stage); any complication, either intraoperative, postoperative within 6 weeks, or at a later stage during follow-up, and its nature; early mortality (death within 30 days); estimated blood loss; rate of conversion to open surgery (for RAS versus CLS) and the reason for conversion; and postoperative pain (VAS or other validated scale).

The selected studies were assessed for methodological quality using the "risk of bias" tool of the Cochrane Collaboration [11]. The method of randomization, allocation concealment, blinding, loss to follow-up, selective outcome reporting, trial funding, and if present other sources of bias were again independently evaluated arbitrated as above.

Statistical analysis

For the main outcome of interest, "use of resources and costs," the mean values, and the standard deviations (SD) were extracted. For the other outcomes, if binary, the number of events was noted. Since the number of RCTs was limited and the used definitions of essential outcome measures were different, additional meta-analysis was not performed.

Results

A flow diagram of the search process is displayed in Fig. 1. The search yielded 272 citations of which 24 underwent full text review after screening of the titles and abstracts. Twelve manuscripts concerning the two same studies were included in the SR after consideration of the full text. Both studies were RCTs comparing laparoscopic to robotic sacrocolpopexy of similar size ($n = 78$; Anger 2014 and Paraiso 2011); the former had hospital cost as a primary outcome measure, whereas in the latter it was operation time. Both studies reported both variables. The characteristics of these studies are summarized in Table 1; the outcomes in Table 2. Required surgeon's experience with RASC prior to the study was similar: surgeons

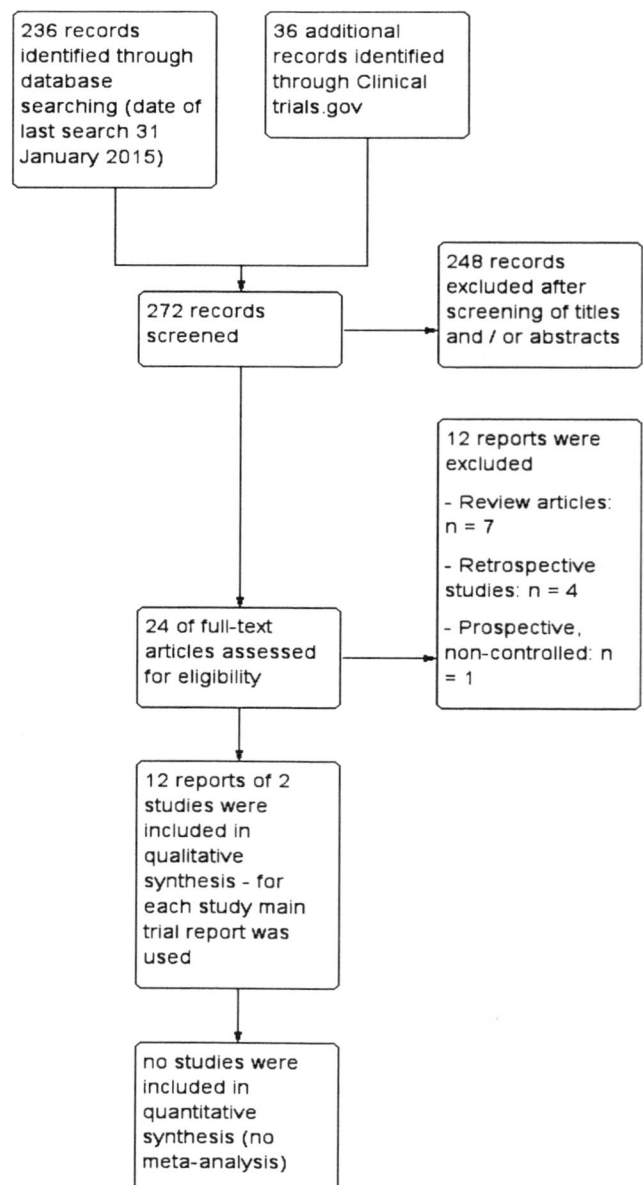

Fig 1 Study flow diagram

Table 1 Study characteristics

Study	Paraiso 2011	Anger 2014
Design	Parallel-group, single-center trial RCT	Two-center, parallel-group RCT
Ethical approval	Yes	Yes
Power calculation	Yes—to detect a 50-min difference in operating time with 90 % power and 5 % type 1 error	Yes—to detect at least US$2500 difference in total charges with 95 % power and 5 % type 1 error
CONSORT statement	Yes	No
Conflict of interest	No conflicts of interest	No conflicts of interest
Participants	Country: USA Setting: Cleveland Clinic Population: women >21 years presenting with posthysterectomy vaginal apex prolapse with POP-Q stage 2–4 desiring surgical management between January 2007 to December 2009 Patients were excluded if not candidates for general anesthesia, underwent a prior sacral colpopexy or rectopexy, had a history of PID, had a BMI >40 kg/m²	Country: USA Setting: University of California-Los Angeles/Cedars-Sinai and Loyola University Medical Centers Population: women with symptomatic pelvic organ prolapse stage II or greater and clinical indication for sacrocolpopexy Patients were excluded if future childbearing, pregnant or pregnancy in the last 12 months, unable to read, write, and comprehend English
Interventions	Sacrocolpopexy using 2 separate 4 × 15 cm pieces of polypropylene mesh. Use of 4 ports for the laparoscopy, 5 for the robotic-assisted laparoscopy in W formation	Sacrocolpopexy with 2 separate pieces of polypropylene mesh and Gore-Tex sutures—surgeon's preference determined brand of the mesh and closure of the retroperitoneal lining
Randomization method	Computer-generated randomization schedule—stratified by surgeon	Computer-based block randomization based on site and need for concurrent hysterectomy randomization on the day of the surgery
Allocation concealment	Use of opaque envelopes	Treatment allocation is uploaded on a password protected website—randomization assignment is revealed to treating surgeon on the day of surgery Under procedure in patient file: laparoscopic sacrocolpopexy per the ACCESS protocol
Blinding	Blinding of research staff and patients	Blinding of patients and research staff for 6 weeks after surgery
Groups comparable	Yes	Yes
Intention-to-treat analysis	Yes	Yes
Follow-up	Up to 1 year	Up to 1 year
Loss to follow-up	4 lost to FU after surgery from LASC 2 from RASC	3/78 before 6 M FU visit
Intervention group	Robotic-assisted sacrocolpopexy (randomized: n = 40—underwent surgery n = 35)	RASC (n = 40)
Control group	Laparoscopic sacrocolpopexy (randomized: n = 38—underwent surgery: n = 33)	LASC (n = 38)
Concomitant surgery	Yes	Yes
Surgical experience	At least 10 robotic procedures	At least 10 procedures of each type
Outcome measures	Primary outcome: operating time Secondary outcomes: postoperative pain, use of NSAIDs, complications, costs, postoperative subjective and objective cure rate	Primary outcome: costs Secondary outcomes: surgical outcomes (blood loss and postoperative pain), POP-Q, symptom severity and QoL, adverse events

were to have performed at least 10 prior robotic procedures. The actual performance was not mentioned in either report. Sacrocolpopexy was performed using two separate pieces of polypropylene mesh. Concomitant procedures were allowed and equally distributed between the two arms in both studies, including retropubic mid-urethral sling and anterior or posterior repairs. Of note is that in Anger's ACCESS trial, 58 % of women underwent a concomitant hysterectomy, whereas in the study by Paraiso only patients with posthysterectomy vault prolapse were included. Other differences at baseline were the setup (single versus two centers) and indication (vault prolapse and/or uterine descent).

The studies also had comparable secondary outcomes which were limited to surgical complications and blood loss, postoperative pain, objective cure rate, and patient satisfaction. Both studies used a blinded computer-based

Table 2 Outcomes

Outcome	Paraiso 2011				Anger 2014		
	LSC ($n=33$)	RASC ($n=35$)	Mean difference	P	LSC ($n=38$)	RASC ($n=40$)	P
Time—sacrocolpopexy	162 ± 47 min	227 ± 47 min	67 (CI 43–89)	<.001	178.4 ± 49.8 min	202.8 ± 46.1 min	.030
Time—total operation operating	199 ± 46 min	265 ± 50 min	66 (43–90)	<.001	225.5 ± 62.3 min	246.5 ± 51.3 min	.110
Costs	∘	∘	∘	∘	US$11,573$\pm$3191	US$19,616$\pm$3135	<.001
- Day of surgery	US$14,342$\pm$2941	US$16,278$\pm$3326	US$1936	.008	US$11,573$\pm$3191	US$12,586$\pm$3315	.160
- Excluding robotics			(448–2,885)				
Costs	∘	∘	∘	∘	US$12,170$\pm$4129	US$20,898$\pm$3386	<.001
- At 6 weeks	∘	∘	∘	∘	US$12,170$\pm$4129	US$13,867$\pm$3386	.060
- Excluding robotics							
Pain	11 days[a]	20 days[a]		<.005[a]	∘	∘	∘
- Use of NSAIDs (days)	28 (2–67)	28 (4–68)		.41	2.6 ± 2.2	3.5 ± 2.1	.044
- VAS at nl activity(wk1)					38.1 ± 15.5	45.4 ± 16.1	.039
- Activity scales (1 wk)							

LSC laparoscopic sacrocolpopexy, *RASC* robotic-assisted sacrocolpopexy, *NSAIDs* nonsteroidal anti-inflammatory drugs, *VAS* visual analog scale, *no data available*, *Excluding robotics* excluding costs of purchase and maintenance costs for robot

[a] Only visual scale (no raw data)

randomization system, hence having low risk for selection bias. Both assessors and patients were blinded to treatment allocation. The data were analyzed on an intention-to-treat basis. In the study by Paraiso, 13 % of the study population ($n=10$) was lost after randomization and prior to surgery.

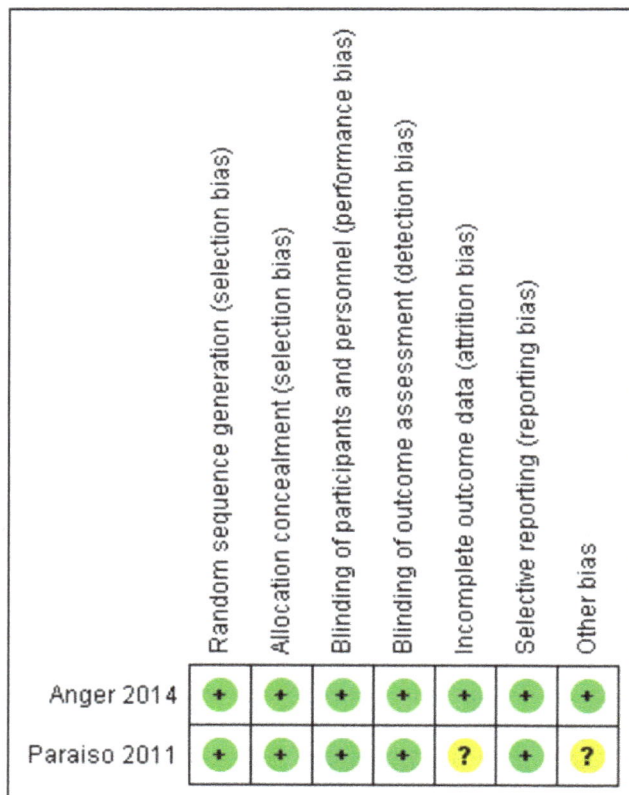

Fig 2 Risk of bias summary: review authors' judgements about each risk of bias item for each included study

Surprisingly, four patients were excluded because they did not meet the criteria, and six others because of patient choice or illness, so attrition bias was considered unclear. Conversely, the attrition bias of the ACCESS trial was low: there were five patients lost to follow-up after the surgery, equally distributed over both treatment arms. The summary of the risk of bias assessment can be found in Fig. 2. Reporting bias is low for both studies; both protocols were also published upfront [12, 13]. Remarkably, the published protocol of the ACCESS trial mentioned initially a follow-up of 1 year postoperatively, yet in the publication a 6-month follow-up is reported on.

Both studies came to different conclusions in terms of the measures initially put forward as primary outcome by either group. In the hands of Paraiso et al., LSC was faster than RASC (199 ± 46 vs. 265 ± 50 min; $p<.001$), yet Anger et al. did not find a difference (225 ± 62.3 vs. 246.5 ± 51.3 min; $p=.110$). Both trials report a significantly higher cost for RASC, yet they use different definitions. The ACCESS breaks down the healthcare costs as those made by the health care provider, first related to the initial procedure, and secondly those related to potential readmissions within 6 weeks. For the surgery-related cost, they report both the purchase of the robot and the maintenance cost as well as its consumables. Eventually, the higher costs in the ACCESS trial (LSC US$11,573$\pm$3191 vs. RASC US$19,616$\pm$3135; $p<.001$) were only due to the higher purchase and maintenance cost of the robot. Excluding those costs, the healthcare cost was actually comparable, with or without concomitant surgery (LSC US$11,573$\pm$3,191 vs. 12,586$\pm$3315; $p=.160$) [14]. This is different for the other study. Firstly, Paraiso does not consider the purchase and maintenance cost of the robot. Even when leaving this contributor to costs, they still find significant higher costs for the RASC (LSC US$14,342$\pm$2941 vs.

RASC $16,278 \pm 3326$; $p = 0.008$). That difference was primarily driven by the higher operating room cost for RASC, and not the costs related to "hospitalization" [12].

In essence therefore, when using similar definitions of operating cost, there were no differences in costs in one but not in the other study. In a nutshell, the operational costs excluding purchase and maintenance were comparable in the former study, but not in the latter. When it comes to investments, purchase costs were not included in one study [12], though were higher when taken into account. The magnitude is as given above, though it is worth noting that the costs of the laparoscopic equipment was not computed by Anger et al., therefore the difference may be exaggerated.

Clinical outcomes were also reported with no difference in complications. In Paraiso et al., three conversions were reported, all in the robotic arm, one to laparotomy, two to LSC. In Anger et al., there were no conversions. Both studies report higher postoperative pain for RASC patients. This persists for only the first week following surgery in the Anger cohort and between three and five weeks for Paraiso, though the scales used were again not comparable. However supporting this observation in Paraiso's study was the extended use of painkillers following RASC (11 days versus 20 days; $p < .005$) [12]. This was not reported by Anger. Efficacy (anatomical outcome) of the procedure was equivalent on short term (6 months [14] or 1 year [12]). The pelvic floor dysfunction and quality of life questionnaires partially overlapped for both studies, yet there were no differences observed again at slightly different time points.

Because of the differences in definitions of essential (primary) outcome measures, we decided not to pool the results for a formal meta-analysis.

Discussion

RASC may be equally effective yet is more expensive

Though efficacy was not a primary outcome in this study, it is reasonable to assume that RASC and LSC are equally efficacious. In reality, it may numerically be very difficult to design a study that would show the opposite. The available randomized trials logically looked at other aspects; one of these being costs. When taking into account the purchase and maintenance costs, the ACCESS trial demonstrates an increased cost when the robot is used [14]. Although the costs of consumables were only reported in one study [12], they are higher than for straight stick LSC. The above is in line with earlier observational studies on the same procedure [15, 16]. Given that hardware and consumable costs are among the principal cost drivers, another result would have been surprising. Other firm contributors are typically operation time and hospital stay, yet they are comparable in one RCT [14] and several observational studies [17, 18] and hence cannot compensate for the increased "material"

costs. This is also in line with randomized studies on other procedures, such as hysterectomy [19], fundoplication [20], and right hemicolectomy [21], as well as the numerous observational studies [22–25]. Obviously, one cannot compare all these studies of different design and quality, and it seems that, roughly spoken, one looks at an excess cost of US$2–3000 [26, 27]. Whether one would come to the same magnitude of excess costs in a European setting or elsewhere remains to be studied, yet, proportionally spoken, it is unlikely that there is a cost model where this difference would not show.

Both studies consistently report more short-term pain, though at later timepoints it is difficult to compare outcomes as different measurement methods were used. This aspect has not been very well studied in observational studies on SC, with one study showing similar levels of postoperative pain [17] or (randomized) studies on other procedures. Park et al. found no significant difference in postoperative pain in a RCT comparing robotic and laparoscopic right hemicolectomy in cancer patients [21]. It is therefore difficult to draw a firm conclusion, though the clinical relevance of increased pain sensation over a very short time with limited increase in pain relief is probably not very important. Further research into the actual cause of a difference in pain may demonstrate the blame does not lay with the robot. For instance, it has been speculated that this may be due to an increased diameter and/or increased tension on the robotic ports, which theoretically can be remediated by further technologic advancements.

The question is how solid one considers the evidence for the above conclusions. First, there are the methodological differences on definition of costs, pain, etc. This is inherent when there are no gold standard methods for this type of research. The two available studies may however be individually criticized as well. One can argue what is the most relevant endpoint to study, but it seems completely acceptable to us to take *cost* as a relevant outcome measure in the current economic situation. Whether the choice for a hospital cost analysis rather than a cost study that looks further than that, is right, may be another point of discussion. It seems however fair to us for a hospital to first do a cost-minimization study as management decisions will be primarily based on the outcomes of such study. *Operation time* is also an acceptable endpoint as this proxy for surgical efficiency bears relevance both to surgeons as well as hospital management. From a methodological viewpoint, it could be argued that it is uncertain whether the surgical skills and experience at the onset of the RCT were comparable for both treatment modalities. Both studies state that a minimum of 10 RASC was required, though actual numbers are lacking. We requested that information, and both authors kindly provided their best estimate, ranging between 10 and 15 for two surgeons and 50 for two other surgeons for the study by Anger et al. For the study by Paraiso et al., one surgeon had a previous experience of 400–500 LSCs and 10 RASCs and the other surgeon had performed about 100 LSCs and 10

RASCs. Nevertheless, even under the "best" circumstances of a very experienced team, it seems not possible to overcome the limitation of an increased cost.

In summary, these two RCTs are the best available evidence and consistently demonstrate higher costs without measurable benefit to the patient. We therefore agree with Steege and Einarsson [10] that stating "robotic is better than conventional surgery" is not supported by high-quality evidence at present. In the absence of any evidence of superiority, is the "problem of how to implement the technology … moot", as the Editorial suggests [10]?

Speculations on future place of robotic in pelvic floor surgery

Nonetheless, this does not mean the robot does not have some assets. Laparoscopic surgeons frequently report discomfort in the neck and upper extremities as well as experience higher stress levels [28–30]. A more static posture during LSC as opposed to open surgery is blamed for this adverse effect [31]. For relatively lengthy operations such as SC (sacrocolpopexy), this may not be a trivial observation. Regardless, this adds to the inherent limited degree of freedom of motion by "straight stick" laparoscopic instruments, which impacts female surgeons more than male and surgeons with smaller hands [30, 32]. Also, in some outdated operating theatres, the inappropriate positioning or limited numbers of monitors may be disturbing [33, 34].

Previously, Tarr et al. studied the ergonomic impact specifically for *sacrocolpopexy* in a prospective cohort of 33 RASC and 53 LSC procedures over a 16-month period [35]. The procedures were performed by a variety of surgeons at different seniority (resident, fellow, attending), though all were previously trained with the studied modalities. As outcome measures, they used a validated five-step score for measuring "Body Part Discomfort" (BPD) in different body regions and the National Aeronautics and Space Administration Task Load Index (NASA-TLI), rating, e.g., mental and physical demands, and effort and frustration with given tasks on a continuous scale. [36]. In a nutshell, this study showed that RASC was associated with lower neck, shoulder, and back discomfort scores [35]. Stress levels, measured by skin conductance level, and heart rate were significantly lower in surgically inexperienced medical students performing tasks with the robot when compared to laparoscopic instrumentation [37]. These findings will need to be validated in a proper RCT and a more homogenous population of surgeons.

Another view is that RASC in the hands of a novice, or of a lesser experienced laparoscopist, is the most safe and effective tool to perform advanced procedures [38]; hence, the economical disadvantages can be ignored. Assuming that one can unequivocally demonstrate that RASC is much easier to be learned than LSC (no study has shown this to our knowledge),

it may be, at a larger scale, the most pragmatic solution for the long and demanding learning process typical for this procedure [8, 39, 40]. Indeed, we have shown that 30 LSCs are required to achieve an operation time within the range of an experienced surgeon, and 60 procedures to obtain similar complication rates [39]. This, combined with the relative low numbers of sacrocolpopexies at each individual training unit, makes adequate training problematic [8]. Robotics in a setting with a double console could be safer and more effective to train junior surgeons. This is however far from certain: one study demonstrated that robotic hysterectomy actually had a longer learning curve ($n = 91$) than what we described for LSC [41]. From a training perspective, one could also follow another strategy and try to shorten the learning process, for instance, by a wider introduction of 3-D LSC [42]. This may require an investment—which is probably less than for a robot—yet will not have the repetitive instrument cost.

For us, there is no doubt that robotic developments boost surgical capacities. Articulation beyond normal manipulation, tremor reduction, and all the other claimed advantages may not be proven; however, these properties, and the improved ergonomics, are a true paradigm shift in surgery. For that alone, the technology warrants further development. Certainly in the field of urogynaecology, for some relatively complex procedures, such as mesh removal, or more novel procedures such as those for urge incontinence, which require bilateral extensive retroperitoneal dissections, there might be a benefit [43].

In conclusion, robotic surgery significantly adds to the costs. To make it sustainable, and to allow further investments in a technology which has not reached its limits, we must move to a more reasonable cost. This can either result from the arrival of a competitor (long expected but not yet a reality) [2] or by negotiating a more reasonable and affordable price either for the hospital [44] or at a higher level. The latter approach has been successfully undertaken in Belgium through negotiation with the medical drug industry [45].

Authors' contribution   GC: protocol development, data extraction, data interpretation, and manuscript writing. JB: protocol development, search strategy development, data extraction, data analysis, manuscript editing. SH: manuscript editing. JV: manuscript editing. BVC: manuscript editing. FVA: manuscript editing. DDR: manuscript editing. IV: manuscript editing. JD: arbitration, data interpretation, manuscript writing/editing.

References

1. van Dam P, Hauspy J, Verkinderen L, Trinh XB, van Dam PJ, Van Looy L, Dirix L (2011) Are costs of robot-assisted surgery warranted for gynecological procedures? Obstet Gynecol Int 2011:973830

2. Iavazzo C, Papadopoulou EK, Gkegkes ID (2014) Cost assessment of robotics in gynecologic surgery: a systematic review. J Obstet Gynaecol Res 40(11):2125–2134

3. Lotan Y (2012) Is robotic surgery cost-effective: no. Curr Opin Urol 22(1):66–69

4. Maher C, Feiner B, Baessler K, Schmid C (2013) Surgical management of pelvic organ prolapse in women. Cochrane Database Syst Rev 4:CD004014

5. Maher CF, Feiner B, DeCuyper EM, Nichlos CJ, Hickey KV, O'Rourke P (2011) Laparoscopic sacral colpopexy versus total vaginal mesh for vaginal vault prolapse: a randomized trial. Am J Obstet Gynecol 204(4):360, e361-367

6. Maher CF, Connelly LB (2012) Cost minimization analysis of laparoscopic sacral colpopexy and total vaginal mesh. Am J Obstet Gynecol 206(5):433, e431-437

7. Freeman RM, Pantazis K, Thomson A, Frappell J, Bombieri L, Moran P, Slack M, Scott P, Waterfield M (2013) A randomised controlled trial of abdominal versus laparoscopic sacrocolpopexy for the treatment of post-hysterectomy vaginal vault prolapse: LAS study. Int Urogynecol J 24(3):377–384

8. Deprest J, Krofta L, Van der Aa F, Milani AL, Den Boon J, Claerhout F, Roovers JP (2014) The challenge of implementing laparoscopic sacrocolpopexy. Int Urogynecol J 25(9):1153–1160

9. Serati M, Bogani G, Sorice P, Braga A, Torella M, Salvatore S, Uccella S, Cromi A, Ghezzi F (2014) Robot-assisted sacrocolpopexy for pelvic organ prolapse: a systematic review and meta-analysis of comparative studies. Eur Urol 66(2):303–318

10. Steege JF, Einarsson JI (2014) Robotics in benign gynecologic surgery: where should we go? Obstet Gynecol 123:1–2

11. Higgins JP, Altman DG, Gotzsche PC, Juni P, Moher D, Oxman AD, Savovic J, Schulz KF, Weeks L, Sterne JA (2011) The Cochrane Collaboration's tool for assessing risk of bias in randomised trials. BMJ 343:d5928

12. Paraiso MF, Jelovsek JE, Frick A, Chen CC, Barber MD (2011) Laparoscopic compared with robotic sacrocolpopexy for vaginal prolapse: a randomized controlled trial. Obstet Gynecol 118(5): 1005–1013

13. Mueller ER, Kenton K, Tarnay C, Brubaker L, Rosenman A, Smith B, Stroupe K, Bresee C, Pantuck A, Schulam P et al (2012) Abdominal Colpopexy: Comparison of Endoscopic Surgical Strategies (ACCESS). Contemp Clin Trials 33(5):1011–1018

14. Anger JT, Mueller ER, Tarnay C, Smith B, Stroupe K, Rosenman A, Brubaker L, Bresee C, Kenton K (2014) Robotic compared with laparoscopic sacrocolpopexy: a randomized controlled trial. Obstet Gynecol 123(1):5–12

15. Tan-Kim J, Menefee SA, Luber KM, Nager CW, Lukacz ES (2011) Robotic-assisted and laparoscopic sacrocolpopexy: comparing operative times, costs and outcomes. Female Pelvic Med Reconstr Surg 17(1):44–49

16. Judd JP, Siddiqui NY, Barnett JC, Visco AG, Havrilesky LJ, Wu JM (2010) Cost-minimization analysis of robotic-assisted, laparoscopic, and abdominal sacrocolpopexy. J Minim Invasive Gynecol 17(4):493–499

17. Seror J, Yates DR, Seringe E, Vaessen C, Bitker MO, Chartier-Kastler E, Roupret M (2012) Prospective comparison of short-term functional outcomes obtained after pure laparoscopic and robot-assisted laparoscopic sacrocolpopexy. World J Urol 30(3): 393–398

18. Antosh DD, Grotzke SA, McDonald MA, Shveiky D, Park AJ, Gutman RE, Sokol AI (2012) Short-term outcomes of robotic versus conventional laparoscopic sacral colpopexy. Female Pelvic Med Reconstr Surg 18(3):158–161

19. Paraiso MF, Ridgeway B, Park AJ, Jelovsek JE, Barber MD, Falcone T, Einarsson JI (2013) A randomized trial comparing conventional and robotically assisted total laparoscopic hysterectomy. Am J Obstet Gynecol 208(5):368, e361-367

20. Morino M, Pellegrino L, Giaccone C, Garrone C, Rebecchi F (2006) Randomized clinical trial of robot-assisted versus laparoscopic Nissen fundoplication. Br J Surg 93(5):553–558

21. Park JS, Choi GS, Park SY, Kim HJ, Ryuk JP (2012) Randomized clinical trial of robot-assisted versus standard laparoscopic right colectomy. Br J Surg 99(9):1219–1226

22. Mirnezami AH, Mirnezami R, Venkatasubramaniam AK, Chandrakumaran K, Cecil TD, Moran BJ (2010) Robotic colorectal surgery: hype or new hope? A systematic review of robotics in colorectal surgery. Colorectal Dis 12(11):1084–1093

23. Bolenz C, Gupta A, Hotze T, Ho R, Cadeddu JA, Roehrborn CG, Lotan Y (2010) Cost comparison of robotic, laparoscopic, and open radical prostatectomy for prostate cancer. Eur Urol 57(3):453–458

24. Finkelstein J, Eckersberger E, Sadri H, Taneja SS, Lepor H, Djavan B (2010) Open versus laparoscopic versus robot-assisted laparoscopic prostatectomy: the European and US experience. Rev Urol 12(1):35–43

25. Breitenstein S, Nocito A, Puhan M, Held U, Weber M, Clavien PA (2008) Robotic-assisted versus laparoscopic cholecystectomy: outcome and cost analyses of a case-matched control study. Ann Surg 247(6):987–993

26. Patel M, O'Sullivan D, Tulikangas PK (2009) A comparison of costs for abdominal, laparoscopic, and robot-assisted sacral colpopexy. Int Urogynecol J Pelvic Floor Dysfunct 20(2):223–228

27. Wright JD, Ananth CV, Lewin SN, Burke WM, Lu YS, Neugut AI, Herzog TJ, Hershman DL (2013) Robotically assisted vs laparoscopic hysterectomy among women with benign gynecologic disease. Jama 309(7):689–698

28. Berguer R, Smith WD, Chung YH (2001) Performing laparoscopic surgery is significantly more stressful for the surgeon than open surgery. Surg Endosc 15(10):1204–1207

29. Park A, Lee G, Seagull FJ, Meenaghan N, Dexter D (2010) Patients benefit while surgeons suffer: an impending epidemic. J Am Coll Surg 210(3):306–313

30. Franasiak J, Ko EM, Kidd J, Secord AA, Bell M, Boggess JF, Gehrig PA (2012) Physical strain and urgent need for ergonomic training among gynecologic oncologists who perform minimally invasive surgery. Gynecol Oncol 126(3):437–442

31. Nguyen NT, Ho HS, Smith WD, Philipps C, Lewis C, De Vera RM, Berguer R (2001) An ergonomic evaluation of surgeons' axial skeletal and upper extremity movements during laparoscopic and open surgery. Am J Surg 182(6):720–724

32. Sutton E, Irvin M, Zeigler C, Lee G, Park A (2014) The ergonomics of women in surgery. Surg Endosc 28(4):1051–1055

33. Berguer R, Forkey DL, Smith WD (2001) The effect of laparoscopic instrument working angle on surgeons' upper extremity workload. Surg Endosc 15(9):1027–1029

34. van Det MJ, Meijerink WJ, Hoff C, Totte ER, Pierie JP (2009) Optimal ergonomics for laparoscopic surgery in minimally invasive surgery suites: a review and guidelines. Surg Endosc 23(6):1279–1285

35. Tarr ME, Brancato SJ, Cunkelman JA, Polcari A, Nutter B, Kenton K (2015) Comparison of postural ergonomics between laparoscopic and robotic sacrocolpopexy: a pilot study. J Minim Invasive Gynecol 22(2):234–238

36. Stefanidis D, Wang F, Korndorffer JR Jr, Dunne JB, Scott DJ (2010) Robotic assistance improves intracorporeal suturing perfor-

mance and safety in the operating room while decreasing operator workload. Surg Endosc 24(2):377–382

37. Hurley AMKPJ, O'Connor L, Dinan TG, Cryan JF, Boylan G, O'Reilly BA (2015) SOS save our surgeons: stress levels reduced by robotic surgery. Gynecol Surg 12(3):197–206

38. Chandra V, Nehra D, Parent R, Woo R, Reyes R, Hernandez-Boussard T, Dutta S (2010) A comparison of laparoscopic and robotic assisted suturing performance by experts and novices. Surgery 147(6):830–839

39. Claerhout F, Verguts J, Werbrouck E, Veldman J, Lewi P, Deprest J (2014) Analysis of the learning process for laparoscopic sacrocolpopexy: identification of challenging steps. Int Urogynecol J 25(9):1185–1191

40. Claerhout F, Roovers JP, Lewi P, Verguts J, De Ridder D, Deprest J (2009) Implementation of laparoscopic sacrocolpopexy—a single centre's experience. Int Urogynecol J Pelvic Floor Dysfunct 20(9): 1119–1125

41. Woelk JL, Casiano ER, Weaver AL, Gostout BS, Trabuco EC, Gebhart JB (2013) The learning curve of robotic hysterectomy. Obstet Gynecol 121(1):87–95

42. Ko JK, Li RH, Cheung VY (2015) Two-dimensional versus three-dimensional laparoscopy: evaluation of physicians' performance and preferenceusing a pelvic trainer. J Minim Invasive Gynecol 22(3):421–427

43. Jager W, Mirenska O, Brugge S (2012) Surgical treatment of mixed and urge urinary incontinence in women. Gynecol Obstet Invest 74(2):157–164

44. White WM, Pickens RB, Elder RF, Firoozi F (2014) Robotic-assisted sacrocolpopexy for pelvic organ prolapse. Urol Clin North Am 41(4):549–557

45. Pauwels K, Huys I, Casteels M, De Nys K, Simoens S (2014) Market access of cancer drugs in European countries: improving resource allocation. Target Oncol 9(2):95–110

29

Minimally invasive management of 14–16-week abdominal ectopic with hemoperitoneum: an emergency laparoscopic procedure

Mohammed Rizk[1] · Haitham Salem[2]

Abstract Since the first laparoscopic cholecystectomy on a pregnant lady in 1991, a plethora of articles and case studies have been published addressing laparoscopy and their role in pregnancy. The Royal College of Obstetricians and Gynecologists Green-top Guidelines recommends laparoscopic surgery as the preferred approach in early ectopic tubal pregnancies. Laparoscopic versus laparotomy management of abdominal ectopic is a traumatic experience both on physical and emotional levels. The case study was a 36-year-old gravida 2 para 0 patient, previously normal pregnant lady, in which the follow-up ultrasound revealed moderate hemoperitoneum at 14–16 weeks of gestation. Upon urgent diagnostic laparoscopy, massive hemoperitoneum was detected despite no clinical signs of hemodynamic instability. Uterus was found to be within the normal measurements consistent with the nonpregnant state. Multiple myomas were clearly seen in the uterine wall. A fetus of 14–16 weeks was detected attached to the colon during formal laparoscopic pelvic and abdominal exploration for ectopic pregnancy. Operative laparoscopy for abdominal ectopic in skillful hands can be considered a feasible management technique carrying all the advantages of a minimally invasive procedure.

Keywords Laparoscopy · Ectopic pregnancy · Minimally invasive surgery

✉ Mohammed Rizk
  mohammed.rizk@gmail.com

[1] Obstetrics & Gynecology Department, Ain Shams University, Cairo, Egypt

[2] Surgery Department, Cairo University, Cairo, Egypt

Introduction

For women in the reproductive age, ectopic pregnancy is one of the most serious conditions to be considered in differential diagnosis of abdominal pain. First described by Wendeler et al. in 1895, Eccyesis or ectopic pregnancy is characterized by implantation of the fertilized ovum in a position other than the uterine cavity [1]. It occurs by a rate of 1–2 % of all pregnancies in developed countries [2]. Eccyesis is generally classified into tubal and nontubal pregnancies. More than 90 % of the abnormal implantation occurs in the Fallopian tube (tubal pregnancies), while the rest (nontubal) might occur at the ovary, cervix, or intra-abdominal [3–5].

In a medical field with extensive scientific advances, ectopic pregnancy remains a major cause of death, particularly during the first trimester (Varma and Gupta [6]). Risk factors include previous ectopic, PID, smoking, multi-parity, previous abortion, tubal surgery, assisted reproductive technology, extremes of age, IUD, and DES exposure in utero [7]. Nitric oxide and low socioeconomic status were also reported as potential risks [8, 9]. However, in up to 50 % of the cases, no risk factors can be identified [10].

The broad spectrum of clinical manifestations with ectopic pregnancy complicates the diagnosis, as they vary from asymptomatic cases to acute abdomen and hemodynamic shock. Most of the cases were initially undiagnosed until complicated with massive hemorrhage or turned into a life-threatening condition. A high index of suspicion with close follow-up is mandatory for early detection of an ectopic pregnancy (Crochet at al. [11]).

Management generally includes medical or surgical methods; both are effective, but the selection depends on clinical situation, localization of ectopic pregnancy, and diagnostic tools. The first successful surgery for an ectopic pregnancy was performed by Robert Lawson Tait in 1883 [12]. Recently,

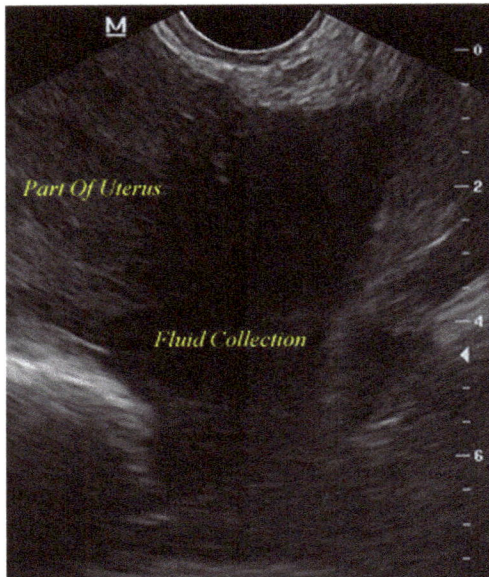

Fig. 1 Ultrasound image in the emergency setting showing the fluid collection in the abdomen and pelvis, with a nongravid uterus

Laparoscopy has experienced numerous changes and developments, replacing to a great extent the traditional laparotomy procedure [13]. Laparoscopic approach has many benefits; it yields less postoperative pain, shorter hospital stay, faster recovery, and better aesthetic results [14, 15].

Although laparoscopy is not indicated for all clinical scenarios, it has become the gold standard for numerous obstetric and gynecological situations [16]. Moreover, unusual types of ectopic are being recently managed with laparoscopic surgery [17].

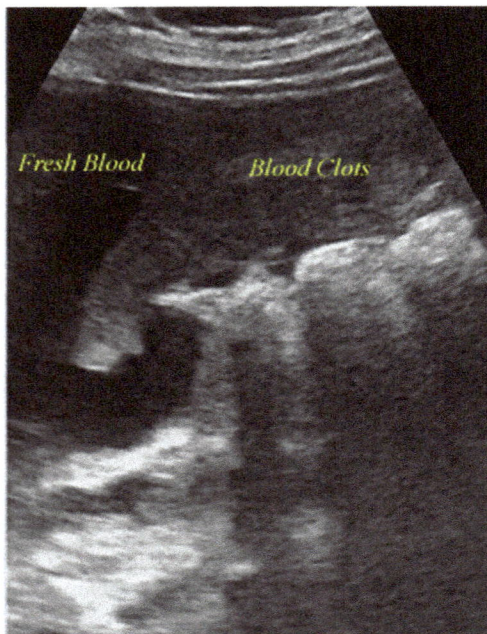

Fig. 2 Ultrasound image showing blood clots and fresh bleeding in the abdomen and pelvis

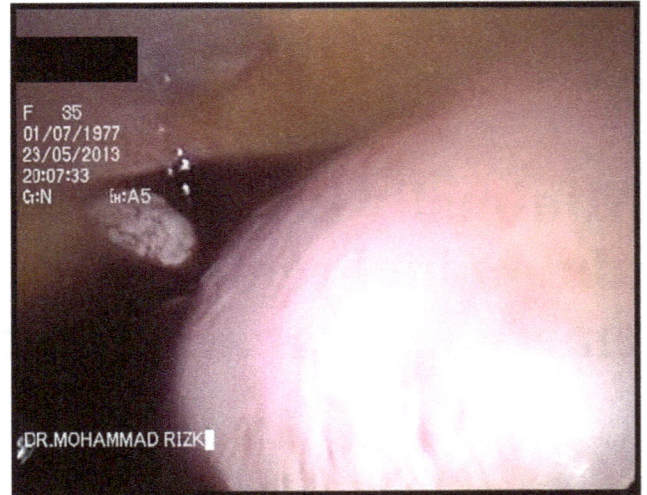

Fig. 3 First look by the laparoscopy camera showing the intra-abdominal collection, with no apparent adnexa

Case

The patient was a 36-year-old Middle Eastern Saudi female, gravida 2 para 0 at 14 weeks and 5 days gestational age based on her last menstrual period. She presented to the emergency department with cramping lower abdominal pain. She has a history of right salpingectomy for previous ectopic pregnancy management. The patient rated her pain as 8 on a severity scale of 10. Physical examination revealed supra-pubic and right lower quadrant tenderness, with no signs of acute peritonitis. She was hemodynamically stable; blood pressure 135/83 mmHg, hemoglobin 10.2 mg/dl, and positive beta hCG. Transvaginal ultrasound revealed no evidence of an intrauterine pregnancy but did show moderate to large amount of complex collection of fluid in the anterior and posterior cul-de-sacs. An ill-defined mass was also noticed; extending slightly to the right of midline (Figs. 1 and 2). These findings were concerning for a ruptured ectopic

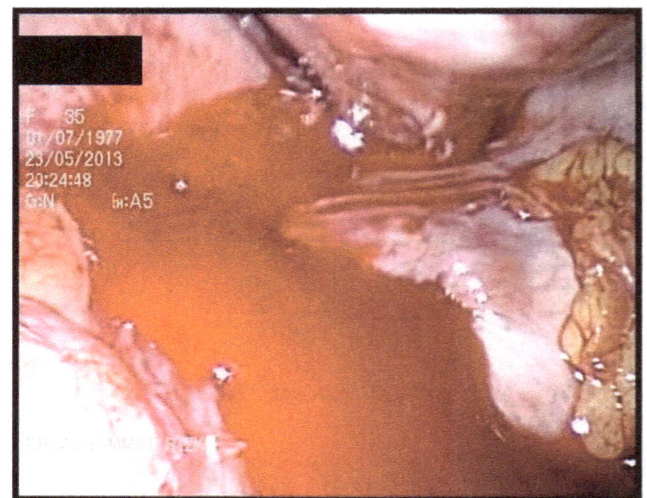

Fig. 4 Exploration showing the intra-abdominal collection

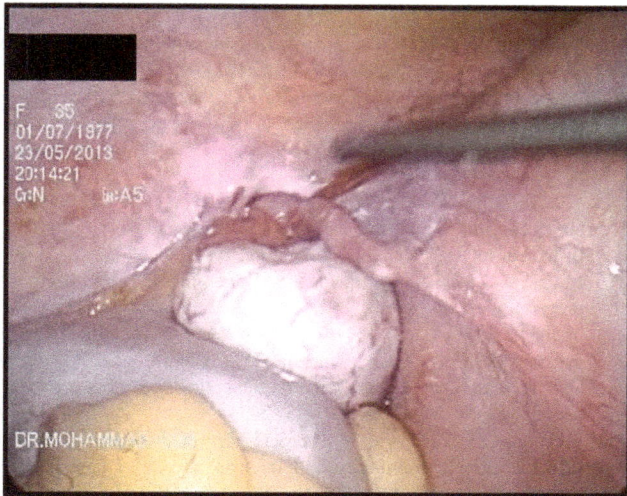

Fig. 5 Ovary and tube after clearing the intra-abdominal collection

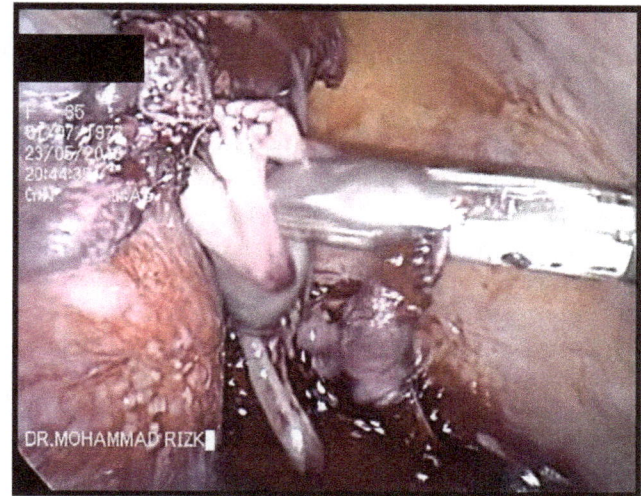

Fig. 7 Peritoneal pregnancy was detected with fetus seen

pregnancy. In light of the patient's symptoms and clinical data, the patient was taken to the operating room for a diagnostic laparoscopy. On inspection, large clots of blood were noticed in the pelvis with active oozing (Figs. 3 and 4). The uterus appeared bulky and malformed by multiple myomas. The left tube and ovary appeared within normal measures (Fig. 5), while the right tube was not present, and the right ovary was detected after aspiration and removal of omental adhesions. An intact corpus luteum was noticed on the left ovary. However, on further abdominal exploration, omental adhesions were noticed near the right ovary (Fig. 6). On inspection, the omentum was found to have a fetus about 14 to 16 weeks (Figs. 7 and 8). At this time, our presumptive diagnosis was an abdominal pregnancy. Adhesiolysis was done with removal of the fetus within an Endobag followed by separation of the omental-placental attachments with partial omentectomy, and then proper hemostasis was achieved. The patient did well postoperatively and was discharged home on postoperative day 1. The patient was given methotrexate in the postoperative period.

Discussion

With an incidence of 1 to 10,000 live births, primary abdominal pregnancy is considered an extremely rare form of ectopic pregnancy [18, 19]. Criteria for omental pregnancy were described in 1942 by Studdiford: normal bilateral fallopian tubes and ovaries, absence of utero-peritoneal fistula, and presence of a pregnancy related to the peritoneal surface exclusively. Our patient here met the diagnostic criteria of Studdiford. Only few reported cases have been treated using laparoscopy in literature [20, 21].

In 1997, a case of primary omental pregnancy diagnosed with laparoscopy at 6-weeks gestational age was described, where a hemorrhagic mass was noticed to be adherent to the omentum close to the left ovary [22]. It was an answer to a previous doubt about the existence of a true omental pregnancy [23]. In 2004, laparoscopic treatment of an abdominal pregnancy was reported, where the gestational sac was noticed in the Douglas pouch [24].

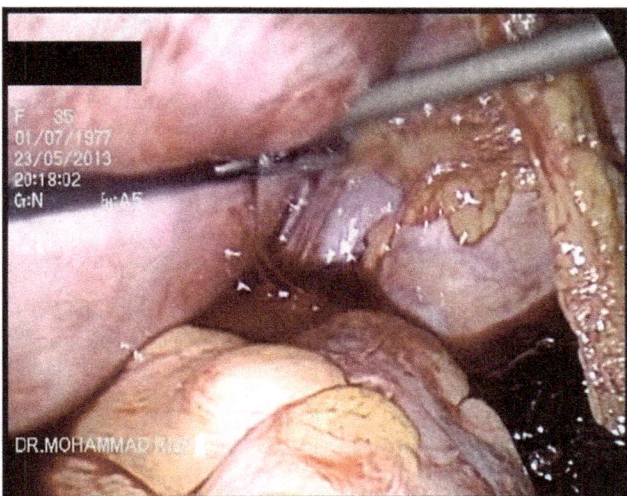

Fig. 6 Adhesiolysis for further exploration

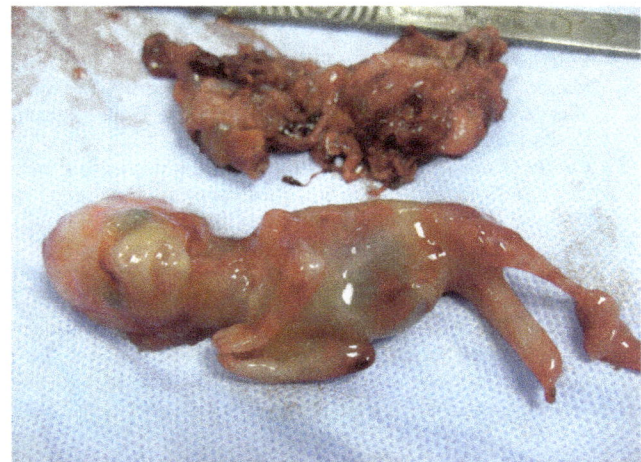

Fig. 8 Fourteen- to 16-week fetus after extraction

Many other reports in the literature describing a hemorrhagic mass with blood clots appeared to be a consistent finding [25, 26]. Hemorrhage is a key factor requiring conversion from laparoscopy to laparotomy [27]. Laparotomy is recommended in most cases due to the risk of significant hemorrhage from the implantation site. Thus, the main stream in literature regarding ectopic pregnancy treatment is usually laparotomy, but with the introduction of laparoscopic surgery, it is now possible to manage these cases with minimally invasive techniques. There are multiple successful case reports of laparoscopic resection of ectopic pregnancies [28, 29]. Massive hemoperitoneum is not an absolute contraindication for laparoscopic management of ectopic pregnancy anymore [16].

Our patient was hemodynamically stable, and hence, we were able to perform laparoscopy without any complications. Although the advanced age of the abdominal pregnancy (14–16 weeks) is not usually treated with a laparoscopic approach, we proved that minimally invasive technique could be a feasible way of management.

Conclusion

Operative laparoscopy for abdominal ectopic in skillful hands can be considered a feasible management technique carrying all the advantages of a minimally invasive procedure.

Compliance with ethical standards All procedures performed in this report were in accordance with the ethical standards of the institutional and/or national research committee and with the Helsinki declaration and its later amendments. Written informed consent was obtained from the patient for publication of this case report and any accompanying images.

References

1. Villegas E, González-Mesa E, Benítez MJ, Luna S, Gómez C, Marsac A, Jiménez J (2014) Tubal ectopic pregnancy two years after laparoscopic supracervical hysterectomy. BMC Womens Health 14:69. doi:10.1186/1472-6874-14-69
2. Kirk E, Bottomley C, Bourne T (2014) Diagnosing ectopic pregnancy and current concepts in the management of pregnancy of unknown location. Hum Reprod Update20(2):250–61
3. Creanga AA, Shapiro-Mendoza CK, Bish CL, Zane S, Berg CJ, Callaghan WM (2011) Trends in ectopic pregnancy mortality in the United States: 1980–2007. Obstet Gynecol 117(4):837–43
4. Kopani F, Rrugia A, Manoku N (2010) Ectopic pregnancy comparison of different treatments. J Prenat Med 4(2):30–4
5. Cecchino GN, AraujoJúnior E, Elito Júnior J (2014) Methotrexate for ectopic pregnancy: when and how. Arch Gynecol Obstet 290(3):417–23
6. Varma R, Gupta J (2009) Tubal ectopic pregnancy. BMJ Clin Evid. Apr 20;2009. pii: 1406
7. Menon S, Sammel M, Vichnin M, Barnhart KT (2007) Risk factors for ectopic pregnancy: a comparison between adults and adolescent women. J PediatrAdolesc Gynecol 20:181–185
8. Al-Azemi M, Refaat B, Amer S, Ola B, Chapman N, Ledger W (2009) "The expression of inducible nitric oxide synthase in the human fallopian tube during the menstrual cycle and in ectopic pregnancy". FertilSteril 94(3):833–840
9. Yuk JS, Kim YJ, Hur JY, Shin JH (2013) Association between socioeconomic status and ectopic pregnancy rate in the Republic of Korea. Int J Gynaecol Obstet 122(2):104–7
10. Majhi AK, Roy N, Karmakar KS, Banerjee PK (2007) Ectopic pregnancy an analysis of 180 cases. J Indian Med Assoc 105(6): 308, 310, 312
11. Crochet JR, Bastian LA, Chireau MV (2013) Does this woman have an ectopic pregnancy?: the rational clinical examination systematic review. JAMA 309(16):1722–9
12. Saranovic M, Vasiljevic M, Prorocic M, Macut ND, Filipovic T (2014) Ectopic pregnancy and laparoscopy. Clin Exp Obstet Gynecol 41(3):276–9
13. Olweny EO, Best SL, Tracy CR, Cadeddu JA (2012) Comparison of outcomes of laparoscopic versus open appendectomy in adults: data from the Nationwide Inpatient Sample (NIS), 2006–2008. Arch Esp Urol 65(3):434–43
14. Khan KS, Wojdyla D, Say L, Gülmezoglu AM, Van Look PF (2006) WHO analysis of causes of maternal death: a systematic review. Lancet 367:1066–1076
15. Wang YL, Weng SS, Huang WC, Su TH (2014) Laparoscopic management of ectopic pregnancies in unusual locations Taiwan. J Obstet Gynecol 53(4):466–70. doi:10.1016/j.tjog.2014.01.004
16. Chaudhary P, Manchanda R, Patil VN (2013) Retrospective study on laparoscopic management of ectopic pregnancy. J ObstetGynaecol India 63(3):173–6. doi:10.1007/s13224-012-0304-z. Epub 2012 Nov 10
17. Yan CM (2010) Laparoscopic management of three rare types of ectopic pregnancy. Hong Kong Med J 16(2):132–6
18. Cunningham G, Leveno KJ, Bloom SL, Hauth JC, Rouse DJ, Sponge CY (2010) "Ectopic pregnancy,". In: Williams Obstetrics, 23rd edn. McGraw-Hill, New York, NY, USA, pp 238–256
19. Atrash HK, Friede A, Hogue CJR (1987) Abdominal pregnancyin the United States: frequency and maternal mortality. Obstet Gynecol 69(3 Pt 1):333–7
20. Studdiford WE (1942) Primary peritoneal pregnancy. Am J Obstet Gynecol 44(3):487–491
21. Watrowski R, Lange A, Möckel J (2015) Primary omental pregnancy with secondary implantation into posterior cul-de-sac: laparoscopic treatment using hemostatic matrix. J Minim Invasive Gynecol 22(3):501–3. doi:10.1016/j.jmig.2014.06.008, Epub 2014 Jun 25
22. Weeks AD, Aagaard J, Bromham D (1997) Laparoscopic management of an abdominal pregnancy. Gynaecol Endosc 6(4):249–250
23. Berghella V, Wolf SC (1996) Does primary omental pregnancy exist? Gynecol Obstet Invest 42(2):133–6
24. Gerli D, Rossetti G, Baiocchi G, Clerici V, Unfer G, Di Renzo C (2004) Early ultrasonographic diagnosis and laparoscopic treatment of abdominal pregnancy. Eur J Obstet Gynecol Reprod Biol 113(1): 103–105
25. Morita Y, Tsutsumi O, Kuramochi K, Momoeda M, Yoshikawa H, Taketani Y (1996) Case report: successful laparoscopic management of primary abdominal pregnancy,". Hum Reprod 11(11): 2546–2547
26. Tsudo T, Harada T, Yoshioka H, Terakawa N (1997) Laparoscopic management of early primary abdominal pregnancy. Obstet Gynecol 90(4):687–688
27. Walid MS, Heaton RL (2010) Diagnosis and laparoscopic treatment of cornual ectopic pregnancy. Ger Med Sci 27:8

30

Natural orifice transluminal endoscopic surgery (NOTES) salpingectomy for ectopic pregnancy: a first series demonstrating how a new surgical technique can be applied in a low-resource setting

Van Peer Sarah[1] · Baekelandt Jan[1]

Abstract This paper demonstrates the feasibility of a salpingectomy for ectopic pregnancy by transvaginal natural orifice transluminal endoscopic surgery (vNOTES). Conventional, reusable laparoscopic instruments were used and inserted through an inexpensive, self-constructed single port device. The self-constructed single port device was made by assembling a surgical glove, a wound protector, one reusable 10-mm trocar and four reusable 5-mm trocars. We report on five patients who underwent a vNOTES salpingectomy between September 2014 and February 2015. All procedures were successfully performed, without conversion to multi-incision laparoscopy or laparotomy. This demonstrates that it is possible to perform a vNOTES salpingectomy without any financial investment in expensive ports, disposable instruments or sealing devices (Video 1). Patient and perioperative data were analysed (Table 1). NOTES salpingectomy is a novel technique requiring further validation. It could be a less invasive alternative to a laparoscopic salpingectomy. A better cosmetic result, by avoiding abdominal incision scars, and less port-related complications, can be expected.

Keywords Transvaginal natural orifice transluminal endoscopic surgery (NOTES) · Single port · Frugal innovation · Tubal pregnancy · Salpingectomy · Low resource · vNOTES

✉ Baekelandt Jan
jan.baekelandt@imelda.be

[1] Department of Obstetrics and Gynaecology, Imelda Hospital Bonheiden, Bonheiden, Belgium

Background

Over the last 20 years, the advantages of laparoscopy in gynaecological surgery, when compared with open surgery, have been accepted worldwide [1]. Less invasive procedures, such as single incision laparoscopic surgery (SILS) [2] and natural orifice transluminal endoscopic surgery (NOTES) [3–5], are a developing field of minimally invasive surgery. NOTES makes use of the natural orifices of the body as surgical channels of endoscopy; transvaginal access is most frequently used for NOTES. This approach makes use of a single incision to introduce a trocar through which all instruments are inserted.

A better cosmetic result, by avoiding abdominal incision scars, and less port-related complications, for example hernia formation, can be expected.

In this report, we aimed to demonstrate the feasibility of a NOTES salpingectomy using only conventional, reusable laparoscopic instruments and an inexpensive, self-constructed single port device that can be quickly and easily assembled. We aimed to demonstrate that there is no need for expensive, commercially available disposable SILS ports, other disposable instruments or sealing devices to perform a safe and equally time-efficient salpingectomy by NOTES.

Material and methods

Patients

Between September 2014 and February 2015, five NOTES salpingectomies were performed for ectopic pregnancy. Ectopic pregnancy was diagnosed based on clinical findings, combined with transvaginal ultrasound and positive serum human chorionic gonadotropin (hCG) level. The NOTES salpingectomies were performed as follows (Video 1). The following patient and perioperative data were collected and retrospectively analysed: patient age, body mass index (BMI), total operating time, serum haemoglobin (Hb) drop, (peri-) operative complications and postoperative pain score. The duration of surgery was defined as the time from incision to the end of closure of the colpotomy.

Surgical technique

The patients were given general anaesthesia and placed in lithotomy position. The lower abdomen and vagina were thoroughly disinfected and draped. A Foley catheter was used to empty the bladder. A 2.5-cm single incision was made in the posterior vaginal fornix. The pouch of Douglas was opened to insert the self-constructed NOTES port. The device was constructed using an Alexis wound protector/retractor (Applied Medical, Rancho Santa Margarita, CA, USA) attached to a size 8 surgical glove (Fig. 1). One finger of the surgical glove was incised to place a 10-mm reusable trocar for CO_2 insufflation and laparoscope insertion. Four 5-mm reusable trocars were placed through the other fingers for insertion of the reusable laparoscopic instruments. We used a standard 0° 10-mm laparoscope. The reusable conventional laparoscopic instruments were a bipolar forceps, a pair of cold scissors, an atraumatic forceps and a suction-irrigation cannula. After placing the patients in Trendelenburg position, CO_2 was insufflated to maintain an adequate pneumoperitoneum.

The diagnosis of a tubal pregnancy could be confirmed during the NOTES procedure in all patients, and both ovaries and contralateral tube were normal. The decision was made to perform a salpingectomy, as demonstrated in the video. After complete resection, the salpinx was extracted through the wound protector into the glove part of the self-constructed port. After haemostasis and rinsing of the peritoneal cavity, the pneumoperitoneum was deflated and the port device removed with the salpinx inside it. The vaginal wall was closed using a resorbable running suture.

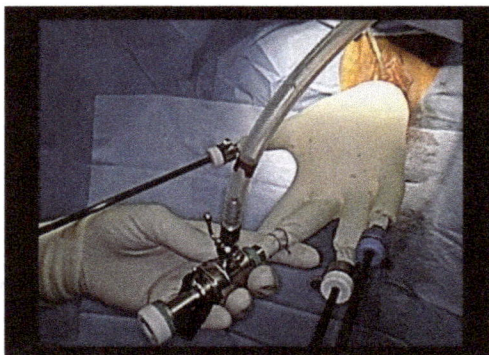

Fig. 1 Conventional, reusable laparoscopic instruments used and inserted through an inexpensive, self-constructed single port device

Parenteral cefazolin and metronidazole were administered preoperatively. As intraoperative analgesia, paracetamol (1000 mg) and ketorolac trometamol (20 mg) were given.

Postoperative pain was assessed using the visual analogue pain scale (VAS) (scoring from 0—no pain, to 10—worst imaginable pain).

Postoperative pain was managed by paracetamol (1000 mg) and ketorolac trometamol (20 mg), followed by oral paracetamol.

Results

Table 1 gives the patient data and operative outcomes. Transvaginal NOTES (vNOTES) for ectopic pregnancy was successfully completed in all patients. No minor or major perior postoperative complications occurred.

The median age of the patients was 29 years (range, 26–32). The median body mass index was 23.76 kg/m^2 (range, 19.6–27). Four patients had had one previous delivery, of which one was by Caesarean section and the other three by normal vaginal delivery. For one patient, the ectopic pregnancy was the first pregnancy.

From incision to vaginal closure, the mean operation time was 33 min. The mean blood loss due to the procedure was 36 cc. The mean drop in haemoglobin level 24 h after the operation was 1.96 g/dl.

In two patients, the ectopic pregnancy ruptured preoperatively causing a haemoperitoneum; in one of these patients, 2 units of packed cells were transfused postoperatively because of a Hb decrease of 5.4 g/dl.

The VAS score 12 h postoperatively was low for all patients, and the median VAS pain scores at 12 h after surgery were 2 (range 1–2).

Discussion

Transvaginal laparoscopy was initially reported as a safe and minimally invasive diagnostic technique in infertility [6]. NOTES is an emerging field in gynaecology, gastrointestinal surgery and urology. The first appendectomy via vNOTES was reported on in 2008 [7]. A randomised study on vNOTES cholecystectomy concluded that transvaginal cholecystectomy can be recommended to future patients as an alternative for a laparoscopic cholecystectomy [8]. In urology, pure vNOTES nephrectomy is found to be technically challenging but feasible [9]. In gynaecology, fertility surgeons were the first to start using transvaginal laparoscopy. Transvaginal hydrolaparoscopy is now used as an outpatient procedure for infertility investigation [10]. It can also be used on an ambulatory basis for reconstructive tubo-ovarian surgery [11]. Experienced laparoscopists are now being advised to consider a

Table 1 Patient characteristics and operative outcomes

Patient	Age (years)	BMI (kg/m^2)	Parity	Operation time (min)	Perioperative findings	Blood loss Haemoperitoneum (cc)	Blood loss Procedure (cc)	Hb decrease (g/dl)
1	28	21.5	1 (VD)	30	Tubal EP Ampullary bleeding	100	20	1.1
2	27	25.5	1 (CS)	35	Tubal EP Ampullary bleeding	75	20	0.7
3	32	19.6	1 (VD)	30	Tubal EP Ruptured	350	50	1.8
4	26	25.2	1 (VD)	50	Tubal EP Ruptured	1400	70	5.4[a]
5	32	27	0	20	Tubal EP Ampullary bleeding	100	20	0.8

[a] 2E packed cells transfused

BMI body mass index, *VD* vaginal delivery, *CS* Caesarean section, *EP* ectopic pregnancy

transition towards fertiloscopy in the diagnostic workup of unexplained infertility, or for the purpose of ovarian drilling [12]. vNOTES can also be used as an approach for adnexal surgery and adhaesiolysis [3–5, 13]. A variety of approaches, including the stomach, oesophagus, bladder and rectum, are being used for NOTES procedures. However, the vast majority of NOTES procedures have been performed transvaginally, as the vagina provides direct access [14].

In this report, vNOTES salpingectomy for tubal pregnancy, unruptured or ruptured, was successfully performed using only conventional, reusable laparoscopic instruments and a self-constructed low-cost NOTES port. The procedures were completed within a reasonable operation time and without complications. No conversion to standard multi-incision laparoscopy or laparotomy was necessary. It was still possible to perform a salpingectomy via vNOTES in a patient with a haemoperitoneum of 1400 ml due to a ruptured ectopic pregnancy. Transvaginal access via a colpotomy was also possible in the two patients who had had no previous vaginal delivery.

Various technical difficulties, such as instrument collision, limited triangulation and reduced tissue traction, are comparable to those for transumbilical SILS and need to be overcome in order to perform vNOTES. These difficulties have been found to be less restricting when compared with SILS, as the colpotomy provides a more flexible entry compared to the infraumbilical fascia opening. Due to camera insertion through the pouch of Douglas, the view through a vNOTES port is opposite to that of a standard laparoscopic view, and this rotation of the surgical field axis required only a brief adaptation period.

Transvaginal NOTES salpingectomy provides a better aesthetic result when compared to a standard laparoscopic salpingectomy as no abdominal incisions are made. Whether patients have less postoperative pain needs to be further assessed in larger studies. A systematic review on vNOTES appendectomies reported a trend towards shorter hospitalisation, quicker recovery, less analgesic requirement and better cosmetic satisfaction [15]. A similar result can be expected for vNOTES salpingectomy. One could argue the possibility of pelvic infection after vaginal surgery, but previous studies have shown that postoperative pelvic infection is unlikely to happen, especially when prophylactic antibiotics are administered [16, 17]. The risk of dyspareunia due to the colpotomy needs to be taken into account. No difference between conventional compared to laparoscopic transvaginal surgery is to be expected, and different studies show the absence of dyspareunia at a mid- and long-term follow-up [16–18]. Sexual abstinence should be recommended for 6 to 8 weeks as is the recommendation for conventional transvaginal surgery [18].

An inexpensive, self-constructed single port device that can quickly and easily be made by any surgeon was used. Combining this self-constructed port device with easily available, conventional and reusable laparoscopic instruments demonstrates that salpingectomy via vNOTES can be performed without increasing the cost of laparoscopic surgery. This poor man's NOTES technique may potentially be applied in a low-resource setting, where only standard basic laparoscopic equipment is available. Besides being less costly, this approach offers other advantages when compared to commercial ports: it makes use of flexible material that enables greater manipulation of instruments, and a greater number and size of instruments can be passed through the incision. Transvaginal NOTES marks the beginning of a new era in the field of endoscopic surgery. NOTES salpingectomy is a novel technique requiring further validation. It could be a less invasive alternative for a laparoscopic salpingectomy.

Funding   No funding was received for this study.

References

1. Nieboer TE, Johnson N, Lethaby A et al (2009) Surgical approach to hysterectomy for benign gynaecological disease. Cochrane Database Syst Rev Issue 3. Art No: CD003677. doi:10.1002/14651858.CD003677.pub4

2. Yang YS, Oh KY, Hur MH, Kim SY, Yim HS (2015) Laparoendoscopic single-site surgery using conventional laparoscopic instruments and glove porttechnique in gynecology: a single surgeon's experience. J Minim Invasive Gynecol 22(1):87–93. doi:10.1016/j.jmig.2014.07.013.

3. Lee CL, Wu KY, Su H et al (2012) Transvaginal natural-orifice transluminal endoscopic surgery (NOTES) in adnexal procedures. J Minim Invasive Gynecol 19(4):509–513

4. Yang YS, Hur MH, Oh KY et al (2013) Transvaginal natural orifice transluminal endoscopic surgery for adnexal masses. J Obstet Gynaecol Res 39(12):1604–1609

5. Ahn KH, Song JY, Kim SH et al (2012) Transvaginal single-port natural orifice transluminal endoscopic surgery for benign uterine adnexal pathologies. J Minim Invasive Gynecol 19(5):631–635

6. Gordts S, Campo R, Puttemans P et al (2008) Transvaginal access: a safe technique for tubo-ovarian exploration in infertility? Review of literature. Gynecol Surg 5:187–191

7. Palanivelu C, Rajan PS, Rangarajan M et al (2008) Transvaginal endoscopic appendectomy in humans: a unique approach to NOTES—world's first report. Surg Endosc 22(5):1343–1347

8. Federlein M, Müller VA, Fritze-Büttner F et al (2014) Transvaginal cholecystectomy: results of a randomized study. Chirurg 85(9):825–832

9. Xue Y, Zou X, Zhang G et al (2015) Transvaginal natural orifice transluminal endoscopic nephrectomy in a series of 63 cases: stepwise transition from hybrid to pure NOTES. Eur Urol Mar 30. doi:10.1016/j.eururo.2015.03.033

10. Gordts S, Campo R, Rombauts L, Brosens I (1998) Transvaginal hydrolaparoscopy as an outpatient procedure for infertility investigation. Hum Reprod 13(1):99–103

11. Gordts S, Campo R, Brosens I (2002) Experience with transvaginal hydrolaparoscopy for reconstructive tubo-ovarian surgery. Reprod Biomed Online 4(Supple 3):72–75

12. Franz M, Ott J, Watrelot A et al (2015) Prospective evaluation of the learning curve of fertiloscopy with and without ovarian drilling. Reprod Biomed Online 30(4):408–414

13. Baekelandt J (2014) Poor man's NOTES: can it be a good approach for adhesiolysis? A first case report with video demonstration. J Minim Invasive Gynecol Nov 10. doi:10.1016/j.jmig.2014.11.001

14. Santos BF, Hungness ES (2011) Natural orifice transluminal endoscopic surgery: progress in humans since white paper. World J Gastroenterol 17:1655–1665

15. Yagci MA, Kayaalp C (2014) Transvaginal appendectomy: a systematic review. J Minim Invasive Surg 2014:384706. doi:10.1155/2014/384706

16. Zornig C, Mofid H, Siemssen L et al (2009) Transvaginal NOTES hybrid cholecystectomy: feasibility results in 68 cases with mid-term follow-up. Endoscopy 41:391–394

17. Lee CL, Wu KY, Su H, Wu PJ, Han CM, Yen CF (2014) Hysterectomy by transvaginal natural orifice transluminal endoscopic surgery (NOTES): a series of 137 patients. J Minim Invasive Gynecol 21(5):818–824

18. Tanaka M, Sagawa T, Yamazaki R, Myojo S, Dohi S, Inoue M (2013) Evaluation of transvaginal peritoneal surgery in young female patients. Surg Endosc 27:2619–2624

31

Does hysteroscopic metroplasty for septate uterus represent a risk factor for adverse outcome during pregnancy and labor?

Nataša Kenda Šuster[1] · Marco Gergolet[2]

Abstract The aim of the study was to evaluate whether hysteroscopic metroplasty for septate uterus represents a risk factor of adverse outcome in pregnancy, during labor, and after delivery. This is a retrospective comparative study of obstetric complications of 99 patients who underwent hysteroscopic metroplasty in a 5-year period (study group) and 4155 women, who gave birth in the same hospital in the same period (control group). No difference in obstetric outcome (preterm labor, hemorrhage before and after delivery, mean weeks of gestation at delivery, mean birth weight, breech presentation, and cesarean section rate) between the two groups has been found. The results of this study suggest that patients who underwent hysteroscopic metroplasty for septate uterus are at no higher risk of adverse obstetric outcome at term and during labor, comparing to the general population. Though vaginal delivery seems to be safe, rare but serious complication, reported by several studies, like uterine rupture during pregnancy or labor, should always be taken into consideration.

Keywords Hysteroscopic metroplasty · Septate uterus · Adverse obstetric outcome · Metroplasty complications

Introduction

Septate uterus is the commonest congenital uterine anomaly and is a known factor of infertility as well as cause of first and

✉ Marco Gergolet
marco.gergolet@gmail.com

[1] Department of Obsterics and Gynecology, University of Ljubljana, Šlajmerjeva 3, 1000 Ljubljana, Slovenia

[2] Casa di Cura Sanatorio Triestino, Via Rossetti 62, 34141 Trieste, Italy

second trimester spontaneous miscarriage and preterm delivery [1–4]. Fetal malpresentation and placentar anomalies have also been reported [5, 6].

Hysteroscopic metroplasty for septate uterus seems to be a simple and relatively safe procedure, but several complications can occur either during the procedure or in subsequent pregnancy and childbirth. In a series of 600 metroplasties, Shveiky reported a 3 % rate of complications, including intra-operative perforations of uterus which occurred in 1 %. Two thirds of complications were related to the cervical dilatation or the insertion of the resectoscope [7]. Agostini analyzed the incidence of early complications in 2116 consecutive operative hysteroscopies. In his series, the rate of perforation resulted to be 1.6 %. After stratifying the data related to the uterine pathology, lysis of synechiae was the procedure with the highest relative risk for perforations, whereas other procedures, such as septa resection, registered a lower incidence of complications. Endometrial ablation, polyp resection, and myoma resection did not cause significant rate of complications whatsoever. Postoperative hemorrhage has been reported in less than 1 % of cases and was mostly self-limiting. The hemorrhage occurred more frequently in case of synechiolisys than in other procedures such as myoma or polyp ablation and septum resection [8]. Complications related to the procedure can manifest during successive pregnancy, labor, and delivery. According to Agostini, patients who underwent hysteroscopic metroplasty are at increased risk for fetal malpresentation at term, low birth weight infants, and delivery by cesarean section [9]. The dilatation of the cervix may disrupt fibers in the cervix which can lead to the cervical-isthmical insufficiency [10]. The incision at the fundus over a security range of 10 mm could cause weakening of the myometrial layer at the fundus, with a subsequent risk for rupture during pregnancy and labor [11]. Perforation of uterus during the procedure and use of monopolar current could represent a predisposing factor for rupture of the uterus during labor [12–14]. On the other hand, cases of uterine rupture after metroplasty have been described independently from used method for septum resection (bipolar or monopolar energy, laser, cold scissors) [12, 14, 15].

The aim of the present study was to verify if hysteroscopic metroplasty for septate uterus represents a risk factor for any minor or severe complication during the subsequent pregnancy and labor.

Materials and methods

Study group consisted of 99 patients who underwent hysteroscopic metroplasty in a 5-year period, between January 2006 to December 2011 at the General Hospital »dr. Franc Derganc« in Nova Gorica, Slovenia, and delivered in the same facility. Labor outcomes of the study group were compared to the labor outcomes of 4155 women (control group) who gave birth in the same period and in the same hospital. Only singleton pregnancies and first delivery after metroplasty were considered. An 8-mm monopolar Karl Storz resectoscope with 1.5 % glycine solution as a distension medium was used. The authors (M.G. and N.K.Š.) performed all the metroplasties. After achieving good visibility, the ostia were taken as orientation points and the procedure was stopped when the fundus was aligned with the tubal ostia or when small arterial blood vessels became visible at the myometrial layer. In order to perform the metroplasty in the early proliferative phase, synchronization of the cycles was done by giving a contraceptive pill for at least 21 days. Five to 7 days after onset of the withdrawal bleeding, the procedure was performed. No intra-operative complication was recorded. All

patients underwent vaginal ultrasound 1 month after surgery to exclude a residual septation. In case of an unclear ultrasound findings, "office" hysteroscopy was carried out. A database file was set up using Microsoft Excel for Windows (Redmond, WA, USA) to facilitate data of entry and retrieval.

Statistical analysis

Data on deliveries and newborns have been obtained from the National Perinatal Informative System of Slovenia (PERIS), a national register including data on deliveries and newborns of all the 13 delivery wards in the Country. SPSS/PC 17.0 program was used for statistical analysis. Student's t test was used for the analysis of quantitative variables; qualitative differences between the two groups were analyzed by the Pearson's χ^2 test.

All procedures followed were in accordance with the ethical standards of the responsible committee on human experimentation (institutional and national) and with the Helsinki Declaration of 1975, as revised in 2000.

The study was observational and retrospective, so an informed consent was not necessary.

Results

In 60 patients (60.6 %), the indication for metroplasty was unexplained primary infertility or prolonged secondary infertility. In 32 (32.3 %) patients, the procedure was performed in course of artificial reproduction technique (ART) workout, which according to data from literature increases the chances of ART success [16, 17]. Data on obstetric outcome are represented in Table 1. Two hundred six (206) patients in the

Table 1 Outcome of pregnancy

Variable	Study group ($n=99$)	Control group ($n=4155$)	p
Preterm delivery total (<37 WG)	8 (8.1 %)	178 (4.4 %)	0.085
Preterm delivery (≤32 WG)	1 (1 %)	17 (0.4 %)	0.366
Mean week of gestation±SD	39.21±2.4	39.47±1.6	0.122
Cesarean section	19 (19.2 %)	59 (15.9 %)	0.371
Mean birth weight (g)±SD	3405±430	3453±466	0.330
Breech presentation	3 (3 %)	161 (3.9 %)	0.666
Placental abruption	1 (1 %)	40 (1 %)	0.962
Placenta praevia	0 (0 %)	3 (0.1 %)	0.782
Early postpartum hemorrhage	2 (2 %)	26 (0.6)	0.090
Uterine atony	2 (2 %)	73 (1.8 %)	0.844
Retained placental fragments	2 (2 %)	41 (1 %)	0.310
Adherent placenta	2 (2 %)	39 (0.9 %)	0.276
Late postpartum hemorrhage	0 (0 %)	5 (0.1 %)	0.730
Uterine rupture	0 (0 %)	2 (0.04)	0.833

WG weeks of gestation

control group have had a previous CS (5.0 %), whereas we recorded two CS out of nine deliveries before metroplasty in the study group. One woman in the study group (1 %) and 17 women in the control group (0.4 %) delivered before 32nd week of gestation (n.s.). Mean week of gestation at delivery was similar in both groups (39.21±2,4 vs. 39.47±1.6 weeks). In the study group, 19 CS were recorded (18.2 %) vs 659 CS in the control group (15.9 %) (n.s.). In the study group, 12 cases of CS were done because of dystocia, 5 cases due to an acute fetal distress, and in 3 cases, the indication was malpresentation (breech presentation), whereas in 2 cases, the indication for CS was a pathological condition of the mother. The rate of breech presentation was similar in both groups (3 vs. 3.9 %). Uterine ruptures were not recorded in the study group, whereas in two cases in the control group, a partial rupture in the previous cesarean section scar were reported during second cesarean section. In both cases, the ruptures were asymptomatic and diagnosed incidentally during the procedure.

The incidences of placental abruption (1 vs. 1 %), early postpartum hemorrhage (2 vs. 0.6 %), uterine atony (2 vs. 1.8 %), retained placental fragments (2 vs. 1 %), adherent placenta (2 vs. 0.9 %), and late postpartum hemorrhage (0 vs. 0.1 %) did not reach the statistical significance.

Discussion

According to numerous papers, septate uterus could be the cause of repeated miscarriage, second trimester pregnancy loss, and fetal malpresentations. Septate uterus is not generally thought to be a cause of infertility, although several papers report a longer time to conceive in this case. Similarly, uterine septum may impair the results of assisted reproductive techniques [18–21].

In a systematic review and meta-analysis of comparative studies, Venetis reported an increased relative risk (RR) for miscarriage in women with congenital uterine anomalies (CUA) compared to women with normal uterus. A higher RR for preterm delivery (2.21), malpresentation at delivery (RR 4.75), low birth weight (RR 1.93), and perinatal mortality rates (RR 2.43) were reported to be significantly higher in women with CUA.

After metroplasty, the probability for spontaneous miscarriage was reduced (RR 0.37) compared with untreated women [22].

A slight but not significant increase of cesarean section rate has been found in the study group. As we already mentioned, this group consisted mainly of infertile women, whose pregnancies are considered frequently at high risk, since obtained after years of infertility or several miscarriages. Subsequently, a more cautious approach to delivery could be a possible explanation for higher incidence of operative delivery. Previous

uterine surgery, uterine septa resection, could also be another indication for CS.

Metroplasties were performed on patients who suffered from previous pregnancy loss or infertility. Several studies reported an increased incidence of premature labor in patients who underwent dilatation and curettage or conceived after a long time of infertility [23, 24]. Though no statistically significant differences have been found between the groups in our study, there was a slight increase of the premature delivery rate in the study group (7.1 %). To compare, the preterm delivery rate in general population varies between 12 to 13 % in the USA and 5 up to 9 % in other developed countries [25].

Agostini reported an incidence of 35 % of breech presentation in patients with a 10-mm residual septum after metroplasty [9]. No differences in the rate of breech presentation between the groups have been found in the present study. Placenta accreta has been reported to be a possible complication of uterine surgery such as hysteroscopic myomectomy and lysis of intra uterine synechiae [26]. No study in the literature reports any case of placenta accreta or increta after metroplasty, and no case has been observed in the present study. According to Sentilhes, uterine surgery using monopolar energy could be a possible factor of weakening of the uterine wall, which could consequently cause uterine rupture during labor. The author concludes that the observation of a security limit of the thickness of the myometrium in case of using monopolar current cannot be enough. In order to avoid uterine rupture, he suggests the use of bipolar energy [27]. According to several studies, uterine perforation during surgery seems to be the most important prognostic risk factor for uterine rupture in pregnancy and during labor [28]. In an extensive review, Valle and Ekpo report different complications in course of surgery. Uterine perforations occurred either in case of using resectoscope or small diameter hysteroscope [29]. Argumentations about higher incidence of surgical complications in case of using resectoscope instead of small diameter scopes with micro scissors or Versapoint seem to be more subjective impressions of some authors rather than evidence-based [10, 30].

Randomized controlled trials are needed to confirm the beneficial effects of metroplasty reported by numerous non-randomized papers [31]. Such trials are in our opinion difficult to carry on, not only because of a relative difficulty to randomize patients but also because of an objective difficulty to design an appropriate study [32].

In the era of internet, women with septate uterus who are aware of dozens of non-randomized publications which confirm the improvement of pregnancy and live birth rates after metroplasty would decline to enter the randomization. Moreover, a multicentre randomized trial would be difficult because of a lack of uniformity in the discrimination between a normal uterine cavity and a small septate uterus. The new ESHRE-ESGE classification on congenital uterine anomalies may result as a helpful tool for reaching more homogeneity in studies especially in the interpretation of uterine cavity imaging, since the terminology "arcuate" uterus has been excluded by this classification [33].

Conclusions

Hysteroscopic metroplasty seems to significantly improve the obstetric outcome in a population of women with previous miscarriage. The procedure seems to be safe when done by skilled surgeons [34, 35].

While waiting for the highest level of evidence, according to prospective and retrospective epidemiological studies, it seems that hysteroscopic resection of uterine septum may improve either the pregnancy outcome or the outcome of ART techniques and may shorten the time to conceive in couples with primary or secondary infertility [18–21, 31, 36].

In experienced hands, the procedure seems not to be harmful for patients and not to threaten the future pregnancy and labor.

References

1. Acién P (1993) Reproductive performance of women with uterine malformations. Hum Reprod 8(1):122–126
2. Homer HA, Li TC, Cooke ID (2000) The septate uterus : a review of management and reproductive outcome. Fertil Steril 73:1–14
3. Tomaževič T, Ban-Frangež H, Ribič-Pucelj M, Premru-Sršen T, Verdenik I (2007) Small uterine septum is an important risk variable for preterm birth. Eur J Obstet Gynecol 135:154–157
4. Gergolet M, Gianaroli L, Kenda Suster N, Verdenik I, Magli MC, Gordts S (2010) Possible role of endometriosis in the aetiology of spontaneous miscarriage in patients with septate uterus. Reprod Biomed Online 21(4):581–585. doi:10.1016/j.rbmo.2010.05.014
5. Stein AL, March CM (1990) Pregnancy outcome in women with Müllerian duct anomalies. J Reprod Med 35(4):411–414
6. Tranquilli AL, Giannubilo SR, Corradetti A (2004) Congenital uterine malformations are associated to increased blood pressure in pregnancy. Hypertens Pregnancy 23(2):191–196
7. Shveiky D, Rojansky N, Revel A, Benshushan A, Laufer N, Shushan A (2007) Complications of hysteroscopic surgery: "Beyond the learning curve". J Minim Invasive Gynecol 14(2): 218–222
8. Agostini A, Cravello L, Bretelle F, Shojai R, Roger V, Blanc B (2002) Risk of uterine perforation during hysteroscopic surgery. J Am Assoc Gynecol Laparosc 9(3):264–267
9. Agostini A, De Guibert F, Salari K, Crochet P, Bretelle F, Gamerre M (2009) Adverse obstetric outcomes at term after hysteroscopic metroplasty. J Minim Invasive Gynecol 16:454–457
10. Litta P, Spiller E, Saccardi C, Ambrosini G, Caserta D, Cosmi E (2008) Resectoscope or Versapoint for hysteroscopic metroplasty. Int J Gynaecol Obstet 101(1):39–42
11. Angell NF, Tan Domingo J, Siddiqi N (2002) Uterine rupture at term after uncomplicated hysteroscopic metroplasty. Obstet Gynecol 100(5 Pt2):1098–1099
12. Tannous W, Hamou J, Henry-Suchet J, Achard B, Lelaidier C, Belaisch-Allart J (1996) Uterine rupture during labour following surgical hysteroscopy. Presse Med 25(4):159–161
13. Sentilhes L, Sergent F, Popovic I, Fournet P, Paquet M, Marpeau L (2004) Factors predictive of uterine rupture after operative hysteroscopy. J Gynecol Obstet Biol Reprod 33:51–55
14. Sentilhes L, Sergent F, Berthier A, Catala L, Descamps P, Marpeau L (2006) Uterine rupture following operative hysteroscopy. Gynecol Obstet Fertil 34(11):1064–1070
15. Homer HA, Li TC, Cooke ID (2000) The septate uterus: a review of management and reproductive outcome. Fertil Steril 73(1):1–14, Review
16. Ban-Frangez H, Tomazevic T, Virant-Klun I, Verdenik I, Ribic-Pucelj M, Bokal EV (2009) The outcome of singleton pregnancies after IVF/ICSI in women before and after hysteroscopic resection of a uterine septum compared to normal controls. Eur J Obstet Gynecol Reprod Biol 146(2):184–187
17. Heinonen PK, Kuismanen K, Ashorn R (2000) Assisted reproduction in women with uterine anomalies. Eur J Obstet Gynecol Reprod Biol 89(2):181–184
18. Grimbizis GF, Camus M, Tarlatzis BC, Bontis JN, Devroey P (2001) Clinical implications of uterine malformations and hysteroscopic treatment results. Hum Reprod Update 7(2):161–174, Review
19. Tomaževič T, Premru-Sršen T, Ribič-Pucelj M, Ban H, Verdenik I, Voger A, Vrtačnik Bokal E, Virant I (1999) Reproductive performance in different grades of uterine anomalies before and after metroplasty by resectoscope. J Am Assoc Gynecol Laparosc(Suppl S56)
20. Pabuçcu R, Gomel V (2004) Reproductive outcome after hysteroscopic metroplasty in women with septate uterus and otherwise unexplained infertility. Fertil Steril 81(6):1675–1678
21. Gergolet M, Campo R, Verdenik I, Kenda Suster N, Gordts S, Gianaroli L (2012) No clinical relevance of the height of fundal indentation in subseptate or arcuate uterus: a prospective study. Reprod Biomed Online 24(5):576–582. doi:10.1016/j.rbmo.2012.01.025
22. Venetis CA, Papadopoulos SP, Campo R, Gordts S, Tarlatzis BC, Grimbizis GF (2014) Clinical implications of congenital uterine anomalies: a meta-analysis of comparative studies. Reprod Biomed Online 29(6):665–683. doi:10.1016/j.rbmo.2014.09.006
23. McCarthy FP, Khashan AS, North RA, Rahma MB, Walker JJ, Baker PN, Dekker G, Poston L, McCowan LM, O'Donoghue K, Kenny LC, SCOPE Consortium (2013) Pregnancy loss managed by cervical dilatation and curettage increases the risk of spontaneous preterm birth. Hum Reprod 28(12):3197–3206
24. Messerlian C, Maclagan L, Basso O (2013) Infertility and the risk of adverse pregnancy outcomes: a systematic review and meta-analysis. Hum Reprod 28(1):125–137. doi:10.1093/humrep/des347
25. Goldenberg RL, Culhane JF, Iams JD, Romero R (2008) Epidemiology and causes of preterm birth. Lancet 371(9606):75–84, Review

26. Al-Serehi A, Mhoyan A, Brown M, Benirschke K, Hull A, Pretotious DH (2008) Placenta accreta: an association with fibroids and Asherman syndrome. J Ultrasound Med 27(11):1623–1628

27. Sentilhes L, Sergent F, Roman H, Verspyck E, Marpeau L (2005) Late complications of operative hysteroscopy: predicting patients at risk of uterine rupture during subsequent pregnancy. Eur J Obstet Gynecol Reprod Biol 120(2):134–138

28. Kayem G, Raiffort C, Legardeur H, Gavard L, Mandelbrot L, Girard G (2012) Specific particularities of uterine scars and their impact on the risk of uterine rupture in case of trial of labor. J Gynecol Obstet Biol Reprod 41(8):753–771. doi:10.1016/j.jgyn.2012.09.033

29. Valle RF, Ekpo GE (2013) Hysteroscopic metroplasty for the septate uterus: review and meta-analysis. J Minim Invasive Gynecol 20(1):22–42. doi:10.1016/j.jmig.2012.09.010

30. Colacurci N, De Franciscis P, Mollo A, Litta P, Perino A, Cobellis L, De Placido G (2007) Small-diameter hysteroscopy with Versapoint versus resectoscopy with a unipolar knife for the treatment of septate uterus: a prospective randomized study. J Minim Invasive Gynecol 14(5):622–627

31. Bosteels J, Weyers S, Puttemans P, Panayotidis C, Van Herendael B, Gomel V, Mol BW, Mathieu C, D'Hooghe T (2010) The effectiveness of hysteroscopy in improving pregnancy rates in subfertile women without other gynaecological symptoms: a systematic review. Hum Reprod Update 16(1):1–11

32. Smit JG, Kasius JC, Eijkemans MJ, Veersema S, Fatemi HM, van EJ S, Campo R, Broekmans FJ (2013) The international agreement study on the diagnosis of the septate uterus at office hysteroscopy in infertile patients. Fertil Steril 99(7):2108–13.e2. doi:10.1016/j.fertnstert.2013.02.027

33. Grimbizis GF, Gordts S, Di Spiezio SA, Brucker S, De Angelis C, Gergolet M, Li TC, Tanos V, Brölmann H, Gianaroli L, Campo R (2013) The ESHRE-ESGE consensus on the classification of female genital tract congenital anomalies. Gynecol Surg 10(3):199–212

34. Paradisi R, Barzanti R, Fabbri R (2014) The techniques and outcomes of hysteroscopic metroplasty. Curr Opin Obstet Gynecol 26(4):295–301

35. Propst AM, Liberman RF, Harlow BL, Ginsburg ES (2000) Complications of hysteroscopic surgery: predicting patients at risk. Obstet Gynecol 96(4):517–520

36. Tomaževič T, Ban-Frangež H, Ribič-Pucelj M, Premru-Sršen T, Verdenik I (2007) Small uterine septum is an important risk variable for preterm birth. Eur J Obstet Gynecol 135:154–157

32

Hysteroscopic morcelation of large type II myoma

Karin Abbink[1] · Sameer Sendy[2] · Tawfig H. Gaafar[3] · Dick C. Schoot[1]

Keywords Hysteroscopic morcelation · Morcelation · Myoma · Fibroids

Introduction

Large uterine submucous fibroids can cause severe clinical symptoms, depending on size and location [1]. The standard technique to remove uterine intracavitary abnormalities is resectoscopy [1]. Electroresection is used to remove polyps, type 0 or I myoma <5 cm diameter, whereas type II myomas are commonly treated in more than one procedure [3, 6].

Hysteroscopic morcelation (HM) is a promising technique to remove myomas. HM reduces tissue by mechanical cutting into small fragments [2–4], whereas subsequent aspiration leads to tissue collection. Several studies indicated successful removal of myomas (type I or 0) and polyps by HM [3]. Consistency of myomas can be a significant factor using morcelation. This communication describes the first successful morcelation of a soft 6-cm type II myoma.

Case

A woman (39 years) visiting the outpatient Gynaecology Clinic[2], complaining of heavy regular menstrual bleeding (HMB), revealed at diagnostic workup a 6-cm submucous uterine fibroid (Fig. 1a, b). Her history included four caesarean sections and a left salpingectomy. Leuprolide acetate showed no benefit. Hysteroscopic removal of the myoma was attempted by using the HM. The patient received misoprostol and antibiotics preoperatively and was counselled for multiple procedures. During an international workshop[2], complete morcelation using HM (TRUCLEAR; Smith and Nephew, Andover, MA, USA) was performed, using a reciprocating 5-mm blade (Fig. 2). Intrauterine pressure of 100 mmHG, a rotary speed of 1400 rpm and a suction of 200 mm Hg was used to morcelate the intracavitary part of the myoma. The remaining intramural part was enucleated and morcelated manoeuvring the stiff blade between the myoma and the capsula. The procedure lasted 15.4 min with 450 cc fluid deficit. Finally, no adherent intracavitary remnants remained (Fig. 1c).

Discussion

This communication describes a complete hysteroscopic morcelation of a soft 6-cm, type II myoma. Studies using HM describe safe resection of type 0 or I myomas [2, 3, 5]. HM is easy to perform, demonstrates less fluid-related complications and shows a shorter learning curve,

✉ Karin Abbink
karinabbink@hotmail.com

[1] Department of Obstetrics and Gynaecology, Catharina Hospital Eindhoven, Michelangelolaan 2, 5623 Eindhoven, The Netherlands

[2] Women's Specialized Hospital, King Fahad Medical City Riyadh, Riyadh, Kingdom of Saudi Arabia

[3] Maternity Hospital, IVF unit, Sulaiman al Habib Medical Complex, Riyadh, Kingdom of Saudi Arabia

Fig. 1 **a** Pre-operative hysteroscopic view of intracavitary part of the myoma (the *arrow* points at the surface of the myoma); **b** US position of myoma in the uterus; the *callipers* indicate the outline of the myoma; **c** post-operative view of the capsule of the enucleated myoma (*arrow* pointing to capsule, small myoma fragment above); **d** all material of the myoma as collected in the tissue trap

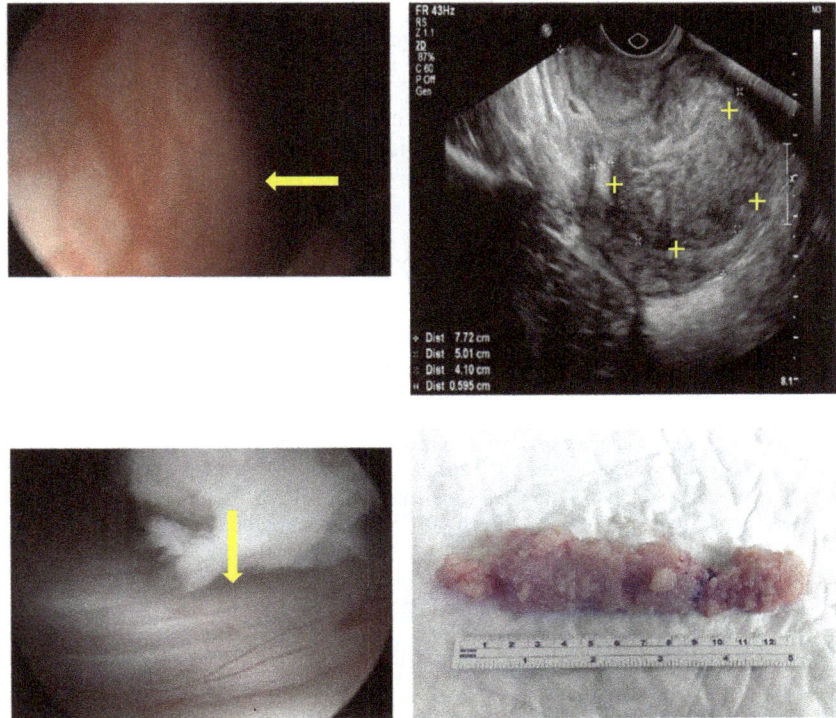

compared to traditional resectoscopes [2, 3, 5]. Significant reduction in operation time may be due to simultaneous aspiration of tissue fragments rather than the removal of each individual fragment by using resectoscopy [1–3]. Risks of complications increase in type II myoma with increased intramural extension [6, 7]. Overall, success rates are lower with higher rates of incomplete resection, post-operative bleeding and reoperation [7].

Probably the soft tissue characteristics led to complete removal in a short operation time, with minimal fluid loss. There is more adaption of tissue into the beak of the device, and larger tissue fragments could

be morcelated. The tip of the device is able to dissect the myoma out of its capsula. Despite the absence of electrical current, no excessive bleeding or other complications occurred which demonstrates the future opportunities of HM.

Furthermore, it could be of importance to examine the consistency of the myoma (e.g. using dynamic sonography and elastography) in the pre-operative assessment prior to hysteroscopic removal.

Morcelation of a type II myoma should be performed in select cases to optimize outcome with notice of the consistency of the myoma.

Fig. 2 TRUCLEAR hysteroscopic morcellator

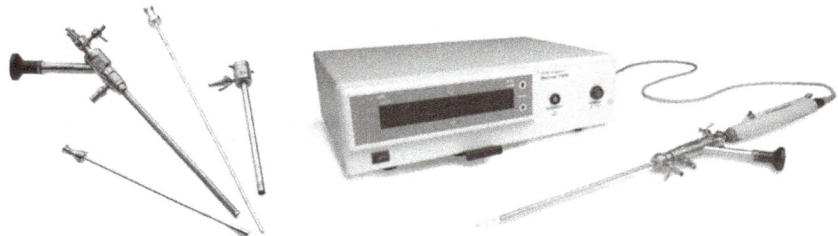

Authors' contribution   Karin Abbink wrote the manuscript. Dick B.C. Schoot collected data and edited the manuscript. Sendy Sameer and Tawfig H. Gaafar collected data.

Informed consent   Informed consent was obtained from the participant included in the study.

References

1. Di Spiezio Sardo et al (2008) Hysteroscopic myomectomy: a comprehensive review of surgical techniques. Hum Reprod Update 14(2):101–119
2. Emanuel et al (2005) The intra uterine morcellator: a new hysteroscopic operation technique to remove intrauterine polyps and myomas. J Minim Invasive Gynecol 12(1):62–66
3. Hamerlynck et al (2011) Clinical implementation of the hysteroscopic morcellator for removal of intrauterine myomas and polyps. A retrospective descriptive study. Gynecol Surg 8(2):193–196
4. Rubino et al (2015) Twelve-month outcomes for patients undergoing hysteroscopic morcellation of uterine polyps and myomas in an office or ambulatory surgical center. J Minim Invasive Gynecol 22(2): 285–290
5. van Dongen et al (2008) Hysteroscopic morcellator for removal of intrauterine polyps and myomas: a randomized controlled pilot study among residents in training. J Minim Invasive Gynecol 15(4):466–471
6. Indman (2006) Hysteroscopic treatment of submucous myomas. Clin Obstet Gynecol 49(4):811–820
7. Wamsteker et al (1993) Transcervical hysteroscopic resection of submucous fibroids for abnormal uterine bleeding: results regarding the degree of intramural extension. Obstet Gynecol 82(5):736–740

33

Effect of salpingectomy, ovarian cystectomy and unilateral salpingo-oopherectomy on ovarian reserve

Oybek Rustamov[1,2] · Monica Krishnan[3,4] · Stephen A Roberts[5] · Cheryl T Fitzgerald[1]

Abstract Pelvic surgery can affect ovarian reserve, but estimates of the potential effect of different surgical procedures are lacking. This study examines the markers of ovarian reserve after different procedures in order to help the provision of informed consent before surgery. Anti-Müllerian hormone (AMH), antral follicle count (AFC) and follicle-stimulating hormone (FSH) of women with a history of salpingectomy, ovarian cystectomy or unilateral salpingo-oophorectomy were compared to those without history of surgery using cross-sectional data adjusting for patient and clinical factors in multivariable regression model. There were 138 women who had had salpingectomy, 36 unilateral salpingo-oopherectomy, 41 cystectomy for ovarian cysts that are other than endometrioma and 40 women had had excision of endometrioma. There was no significant difference in AMH (9 %; $p = 0.33$), AFC (-2 %; $p = 0.59$) or FSH (-14 %; $p = 0.21$) in women with a history of salpingectomy compared to women without surgery. Women with a history of unilateral salpingo-oophorectomy were found to have significantly lower AMH (-54 %; $p = 0.001$). These women also had lower AFC (-28 %; $p = 0.34$) and higher FSH (14 %; $p = 0.06$), the effect of which did not reach statistical significance. The study did not find any significant associations between a history of cystectomy, for disease other than endometrioma and AMH (7 %; $p = 0.62$), AFC (13 %; $p = 0.18$) or FSH. (11 %; $p = 0.16$). Women with a history of cystectomy for ovarian endometrioma had 66 % lower AMH ($p = 0.002$). Surgery for endometrioma did not significantly affect AFC (14 %; $p = 0.22$) or FSH (10 %; $p = 0.28$). Salpingo-oopherectomy and cystectomy for endometrioma cause a significant reduction in AMH levels. Neither salpingectomy nor cystectomy for cysts other than endometrioma has appreciable effects on ovarian reserve.

Keywords Salpingectomy · Ovarian cystectomy · Salpingo-oopherectomy · Ovarian reserve · AMH · AFC · FSH

✉ Oybek Rustamov
oybek_rustamov@yahoo.co.uk

1 Department of Reproductive Medicine, St Mary's Hospital, Manchester Academic Health Science Centre (MAHSC), Central Manchester University Hospital NHS Foundation Trust, Manchester M13 0JH, UK

2 Present address: Aberdeen Maternity Hospital, University of Aberdeen, Aberdeen AB25 2ZN, UK

3 Present address: Sheffield Teaching Hospitals, Royal Hallamshire Hospital, Sheffield S10 2JF, UK

4 Manchester Royal Infirmary, Central Manchester University Hospitals NHS Foundation Trust, Manchester M13 9WL, UK

5 Centre for Biostatistics, Institute of Population Health, Manchester Academic Health Science Centre (MAHSC), University of Manchester, Manchester M13 9PL, UK

Introduction

Human ovarian reserve is determined by the size of oocyte pool at birth and an age-related decline in oocyte numbers thereafter. Both of these processes are largely under the influence of genetic factors, and to date, no effective interventions are available to improve physiological ovarian reserve [1]. However, various other environmental, pathological and iatrogenic factors appear to play a role, and consequently, it may be influenced either directly or indirectly. The use of chemotherapeutic agents, certain radio-therapeutic modalities and surgical interventions that damage the ovarian parenchyma can cause substantial damage to ovarian reserve [2, 3]. Estimation of the effect of each of these interventions is of importance in identifying lesser ootoxic treatment modalities.

Age is the main determinant of the number of non-growing follicles, accounting for 84 % of its variation. [4]. However, biomarkers that allow direct assessment of dynamics of growing follicles, anti-Müllerian hormone (AMH) and antral follicle count (AFC) may provide more accurate estimation of ovarian reserve [5]. Although these markers only reflect folliculogenesis of already recruited growing follicles, there appears to be a good correlation between their measurements and histologically determined total ovarian reserve [4]. Thus, the biomarkers can be utilised for the estimation of the effect of the above adverse factors on the primordial oocyte pool.

Surgical interventions that lead to disruption of the blood supply to the ovaries or involve direct damage to ovarian tissue may be expected to lead to a reduction in the primordial follicle pool. Indeed, a number of studies have reported an association between surgical interventions to the ovaries and a reduction in ovarian reserve [3]. However, given that both the underlying disease and surgery may affect ovarian reserve, disentanglement of the individual effects of these factors may be challenging and requires careful analysis. Here, we present a study that, in as far as is possible in cross-sectional data, intended to estimate the effect of tubal and ovarian surgery on ovarian reserve independently of underlying disease.

Methods

The effect of salpingectomy, ovarian cystectomy and unilateral salpingo-oopherectomy on ovarian reserve was studied using serum biomarkers AMH, AFC and follicle-stimulating hormone (FSH) in a large cross-sectional study of patients referred for infertility management.

Population

All women between ages of 20 to 45 who were referred to the Women's Outpatient Department and the Reproductive Medicine Department of Central Manchester University Hospitals NHS Foundation Trust for management of infertility between 1 September 2008 and 16 November 2010 and had AMH measurement using the DSL assay ((DSL, Active MIS/AMH ELISA; Diagnostic Systems Laboratories, Webster, TX) were included. We excluded patients referred for fertility preservation and those with a diagnosis of polycystic ovaries (PCO) on transvaginal ultrasound scan which was defined as volume of one or both ovaries more than 10 ml. Patients with haemolysed AMH and/or FSH samples were not included in the analysis of these markers.

Measurement of AMH

Blood samples for AMH were taken without regard to the day of women's menstrual cycle. Serum samples were separated within 2 h of venipuncture in the Biochemistry Laboratory of our hospital and frozen at −20 °C until analysed in batches using the enzymatically amplified two-site immunoassay (DSL, Active MIS/AMH ELISA; Diagnostic Systems Laboratories, Webster, TX). All samples were processed strictly according to the manufacturer's recommendations. The working range of the assay was up to 100 pmol/L and a minimum detection limit was 0.63 pmol/L. The intra-assay coefficient of variation (CV) ($n = 16$) was 3.9 % (at 10 pmol/l) and 2.9 % (at 56 pmol/l). The inter-assay CV ($n = 60$) was 4.7 % (at 10 pmol/l) and 4.9 % (at 56 pmol/l).

Measurement of FSH

Women had measurement of basal FSH, luteinizing hormone (LH) and oestradiol levels (E2) during early follicular phase (days 2–5) of their menstrual cycle as part of their initial workup. Blood samples were transported to the Biochemistry Laboratory within 2 h of venipuncture for sample processing and analysis. Specific immunoassay kits (Cobas, Roche Diagnostics, Mannheim, Germany) and an autoanalyser platform were used (Roche Modular Analytics E170, Roche, USA) for analysis of FSH. The intra-assay CV was 6.0 % and inter-assay CV was 6.8 %.

Measurement of AFC

Measurement of AFC was conducted in patients referred for assisted conception. The department used a stringent methodology for the assessment of AFC, which consists of counting all antral follicles measuring 2–6 mm in longitudinal and transverse cross sections of both ovaries using transvaginal ultrasound scanning (Toshiba Nemio F2534312) at early follicular phase of the menstrual cycle. The AFC with the closest date to AMH measurement was selected. The ultrasound assessments were conducted by a number of qualified sonographers, who used the same methodology for the measurement of AFC.

Definitions and groups

Women's body mass index (BMI) was categorised using standard NHS reference ranges: Underweight (<18.5), Normal (18.5–24.9), Overweight (25–29.9) and Obese (30–40) [8]). The causes of infertility were established by searching the referral letters, clinical notes and letters generated following clinic consultations. Women with a history of bilateral tubal block, which was confirmed by laparoscopic dye test, and patients with a history of bilateral salpingectomy were categorised as having severe tubal factor infertility. Women with unilateral tubal patency or unilateral salpingectomy were categorised as having mild tubal factor infertility. Severe male factor infertility was defined as azoospermia or severe oligospermia (<1 mln sperm sample) and partners with abnormal sperm count that do not meet the above criteria being classified as having mild male factor infertility.

Patients with reproductive surgery were categorised as having a history of salpingectomy, unilateral salpingo-oopherectomy, cystectomy for ovarian cysts other than ovarian endometrioma and cystectomy for endometrioma. In our department, stripping of cyst wall with subsequent diathermy of bleeding areas of the cyst bed is the standard method for excision of endometriotic cyst. However, the dataset did not contain data on surgical techniques and, therefore, we were not able to investigate the effect of specific surgical procedures.

Statistical analysis

A multivariable regression model that included age, ethnicity, endometriosis, presence of ovarian endometrioma, causes of infertility, and tubal and ovarian surgery was fitted to the logarithm of each of the ovarian reserve markers: AMH, AFC and FSH. The age on the day of the measurement of each of the marker of ovarian reserve (AMH, AFC and FSH) was included in the model as a quadratic function following centering to 30 years of age. Preliminary analysis of AMH, AFC and FSH indicated that logarithmically transformed values with a quadratic age term provided adequate fits. Differences between the groups were considered significant at $p < 0.05$. Interactions between all explanatory variables were tested at a significance level of 0.01.

Results

In total, 3179 women were included in the study. The AMH measurements of 66 women were excluded due to haemolysed samples or delay in processing the samples, leaving 3113 women for analysis. Of women, 1934 had AFC and 2580 had FSH. The mean (±SD) age, AMH, AFC and FSH of patients were 32.8 ± 4.5, 17.3 ± 14.8, 13.9 ± 6.2 and 8.0 ± 7.5, respectively. There were 138 women who had unilateral or bilateral salpingectomy, 36 women with a history of unilateral salpingo-oopherectomy, 41 women with a history of cystectomy for ovarian cysts other than endometrioma and 40 women had cystectomy for endometrioma. The results of the regression analysis on the effect of reproductive surgery on AMH, AFC and FSH are shown in Table 1.

The analysis did not find any significant differences in AMH (increase of 9 %; $p = 0.33$), AFC (−2 %; $p = 0.59$) and FSH (−14 %; $p = 0.21$) between women with a history of

Table 1 Multivariable regression analysis

	Number	Coef	95 % CI	p
Salpingectomy				
AMH	2128	0.094	−0.097, 0.285	0.333
AFC	1697	−0.027	−0.126, 0.072	0.595
FSH	1929	−0.056	−0.143, 0.032	0.210
Oopherectomy				
AMH	3049	−0.540	−0.868, −0.213	**0.001**
AFC	1946	−0.280	−0.857, 0.298	0.342
FSH	2546	0.139	−0.006, 0.284	0.060
Cystectomy other				
AMH	2128	0.075	−0.226, 0.376	0.626
AFC	1697	0.130	−0.064, 0.323	0.189
FSH	1929	0.110	−0.044, 0.265	0.161
Cystectomy endometrioma				
AMH	2128	−0.667	−1.081, −0.252	**0.002**
AFC	1697	0.144	−0.089, 0.376	0.225
FSH	1929	0.103	−0.084, 0.290	0.281

The fitted coefficient (log difference between the group indicated and all other patients), 95 % confidence interval and associated p value adjusted for age, ethnicity causes of infertility, endometriosis (without endometrioma) and endometrioma

Statistically significant values ($p<0.005$) are provided in bold

salpingectomy and those without surgery (Table 1). Women with a history of unilateral salpingo-oopherectomy were found to have significantly lower AMH (−54 %; $p = 0.001$) and AFC (−28 %; $p = 0.34$) and increased FSH (14 %; $p = 0.06$), and the effect on AMH reached statistical significance (Table 1). The study did not find a significant association between previous history of ovarian cystectomy that was for disease other than endometrioma and AMH (7 %; $p = 0.62$), AFC (13 %; $p = 0.18$) or FSH (11 %; $p = 0.16$) (Table 1). Women with a history of ovarian cystectomy for endometrioma had 66 % lower AMH ($p = 0.002$) levels but the effects on AFC (14 %; $p = 0.22$) and FSH (10 %; $p = 0.28$) were not significant (Table 1).

Discussion

In salpingectomy, tubal and ovarian branches of uterine arteries are often excised alongside the mesosalpynx and, hence, it is believed that disruption to blood supply to ovaries may lead to reduction of ovarian reserve. However, in our study, we did not observe an appreciable association between salpingectomy and any of the biomarkers of ovarian reserve suggesting this surgery does not affect ovarian reserve. These findings are supported by a longitudinal study that assessed the effect of tubal dissection to AMH, AFC and FSH ($n = 49$) [6]. There were no differences between preoperative and 3-month postoperative measurements with median AMH (1.5

vs. 1.4; $p = 0.07$), AFC (8.4 ± 3.7 vs. 7.9 ± 4.1; $p = 0.09$), FSH (7.6 ± 2.1 vs. 7.7 ± 2.1; $p = 0.10$). Silva et al. assessed the effect of tubal ligation ($n = 52$) in longer term postoperative period (1 year) and reported that median AMH (1.43, IQR 0.63–2.62 vs. 1.30, IQR 0.53–2.85; $p = 0.23$) and mean AFC (8, IQR 5–14 vs. 11, IQR 7–15; $p = 0.12$) did not change significantly [7]. Thus, our results along with other published evidence suggest that salpingectomy or tubal division does not have an adverse effect on ovarian reserve. Therefore, advising salpingectomy for various indications, including treatment of tubal pathology, sterilisation or opportunistic procedure as part of risk reduction strategy in ovarian carcinoma appears to be safe with regard to preserving ovarian reserve.

Although salpingo-oophorectomy is rare in women of reproductive age, significant ovarian pathologies and acute diseases such as ovarian torsion may necessitate unilateral salpingo-oophorectomy. There is plausible causative relationship between this surgery and ovarian reserve, although to our knowledge there is no previous published evidence. We found that women with history of unilateral salpingo-oophorectomy have significantly lower AMH (−54 %) suggesting the surgery has considerable negative impact on ovarian reserve measured with this biomarker. Similarly, the patients with a history of salpingo-oophorectomy had considerably higher FSH (13 %) and lower (−24 %) AFC. However, these did not reach statistical significance which may be due to small sample size and relative poor discriminatory power of AFC and FSH compared to that of AMH. The important clinical question in the management of patients with salpingo-oophorectomy is whether these patients have comparable reproductive lifespan or experience accelerated loss of oocytes resulting in premature loss of fertility, as this would allow appropriate preoperative counseling of patients regarding the long-term effect of the surgery on fertility and age at menopause. There is a need for studies with a larger number of patients, preferably using long-term longitudinal data, to investigate this question.

In women with a history of ovarian cystectomy for cysts other than those due to endometrioma, we did not observe any significant association between surgery and markers of ovarian reserve. However, women that had ovarian cystectomy for endometrioma appear to have significantly lower AMH (−66 %) compared to those without a history of surgery.

During the last few years, a number of studies have assessed the effect of excision of endometrioma on AMH [8–10]. The studies have been summarised by a recent systematic review, which concluded that excision of endometrioma results in damage to ovarian reserve [3]. Further studies evaluated the mechanism of damage, and these suggest that coagulation for the purpose of hemostasis as well as stripping of the cyst wall may cause direct damage to ovarian reserve. Sonmezer et al. compared the effect of diathermy coagulation ($n = 15$) for hemostasis compared to the use of hemostatic matrix ($n = 13$) in a randomised controlled trial and reported that the use of diathermy coagulation is associated with significantly lower AMH measurements (1.64 ± 0.93 vs. 2.72 ± 1.49 ng/mL) in the first postoperative month [11].

Similarly, stripping of the cyst wall also appears to have a detrimental effect on ovarian reserve due to inadvertent removal of ovarian tissue [12]. Using histological data, Roman et al. demonstrated that normal ovarian tissue was removed in 97 % specimens of surgically removed endometriomata [13]. Furthermore, it appears that ovarian cortex containing endometrioma appears to have significantly reduced density compared to normal ovarian cortex, and therefore, loss of oocyte containing normal ovarian cortex may be unavoidable in cystectomy for endometrioma [14]. Matsuzaki et al. conducted a histological assessment of cystectomy specimens and found that normal ovarian tissue adjacent to cyst wall was found in 58 % (71/121) of patients with endometrioma, whereas normal ovarian tissue was excised in 5.4 % (3/56) following cystectomy for other benign cysts [15]. Donnez et al. reported the use of combined stripping and vaporization

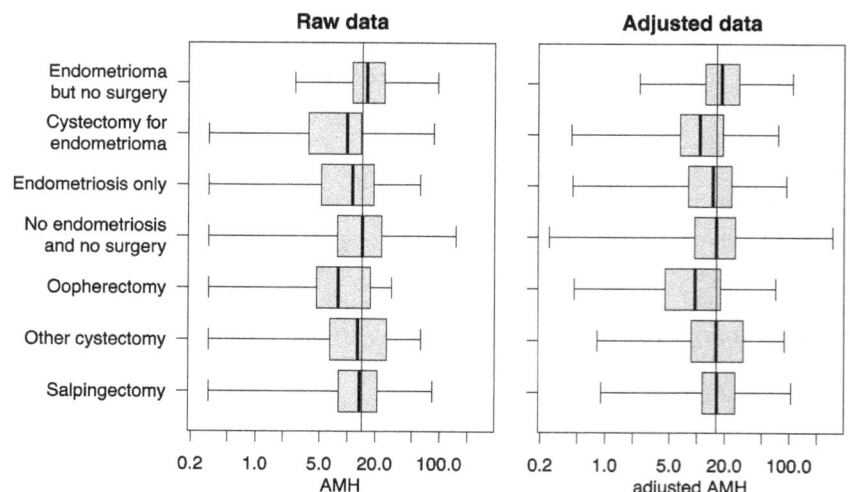

Fig. 1 AMH by treatment groups. *Left hand panel* shows the raw data AMH measurement (in pmol/L) and the right hand panel the AMH adjusted for age, ethnicity, causes of infertility, endometriosis, endometrioma and surgery using the multivariable regression model for the various treatment groups

technique was safe with regard to protecting an ovarian reserve [16]. More recently, Ata et al. reported that mean decline of AMH levels was less in suturing and haemostatic sealent technique compared to bipolar desiccation suggesting energy sources may have more detrimental effect on ovarian reserve [17].

Interestingly, contrary to AMH levels, the surgery does not seem to affect AFC measurements. A recent systematic review of 13 studies reported that AFC did not change following excision of endometrioma compared to that of prior surgery [18]. Similarly, our data did not show a significant difference in AFC measurements in patients with a history of excision of endometrioma, whilst AMH measurements of the patients with surgery was significantly (66 %) lower. This suggests that either (a) there is increased expression of AMH in the presence of endometrioma and hence the dramatic decline following cystectomy or (b) the performance characteristics of AFC is not sufficiently precise for the detection of change between the measurements. We believe exploration of these questions further may improve our understanding of the pathophysiology of ovarian endometriosis and performance of the markers of ovarian reserve in the presence of the disease.

In summary, in our study, women with a history of cystectomy for endometrioma had significantly lower AMH, whilst those had cystectomy for other benign cysts do not appear to have lower AMH. In view of our findings and other published research evidence, it seems clear that cystectomy for endometrioma results in a significant reduction in AMH levels.

Strengths and limitations

The published studies have used longitudinal data comparing biomarkers before and after cystectomy and provide reliable estimates on the effect of the intervention on ovarian reserve. However, data on the effect of salpingectomy and unilateral salpingo-oopherectomy is lacking. In addition to a reevaluation of the effect of cystectomy, this study has assessed the impact of salpingectomy and unilateral salpingo-oopherectomy on markers of ovarian reserve. In contrast to published studies, this study employed analysis of cross-sectional data. Although we have adjusted for all the measured confounders, we cannot be certain that all relevant factors have been included and the apparent effects of surgery here may be causally related to some unmeasured factor related to the decision whether or not to intervene surgically. In patients with a history of cystectomy for endometrioma, we estimated independent effects of pathology and surgery providing important data for preoperative counseling.

It is important to note that the study evaluated the effect of surgery using retrospective data which has limitations due variation in recording of surgical history and missing data. Recent studies showed that AMH measurements may be prone to an inaccuracy due to methodological issues [19, 20]. However, this appears to be largely confined to initial Gen II AMH Assay [20, 21]. The study employed the data obtained using first-generation DSL AMH assay, which appears to provide more reproducible measurements [20, 22].

It is important to note although the effects are significant in a population level, there is considerable variation between individuals in the effects of surgery (Fig. 1). It is not clear whether this variability represents measurement error arising from the assays and sampling procedures, or true inter-individual differences in the effects between women. Thus, clinicians should exercise caution in predicting the effect of surgery on the ovarian reserve of individual patients.

Conclusion

This multivariable regression analysis of retrospectively collected cross-sectional data suggests that neither salpingectomy nor ovarian cystectomy for cysts other than endometrioma has an appreciable effect on ovarian reserve determined by AMH, AFC and FSH. In contrast, salpingo-oopherectomy and ovarian cystectomy for endometrioma appear to have a significant detrimental impact on ovarian reserve. On the basis of findings of this study and other published studies, women undergoing reproductive surgery should be counseled with regard to the potential adverse effect of the surgery on their ovarian reserve.

Acknowledgments The authors would like to thank colleagues Dr. Greg Horne (Senior Clinical Embryologist), Ann Hinchliffe (Clinical Biochemistry Department) and Helen Shackleton (Information Operations Manager) for their help in obtaining datasets for the study.

Author contributions OR prepared the dataset, conducted the statistical analysis and prepared the manuscript. MK assisted in data extraction and contributed to the discussion and the review of the manuscript. SR and CF oversaw and supervised the preparation of dataset, statistical analysis, contributed to the discussion and reviewed the manuscript.

Compliance with ethical standards Ethical approval for collation and use of already collected patient data was obtained from Ethics Committee.

Grant support No funding was sought for this study.

References

1. Schuh-Huerta SM, Johnson NA, Rosen MP, Sternfeld B, Cedars MI, Reijo Pera RA (2012a) Genetic variants and environmental factors associated with hormonal markers of ovarian reserve in Caucasian and African American women. Hum Reprod 27:594–608

2. Nielsen SN, Andersen AN, Schmidt KT, Rechnitzer C, Schmiegelow K, Bentzen JG, Larsen EC (2013) Reprod BioMed Online 27(2):192–200

3. Somigliana E, Berlanda N, Benaglia L, Viganò P, Vercellini P, Fedele L (2012) Surgical excision of endometriomas and ovarian reserve: a systematic review on serum antimüllerian hormone level modifications. Fertil Steril 98(6):1531–1538

4. Hansen KR, Hodnett GM, Knowlton N, Craig LB (2011) Correlation of ovarian reserve tests with histologically determined primordial follicle number. Fertil Steril 95:170–175

5. van Disseldorp J, Kwee C.B.L. J, C.W.N L, M.J.C E, Broekmans FJ (2010) Comparison of inter- and intra-cycle variability of anti-Müllerian hormone and antral follicle counts. Hum Reprod 25:221–227

6. Ercan CM, Sakinci M, Coksuer H, Keskin U, Tapan S, Ergun A. Ovarian reserve testing before and after laparoscopic tubal bipolar electrodesiccation and transection. Eur J Obstet Gynecol Reprod Biol 2013

7. Silva AL, Ré C, Dietrich C, Fuhrmeister IP, Pimentel A, Corleta HV (2013) Impact of tubal ligation on ovarian reserve as measured by anti-Müllerian hormone levels: a prospective cohort study. Contraception 88(6):700–705

8. Chang HJ, Han SH, Lee JR, Jee BC, Lee BI, Suh CS, et al. (2010) Impact of laparoscopic cystectomy on ovarian reserve: serial changes of serum anti-Mullerian hormone levels. Fertil Steril 94:343–349

9. Ercan CM, Sakinci M, Duru NK, Alanbay I, Karasahin KE, Baser I (2010) Antimullerian hormone levels after laparoscopic endometrioma stripping surgery. Gynecol Endocrinol 26:468–472

10. Lee DY, Young Kim N, Jae Kim M, Yoon BK, Choi D (2011) Effects of laparoscopic surgery on serum anti-M€ullerian hormone levels in reproductive-aged women with endometrioma. Gynecol Endocrinol 27:733–736

11. Sönmezer M, Taşkın S, Gemici A, Kahraman K, Özmen B, Berker B, Atabekoğlu C (2013) Can ovarian damage be reduced using hemostatic matrix during laparoscopic endometrioma surgery? A prospective, randomized study. Arch Gynecol Obstet 287(6):1251–1257

12. Donnez J, Nisolle M, Gillet N, Smets M, Bassil S, Casanas-Roux F (1996) Large ovarian endometriomas. Hum Reprod 11:641–646

13. Roman H, Tarta O, Pura I, Opris I, Bourdel N, Marpeau L, et al. (2010) Direct proportional relationship between endometrioma size and ovarian parenchyma inadvertently removed during cystectomy, and its implication on the management of enlarged endometriomas. Hum Reprod 25:1428–1432

14. Sanchez A, P. Viganò, Somigliana E, Panina-Bordignon P. Vercellini and Candiani M. The distinguishing cellular and molecular features of the endometriotic ovarian cyst: from pathophysiology to the potential endometrioma-mediated damage to the ovary, Hum. Reprod. Update (2014).

15. Matsouzaki S, Houlle C, Darcha S, Pouly JL, Mage G, Canis M (2009) Analysis of risk factors for the removal of normal ovarian tissue during laparoscopic cystectomy for ovarian endometriosis. Hum Reprod 24:1402–1406

16. Donnez J, Lousse JC, Jadoul P, Donnez O, Squifflet J (2010) Laparoscopic management of endometriomas using a combined technique of excisional (cystectomy) and ablative surgery. Fertil Steril 94:28–32

17. Ata B, Turkgeldi E, Seyhan A, Urman B. Effect of hemostatic method on ovarian reserve following laparoscopic endometrioma excision; comparison of suture, hemostatic sealant, and bipolar dessication. A systematic review and meta-analysis. J Minim Invasive Gynecol. 2015; 22(3):363–722010; 94(1):28–32.

18. Muzii L, Di Tucci C, Di Feliciantonio M, Marchetti C, Perniola G, Panici PB (2014) The effect of surgery for endometrioma on ovarian reserve evaluated by antral follicle count: a systematic review and meta-analysis. Hum Reprod 29(10):2190–2198

19. Rustamov O, Smith A, Roberts SA, Yates AP, Fitzgerald C, Krishnan M, Nardo LG, Pemberton PW (2012) Anti-Mullerian hormone: poor assay reproducibility in a large cohort of subjects suggests sample instability. Hum Reprod 27:3085–3091

20. Rustamov O, Smith A, Roberts S, Yates A, Fitzgerald C, Krishnan M, Nardo L, Pemberton P (2014) The measurement of Anti-Müllerian hormone: a critical appraisal. J Clin Endocrinol Metab J Clin Endocrinol, Metab 99:723–732

21. Craciunas L, Roberts SA, Yates AP, Smith A, Fitzgerald C, Pemberton PW (2015) Modification of the Beckman-Coulter second-generation enzyme-linked immunosorbent assay protocol improves the reliability of serum antimüllerian hormone measurement. Fertil Steril 103(2):554–559

22. Rustamov O, Pemberton PW, Roberts SA, Smith A, Yates AP, Patchava SD, Nardo LG (2011) The reproducibility of serum anti-Müllerian hormone in subfertile women: within and between patient variability. Fertil Steril 95:11

34

Retention of laparoscopic psychomotor skills after a structured training program depends on the quality of the training and on the complexity of the task

Carlos Roger Molinas[1,2] · Rudi Campo[2]

Abstract This follow-up RCT was conducted to evaluate laparoscopic psychomotor skills retention after finishing a structured training program. In a first study, 80 gynecologists were randomly allocated to four groups to follow different training programs for hand-eye coordination (task 1) with the dominant hand (task 1-a) and the non-dominant hand (task 1-b) and laparoscopic intra-corporeal knot tying (task 2) in the Laparoscopic Skills Testing and Training (LASTT) model. First, baseline skills were tested (T1). Then, participants trained task 1 (G1: 1-a and 1-b, G2: 1-a only, G3 and G4: none) and then task 2 (all groups but G4). After training all groups were tested again to evaluate skills acquisition (T2). For this study, 2 years after a resting period, 73 participants were recruited and tested again to evaluate skills retention (T3). All groups had comparable skills at T1 for all tasks. At T2, G1, G2, and G3 improved their skills, but the level of improvement was different (G1 = G2 > G3 > G4 for task 1; G1 = G2 = G3 > G4 for task 2). At T3, all groups retained their task 1 skills at the same level than at T2. For task 2, however, a skill decay was already noticed for G2 and G3, being G1 the only group that retained their skills at the post-training level. Training improves laparoscopic skills, which can be retained over time depending on the comprehensiveness of the training program and on the complexity of the task. For high complexity tasks, full training is advisable for both skills acquisition and retention.

Keywords Laparoscopy · Training · Psychomotor · Intra-corporeal knot tying · Skills acquisition · Skills retention · LASTT model

Introduction

The ideal method for training in laparoscopic surgery is an issue of continuous debate and research. Although the classic apprentice-tutor model is still widely used, general agreement exists upon the importance of acquiring laparoscopic skills outside the operating room for ethical and practical reasons, such as the reduction of the operating time and the complications rates [1–5].

To facilitate the training and assessment of three specific basic laparoscopic psychomotor skills (i.e., camera navigation, hand-eye coordination, and bimanual coordination), the European Academy of Gynecological Surgery has developed an inanimate box model (i.e., the Laparoscopic Skills Testing and Training (LASTT) model) and demonstrated its feasibility, its face validity (the realism of the method), and its construct validity (the ability of the method to differentiate between novices and experts) [6, 7].

It has also been demonstrated in this model that training of basic laparoscopic psychomotor skills, specifically hand-eye coordination, facilitates the acquisition of more advanced skills, such as laparoscopic intra-corporeal knot tying [8]. Indeed, in contrast with trainees who did not follow the complete training program, trainees who trained hand-eye coordination with both the dominant hand (DH) and the non-dominant hand (NDH) registered a better starting level [8] and a shorten learning curve of laparoscopic intra-corporeal knot tying (unpublished observations).

In addition to laparoscopic psychomotor skills acquisition, the capacity to retain both basic and advanced skills is of

✉ Carlos Roger Molinas
roger.molinas@neolife.com.py

[1] Neolife Medicina y Cirugía Reproductiva, Avenida Brasilia 760, 1434 Asunción, Paraguay

[2] European Academy of Gynaecological Surgery, Leuven, Belgium

outmost importance for defining an efficient laparoscopic training program. Some studies have already addressed this in different populations, using different models and scoring systems for both training and testing, and after different time points. The reported results are very consistent indicating that most skill remained better than at baseline. It is not sufficiently clear, however, the reasons why only some of them are retained at the post-training levels whereas some start deteriorating very soon [9–13].

This study was designed to evaluate the specific effect of different types of structured training programs upon laparoscopic psychomotor skills retention after a resting period of 2 years.

Materials and methods

Participants and venue

The study was carried out in 2009 in the Centro Médico La Costa in Asunción, Paraguay, and intended to include the 60 gynecologists who had previously participated in a study aimed to evaluate laparoscopic skills acquisition, as reported previously [8], and the 20 gynecologists who were also recruited at that time specifically for the aims of this study on skills retention. These gynecologists had at that time sufficient experience in open and vaginal surgery but little or no experience in laparoscopic surgery (level 0–1 of the European Society of Gynecological Endoscopy classification) [6]. Participants who practice laparoscopic surgery or skills training between the previous and this study were excluded. A total of 73 participants were recruited for this study and their age, gender, training status (i.e., residents or specialists), and dominant hand side were recorded (Fig. 1). The remaining seven participants were not eligible for this study because they became experts in laparoscopy ($n = 3$) or were no longer accessible due to geographical limitations ($n = 4$).

Instruments, materials, and tasks

The LASTT model, with the relevant materials for different tasks, was inserted into the Szabo trainer box (Karl Storz, Tutlingen, Germany). The tasks were performed with standard laparoscopic instruments (10 mm 0° optic, 5 mm Kelly dissection forceps, 5 mm Koh needle holders), and the optic was connected to an all-in-one (monitor, light source, and video camera) laparoscopic tower (Karl Storz, Tutlingen, Germany).

Task 1 (hand-eye coordination) Participants navigated a camera with a 0° optic and grasped and transported six objects to six targets as described previously [8]. Briefly, they stood behind the trainer box in the midline. The optic was introduced through a midline port and the Kelly forceps through

a lower and lateral port, to the right or the left according to the hand being evaluated. The Kelly forceps was held with the hand being evaluated and the camera with the contralateral hand. Participants were allowed to start the task when the first target and tip of the Kelly forceps were shown on the screen (start time). The matched targets (10 × 1 mm nails) and objects (5 × 4 mm open cylinders) were identifiable by color. The first object was grasped and transported to its target. Only when they succeeded in introducing the first cylinder into the first nail were they allowed to continue with the others in a fixed order. The task was executed and scored with both the DH (task 1-a) the NDH (task 1-b). The time for each repetition was limited to 600 s. The task finished either when the last object was transported to its target or when the time limit expired.

Task 2 (laparoscopic intra-corporeal knot tying) Participants performed an intra-corporeal knot tying as described previously [8]. Briefly, they stood to the left of the trainer box. A soft pad with two pre-mounted sutures (vicryl 2-0, 20 cm length), 1 cm between entry and exit sites, and tails equally distributed at both sites was fitted in the Szabo trainer box in a horizontal position. The optic was introduced through a midline port and the needle holders through lower and lateral ports. The camera was fixed at a distance that allowed visualization of the entire operating field, and the needle holders were held with the relevant hands. The tip of the thread was grasped with the left needle holder, and the thread was pulled through the pad, leaving a 2-cm tail on the opposite side. Then, a double counter-clockwise knot was made, followed by a single clockwise knot and finally by a single counter-clockwise knot. The time for each repetition was limited to 600 s. The task finished either when the participant considered he/she completed the knot or when the time limit had expired. Then, the tutor performed a quality control, and only the flat and square knots were considered correctly performed.

Scoring system

The measurement of the tasks was based on the time to correct performed exercise (TCPE), which reflects errors and economy of movements in the result and as such engages and accuracy assurance. Thus, when the task was successfully accomplished within the time limit, the score was the time actually used to execute the task, ranging from 1 to 600. However, if for any reason the task could not be successfully accomplished within the time limit, a penalty score of 1200 was established.

Experimental design

At the time of the first study, 80 participants were randomly allocated to four different groups (G), according to the training program to be performed. Participants allocated to G4 were recruited specifically for the aims of this skills retention study,

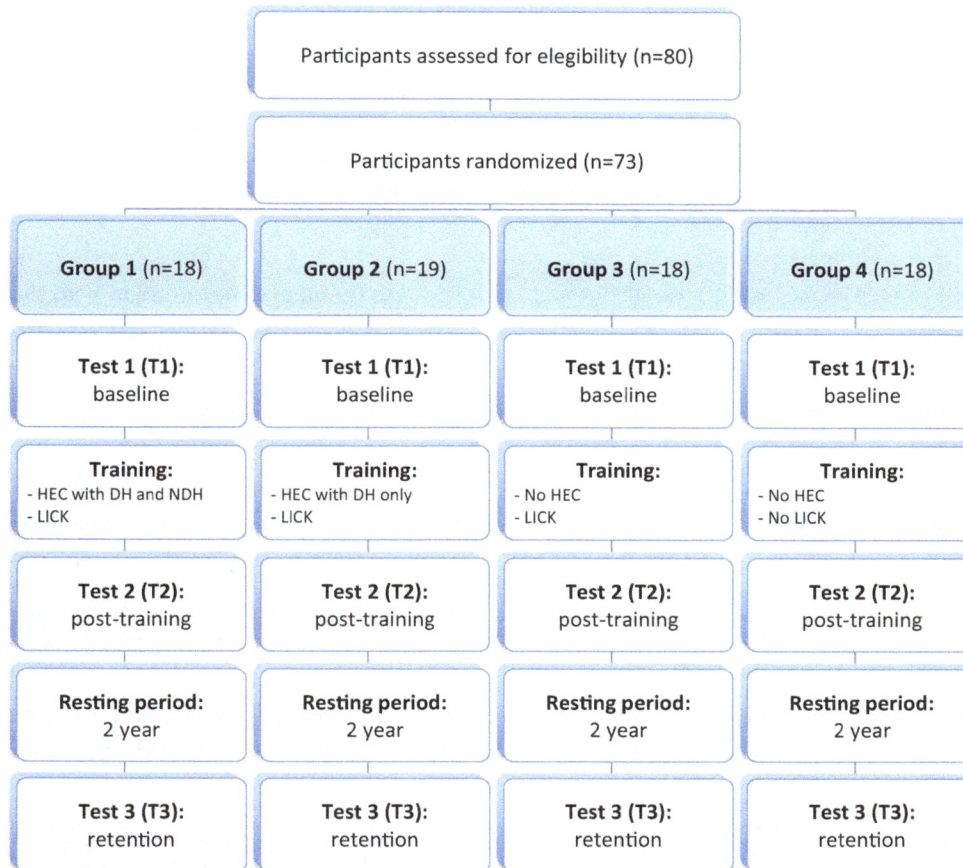

Fig. 1 Flowchart of participation. *HEC* ham-eye coordination, *DH* dominant hand, *NDH* non-dominant hand, *LICK* laparoscopic intra-corporeal knot tying

and therefore, they were disregarded for the first study about skills acquisition [8]. For the aims of the present study, 73 participants could be recruited again, remained all of them in the group originally assigned (Fig. 1).

To evaluate the baseline levels, all tasks were tested before training (T1) in sessions organized specifically for this aim. The test session started with detailed explanation and video demonstrations of the different tasks, and then, each participant performed three repetitions of task 1-a, task 1-b, and task 2. For each task, the average of the triplicate observations was used for statistical analysis [8].

Then, the assigned training program started. Training sessions of 1.5 h each were performed every 1 to 3 days, being approximately 1 month the average duration of the program [8]. In G1, the training program consisted in 60 repetitions of task 1-a and 60 repetitions of task 1-b in alternating order, followed by 60 repetitions of task 2. In G2, the training program consisted in 60 repetitions of task 1-a, followed by 60 repetitions of task 2. In G3, the training program consisted in 60 repetitions of task 2 directly, without any previous training for task 1. In G4, participants did not perform any training, not for task 1 nor for task 2.

To evaluate skills acquisition, the tasks were tested immediately after training (T2) in the same manner than for T1. The average duration in between T1 and T2 was 30 days.

To evaluate skills retention, after the sole effect of the exposition determined by this study, participants did not practice any type of laparoscopic procedure (no lab training nor surgery) and the tasks were tested again (T3) after a 2-year resting period in the same manner than for T1 and T2.

Statistics

For evaluating the scores of all tasks (continuous variables), non-parametric tests were used because data were not normally distributed. Therefore, unless otherwise indicated, all data are presented as median (interquartile range). For G1, G2, and G3, scores before and after training were already reported in a previous study [8]. For statistical analysis of the present study, only the data of participants enrolled in both studies were included (i.e., data of participants of the previous study who did not participate in this study were excluded).

All statistical comparisons were performed using the GraphPad Prism Software, and two-tailed P values <0.05 were considered significant.

Intergroup differences at T1, T2, and T3 were evaluated with Kruskal-Wallis test and Dunn's multiple comparison tests, whereas intra-group differences at the three time points were evaluated with Friedman test and Dunn's multiple comparison tests. Intra-group differences between DH (task 1-a) and NDH (task 1-b) were evaluated with Wilcoxon test.

Results

A total of 73 participants (G1 $n = 18$, G2 $n = 19$, G3 $n = 18$, G4 $n = 18$) were recruited (Fig. 1). All participants performed all assigned tasks, and their demographics (i.e., age, gender, training status, and DH side) were comparable and reported in Table 1.

Task 1-a (hand-eye coordination with the DH)

At T1, all groups had comparable scores, being 223 (174–279) for G1, 223 (112–350) for G2, 215 (162–266) for G3, and 194 (165–260) for G4 (all comparisons NS).

At T2, all groups that performed some kind of training improved their scores, being 44 (37–48) for G1 ($P < 0.0001$), 42 (37–51) for G2 ($P < 0.0001$), and 75 (62–95) for G3 ($P < 0.0001$), whereas G4 did not show any improvement and scored 201 (171–253) (NS). G1 scored similar than G2 (NS) and better than G3 ($P = 0.001$) and G4 ($P < 0.0001$). G2 scored better than G3 ($P = 0.004$) and G4 ($P < 0.0001$). G3 scored better than G4 ($P = 0.03$).

At T3, all groups retained their skills almost at the same level than at T2, being 60 (39–63) for G1 (NS), 55 (48–64) for G2 (NS), and 87 (79–98) for G3 (NS), whereas G4 showed a slight improvement scoring 160 (107–182) ($P = 0.02$). Also,

the intergroup differences detected at the end of the training program remains comparable at T3, G1 scoring similar than G2 (NS) and better than G3 ($P = 0.001$) and G4 ($P < 0.0001$) and G2 scoring better than G3 ($P = 0.001$) and G4 ($P < 0.0001$). However, due to the slight improvement in G4, differences between G3 and G4 were no longer significant (NS) (Fig. 2).

Task 1-b (hand-eye coordination with the NDH)

At T1, all groups had comparable scores, being 342 (277–484) for G1, 343 (196–561) for G2, 358 (210–476) for G3, and 310 (205–730) for G4 (all comparisons NS).

At T2, all groups that performed some kind of training improved their scores, being 54 (45–63) for G1 ($P < 0.0001$), 71 (59–81) for G2 ($P < 0.0001$), and 92 (83–143) for G3 ($P < 0.0001$), whereas G4 did not show any improvement and scored 283 (202–364) (NS). G1 scored similar than G2 (NS) and better than G3 ($P = 0.0001$) and G4 ($P < 0.0001$). G2 scored similar than G3 (NS) and better than G4 ($P < 0.0001$). G3 scored better than G4 ($P = 0.02$).

At T3, all groups retained their skills at the same level than at T2, being 67 (54–78) for G1 (NS), 90 (65–102) for G2 (NS), 100 (95–123) for G3 (NS), and 239 (206–327) for G4 (NS). Also, the intergroup differences detected at the end of the training program remains comparable at T3, G1 scoring similar than G2 (NS) and better than G3 ($P = 0.001$) and G4 ($P < 0.0001$), G2 scoring similar than G3 (NS) and better than G4 ($P < 0.0001$), and G3 scoring better than G4 ($P = 0.005$) (Fig. 3).

DH vs. NDH for hand-eye coordination

At all times points, all groups scored better for the DH than for the NDH (G1 $P = 0.0001$, $P = 0.0003$, $P < 0.0001$; G2 $P = 0.01$, $P < 0.0001$, $P < 0.0001$; G3 $P = 0.0003$, $P < 0.0001$,

Table 1 Participants' demographics

	Groups			
	G1 ($n = 18$)	G2 ($n = 19$)	G3 ($n = 18$)	G4 ($n = 18$)
Age (median and range in years)	31 (28–47)	30 (28–39)	34 (29–47)	32 (28–45)
Gender (%)				
• Male	10 (55 %)	9 (50 %)	9 (50 %)	9 (50 %)
• Female	8 (45 %)	10 (50 %)	9 (50 %)	9 (50 %)
Training status (%)				
• Residents	8 (45 %)	11 (58 %)	8 (45 %)	7 (39 %)
• Specialists	10 (55 %)	8 (42 %)	10 (55 %)	11 (61 %)
Dominant hand side				
• Right	17 (94 %)	17 (89 %)	17 (94 %)	17 (94 %)
• Left	1 (6 %)	2 (11 %)	1 (6 %)	1 (6 %)

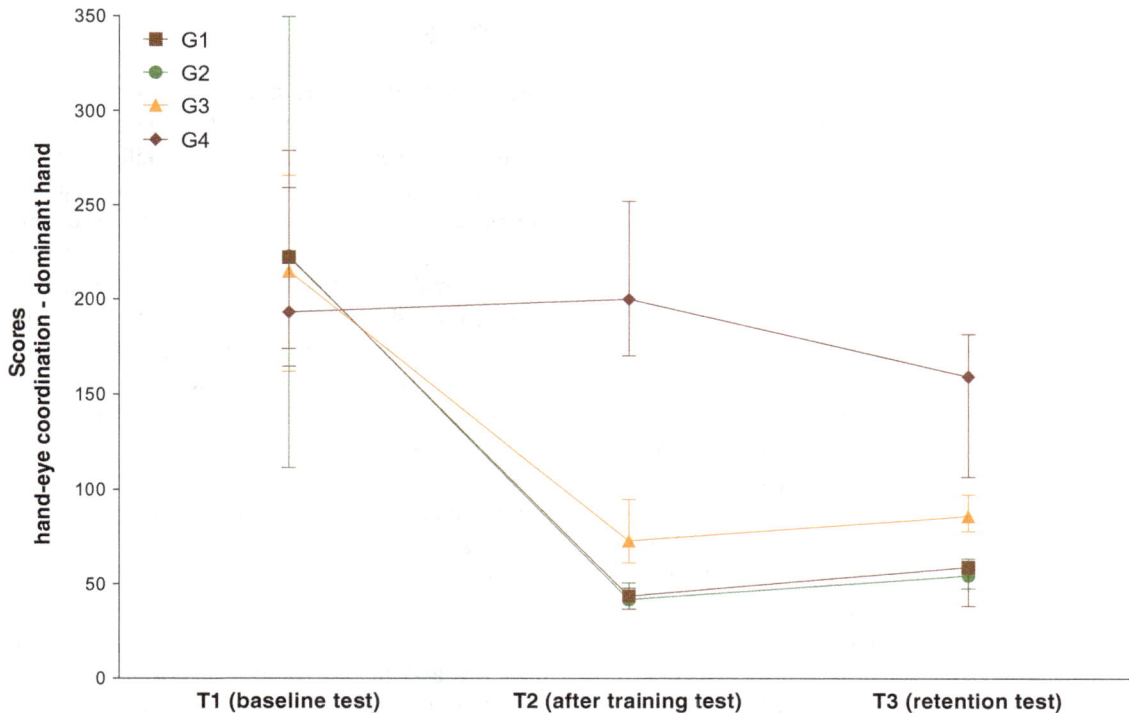

Fig. 2 Skills for hand-eye coordination with the dominant hand (task 1-a). Participants were randomly allocated to different groups according to the training program (G1, G2, G3, and G4), and the skills were measured before training to evaluate the baseline levels (T1), immediately after training to evaluate skills acquisition (T2), and 2 years later to evaluate skills retention (T3). Median (interquartile range) scores are presented

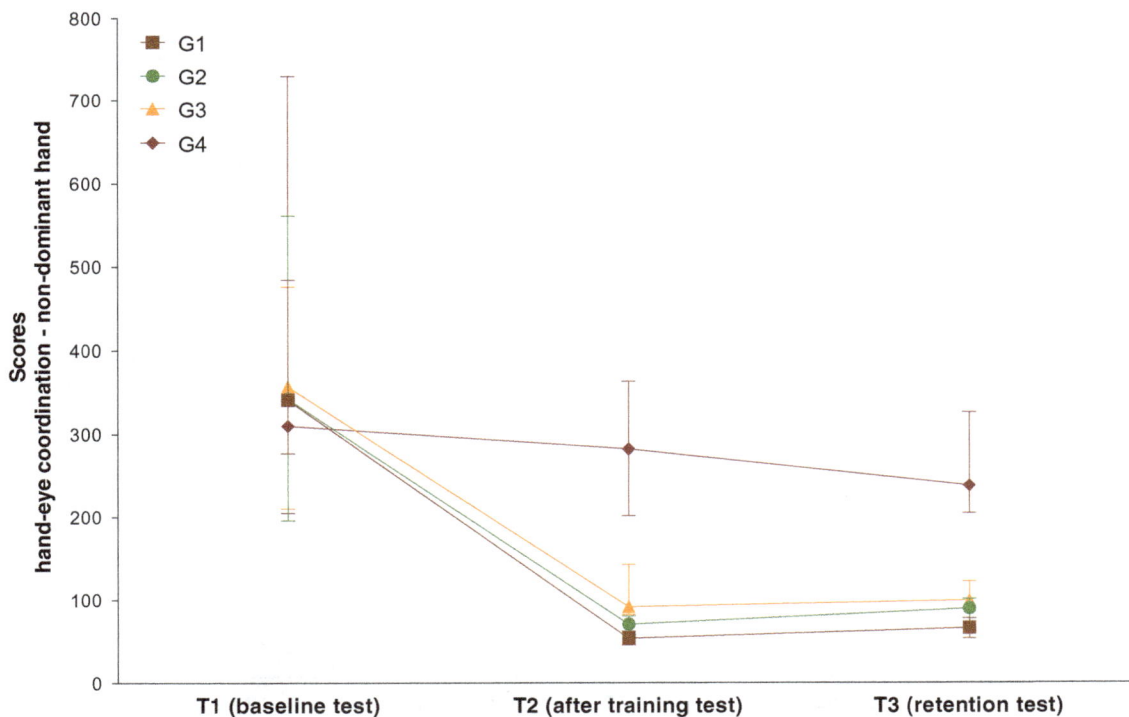

Fig. 3 Skills for hand-eye coordination with the non-dominant hand (task 1-b). Participants were randomly allocated to different groups according to the training program (G1, G2, G3, and G4), and the skills were measured before training to evaluate the baseline levels (T1), immediately after training to evaluate skills acquisition (T2), and 2 years later to evaluate skills retention (T3). Median (interquartile range) scores are presented

$P < 0.0001$; and G4 $P < 0.0001$, $P < 0.0001$, $P < 0.0001$, at T1, T2, and T3, respectively).

Task 2 (laparoscopic intra-corporeal knot tying)

At T1, all groups had comparable scores, being 334 (231–1200) for G1, 250 (208–1200) for G2, 326 (202–1200) for G3, and 477 (341–1200) for G4 (all comparisons NS).

At T2, all groups that performed some kind of training improved their scores, being 32 (26–37) for G1 ($P < 0.0001$), 32 (28–44) for G2 ($P < 0.0001$), and 35 (31–37) for G3 ($P < 0.0001$), whereas G4 did not show any improvement and scored 459 (425–749) (NS). G1, G2, and G3 had comparable scores (NS), scoring the three groups better than G4 ($P < 0.0001$, $P < 0.0001$, $P < 0.0001$).

At T3, G1 scored 51 (40–65), retaining the skills at the same level than at T2 (NS). G2 scored 62 (44–88) and G3 scored 74 (64–88), both groups scoring slightly worse than at T2 ($P = 0.01$, $P = 0.008$). G4 scored 457 (374–578) without any improvement in comparison with T2 (NS). Also, the intergroup differences detected at the end of the training program remains comparable at T3, having G1, G2, and G3 similar scores (NS), all of them better than G4 ($P < 0.0001$, $P < 0.0001$, $P = 0.0005$) (Fig. 4).

Discussion

The general aim of this study was to evaluate laparoscopic skills retention after a structured training program. The specific objectives were to assess whether skill retention varies according to the training program and the laparoscopic task complexity. To evaluate the former, we used four different training programs and hypothesized that the program assigned to G1 would determine better results, whereas the program assigned to G4 would determine poorer results. To evaluate the latter, we used basic and advanced tasks and hypothesized that hand-eye coordination with the DH would be the easier to retain, whereas intra-corporeal knot tying would be the more difficult to retain.

Our data demonstrate that after a 2-year resting period, and without practicing any laparoscopic surgery o skill training, participants retained to a large extent the skills registered at the end of the training programs and that although some skill decay was noticed, they remained significantly better than at baseline. The level of retention, however, varied according to the group and the task analyzed, confirming our hypothesis.

Indeed, G1 had the better improvement after training (T2 vs. T1) and was able to retain the skills of the three tasks at the same level than 2 years earlier (T3 vs. T2), indicating the relevance of a comprehensive training for skills acquisition

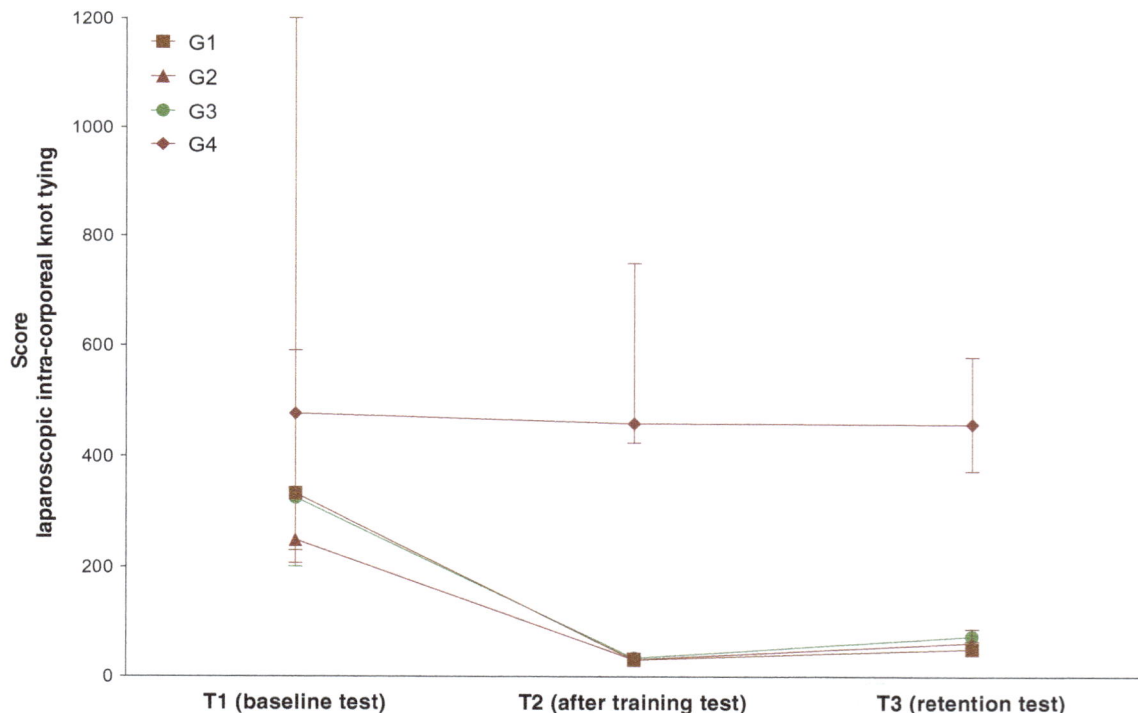

Fig. 4 Skills for laparoscopic intra-corporeal knot tying (task 2). Participants were randomly allocated to different groups according to the training program (G1, G2, G3, and G4), and the skills were measured before training to evaluate the baseline levels (T1), immediately after training to evaluate skills acquisition (T2), and 2 years later to evaluate skills retention (T3). Median (interquartile range) scores are presented

and retention. G4, however, did not show any improvement after training (T2 vs. T1), maintaining the sub-optimal skills execution in this study (T3 vs. T2) for more difficult tasks. For easiest task, however, a slight but significant improvement was observed, indicating a learning effect after few repetitions. G2 and G3 were in between the previous groups and had a significant improvement after training (T2 vs. T1). This was observed for trained and non-trained tasks, suggesting that intra-corporeal knot tying training may compensate to some extent the lack of hand-eye coordination training. Interestingly, both G2 and G3 were able to retain the hand-eye coordination skills, but not the intra-corporeal knot tying skills, at the same level than 2 years earlier, suggesting that retention of most difficult tasks may require more training.

Our data are consistent with the reports of other studies, but we must be cautious for general conclusions because the studies evaluating skills retentions differ significantly in study populations, training and tests programs/models, resting period, scoring systems, coaching and feedback, etc., as discussed in detail below.

Akdemir et al. evaluated skills retention in 11 first-year gynecology residents (without experience in laparoscopy) 6 months after a training program [9]. Although a matched control group was included for skills acquisition evaluation, there was no control group for skills retention evaluation. The 5-week program consisted in lectures (week 1) and 1-h practice session per week on a box trainer (weeks 2–5). The tasks performed in this box were well described, but the number of repetitions and the level of proficiency acquired were not reported. The baseline, post-training, and retention tests were done in another model (salpingectomy on the LapSim), and time, economy (path lengths and angular path), and error (blood loss and ovarian damage) were measured. The study concluded that the skills suffered a slight (angular path) or significant (time and path length) deterioration although they remained significantly better than at baseline [9].

Bonrath et al. evaluated skills retention in 36 medical students (without experience in laparoscopy) 6 or 11 weeks after a training program [10]. The 5-day program consisted in tutorials (day 1), baseline test (day 2), training (days 3–4), and post-training test (day 5). Participants, working in fixed pairs and accompanied by an expert for individual coaching, performed 4 cycles of nine tasks (navigation, grasping, transfer, positioning, cutting, loop tie, extra-corporal and intra-corporal knot tying and clipping) in a box trainer. The skills retention was evaluated after different time points (6 and 11 weeks) but unfortunately in two different groups. For testing purposes, time and errors of the same tasks performed during training were scored. The study concluded that skills are retained for at least 6 weeks and that deterioration, especially of the difficult tasks, started around 11 weeks [10].

Magaard et al. evaluated skills retention in a cohort of novices ($n = 9$) and experts ($n = 10$) 6 and 18 months after a training program [11]. The program (salpingectomy on the LapSim) consisted in 10 sessions (sessions 1–3: familiarization with the simulator, session 4: baseline test, sessions 5–9: training, session 10: after training test). The retention skills tests were done in the same model and time; economy and error ("bleeding") were measured. The novices were tested after 6 and 18 months, and the experts only after 6 months. The study reported different performance for novices and experts. For novices, the skills were retained after 6 months, but they return back to the pre-training level after 18 months [11]. For experts, it seemed that the training program had no effect at all since they showed a constant performance from the baseline test up to the retention test at 6 months.

Hiemstra et al. evaluated skills retention in seven novices 1 year after a training program [12]. The seven-session program consisted in a baseline test (session 1), once a week training (sessions 2–6), and a final test (session 7). Participants performed five tasks on a box trainer (pipe cleaner, placing rubber band, placing beads, cutting circle, and intra-corporeal knot tying). Scores for speed and precision were measured. The retention test was performed in the same model. The study concluded that most basic skills acquired during a short training program sustain over time and that although some showed deterioration after 1 year, all skills remained better than before training [12].

De Win et al. evaluated skills retention in 145 medical students 1 and 6 months after different training programs [13]. Participants were randomly allocated to different groups according to training frequency (three sessions daily, two sessions daily, one session daily, one session on alternative days, one session per week, one session per week with optional additional practice in between sessions). All groups underwent six training sessions of 1.5 h each, consisting in three basic tasks (thumbnail, paperclip, needle rotation) to learn intra-corporeal suturing (session 1), needle positioning and penetration (session 2), and suturing (sessions 3–6). For the post-training and the retention tests, a 5-cm chicken-skin incision model was used and time was scored. The study concluded that once daily, 1.5-h session seems most beneficial for acquiring and for retaining intra-corporeal endoscopic suturing [13].

To a certain extent, our study counteract the limitations of these studies and extent their observations in several aspects. First, we enrolled a larger study population than most other studies. Second, our study comprises a longer resting period and ascertains that participants did not practice laparoscopic surgery or skill training during the 2-year resting period. Third, our study evaluates and discriminates between tasks of different levels of difficulties. Fourth, our study ascertains that during the skills acquisition phase, training was long enough to reach the plateau of the learning curve, in contrast with other studies in which participants were just briefly exposed to a task or allowed to practice it for a short period.

To be able to accomplish our objectives, the major challenge was to recruit the same participants of a study carried out 2-year earlier to evaluate skills acquisition. At that time, we recruited gynecologists with sufficient experience in open and vaginal surgery but without experience in laparoscopy. In order to avoid any confounding effect of additional training in laparoscopy, only those who did not performed any laparoscopic procedure during the resting period were included in the present study. This challenge was achieved because we were able to recruit 91.25 % of the participants of the previous study (90 % in G1, G3, and G4 and 95 % in G2), who were obviously 2 years older and some of them with other training status (many residents became specialists). Today, when gynecological laparoscopic surgery became a routine procedure in daily practice, this study population is no longer available worldwide. In our setting, however, this was still not the case; residents and specialists being exposed only to the tools and experience offered by the study design and hence being them a unique population for studying a variety of parameters that can affect training in laparoscopy. We are fully aware that this situation is difficult to reproduce and that might not be clinically realistic, because in most scenarios, an intensive 1-month training will not be followed by a 2-year period without exposure to laparoscopic surgery. On the contrary, one would be encouraged to apply one's surgical training in the operating room to solidify hand memory and to advance one's skills.

In conclusion, our study demonstrates that when using the European Academy of Gynecological Surgery inanimate box model, LASTT, laparoscopic skills retention depends on the quality of the previous training program and on the task complexity, suggesting that a comprehensive training is advisable to acquire and to retain laparoscopic skills. This indicates that laparoscopic psychomotor skills are comparable to swimming or cycling in the sense that they can be retained for longer periods of time once achieved proficiency. It remains unclear, however, the ideal method for a faster skills acquisition, which will require the evaluation of the characteristics of the learning curves of both basic and advanced laparoscopic skills, as well as the evaluation of other potential influencing factors, such as tutor feedback [14] and the additive effect of training others basic skills (e.g., camera navigation, bimanual coordination). And more importantly, it also remains to be demonstrated the predictive validity of these training models.

Acknowledgments We would like to thank the Centro Médico La Costa for offering their facilities for the study to be performed, Mrs. Alicia Amarilla and Mrs. Florence Vandenberghe for her support in collecting the data and writing the manuscript, respectively, and specially to all gynecologists who actively participated in the study. We also would like to thank Karl Storz for providing the instruments and materials used in the study.

Authors' contribution CR Molinas: protocol/project development, data collection and management, and data analysis Manuscript writing/editing.

R Campo: protocol/project development and manuscript writing/editing.

Compliance with ethical standards

Funding This study did not receive any funding and was funded by the authors' own resources.

References

1. Subramonian K, DeSylva S, Bishai P, Thompson P, Muir G (2004) Acquiring surgical skills: a comparative study of open versus laparoscopic surgery. Eur Urol 45:346–351
2. Korndorffer JR, Stefanidis D, Scott DJ (2006) Laparoscopic skills laboratories: current assessment and a call for resident training standards. Am J Surg 191:17–22
3. Munz Y, Kumar BD, Moorthy K, Bann S, Darzi A (2004) Laparoscopic virtual reality and box trainers: is one superior to the other? Surg Endosc 18:485–494
4. Korndorffer JR, Dunne JB, Sierra R, Stefanidis D, Touchard CL, Scott DJ (2005) Simulator training for laparoscopic suturing using performance goals translates to the operating room. J Am Coll Surg 201:23–29
5. Aggarwal R, Hance J, Undre S, Ratnasothy J, Moorthy K, Chang A, Darzi A (2006) Training junior operative residents in laparoscopic suturing is feasible and efficacious. Surgery 139:729–734
6. Molinas CR, De Win G, Ritter O, Keckstein J, Miserez M, Campo R (2008) Feasibility and construct validity of a novel laparoscopic skills testing and training model. Gynecol Surg 5:281–290
7. Campo R, Resing C, Van Belle Y, Nassif J, O'Donovan P, Molinas CR (2010) A valid model for testing and training laparoscopic pshycomotor skills. Gynecol Surg 7:133–141
8. Molinas CR, Campo R (2010) Defining a structured training program for acquiring basic and advanced laparoscopic psychomotor skills in a simulator. Gynecol Surg 7:427–435
9. Akdemir A, Zeybek B, Ergenoglu AM, Yeniel AO, Sendag F (2014) Effect of spaced training with a box trainer on the acquisition and retention of basic laparoscopic skills. Int J Gynaecol Obstet 127:309–313
10. Bonrath EM, Weber BK, Fritz M, Mees ST, Wolters HH, Senninger N, Rijcken E (2012) Laparoscopic simulation training: testing for skill acquisition and retention. Surgery 152:12–20
11. Maagaard M, Sorensen JL, Oestergaard J, Dalsgaard T, Grantcharov TP, Ottesen BS, Larsen CR (2011) Retention of laparoscopic procedural skills acquired on a virtual-reality surgical trainer. Surg Endosc 25:722–727
12. Hiemstra E, Kolkman W, Van De Put MA, Jansen FW (2009) Retention of basic laparoscopic skills after a structured training program. Gynecol Surg 6:229–335
13. De Win G, Van Bruwaene S, De Ridder D, Miserez M (2013) The optimal frequency of endoscopic skill labs for training and skill retention on suturing: a randomized controlled trial. J Surg Educ 70:384–393
14. Schaafsma BE, Hiemstra E, Dankelman J, Jansen FW (2009) Feedback in laparoscopic skills acquisition: an observational study during a basic skills training course. Gynecol Surg 6:339–343

35

Gynaecological endoscopic surgical education and assessment. A diploma programme in gynaecological endoscopic surgery

Rudi Campo[1,2,3,4] · Arnaud Wattiez[1,2,3] · Vasilis Tanos[2,3] · Attilio Di Spiezio Sardo[3] · Grigoris Grimbizis[3] · Diethelm Wallwiener[2,5] · Sara Brucker[3,5] · Marco Puga[2] · Roger Molinas[2] · Peter O'Donovan[2,3] · Jan Deprest[3,6] · Yves Van Belle[2] · Ann Lissens[2,6,7] · Anja Herrmann[8] · Mahmood Tahir[4] · Chiara Benedetto[4] · Igno Siebert[9] · Benoit Rabischong[10] · Rudy Leon De Wilde[3,8]

Abstract In recent years, training and education in endoscopic surgery has been critically reviewed. Clinicians, both surgeons as gynaecologist who perform endoscopic surgery without proper training of the specific psychomotor skills, are at higher risk to increased patient morbidity and mortality. Although the apprentice-tutor model has long been a successful approach for training of surgeons, recently, clinicians have recognised that endoscopic surgery requires an important training phase outside the operating theatre. The Gynaecological Endoscopic Surgical Education and Assessment programme (GESEA) recognises the necessity of this structured approach and implements two separated stages in its learning strategy. In the first stage, a skill certificate on theoretical knowledge and specific practical psychomotor skills is acquired through a high-stake exam; in the second stage, a clinical programme is completed to achieve surgical competence and receive the corresponding diploma. Three diplomas can be awarded: (a) the Bachelor in Endoscopy, (b) the Minimally Invasive Gynaecological Surgeon (MIGS) and (c) the Master level. The Master level is sub-divided into two separate diplomas: the Master in Laparoscopic Pelvic Surgery and the Master in Hysteroscopy. The complexity of modern surgery has increased the demands and challenges to surgical education and the quality control. This programme is based on the best available scientific evidence, and it counteracts the problem of the traditional surgical apprentice-tutor model. It is seen as a major step toward standardisation of endoscopic surgical training in general.

Keywords Laparoscopy · Hysteroscopy · Practical skills · Education · Endoscopic surgery

Introduction

In recent years, training and education in endoscopic surgery has been critically reviewed [1, 2]. Laparoscopy has gained

The article was published in the *European Journal of Obstetrics & Gynecology and Reproductive Biology* and it has been reproduced in the *Gynecological Surgery* with the permission from Elsevier

✉ Rudi Campo
Rudi.Campo@lifeleuven.be

1 Life Expert Centre, Schipvaartstraat 2 Bus 4, 3000 Leuven, Belgium

2 European Academy for Gynaecological Surgery, Diestsevest 43/0001, 3000 Leuven, Belgium

3 European Society for Gynaecological Endoscopy, Diestsevest 43/0001, 3000 Leuven, Belgium

4 European Board and College of Obstetrics and Gynaecology, Brussels, Belgium

5 Department of Women's Health, University Hospital Tuebingen, Calwerstraat 7, 72077 Tuebingen, Germany

6 Center for Surgical Technologies, Leuven, Belgium

7 University Hospitals Leuven, Leuven, Belgium

8 Pius-Hospital Oldenburg, Department of Gynecology, Obstetrics and Gynaecological Oncology, Carlvon Ossietzky University, Georgstraße 12, 26121 Oldenburg, Germany

9 African Endoscopic Training Academy, Cape Town, South Africa

10 International Centre for Endoscopic Surgery, Clermont-Ferrand, France

wider acceptance within the surgical community as a preferred tool and became the golden standard, instead of laparotomy, for diagnosis and treatment of many diseases [1, 2]. Laparoscopic procedures provide higher surgical competence and improved patient outcome [3, 4] coherent with a reduction in blood loss, postoperative pain, infection rates and hospital stays [5, 6]. However, laparoscopic procedures are not commonly applied in complex procedures, because only a minority of surgeons possess advanced laparoscopic skills [7].

An endoscopic surgeon ideally must possess theoretical background of anatomy, pathology, treatment options, surgical techniques and adequate practical laparoscopic psychomotor skills (LPS) [8], including laparoscopic camera navigation (LCN), hand-eye coordination (HEC) and bi-manual coordination (BMC), prior to enter the in-operating room (OR) training programme. Laparoscopic skills are difficult to learn. In particular, laparoscopy requires excellent HEC on a 2D screen and counterintuitive movements for manipulating instruments [2].

Surgical competence can only be acquired if the in-OR teaching is performed by a highly skilled surgeon and is characterised by a continuous learning process. The apprentice first observes the procedure then assists the surgeon and finally operates under guidance. However, in endoscopic and more specific in laparoscopic surgery, the surgical training must be preceded by structured dry skill lap training with the acquisition of the specific LPS. The learning characteristics of LPS in contrary to the surgical competence do not require constant supervision from a highly skilled surgeon but relies on repetitive practise, and once gained, these abilities are retained over a long period of time (unpublished observations) [9–13].

Clinicians, both surgeons as gynaecologist who perform endoscopic surgery without proper training of the specific psychomotor skills, are at higher risk to increased patient morbidity and mortality [14–16]. Although the apprentice-tutor model has long been a successful approach for training of surgeons, recently, clinicians have concluded that endoscopic surgery requires an important training phase outside the operating theatre.

The Gynaecological Endoscopic Surgical Education and Assessment (GESEA) recognises the necessity of this structured approach and implements two assessment stages in its learning strategy. In the first stage, a skill certificate on theoretical knowledge and specific practical psychomotor skills is acquired through a high-stake exam; in the second stage, a clinical programme is completed to achieve surgical competence and receive the corresponding diploma (Fig. 1) [17–23].

Three diplomas can be awarded: (a) the Bachelor in Endoscopy, (b) the Minimally Invasive Gynaecological Surgeon (MIGS) and (c) the Master level. The Master level is sub-divided into two separate diplomas: the Master in Laparoscopic Pelvic Surgery and the Master in Hysteroscopy (Fig. 2) [17–23].

The European Society for Gynaecological Endoscopy (ESGE) is responsible for the diploma in collaboration with the European Board and College of Obstetrics and Gynaecology (EBCOG) [21]. +he Academy is the notified body for the high-stake exam and for issuing +he Academy skill certificate (Fig. 1) [20].

The complexity of modern surgery has increased the demands and challenges to surgical education and the quality control. This programme is based on the best available scientific evidence, and it counteracts the problem of the traditional surgical apprentice-tutor model. It is seen as a major step toward standardisation of endoscopic surgical training in general.

Training

Prior to enter the in-OR training, a theoretical and practical programme with self-evaluation modules is defined.

An online teaching programme is provided to train and test the theoretical knowledge (www.websurg.com/winners/). This programme offers a set of peer-reviewed tutorials and the possibility of self-assessment by means of five multiple choice questions (MCQ's) randomly chosen from a pool after each tutorial section. When these MCQ's are correctly answered, then the topic is approved. As the MCQ's are not correctly answered, a new set of five MCQ's is provided [24–29]. Only when all topics for a specific level have been passed, then the participant can be considered as a candidate for +he Academy certification.

+he Academy has developed a series of tools and methods for training and testing of practical endoscopic skills: the Laparoscopic Skills Training and Testing model (LASTT), the Suturing Training and Testing model (SUTT) and the Hysteroscopic Training and Testing model (HYSTT) [21].

The LASTT model can be used as an insert in a conventional trainer box and comprises three different exercises that aim to train and evaluate three specific LPS: LCN, HEC and BMC. The result of an exercise is expressed in time to correct performed exercise [18]. Construct, content and face validity of those exercises have been published [30, 31].

The SUTT model has been developed to train and test more complex and fine LPS like needle manipulation, intracorporeal knotting, cutting and tissue approximation using both dominant and non-dominant hands. These exercises are performed in a pelvic trainer with a 0° 10-mm optic and two needle holders.

The HYSTT model represents the spatial distribution and orientation of the different planes and angles of a normal uterus. Here a 2.9-mm 30° optic is used and two exercises are defined to train and test camera navigation and HEC.

The results of each exercise are reported on an online scoring platform providing the surgeon his position in the

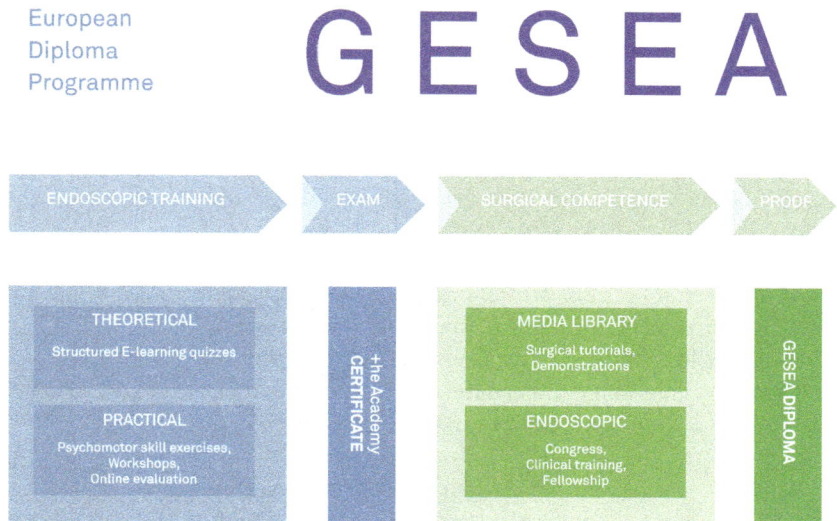

Fig. 1 The Gynaecological Endoscopic Surgical Education and Assessment (GESEA) structured learning and validation path

European Diploma Programme

GESEA

ENDOSCOPIC TRAINING → EXAM → SURGICAL COMPETENCE → PROOF

THEORETICAL
Structured E-learning quizzes

PRACTICAL
Psychomotor skill exercises, Workshops, Online evaluation

+he Academy CERTIFICATE

MEDIA LIBRARY
Surgical tutorials, Demonstrations

ENDOSCOPIC
Congress, Clinical training, Fellowship

GESEA DIPLOMA

benchmark population and an allocation to the excellent, fair and room for improvement group.

Certificate

To validate the knowledge and endoscopic practical psychomotor skills, +he Academy has developed a high-stake exam.

The theoretical exam consists of 50 MCQ's to evaluate the knowledge of the individual in the specific areas of expertise according to the level. The practical exam consists of the three LASTT exercises, the level corresponding SUTT and HYSTT

exercises, which are performed in a standardised environment supervised by a director of examination and one accredited mentor for each working station.

The exam is performed at international congresses and in an accredited GESEA diploma centre. Within 14 days, the participant receives the global result as a pass, by receiving +he Academy skill certificate, or a fail (Fig. 1). No detailed information as regards the scores of the different tests is provided. If the mentee fails the exam, then the total exam has to be repeated. In case of dispute, the mentee can address a complaint to the exam appeal commission.

Fig. 2 The three proficiency levels of the GESEA programme

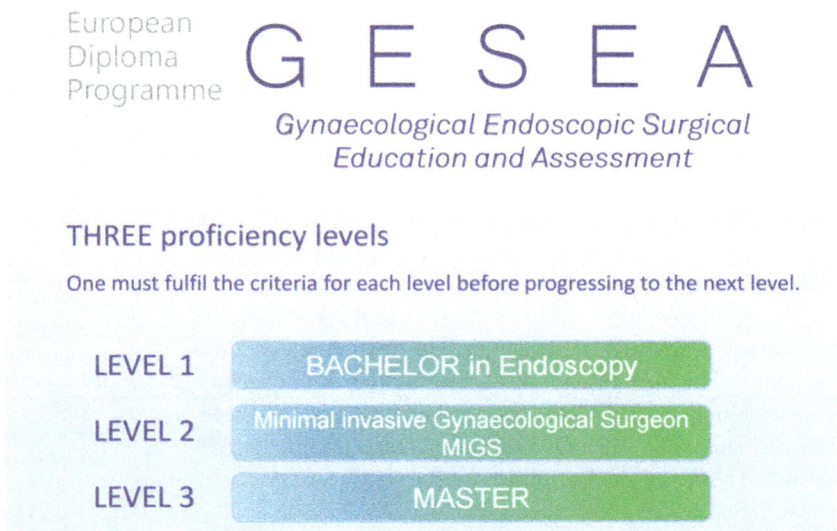

European Diploma Programme

GESEA

Gynaecological Endoscopic Surgical Education and Assessment

THREE proficiency levels

One must fulfil the criteria for each level before progressing to the next level.

LEVEL 1 — BACHELOR in Endoscopy

LEVEL 2 — Minimal invasive Gynaecological Surgeon MIGS

LEVEL 3 — MASTER

Diploma of surgical competence

Each level of the GESEA curriculum results in a diploma (Fig. 1); the Bachelor, Minimal Invasive Gynaecological surgeon and Master diploma (Fig. 2).

The bachelor diploma, specifically designed for residents or endoscopists who carried out less than 200 interventions, can be viewed as a prerequisite to starting the in-OR clinical training in endoscopic surgery. Requirements for this diploma are +he Academy Bachelor skill certificate, exposure as an observer to at least 30 endoscopic procedures and proof of attendance of a recognised endoscopic congress or workshop.

Requirements for the MIGS diploma are +he Academy MIGS skill certificate, proof of a predefined surgical clinical curriculum in laparoscopy and hysteroscopy in a period of max. 5 years, 50 CME/CPD points of endoscopic congresses or workshops and 20 ESGE educational points including scientific contribution (e.g. publication), mentorship, etc.

The Master diploma can be achieved separately for laparoscopy and hysteroscopy, which follows the same flow chart as the MIGS diploma.

Conclusion

The endoscopic approach to surgical patient care has a different dimension in the learning process in comparison to the traditional 'open' surgery. The specialised equipment and instrumentation require a different set of technical skills and organisation of the surgical team [28].

Professional organisations are responsible for setting the standards for training the next generation of specialists to ensure patient safety. The training programme should be standardised, include objective metrics of validation, offer universal accessibility and provide credentials to confirm successful training [23–28].

The innovative approach of the GESEA programme has acknowledged the need for different skills with different learning paths. Surgical knowledge and practical skill performance are evaluated with objective methods. However, the criteria for acquiring the GESEA diplomas are related to performance, continuous medical education and professional development.

The GESEA programme follows minimal standards and provides a structured training path for the endoscopy surgeons. This programme provides training in endoscopic procedures with built-in safety and the best possible surgical outcome. GESEA criteria increase the quality of the one-to-one clinical training programme in endoscopic procedures for all stakeholders [17–23].

Full article is available on www.ebcog.org and www.esge.org.

References

1. Antoniou SA, Antoniou GA, Koutras C, Antoniou AI (2012) Endoscopy and laparoscopy: a historical aspect of medical terminology. Surg Endosc 26:3650–3654
2. De Win G, Van Bruwaene S, Kulkarni J, Van Calster B, Aggarwal R, Allen C, Lissens A, De Ridder D, Miserez M (2015) An evidence based laparoscopic simulation curriculum shortens the clinical learning curve and reduces surgical adverse events. BJS 102:110–110
3. He H, Zeng D, Ou H, Tang Y, Li J, Zhong H (2013) Laparoscopic treatment of endometrial cancer: systematic review. J Minim Invasive Gynecol 20(4):413–423
4. Okholm C, Goetze JP, Svendsen LB, Achiam MP (2014) Inflammatory response in laparoscopic vs. open surgery for gastric cancer. Scand J Gastroenterol 49(9):1027–1034
5. Nieboer TE, Johnson N, Lethaby A, et al. (2009) Surgical approach to hysterectomy for benign gynaecological disease. Cochrane Database Syst Rev Issue 3:CD003677
6. Medeiros LR, Rosa DD, Bozzetti MC, et al. (2009) Laparoscopy versus laparotomy for benign ovarian tumour. Cochrane Database Syst Rev Issue 2:CD004751
7. De Win G, Everaerts W, De Ridder D, Peeraer G (2015) Laparoscopy training in Belgium: results from a nationwide survey, in urology, gynecology, and general surgery residents. Adv Med Educ Pract 6:55–63
8. Sinitsky DM, Fernando B, Berlingieri P (2012) Establishing a curriculum for the acquisition of laparoscopic psychomotor skills in the virtual reality environment. Am J Surg 204(3):367–376
9. Molinas CR, Campo R (2016) Laparoscopic skills retention after a structured training programme. doi:10.1007/s10397-016-0962-4
10. Aggarwal R, Tully A, Grantcharov T, Larsen CR, Miskry T, Farthing A, Darzi A (2006) Virtual reality simulation training can improve technical skills during laparoscopic salpingectomy for ectopic pregnancy. BJOG 113:1382–1387
11. Ascher-Walsh CJ, Capes T (2007) An evaluation of the resident learning curve in performing laparoscopic supracervical hysterectomies as compared with patient outcome: five-year experience. J Minim Invasive Gynecol 14:719–723
12. Simons AJ, Anthone GJ, Ortega AE, Franklin M, Fleshman J, Geis WP, Beart RW (1995) Laparoscopic-assisted colectomy learning curve. Dis Colon Rectum 38:600–603
13. Ghomi A, Littmann P, Prasad A, Einarsson JL (2007) Assessing the learning curve for laparoscopic supracervical hysterectomy. JSLS 11:190–194
14. Van Der Wal G. (2007) Risico's minimaal invasieve chirurgie onderschat. http://www.igz.nl/zoekresultaten.aspx?q=laparoscopische%20operaties. Accessed 15 Dec 2015
15. Tijam IM, Persoon M, Hendrikx AJ, Muijtjens AM, Witjes JA, Scherpbier AJ (2012) Program for laparoscopic urologic skills: a newly developed and validated educational program. Urology 79(4):815–820
16. Stefanidis D, Acker C, Heniford BT (2008) Proficiency-based laparoscopic simulator training leads to improved operating room skill that is resistant to decay. Surg Innov 15(1):69–73
17. Campo R, Molinas CR, De Wilde RL, et al. (2012) Are you good enough for your patients? The European certification model in laparoscopic surgery. Facts Views Vis Obgyn 4:95–101
18. Campo R, Wattiez A, De Wilde RL, Molinas CR (2012) Training in laparoscopic surgery: from the LAB to the OR. Zdrav Var 51:285–298
19. Campo R, Reising C, Belle Y, Nassif J, O'Donovan P, Molinas CR (2010) A valid model for testing and training laparoscopic psychomotor skills. Gynecol Surg 7:133–141

20. The European Academy of Gynaecological Surgery. Courses, tools, certification. http://www.europeanacademy.org/Gynaecological_Surgery.html. Accessed 15 Dec 2015

21. European Board and College of Obstetrics & Gynaecology (EBCOG) (2014) Standards of Care for Women's Health in Europe- Gynaecological Services: accessible at (www.ebcog.eu)

22. Molinas CR, Campo R (2010) Defining a structured training program for acquiring basic and advanced laparoscopic psychomotor skills in a simulator. Gynecol Surg 7:427–435

23. Campo R, Puga M, Meier Furst R, Wattiez A, De Wilde RL (2014) Excellence needs training "Certified programme in endoscopic surgery". Facts Views Vis Obgyn 6(4):240–244

24. Carneson J, Delpierre G, Masters K. Designing and managing multiple-choice questions: appendix B, designing MCQs—do's and don'ts. http://www.uct.ac.za/projects/cbe/mcqman/mcqappb.html. Accessed 17 Mar 2015

25. Haladyna TM, Mahwah NJ (1999) Developing and validating multiple-choice test items. Lauwrence Erlbaum Associates

26. Haladyna TM (1989) Taxonomy of multiple-choice item-writing rules. Appl Meas Educ 2:37–50

27. Jacobs LC (2008) How to write better tests: a handbook for improving test construction skills. http://www.iub.edu/~best/pdf_docs/better_tests.pdf. Accessed 27 Dec 2014

28. Marshall JC, Hales LW (1971) Classroom test construction. Addison-Wesley, Reading

29. University of Oregon teaching effectiveness program. Writing multiple-choice questions that demand critical thinking. http://tep.uoregon.edu/resources/assessment/multiplechoicequestions/mc4critthink.html. Accessed 27 Dec 2014

30. Molinas CR, De Win G, Ritter O, Keckstein J, Miserez M, Campo R (2008) Feasibility and construct validity of a novel laparoscopic skills testing and training model. Gynecol Surg 5(4):281–290

31. Munz Y, Kumar BD, Moorthy K, Bann S, Darzi A (2004) Laparoscopic virtual reality and box trainers: is one superior to the other? Surg Endosc 18:485–494

32. Molinas CR and Campo R. Laparoscopic skills retention after a structured training programme. Submitted

36

Deep infiltrating endometriosis affecting the urinary tract—surgical treatment and fertility outcomes in 2004–2013

Liisu Saavalainen[1] · Oskari Heikinheimo[1] · Aila Tiitinen[1] · Päivi Härkki[1]

Abstract Urinary tract endometriosis (UTE) is a rare form of deep infiltrating endometriosis. We studied the operative treatment of UTE and evaluated postoperative recurrences and fertility outcomes. This is a retrospective cohort study of 53 women who underwent operative treatment for UTE in 2004–2013 at Helsinki University Hospital, and were followed-up until the end of 2014. The data were gathered from the hospital's electronic database. The main outcome measures were complications, reoperations, postoperative pregnancies, and deliveries. Preoperative diagnosis was accurate in 72 % with bladder endometriosis and in 93 % with ureteral disease. Thirty-one (58 %) of the 53 operations were performed via laparoscopy. Postoperative complications requiring re-intervention occurred in five cases (9 %). Five reoperations were performed in four cases due to endometriosis recurrence, only two due to recurrence of UTE (4 %). Twenty-eight women wished for pregnancy; 18 (64 %) of them conceived. Infertility treatment was needed in 20 (71 %) cases. Twelve (75 %) women delivered via cesarean section; intraoperative difficulties occurred in ten (83 %). The complication rate with UTE operations is acceptable and recurrences are rare. Infertility is common, but 57 % of those who wished for a child succeeded. A majority of the deliveries involved unplanned and complicated cesarean section.

Keywords Endometriosis · Bladder · Fertility · Ureter · Urinary tract

✉ Päivi Härkki
paivi.harkki@hus.fi

[1] Department of Obstetrics and Gynecology, University of Helsinki and Helsinki University Hospital, Sofianlehdonkatu 5, PO Box 610, FI-00029 HUS Helsinki, Finland

Background

Urinary tract endometriosis (UTE) is a form of deep infiltrating endometriosis (DIE) affecting 0.3–12 % of all women suffering from endometriosis [1, 2] and 14–20 % of all DIE patients [3]. According to the latest article, 52 % of DIE patients may suffer from UTE [3]. Of the various forms of UTE, bladder endometriosis is the most common (85 %), followed by that of the ureter (9 %), kidney (4 %), and urethra (2 %) [1].

Regarding symptomatology, 70 % of patients with bladder endometriosis suffer from urinary frequency, urgency, and dysuria, and 20–35 % from hematuria. When endometriosis involves the ureters, there often are no symptoms, which might lead to silent loss of renal function [2]. The risk of ureteral endometriosis increases if a rectovaginal nodule is larger than 3 cm [3–5]. Thus, urinary tract ultrasonography, urography, or magnetic resonance imaging (MRI) is recommended when planning surgery for DIE [6, 7].

The treatment of choice for severe DIE not responding to medication is surgery, i.e., complete resection of all endometriotic lesions including possible bladder, ureteral, and bowel lesions. Surgical treatment results in good pain relief for a long time [8] and 90 % of patients are satisfied [9]. Surgery is the first option in cases of UTE-related hydronephrosis. Moreover, it has been suggested that the recurrence rate of bladder endometriosis is lower than that seen in connection with other forms of endometriosis [10].

However, unlike pelvic pain, there is no consensus concerning the first-line treatment of infertility (surgery vs. assisted reproduction techniques (ART)) in DIE patients. According to the ESHRE guidelines, there is not enough evidence to propose surgery before ART [11]. In addition, there are conflicting results on impact of endometriosis on infertility: presence of endometrioma may [12] or may not [13, 14] reduce ovarian reserve and even the presence of DIE may have an impact on ovarian function [15, 16]. On the other hand, surgery of ovarian endometrioma may [17] or may not [18] have a negative impact on ovarian reserve, and surgery of DIE may [19, 20] or may not improve fertility [21, 22]. Nevertheless, these operations carry a high risk of complications [9]. Even though fertility is often unaffected by such complications, pregnancy rates are lower after bowel versus urinary tract complications [23]. After repeated operations, fertility is further diminished [24, 25]. On the other hand, delaying surgery may lead to prolonged painful complaints during ART and eventually to more difficult surgery [26]. Finally, infertility is multifactorial in endometriosis patients and the choice of treatment is individual.

The aims of the present study were to evaluate the outcome of operative treatment of UTE, to study factors affecting postoperative fertility, and to analyze the course of postoperative pregnancies.

Methods

During a 10-year period from January 2004 to December 2013, a total of 53 women underwent surgical treatment for UTE at our department. The department is a tertiary referral hospital and also one of the referral centers for patients with severe endometriosis. During the study period, we also operated altogether 400 women with DIE of the rectovaginal septum; 182 of those involved colorectal resection and 70 % of the bowel procedures were performed laparoscopically. Patient records in the hospital district of Helsinki and Uusimaa (HUS) are electronic, and therefore all operations, complications, and reoperations can be identified and the data retrieved. The patients were identified on the basis of diagnosis and specific surgical codes. In this study, we included all bladder resections for endometriosis with or without concomitant procedures and all ureteroneocystostomies (UNC) for severe ureteral endometriosis. Extrinsic ureteral endometriotic nodules were completely resected around the ureters without UNC among six patients in connection with operation of bladder endometriosis. Unfortunately, we are missing the most of those patients with ureterolysis associated with DIE in the rectovaginal septum not connected with bladder endometriosis as a result of a lack of specific surgical code. Thus, these patients are not included as a separate group in the present study.

Before initiation of this study, Institutional Review Board approval was obtained (21.3.2013). The ethics committee of the Hospital District of Helsinki and Uusimaa approved the study protocol (28/13/03/03/2013).

Operative techniques

The patients were often approached by a multidisciplinary team. Gynecologists were experienced in advanced laparoscopic surgery with the aid of one assistant. All bladder resections were performed by a gynecologist. All UNCs were performed together with a urologist. A gastrointestinal surgeon was involved if bowel endometriosis was to be treated. One gynecologist (P.H.) performed 43 (78 %) of all the operations. In 33 (62 %) cases, either a urologist (in 23 operations) or/and a gastrointestinal surgeon (in 22 operations) was present. The same urologist was present in 11 and the same gastrointestinal surgeon in 14 of all the operations.

Partial cystectomy was performed either via laparoscopy ($n = 31$) or laparotomy ($n = 12$). Bladder nodules were separated from the anterior wall of the uterus and complete excision of these nodules was carried out. The bladder was sutured in most cases in a single layer with continuous resorbable sutures and a bladder catheter was left in place for 10 days postoperatively. Ureteral stents were used only in cases of ureteral proximity. Full-thickness bladder resection was carried out except for two cases where the nodule was mobilized and excised without opening the mucosal layer of the bladder wall.

To perform ureteral shaving in association with bladder operation, the ureter was freed from all fibrotic tissue and the endometriotic nodule was removed laparoscopically.

Ureteral stenting was always carried out either via cystoscopy or cystostomy during UNC procedures when endometriosis involved the ureters. All cases of ureteral reimplantation with UNC ($n = 13$) were performed via laparotomy with a urologist. Large endometriotic nodules affecting the ureters were excised; the ureter was cut above the nodule and reimplanted into the bladder. Ureteral stents were left in place for 4 to 6 weeks and bladder catheters for 10 days.

Prophylactic antibiotics were given to all—a combination of cefuroxime (1.5/g) and metronidazole (0.5/g) intravenously in 34 (64 %) cases and cefuroxime (1.5 /g) intravenously in 15 (28 %). Peroral antibiotics were continued as long as a catheter was in a bladder or ureter. Low-molecular-weight heparin was used after 33 (62 %) operations. Patients were discharged with a bladder catheter and visited hospital for its removal after routine cystography.

Follow-up and data collection

After surgery, the women were followed-up with a scheduled visit at 1–2 months postoperatively. Symptoms of pain, urinary and bowel function were inquired at the time of the visit without validated questionnaires or urodynamic examinations. Data concerning demographic characteristics, as well as pre-, per-, and postoperative data were collected retrospectively from the electronic patient files. The follow-up period was until the end of 2014.

Complications were graded according to the Clavien–Dindo classification system as follows: I, minor complications not requiring medical or surgical intervention; II, complications requiring pharmacological treatment or blood transfusion; III, complications requiring re-intervention; IV, life-threatening complications, and V, death [27].

Recurrences were defined as cases requiring a new operation. We also assessed the factors associated with postoperative fertility among women younger than 43 years of age at the time of operation. All pregnancies and deliveries, but not biochemical pregnancies, were analyzed.

Statistical analysis

Statistical analysis was performed by using the Statistical Package for the Social Sciences (SPSS) version 21.0 for Windows. The chi-square test and Fisher's exact two-sided test were used as necessary. Means were compared by using Student's t test. Differences were considered statistically significant if $p < 0.05$.

Findings

Demographics and preoperative data

During the study period, 53 women underwent surgery for UTE. The patients were referred to the clinic because of a known history of DIE or symptoms typical of UTE such as dysuria, urinary urgency, or hematuria, or because of radiological findings such as hydronephrosis. Infertility was not the main indication for operative management in any case.

The characteristics of the study patients are summarized in Table 1. Altogether, 31 (58 %) women had preoperative urinary symptoms, with macroscopic hematuria in seven (13 %) patients. Every patient was examined by means of vaginal

Table 1 Patients characteristics and their preoperative data ($n = 53$)

Variable	Number	Percent
Age (years (mean, SD))	35.0	4.4
BMI (kg/m^2 (mean, SD))	23.1	3.7
Smoking	10	19
History of previous pregnancy	11	21
Nulliparous	47	89
History of infertility	28	53
Previous operative treatment due to endometriosis	24	45
Preoperative hormonal treatment	23	43
Preoperative symptoms		
Dysmenorrhea	48	91
Dysuria, pollakisuria, and/or hematuria	31	58
Dyschezia and/or hematemesis	20	38
Dyspareunia	21	40

Data are shown as n (%) unless stated otherwise. ($n = 53$)

gynecological ultrasonography. Preoperatively, magnetic resonance imaging (MRI) was performed in 33 (62 %) patients and computed tomography (CT) in eight (15 %). In 13 (25 %) cases, there were no preoperative imaging examinations concerning the ureters or kidneys. Altogether, 13 cystoscopies were performed preoperatively. Preoperative diagnosis was accurate in 31 (72 %) cases concerning bladder endometriosis and in 13 (93 %) cases concerning ureteral disease.

The patients were divided into three groups as follows: Group A: patients with isolated bladder endometriosis excluding DIE elsewhere ($n = 8$) (procedures performed: isolated partial cystectomy or shaving (two patients)). Group B: bladder endometriosis associated with other types of endometriosis but no intrinsic ureteral lesions ($n = 31$) (procedures: partial cystectomy with concomitant procedures excluding UNC). Group C: severe ureteral endometriosis associated with other types of endometriosis ($n = 14$) (procedures: UNC with concomitant procedures including partial cystectomy (three patients) and nephrectomy (one patient)). The diagnosis of endometriosis was confirmed by histology in each case.

Operative data

Thirty-one (58 %) of the 53 operations were performed via laparoscopy. The mean (±SD) operative time in laparoscopic procedures was 146 ± 61 min and blood loss was 73 ± 122 ml. Corresponding figures were 225 ± 81 min and 1567 ± 1107 ml in procedures performed via laparotomy. As the difficulty of the operations increased from Group A to Group C, the proportion of laparotomies as well as the length of operating time increased (Table 2). The length of sick leave was 26 ± 16 days vs. 58 ± 67 days in procedures performed via laparoscopy vs. laparotomy, respectively.

There were a total of 170 concomitant procedures, which varied from superficial electrocoagulation to nephrectomy (Table 3). The mean number of concomitant procedures in the operations performed via laparoscopy was 2.5 and 4.1 in those performed via laparotomy.

The bladder operations were mostly partial cystectomies ($n = 41$, groups A, B, and C), and shaving of the endometriotic nodule was performed twice (group A). Seventy-two percent of them were operated upon via laparoscopy; laparotomy was chosen in connection with several DIE lesions. All cases of isolated bladder endometriosis (group A) and concomitant six cases of ureteral shavings were operated laparoscopically (group B). The median size of the bladder nodules was 3 cm (range 2–4 cm) and their locations were in the bladder dome in 17 (40 %), the posterior wall in 24 (56 %), and the trigone in two (5 %) of the cases.

Table 2 Perioperative and postoperative data

Variables	Group A (n = 8)	Group B (n = 31)	Group C (n = 14)	Total (n = 53)
Laparoscopy	8 (100)	23 (74)	0 (0)	31 (58)
Three or more concomitant procedures	0 (0)	10 (32)	10 (71)	20 (38)
Operation time (min, SD)	123 (41)	164 (63)	249 (89)	180 (80)
Blood loss (ml, SD)	88 (170)	465 (853)	1773 (1094)	734 (1048)
Hospital stay (days, SD)	2.3 (1.0)	3.9 (2.3)	8.5 (5.7)	4.9 (4.1)
Women who wished for a child	6 (75)	13 (42)	9 (64)	28 (53)
Women treated with ART	3 (50)	9 (69)	8 (89)	20 (71)
Women who conceived	4 (67)	8 (62)	6 (67)	18 (64)
Conceived spontaneously	1 (17)	4 (31)	1 (11)	6 (21)
Women who delivered	3 (50)	8 (62)	5 (56)	16 (57)

Data are shown as n (%) unless stated otherwise

Group A: isolated partial cystectomy

Group B: partial cystectomy with concomitant procedures excluding UNC

Group C: UNC with concomitant procedures including partial cystectomy

In group C, UNC was performed 13 times, twice bilaterally. One concomitant nephrectomy was performed because of a silent kidney with resection of ureteral endometriosis in pelvis. Indications for UNC were moderate hydronephrosis (n = 5, one bilateral), severe hydronephrosis with diminished renal function (n = 6, one bilateral), persisting large nodule after ureteral shaving done twice (n = 1), and silent kidney

Table 3 Concomitant procedures

Variable	Number	Percent
Rectovaginal resection (other than sacrouterine ligaments only)	32	60
Bowel resection	21	40
Vaginal resection	17	32
Electroresection, puncture, or enucleation of endometrioma(s) in the ovaries	17	32
Parametrial resection	16	30
Cystoscopy	13	25
Electrocoagulation of peritoneal endometriosis	10	19
Chromopertubation	9	17
Salpingo-oophorectomy (unilateral in 3, bilateral in 5)	8	15
Resection of sacrouterine ligaments[a]	8	15
Shaving of ureteral endometriosis	6	11
Hysterectomy	6	11
Protective ileostomy	4	8
Hysteroscopy	2	4
Nephrectomy	1	2
Total	170	

Data are shown as n (%)

[a] Counted as a procedure when no rectovaginal resection was carried out

(n = 1). All UNC operations were performed via laparotomy with the aid of a urologist. UNC was done to the left side eight times, right side three times, and bilaterally twice. Histological examination revealed intrinsic endometriosis of the ureter in one case, whereas in ten cases the disease was extrinsic or the specimen was taken from surrounding tissue not including the ureter.

During all the UTE operations, grade I complications occurred in two (4 %) and grade II complications in 21 (40 %) women. None of the complications occurred after operations on isolated bladder endometriosis (group A). In group B, three minor bladder leakages were discovered during routine cystography 10 days after the laparoscopic procedure and therefore bladder catheter was kept for another 2 weeks and removed after normal re-cystography in all three patients. In group C, one patient had urinary leakage from the bladder to the vagina and rectum on the 18th postoperative day after combined bladder and colorectal resection, protective ileostomy, and UNC via laparotomy. Cystography had been normal the day before and bladder catheter had been removed. No fistula was detected during CT urography but leakage came to an end following insertion of a new bladder catheter. After 2 weeks with this catheter, cystography and cystoscopy were normal and leakage vanished. The most common complication was hemorrhage and altogether 16 women in groups B and C received blood transfusions after the operations performed via laparotomy.

There were five (9 %) grade III complications: three reoperations were performed after laparoscopy and two after laparotomy. In group B, one perforation of the ileum occurred after laparoscopic bladder resection with severe bowel adhesions. Ileal resection was performed on the second postoperative day. One UNC was done after ureteral lesion caused by electrocoagulation during laparoscopic resection of the bladder, rectum, and rectovaginal nodule. In addition, infection and rupture of bladder sutures occurred on the 14th postoperative day after laparoscopic bladder and rectovaginal nodule resection and re-suturation was performed. In group C, there was one fascial rupture and one postoperative hemorrhage with abscess formation requiring re-laparotomy. There were no life-threatening complications (grade IV), or complications resulting in death (grade V). Postoperative complications requiring re-intervention occurred in 9.7 % of the cases operated via laparoscopy and 9.1 % via laparotomy. Complications are shown in Table 4.

Follow-up data

Fifty patients (94 %) attended the follow-up visit 1–2 months postoperatively; 100 % in group A, 90 % in group B, and 100 % in group C. Altogether, 12 patients (12/50, 24 %) had some urinary problems at this time. One patient in group A (1/8, 13 %) had transient mild urgency. Eight patients had mild urinary problems in group B (8/28, 29 % (four dysuria, one urgency, one incontinence, two lower urinary tract infections)). In addition, one patient in group B had several problems (long-lasting postoperative pain, hematuria, and re-hydronephrosis) following shaving of bladder and ureteral endometriosis, and UNC was performed 10 months later.

Finally, two patients in group C (2/14, 14 %) had some problems at the follow-up visit. One patient continued to have pyelonephritis from the preoperative to postoperative period. The other patient had persisting pain after UNC which she had had already preoperatively and bladder atony for 4 months requiring self-catheterization; urodynamic studies were normal after 4 months. She was admitted to the pain clinic and eventually underwent hysterectomy 4 years later. These follow-up urinary problems are not included in postoperative complications in Table 4.

The mean overall length of follow-up time was 5.1 years (range 1.1–10.4 years). Two women were lost to follow-up time since they moved to another hospital district; two women were followed only 2.5 and 3 years. Five reoperations were performed among four (8 %) women because of recurrence of endometriosis. Only two of them (4 %) had recurrence of UTE. One patient needed a partial bladder resection 21 months after a shaving operation of the bladder endometriosis. The other patient had undergone previous shaving operation of ureteral endometriosis before an index operation: shaving of the bladder and ureteral nodules, resection of sacrouterine ligament endometriosis, enucleation of bilateral endometrioma, and appendectomy. After 10 months, she had recurrent hydronephrosis and UNC was performed successfully.

Table 4 Complications classified in grades I–V

		Complication (n)	Cure
Group A	Grade I–V	–	–
Group B	Grade I	Minor symptoms (postoperative pain) (2)	Hospital stay and follow-up
	Grade II	Intraoperative hemorrhage (3), with symptoms of ileus (2)	Blood transfusion, conservative care
		Hydronephrosis (1)	Ureteral catheter
		Postoperative infection (2)	Antibiotics and follow-up
		Minor bladder leakage in cystography (3)	Extended use of bladder catheter
	Grade III	Perforation of ileum (1)	Ileal resection
		Leakage from ureter with ileus (1)	Ureteroneocystostomy
		Rupture of bladder suture (1)	Bladder suturing
	Grade IV–V	–	–
Group C	Grade I	–	–
	Grade II	Intraoperative hemorrhage (7), symptoms of ileus (1), and infection (1)	Blood transfusion, conservative care, antibiotics
		Leakage from bladder to vagina and rectum, and intraoperative hemorrhage (1)	Extended use of bladder catheter, blood transfusion
	Grade III	Postoperative rupture of fascial sutures, and intraoperative hemorrhage (1)	Fascial resuturing
		Postoperative hemorrhage and abscess (1)	Evacuation of hemorrhage
	Grade IV–V	–	–

Classification of surgical complications according to Dindo et al. [6]

Group A: isolated partial cystectomy

Group B: partial cystectomy with concomitant procedures excluding UNC

Group C: UNC with concomitant procedures including partial cystectomy and nephrectomy

Postoperative fertility

Twenty-eight (53 %) of the 53 women had a wish for pregnancy after the operative treatment of UTE. Two women were to lost to follow-up during the follow-up time. Eighteen women conceived, i.e., 64 % of those who wished for a child (Fig. 1). Analysis of multiple variables revealed no statistically significant difference between the women who conceived vs. those who did not (Table 5).

There were a total of 26 pregnancies, resulting in 19 deliveries (including one twin pregnancy), four miscarriages, and one extrauterine pregnancy. Two pregnancies were ongoing in the third trimester at the end of the follow-up period. Seven (27 %) pregnancies were spontaneous, whereas ART was needed in 19 (73 %) cases, two of them with ovum donation. Altogether, 20 children were born to 16 mothers, and 57 % of those who wished for a child gave birth. The mean (±SD) time from UTE operation to delivery of the first child was 2.5 ± 1.4 years.

The rate of pregnancy complications was high; 10 (63 %) of the 16 first pregnancies required antenatal follow-up or treatment. There were three cases of hemorrhage due to partial placental abruption or total placental previa, three cases of hypertension or preeclampsia, and one case of symptomatic hydronephrosis.

Four of the first deliveries (25 %, 4/16) were vaginal, all among women belonging to Group B. However, 12 (75 %) were via cesarean section, most (75 %) involving emergency procedures for various reasons. The mean (±SD) duration of the cesarean section was 67 min (±31 min), and blood loss was 2400 ml (±2050 ml) with no difference between the groups. Similarly, there were intraoperative difficulties in 10 (83 %) cases: 6 cases (i.e., 50 %) of severe adhesions, four cases of difficulties with extraction of the neonate, 2 cases of bladder laceration, 1 case of uterine atony, and 1 case of difficult placental retrieval. None of the women concerned had had severe complications during their UTE operations. Both women with bladder injuries had undergone partial cystectomy because of bladder endometriosis (group B).

The average weight of the first full-term infants (n = 14) was 3.3 kg (SD 0.48 kg), Apgar scores at 5 min were seven or

more in all cases, and cord blood pH was on average 7.25 (7.06–7.37). There were three preterm deliveries (19 %) and these neonates were also healthy.

Conclusions

We found that the UTE operations were usually associated with other DIE lesions making them demanding; isolated bladder and ureteral endometriosis were rare. However, the rate of postoperative complications was acceptable and the recurrence rate was low. The women conceived better than expected according to the results of previous studies concerning DIE other than UTE [28–30], but needed infertility treatment. On the other hand, the pregnancies and deliveries were complicated, and the high rate of complicated cesarean deliveries was particularly worrying.

The patients with UTE were typical endometriosis patients—on average nonsmoking, normal-weight 35-year-old women with a wish for a child and thus no current use of hormonal medication. Nine out of 10 patients suffered from dysmenorrhea and more than half suffered from symptoms suggestive of UTE. As in other studies [7, 10, 31–35], almost half of our patients had a history of previous endometriosis surgery. This might indicate that the delay in reaching the correct diagnosis and getting to the referral center is long.

Urinary tract symptoms occurred in almost three quarters of the patients with bladder endometriosis, and severe pain in nearly half of the patients with ureteral endometriosis. Bladder endometriosis was not suspected preoperatively in nearly a third of the patients; only two of them had urinary tract symptoms and they all suffered from severe DIE. MRI was performed in two thirds of the patients and the preoperative diagnosis was correct in more than 70 % of the cases. Ureteral disease was undiagnosed only once with UNC patients when hydronephrosis was not noticed in MRI [3]. Nowadays, preoperative assessment to localize all DIE lesions is recommended to decide the surgical approach and to plan a multidisciplinary team work. Our preoperative examinations include nowadays thorough ultrasound mapping of the pelvis [36] and MRI to diagnose all DIE lesions and even asymptomatic DIE lesions before renal function is impaired.

Half of all our operations were performed via laparoscopy. A similar rate has been reported in previous studies, in which many concomitant procedures have also been performed [5, 6, 34] but there are also reports where all or almost all urinary tract operations have been performed laparoscopically [3, 7, 10, 32, 37, 38]. All our isolated bladder resections and associated ureteral shavings were done laparoscopically as in many other series [10, 35, 39, 40] but with increasing amount of concomitant procedures also the proportion of laparotomies increased. Further, in contrast to some other studies [24, 41–43], none of the UNCs were performed via laparoscopy

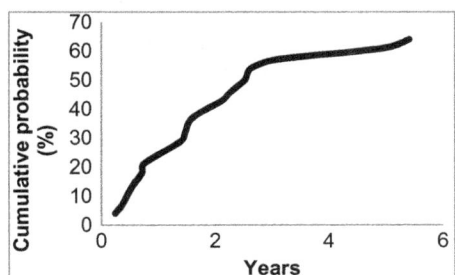

Fig. 1 Number of women who conceived, i.e., 64 % of those who wished for a child

Table 5 Characteristics of women wishing to conceive

Variable	Women who did not conceive ($n = 10$)	Women who conceived ($n = 18$)	p value	Spontaneous pregnancy ($n = 6$)
Age (years, SD)	33.8 (4.6)	33.0 (3.1)	0.549	34.6 (3.5)
BMI (kg/m^2, SD)	23.1 (3.2)	22.1 (2.4)	0.389	21.1 (2.8)
Smoking	2 (20)	0 (0)	0.119	0 (0)
Previously gravid	1 (10)	4 (27)	0.745	2 (33)
Previous deliveries	0 (0)	3 (17)	0.393	1 (17)
Previous infertility	7 (70)	11 (61)	0.703	3 (50)
Previous operations due to endometriosis	6 (60)	3 (17)	0.100	0 (0)
Type of endometriosis			0.961	
Group A	2 (20)	4 (27)		1 (17)
Group B	5 (50)	8 (44)		4 (67)
Group C	3 (30)	6 (33)		1 (17)
Laparoscopy	5 (50)	10 (56)	0.544	5 (83)
Bowel resection	4 (40)	8 (44)	1.000	2 (33)
Hydronephrosis	2 (20)	6 (33)	0.669	1 (17)
Status of ovaries after operation			0.399	
No procedures	6 (60)	10 (56)		4 (67)
To one ovary	1 (10)	4 (22)		2 (33)
To both ovaries	0 (0)	2 (11)		0 (0)
Frequent procedures	3 (30)	2 (11)		0 (09
Major complications			0.341	
Grade I	1 (10)	0 (0)		0 (0)
Grade II	5 (50)	6 (33)		2 (33)
Grade III	0 (0)	1 (6)		0 (0)
Grade IV	0 (0)	0 (0)		0 (0)
Follow-up time (years, SD)	5.2 (3.3)	5.5 (2.4)	0.767	4.2 (1.6)

Data are shown as n (%) unless stated otherwise

in our series as our urologist are not yet so familiar with advanced laparoscopy.

As there is no specific procedure code for ureterolysis, we were unable to retrieve all ureteral shaving operations performed in connection with DIE of the rectovaginal septum. The indications for UNC in our study were moderate or severe hydronephrosis with or without decrease in the kidney function, silent kidney, and reoperation in which ureterolysis could not be performed. Preoperative differentiation between intrinsic and extrinsic ureteral endometriosis is not always easy. Extrinsic type of ureteral endometriosis is more common and endometriosis lesion invades only to the ureteral adventitia or surrounding connective tissue without hydronephrosis. This type of endometriosis can be treated by ureteral shaving but the recurrence rate varies from 20 to 33 % [3]. Intrinsic type of ureteral endometriosis represents around 20 % of cases and lesion infiltrates to the muscular layer of the ureter. This type of endometriosis with moderate or severe hydronephrosis often needs ureteral resection and reanatomosis or reimplantation. It is controversial what kind of operation is needed in case of hydronephroses and diminished renal function [3].

Large endometriotic nodule and severe hydronephrosis are risk factors for adverse outcome and might be indications for ureteral resection [35]. In our study, UNC was chosen as endometriotic lesions were large, situated near the bladder wall, or caused hydronephrosis but most of the lesions were extrinsic by histology. It means that in theory ureterolysis via ureteral shaving could have been performed more often [31, 44]. In the future, we aim to increase the proportion of laparoscopic surgery in UTE as in many other referral centers.

UTE cannot be discussed without taking the other aspects of DIE affecting the symptoms and operations into consideration. As expected, the operations in our study were difficult and concomitant procedures were numerous. Also, the rate of bowel resection was higher (i.e., 40 %) than in some studies [6, 32, 33, 39, 43]. However, some of the previous studies have included patients with only isolated bladder endometriosis or cases where only ureteral endometriosis has been operated upon [6, 38]. Moreover, collaboration of different specialists is not commonly reported, even though the purpose is complete resection of all endometriotic lesions in the same operation. In Finland, multidisciplinary approach is recommended [31, 43, 45] in contrast to some other countries where gynecologist commonly perform urinary and gastrointestinal surgery on their own [3, 38]. In our study, a second specialist, either a urologist or a gastrointestinal surgeon, attended the operation in more than 60 % of the cases.

The rate and type of complications was in line with those reported in previous studies [5, 31, 33]. The most typical complication was intraoperative hemorrhage of over 1000 ml, but this only occurred during laparotomies. The amount of intraoperative bleeding is rarely reported in other studies. Altogether, 53 % had some problems postoperatively; most of them were minor. However, 9 % of women needed a reoperation for complications: perforation of the ileum after adhesiolysis, ureteral lesion caused by electrocoagulation in connection with bowel resection, rupture of bladder sutures, rupture of fascial sutures, and intra-abdominal abscess. There was no difference in complications needing a re-intervention between laparoscopy or laparotomy. Three bladder leakages were discovered in routine cystography before removal of a bladder catheter and leakage was cured with prolonged use of the catheter. In addition, urine leakage from the bladder to the vagina and rectum 1 day after the removal of a bladder catheter was cured with extended use of a catheter whereas one postoperative hydronephrosis was treated with a ureteral stent.

Ninety-four percent of women attended the follow-up visit, 76 % of them were asymptomatic and only one patient needed temporary self-catheterization after removal of the bladder catheter. Twenty-four percent of women had some problems at 1–2 months postoperatively but only 4 % (2/50) were severe. The long-term follow-up was 5.1 years and two women were lost after moving elsewhere. The recurrence rate of UTE following surgery was 4 %, which is comparable with that in previous studies [6, 10, 33–35]. Thus, it has been suggested that recurrences are less common after surgery for UTE than for other forms of endometriosis [10].

Fertility has been studied more widely among DIE than UTE patients. As infertility was affecting over half of our patients preoperatively, we consider that reporting postoperative pregnancy rates is important. Only a few studies have involved assessment of fertility following surgical treatment of UTE and to our knowledge there are no previous studies of pregnancy complications or deliveries. A cohort study of 109 women reported postsurgical fertility after laparoscopic excision of ureteral endometriosis, demonstrating a total of 26 pregnancies in 20 women (56 %), among the 36 women who wished to conceive [35]. In studies concerning fertility after operative treatment of rectovaginal endometriosis, the postoperative pregnancy rate has ranged between 19 and 65 % among all patients [28–30, 46], and among patients with a history of infertility, between 10 and 58 % [28, 30, 45, 46]. In our study, the corresponding figures were 64 and 61 %. Moreover, live birth rates were 56 and 61 %, which is very encouraging. As ART was needed in most cases, these figures

might also reflect the development of infertility treatments, as also suggested in connection with a national Danish cohort study [47]. Remarkably, in two cases treatment with donated oocytes was used, although in one of these cases several procedures involving both ovaries were performed.

Analysis of multiple pre- and perioperative factors did not reveal any differences between women who eventually conceived vs. those who did not. This is in contrast to the results of previous studies, in which concurrent adenomyosis or hydronephrosis [35], older woman or high ASRM scores [48], or surgical treatment by means of laparotomy [28, 46] has been associated with lower postoperative pregnancy rates among women with DIE. Unfortunately, we do not have data on the incidence of adenomyosis in our patients. In our study, only one spontaneous pregnancy occurred after laparotomy and five spontaneous pregnancies occurred after laparoscopy.

To our knowledge, no previous study has been carried out to assess the incidence of pregnancy or delivery complications among women who have undergone operation for UTE. A high rate, up to three quarters of all pregnancies and deliveries in our series, were complicated. In a large Swedish registry-based study, all forms of endometriosis were found to be associated with increased risks of preeclampsia, antepartum hemorrhage, and preterm birth as well as an increase in the rate of cesarean delivery [49]. Moreover, rectovaginal endometriosis has been associated with a risk of placenta previa [30]. Thus, our results on the rate of complicated delivery are in line with those concerning endometriosis in general or DIE [30, 49], with the exception that the rate of cesarean delivery was even higher. In addition, the majority of these deliveries ended as emergency operations, hemorrhage exceeding 1500 ml occurred in more than half of the cases and intraoperative problems occurred in 80 % of the cesarean deliveries. All these figures are several-fold greater than those reported in connection with cesarean sections overall in Finland [50]. As the number of cesarean deliveries was limited, we did not see a significant correlation between various perioperative factors in the primary operation (such as blood loss) and the risk of emergency or complicated cesarean section. In our series, bladder was opened in all except two patients either due to resection of bladder endometriosis or in connection with UNC procedure. Postoperative adhesions could in theory make cesarean sections more difficult. Hence, according to this study, both pregnancy and delivery complications were common after operative treatment of UTE.

Our study has limitations. In this retrospective case series, the number of patients is small, which is a common problem in connection with this form of endometriosis. Operative skills of our gynecologists may not be as good as in larger laparoscopic centers. However, the retrospective nature of the study does not impair its validity, as we had good access to all follow-up data including the postoperative pregnancies and their outcomes. Also, the follow-up time is one of the longest [32, 33].

In conclusion, with the use of preoperative imaging, planning, and multidisciplinary team work, the complication and recurrence rates of operatively treated UTE are acceptable. Two thirds of the women who wished for pregnancy conceived, but mostly by means of ART. However, pregnancies and deliveries following UTE surgery may carry a risk of complications. Thus, centralizing the overall care of UTE patients to a few referral centers seems justified.

Acknowledgments This study was supported by Helsinki University Central Hospital Research funds.

The authors would like to thank Arja-Riitta Pauna for radiological consultation and Maarit Mentula for her kind advice with the statistics.

Authors' contribution L Saavalainen performed data collection and managing, data analysis, and manuscript writing. O Heikinheimo was responsible for project development, data analysis, and manuscript editing. A Tiitinen was responsible for project development and manuscript editing. P Härkki was responsible for project development, data managing, data analysis, and manuscript editing.

Compliance with ethical standards

Informed consent For this kind of electronic data-based study, informed consent is not required in Finland.

Human studies This article does not contain any studies with human participants performed by any of the authors.

References

1. Maccagnano C, Pellucchi F, Rocchini L, Ghezzi M, Scattoni V, Montorsi F, Rigatti P, Colombo R (2012) Diagnosis and treatment of bladder endometriosis: state of the art. Urol Int 89:249–258. doi:10.1159/000339519

2. Maccagnano C, Pellucchi F, Rocchini L, Ghezzi M, Scattoni V, Montorsi F, Rigatti P, Colombo R (2013) Ureteral endometriosis: proposal for a diagnostic and therapeutic algorithm with a review of the literature. Urol Int 91:1–9. doi:10.1159/000345140

3. Knabben L, Imboden S, Fellmann B, Nirgianakis K, Kuhn A, Mueller MD (2015) Urinary tract endometriosis in patients with deep infiltrating endometriosis: prevalence, symptoms, management, and proposal for a new clinical classification. Fertil Steril 103:147–152

4. Donnez J, Nisolle M, Squifflet J (2002) Ureteral endometriosis: a complication of rectovaginal endometriotic (adenomyotic) nodules. Fertil Steril 77:32–37. doi:10.1016/S0015-0282(01)02921-1

5. Kjer JJ, Kristensen J, Hartwell D, Jensen MA (2014) Full-thickness endometriosis of the bladder: report of 31 cases. Eur J Obstet Gynecol Reprod Biol 176:31–33. doi:10.1016/j.ejogrb.2014.02.018

6. Antonelli A, Simeone C, Zani D, Sacconi T, Minini G, Canossi E, Cunico S (2006) Clinical aspects and surgical treatment of urinary tract endometriosis: our experience with 31 cases. Eur Urol 49: 1093–1098. doi:10.1016/j.eururo.2006.03.037

7. Bosev D, Nicoll LM, Bhagan L, Lemyre M, Payne CK, Gill H, Nezhat C (2009) Laparoscopic management of ureteral endometriosis: the Stanford University hospital experience with 96 consecutive cases. J Urol 182:2748–2752. doi:10.1016/j.juro.2009.08.019

8. Roman H, Vassilieff M, Gourcerol G, Savoye G, Leroi AM, Marpeau L, Michot F, Tuech JJ (2011) Surgical management of deep infiltrating endometriosis of the rectum: pleading for a symptom-guided approach. Hum Reprod 26:274–281. doi:10.1093/humrep/deq332

9. Payá V, Hidalgo-Mora J, Diaz-Garcia C, Pellier A (2011) Surgical treatment of rectovaginal endometriosis with rectal involvement. Gynecol Surg 8:269–277

10. Seracchioli R, Mabrouk M, Montanari G, Manuzzi L, Concetti S, Venturoli S (2010) Conservative laparoscopic management of urinary tract endometriosis (UTE): surgical outcome and long-term follow-up. Fertil Steril 94:856–861. doi:10.1016/j.fertnstert.2009.04.019

11. Dunselman GAJ, Vermeulen N, Becker C, Calhaz-Jorge C, D'Hooghe T, De Bie B, Heikinheimo O, Horne AW, Kiesel L, Nap A, Prentice A, Saridogan E, Soriano D, Nelen W (2014) ESHRE guideline: management of women with endometriosis. Hum Reprod 29:400–412. doi:10.1093/humrep/det457

12. Gupta S, Agarwall A, Agarwal R, Ricardo Loret de Mola J (2006) Impact of ovarian endometrioma on assisted reproduction outcomes. Reprod Biomed 13:349–360

13. Benaglia L, Pasin R, Somigliana E, Vercellini P, Ragni G, Fedele L (2011) Unoperated ovarian endometriomas and responsiveness to hyperstimulation. Hum Reprod 26:1356–1361. doi:10.1093/humrep/der097

14. Ruiz-Flores FJ, Garcia-Velasco JA (2012) Is there a benefit for surgery in endometrioma-associated infertility? Curr Opin Obstet Gynecol 24:136–140. doi:10.1097/GCO.0b013e32835175d9

15. Papaleo E, Ottolina J, Vigano P, Brigante C, Marsiglio E, De Michele F, Candiani M (2011) Deep pelvic endometriosis negatively affects ovarian reserve and the number of oocytes retrieved for in vitro fertilization. Acta Obstet Gynecol Scand 90:878–884. doi:10.1111/j.1600-0412.2011.01161.x

16. Ballester M, Oppenheimer A, d'Argent EM, Touboul C, Antoine J, Nisolle M, Darai E (2012) Deep infiltrating endometriosis is a determinant factor of cumulative pregnancy rate after intracytoplasmic sperm injection/in vitro fertilization cycles in patients with endometriomas. Fertil Steril 97:367–3U2. doi:10.1016/j.fertnstert.2011.11.022

17. Somigliana E, Berlanda N, Benaglia L, Vigano P, Vercellini P, Fedele L (2012) Surgical excision of endometriomas and ovarian reserve: a systematic review on serum antimullerian hormone level modifications. Fertil Steril 98:1531–1538. doi:10.1016/j.fertnstert.2012.08.009

18. Muzii L, Di Tucci C, Di Feliciantonio M, Marchetti C, Perniola G, PB P (2014) The effect of surgery for endometrioma on ovarian reserve evaluated by antral follicle count: a systematic review and meta-analysis. Hum Reprod 29:2190–2198. doi:10.1093/humrep/deu199

19. Stepniewska A, Pomini P, Bruni F, Mereu L, Ruffo G, Ceccaroni M, Scioscia M, Guerriero M, Minelli L (2009) Laparoscopic treatment of bowel endometriosis in infertile women. Hum Reprod 24: 1619–1625. doi:10.1093/humrep/dep083

20. Bianchi PHM, Pereira RMA, Zanatta A, Alegretti JR, Motta ELA, Serafini PC (2009) Extensive excision of deep infiltrative endometriosis before in vitro fertilization significantly improves pregnancy rates. J Minim Invasive Gynecol 16:174–180. doi:10.1016/j.jmig.2008.12.009

21. Douay-Hauser N, Yazbeck C, Walker F, Luton D, Madelenat P, Koskas M (2011) Infertile women with deep and intraperitoneal endometriosis: comparison of fertility outcome according to the extent of surgery. J Minim Invasive Gynecol 18:622–628. doi:10.1016/j.jmig.2011.06.004

22. Vercellini P, Pietropaolo G, De Giorgi O, Daguati R, Pasin R, Crosignani PG (2006) Reproductive performance in infertile women with rectovaginal endometriosis: is surgery worthwhile? Obstet Gynecol 195:1303–1310. doi:10.1016/j.ajog.2006.03.068

23. Kondo W, Darai E, Yazbeck C, Panel P, Tamburro S, Dubuisson J, Jardon K, Mage G, Madelenat P, Canis M (2011) Do patients manage to achieve pregnancy after a major complication of deeply infiltrating endometriosis resection? Eur J Obstet Gynecol Reprod Biol 154:196–199. doi:10.1016/j.ejogrb.2010.09.007

24. Berlanda N, Vercellini P, Fedele L (2010) The outcomes of repeat surgery for recurrent symptomatic endometriosis. Curr Opin Obstet Gynecol 22:320–325. doi:10.1097/GCO.0b013e32833bea15

25. Vercellini P, Somigliana E, Daguati R, Barbara G, Abbiati A, Fedele L (2009) The second time around: reproductive performance after repetitive versus primary surgery for endometriosis. Fertil Steril 92:1253–1255. doi:10.1016/j.fertnstert.2009.04.037

26. Roman H (2015) Colorectal endometriosis and pregnancy wish: why doing primary surgery. Front Biosci 7:83–93

27. Dindo D, Demartines N, Clavien P (2004) Classification of surgical complications—a new proposal with evaluation in a cohort of 6336 patients and results of a survey. Ann Surg 240:205–213. doi:10.1097/01.sla.0000133083.54934.ae

28. Darai E, Lesieur B, Dubernard G, Rouzier R, Bazot M, Ballester M (2011) Fertility after colorectal resection for endometriosis: results of a prospective study comparing laparoscopy with open surgery. Fertil Steril 95:1903–1908. doi:10.1016/j.fertnstert.2011.02.018

29. Tarjanne S, Heikinheimo O, Mentula M, Harkki P (2015) Complications and long-term follow-up on colorectal resections in the treatment of deep infiltrating endometriosis extending to bowel wall. Acta Obstet Gynecol Scand 94:72–79. doi:10.1111/aogs.12515

30. Vercellini P, Parazzini F, Pietropaolo G, Cipriani S, Frattaruolo MP, Fedele L (2012) Pregnancy outcome in women with peritoneal, ovarian and rectovaginal endometriosis: a retrospective cohort study. BJOP 119:1538–1543. doi:10.1111/j.1471-0528.2012.03466.x

31. Rozsnyai F, Roman H, Resch B, Dugardin F, Berrocal J, Descargues G, Schmied R, Boukerrou M, Marpeau L, CIRENDO Study Grp (2011) Outcomes of surgical management of deep infiltrating endometriosis of the ureter and urinary bladder. JSLS 15:439–447. doi:10.4293/108680811X13176785203798

32. Schonman R, Dotan Z, Weintraub AY, Bibi G, Eisenberg VH, Seidman DS, Goldenberg M, Soriano D (2013) Deep endometriosis inflicting the bladder: long-term outcomes of surgical management. Arch Gynecol Obstet 288:1323–1328. doi:10.1007/s00404-013-2917-6

33. Chapron C, Bourret A, Chopin N, Dousset B, Leconte M, Amsellem-Ouazana D, de Ziegler D, Borghese B (2010) Surgery for bladder endometriosis: long-term results and concomitant management of associated posterior deep lesions. Hum Reprod 25:884–889. doi:10.1093/humrep/deq017

34. Fedele L, Bianchi SF, Zanconato G, Bergamini V, Berlanda N, Carmignani L (2005) Long-term follow-up after conservative surgery for bladder endometriosis. Fertil Steril 83:1729–1733. doi:10.1016/j.fertnstert.2004.12.047

35. Uccella S, Cromi A, Casarin J, Bogani G, Pinelli C, Serati M, Ghezzi F (2014) Laparoscopy for ureteral endometriosis: surgical details, long-term follow-up, and fertility outcomes. Fertil Steril 102:160- +. doi:10.1016/j.fertnstert.2014.03.055

36. Exacoustos C, Malzoni M, Di Giovanni A, Lazzeri L, Tosti C, Petraglia F, Zupi E (2014) Ultrasound mapping system for the surgical management of deep infiltrating endometriosis. Fertil Steril 102:143- +. doi:10.1016/j.fertnstert.2014.03.043

37. Ghezzi F, Cromi A, Bergamini V, Serati M, Sacco A, Mueller MD (2006) Outcome of laparoscopic ureterolysis for ureteral endometriosis. Fertil Steril 86:418–422. doi:10.1016/j.fertnstert.2005.12.071

38. Frenna V, Santos L, Ohana E, Bailey C, Wattiez A (2007) Laparoscopic management of ureteral endometriosis: our experience. J Minim Invasive Gynecol 14:169–171. doi:10.1016/j.jmig.2006.09.009

39. Kovoor E, Nassif J, Miranda-Mendoza I, Wattiez A (2010) Endometriosis of bladder: outcomes after laparoscopic surgery. J Minim Invasive Gynecol 17:600–604. doi:10.1016/j.jmig.2010.05.008

40. Nezhat C, Nezhat F, Nezhat CH, Nasserbakht F, Rosati M, Seidman DS (1996) Urinary tract endometriosis treated by laparoscopy. Fertil Steril 66:920–924

41. Mereu L, Gagliardi ML, Clarizia R, Mainardi P, Landi S, Minelli L (2010) Laparoscopic management of ureteral endometriosis in case of moderate-severe hydroureteronephrosis. Fertil Steril 93:46–51. doi:10.1016/j.fertnstert.2008.09.076

42. Stepniewska A, Grosso G, Molon A, Caleffi G, Perin E, Scioscia M, Mainardi P, Minelli L (2011) Ureteral endometriosis: clinical and radiological follow-up after laparoscopic ureterocystoneostomy. Hum Reprod 26:112–116. doi:10.1093/humrep/deq293

43. Schonman R, Dotan Z, Weintraub AY, Goldenberg M, Seidman DS, Schiff E, Soriano D (2013) Long-term follow-up after ureteral reimplantation in patients with severe deep infiltrating endometriosis. Eur J Obstet Gynecol Reprod Biol 171:146–149. doi:10.1016/j.ejogrb.2013.08.027

44. Miranda-Mendoza I, Kovoor E, Nassif J, Ferreira H, Wattiez A (2012) Laparoscopic surgery for severe ureteric endometriosis. Eur J Obstet Gynecol Reprod Biol 165:275–279. doi:10.1016/j.ejogrb.2012.07.002

45. Stepniewska A, Pomini P, Scioscia M, Mereu L, Ruffo G, Minelli L (2010) Fertility and clinical outcome after bowel resection in infertile women with endometriosis. Reprod BioMed Online 20:602–609. doi:10.1016/j.rbmo.2009.12.029

46. Ferrero S, Anserini P, Abbamonte LH, Ragni N, Camerini G, Remorgida V (2009) Fertility after bowel resection for endometriosis. Fertil Steril 92:41–46. doi:10.1016/j.fertnstert.2008.04.070

47. Hansen MVH, Dalsgaard T, Hartwell D, Skovlund CW, Lidegaard O (2014) Reproductive prognosis in endometriosis. A national cohort study. Acta Obstet Gynecol Scand 93:483–489. doi:10.1111/aogs.12373

48. Darai E, Carbonnel M, Dubernard G, Lavoue V, Coutant C, Bazot M, Ballester M (2010) Determinant factors of fertility outcomes after laparoscopic colorectal resection for endometriosis. Eur J Obstet Gynecol Reprod Biol 149:210–214. doi:10.1016/j.ejogrb.2009.12.032

49. Stephansson O, Kieler H, Granath F, Falconer H (2009) Endometriosis, assisted reproduction technology, and risk of adverse pregnancy outcome. Hum Reprod 24:2341–2347. doi:10.1093/humrep/dep186

50. Pallasmaa N, Ekblad U, Aitokallio-Tallberg A, Uotila J, Raudaskoski T, Ulander V, Hurme S (2010) Cesarean delivery in Finland: maternal complications and obstetric risk factors. Acta Obstet Gynecol Scand 89:896–902. doi:10.3109/00016349.2010.487893

37

Ergonomics of laparoscopic graspers and the importance of haptic feedback: the surgeons' perspective

Chantal C. J. Alleblas[1] · Michel P. H. Vleugels[2] · Theodoor E. Nieboer[1]

Abstract Haptic feedback is drastically reduced in laparoscopic surgery compared to open surgery. Introducing enhanced haptic feedback in laparoscopic instruments might well improve surgical safety and efficiency. In the design process of a laparoscopic grasper with enhanced haptic feedback, handle design should be addressed to strive for optimal usability and comfort. Additionally, the surgeons' perspective on the potential benefits of haptic feedback should be assessed to ascertain the clinical interest of enhanced haptic feedback. A questionnaire was designed to determine surgeons' use and preferences for laparoscopic instruments and expectations about enhanced haptic feedback. Surgeons were also asked whether they experience physical complaints related to laparoscopic instruments. The questionnaire was distributed to a group of laparoscopic surgeons based in Europe. From the 279 contacted subjects, 98 completed the questionnaire (response rate 35 %). Of all respondents, 77 % reported physical complaints directly attributable to the use of laparoscopic instruments. No evident similarity in the main preference for graspers was found, either with or without haptic feedback. According to respondents, the added value of haptic feedback could be of particular use in feeling differences in tissue consistencies, feeling the applied pressure, locating a tumor or enlarged lymph node, feeling arterial pulse, and limiting strain in the surgeon's hand. This study stresses that the high prevalence of physical complaints directly related to laparoscopic

instruments among laparoscopic surgeons is still relevant. Furthermore, the potential benefits of enhanced haptic feedback in laparoscopic surgery are recognized by laparoscopic specialists. Therefore, haptic feedback is considered an unmet need in laparoscopy.

Keywords Laparoscopy · Ergonomics · Human-product interaction · Haptic feedback

Background

In laparoscopic surgery, haptic feedback should enable surgeons to perceive interaction forces between instrument and tissue. This is beneficial information regarding accurate regulation of tissue manipulation forces and recognition of tissue characteristics. In open surgery, the surgeon is able to manipulate tissue directly with the gloved hand; i.e., the surgeon directly perceives haptic feedback. In contrast, during laparoscopy, the surgeon can only manipulate tissue indirectly due to the interference of instruments, which are inserted through small incisions. Consequently, haptic feedback is drastically reduced in laparoscopic surgery compared to open abdominal surgery. This is mainly caused by the friction within instruments and dynamic properties of the laparoscopic surgical setup [1, 2]. Introducing enhanced haptic feedback in laparoscopic instruments might well be beneficial for surgical safety and efficiency.

The results of several (pre)clinical studies show that haptic feedback is deficient in laparoscopic surgery [3–5]. Moreover, intra-operative complications appear to be often the result of intentional actions, resulting in unintentional outcomes, caused by visual misperception [6–8]. Additionally, surgical specialists have identified technology as one of the most important risk domains for patient safety [9]. Tholey et al. found that the availability of both visual and haptic feedback leads to

✉ Chantal C. J. Alleblas
  chantal.alleblas@radboudumc.nl

[1] Department of Obstetrics and Gynecology, Radboud University Medical Center, P.O. Box 9101, 6500HB Nijmegen, The Netherlands

[2] Department of Obstetrics and Gynecology, Riverland Hospital, Tiel, The Netherlands

Table 1 Demographic information

Characteristics	Data	
	Mean	Standard deviation
Age in years	45.5	8.9
Glove size (general)	7.4	0.6
Glove size (men)	7.6	0.4
Glove size (women)	6.8	0.4
Years of experience	17.7	8.5
Years of experience in endoscopy	13.5	8.2
Endoscopic procedures per month	16.5	14.2

better tissue characterization than exclusively visual or haptic feedback [10]. Previous studies argue for the implementation of enhanced haptic feedback to increase efficiency in terms of more successful grasping actions [11] and accurate control over the instrument-tissue interaction forces [12]. Two recently published literature reviews provide an overview of studies that have been performed regarding haptic feedback in minimally invasive surgery [2, 13]. The authors conclude that both patients and surgeons may well benefit from enhanced haptic feedback in minimally invasive surgical equipment. Although several technological efforts have been made in artificial settings, it is argued that a clinically driven approach should be deployed for a feasible application in surgical practice [14].

Laparoscopic instruments are known to cause physical discomfort [15, 16] and, moreover, to cause injuries especially affecting the thumbs [17, 18]. Furthermore, almost all laparoscopic handles come with the adage "one size fits all" whereas small hand size is a known risk factor for experiencing physical discomfort and difficulties in the use of laparoscopic instruments [19–21]. Instrument handles are the most important physical interface for laparoscopic surgeons [22]. To strive for optimal usability and comfort, handle design should be specifically addressed during the design process of new types of surgical instruments.

Related to the development of a laparoscopic haptic feedback grasper [23], the tools that are already used in laparoscopy need to be evaluated. The involvement of end users in the design process is indispensible for suitability, safety, and acceptance [24, 25]. Therefore, the aim of this study was to perform an evaluation of expert opinions regarding handle designs of currently used laparoscopic gaspers and to determine surgeons' needs and expectations regarding haptic feedback instruments.

Methods

A questionnaire was designed to determine the surgeons' current use of instruments, their physical complaints related to instrument use, as well as their needs and preferences for laparoscopic instruments. Furthermore, we aimed to identify expectations regarding haptic feedback in future instrument developments. The survey was distributed among attendees of the 23rd annual congress of the European Society for Gynecological Endoscopy (September 2014) and the annual meeting of the Dutch Working Group for Gynecological Endoscopy (October 2014). Additionally, an online version was distributed among the members of the Dutch Society of Endoscopic Surgery (January 2015). The questionnaire was accompanied with an explanation of the aim and was subdivided into categories concerning demographics, physical complaints related to laparoscopic instrument use, handgrip assessment of currently used laparoscopic graspers, preferences for handle designs, and expectations regarding implementation of haptic feedback in laparoscopic surgery. Questions and answer options are presented in the Appendix. A descriptive data analysis was performed with SPSS software, version 22.

Findings

Demographics

A total of 279 subjects were contacted. The number of returned questionnaires was 98 (response rate 35 %), among which were 63 gynecologists, 27 general surgeons, 4

Fig. 1 Prevalence of physical complaints in the upper extremities (directly attributable to the use of laparoscopic instruments)

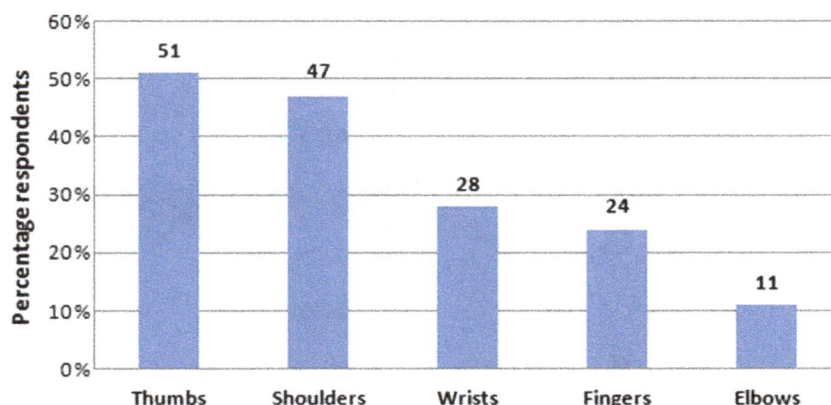

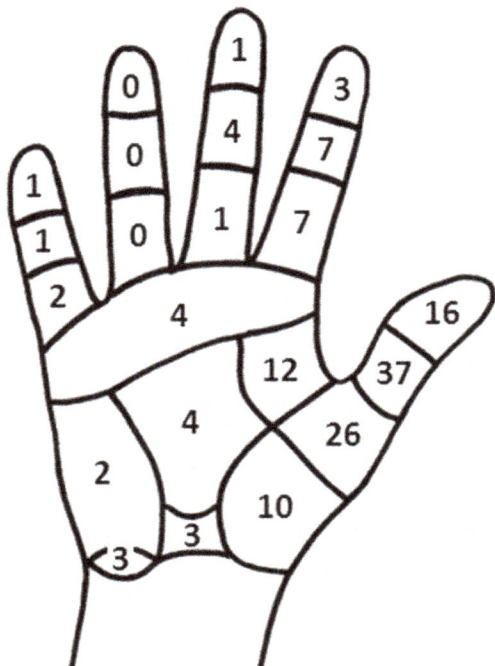

Fig. 2 Hand map [26] including the frequency of reported areas of discomfort due to pressure caused by instruments

urologists, 2 pediatric surgeons, and 2 medical technicians. The majority of respondents were male (68 %). Four respondents were left-handed, and 9 respondents were ambidextrous. All respondents worked in Europe of which the majority was established in The Netherlands (86 %). Table 1 presents the additional demographic data.

Physical complaints

Overall, 77 % of the surgeons reported physical complaints directly attributable to the use of laparoscopic instruments. Figure 1 illustrates the prevalence of physical complaints as indicated for specific parts of the upper extremities. The frequency of discomfort in the palm of the hand from pressure caused by instruments as indicated by the surgeons is illustrated in Fig. 2 [26].

Handgrip assessment

Handles including indicated use and preferences by respondents are shown in Fig. 3. The long-lever pistol grip was most commonly used. When combined, 99 % of respondents indicated that they used at least one of the two types of scissors handles. Respondents were asked in what percentage of laparoscopic procedures they used each handle type. A total of 24 % respondents indicated that they used the back-hinged scissors handle during all procedures. For the front-hinged scissors handle, this was 32 %. Less often used as standard equipment was the in-line handle (4 %) and the long-lever pistol grip (12 %), whereas the short-lever pistol grip was never reported to be used in all procedures. When specifically asked what kind of handle would be preferred for a haptic feedback instrument, the front-hinged scissors handle and the long-lever pistol grip were most frequently chosen. Regarding the usability of handgrips, three aspects including functionality, comfort, and freedom of movement were assessed on a 7-point Likert scale. The long-lever pistol grip scored the highest on all the three aspects (Table 2).

Two extra user features were evaluated. Respondents were asked to estimate what percentage of time they positioned their index finger forward on the rotation knob of the handle. The majority (48 %) of respondents reported to adopt this grip during less than a quarter of the overall procedure time, and 16 % reported to adopt this grip for over 75 % of the procedure time. Furthermore, 51 % of respondents indicated to control a scissors handle by means of a so-called "palm grip" as illustrated in Fig. 4. The most frequently reported reasons to do this were as follows: in case of more static surgical steps, in case the application of more force is necessary, or in order to relieve strain or pressure on the thumb.

Haptic feedback

To estimate the added value of haptic feedback in clinical scenarios, respondents were asked to assess nine scenarios on a 6-point Likert scale where 0 means "not useful" and 5 means "very

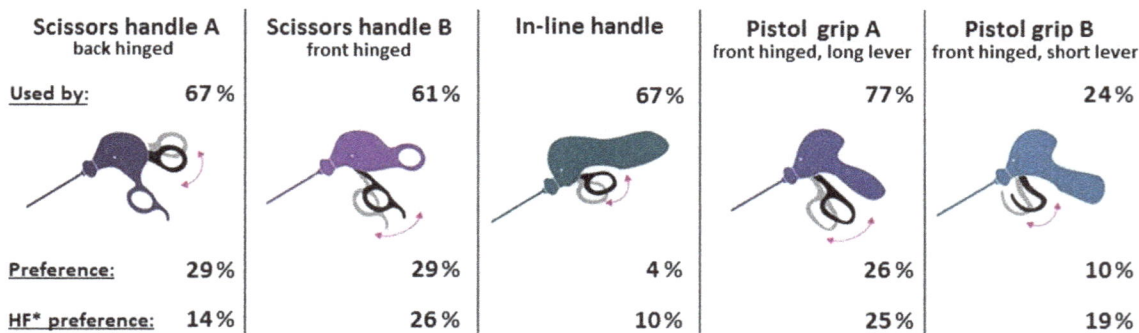

Scissors handle A back hinged	Scissors handle B front hinged	In-line handle	Pistol grip A front hinged, long lever	Pistol grip B front hinged, short lever
Used by: 67 %	61%	67%	77%	24%
Preference: 29%	29%	4%	26%	10%
HF* preference: 14%	26%	10%	25%	19%

Fig. 3 Presented handles for assessment including use and preferences for current use and future haptic feedback instruments. *HF* haptic feedback

Table 2 Handgrip usability assessment

Handle	Functionality	Comfort	Freedom of movement
Scissors handle A	4.4 ± 1.8	3.8 ± 1.7	4.1 ± 1.5
Scissors handle B	5.0 ± 1.4	4.6 ± 1.4	4.9 ± 1.3
In-line handle	4.0 ± 1.6	4.6 ± 1.5	4.7 ± 1.6
Pistol grip A	5.3 ± 1.4	5.3 ± 1.4	5.0 ± 1.3
Pistol grip B	4.5 ± 1.8	4.6 ± 1.7	4.4 + 1.6

For illustrations of the handle types, see Fig. 3. Assessment was based on a 7-point Likert scale where 1 means "the worst" and 7 means "the best" for the constructs' functionality and freedom of movement. Comfort was assessed on a 7-point Likert scale where 1 means "very uncomfortable" and 7 means "very comfortable"

useful" for clinical practice. The results are presented in Table 3. The possibility to feel differences in tissue consistencies and the ability to feel how much pressure is being applied were expected to be the most promising outcomes of integrated haptic feedback. Reduction of operation time and reduction of conversions to open surgery were least expected be a consequence of enhanced haptic feedback.

Discussion

In this study, expert experiences and opinions regarding handle designs of laparoscopic graspers and regarding implementation of enhanced haptic feedback were evaluated. This study shows, with a prevalence of 77 %, that physical complaints related to the use of laparoscopic instruments are commonly experienced. Whereas direct questioning revealed no similar handgrip preference among the surgical specialists, the handgrip usability assessment results favored the long-lever pistol grip design. Furthermore, the results regarding the utility assessment of haptic feedback show clinical support for the implementation of enhanced haptic feedback in laparoscopic graspers.

Exposure to risk factors for developing physical complaints should obviously be avoided. In the context of laparoscopic instrument use, these risk factors involve adverse postures and motions of the upper extremities, adverse force exertion and excessive local pressure, or friction in the contact surface between instrument and hand [27]. Other risk factors, including precise working and repetitive movements, are apparently inherent to tasks that are to be performed during laparoscopic surgery. However, these factors can also be reinforced by suboptimal surgical instrument design [11].

Respondents did not show evident similarity in their main preference for graspers, either with or without haptic feedback. However, the long-lever pistol grip was best appraised in the usability assessment. Fifty-one percent of the respondents do sometimes control a scissors handle by means of a so-called palm grip, which approaches the hand posture when controlling a pistol grip. Moreover, our results emphasize that discomfort as a result of contact pressure is frequently experienced in the thumb and thenar area. Based on the indicated use of instruments, we concluded that this pressure-induced discomfort is a result from the use of scissors handles. Additionally, two recent studies also reported clinical support for a pistol-grip handle design. A pistol grip would specifically meet the need to alleviate contact stress during instrument control [28, 29]. In summary, these results suggest that a haptic feedback grasper is best equipped with a pistol grip.

As mentioned in the "Background" section, laparoscopic handles usually come with the adage "one size fits all." A laparoscopic stapler generally comes with a long-lever pistol grip. Sutton et al. reported that the handles of these devices are too big for a certain group of surgeons, particularly women, who have significantly smaller hands than men [19]. Therefore, two or more sizes should be considered to ascertain suitability for the whole range of end users.

The potential benefits which haptic feedback yields are acknowledged by the respondents. More specifically, according to laparoscopic specialists, enhanced haptic feedback could be of particular use in feeling differences in tissue consistencies, feeling how much pressure is being applied, locating a tumor or enlarged lymph node, feeling arterial pulse, and enhanced instrument ergonomics in terms of limiting the force on the surgeons' hand.

This study provides directives for the handle design of a haptic feedback grasper. As suggested by Matern et al. during the design process of surgical instruments, muscle activity and task performance under dynamic conditions should be considered [30]. Based on the results of the questionnaire and the principles of haptic feedback, we may hypothesize that haptic feedback is an unmet need in laparoscopic surgery. Along with the development of such a device, the assessed scenarios should be examined in (pre-)clinical experimental research.

Rather than a direct assessment of readily available instruments, this assessment was based on pictures which can be considered as a limitation of our study. A large group of respondents report to use a front-hinged scissors handle, whereas the vast

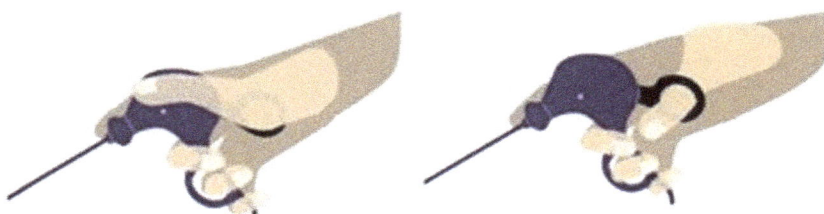

Fig. 4 Illustration of the palm grip (*left*) versus the usual grip (*right*)

Table 3 Assessment of the utility of haptic feedback in clinical scenarios

Scenario	Mean ± SD[a]
Feeling differences in tissue consistencies	3.5 ± 1.5
Locating a tumor or enlarged lymph node	3.2 ± 1.7
Feeling arterial pulse	2.7 ± 1.6
Feeling how much pressure is being applied	3.6 ± 1.4
Limiting the force on the surgeons' hand	3.4 ± 1.5
Lowering the time to complete surgery	2.4 ± 1.7
Reducing complications	3.2 ± 1.6
Reduction of conversions to open surgery	2.1 ± 1.6
Performing laparoscopy instead of open surgery	2.4 ± 1.7

[a] Assessment based on a 6-point Likert scale ranging from 0 to 5 and presented as mean ± SD

majority of scissors handles used are equipped with back-hinged actuation. We might consider this an artifact of the used method, but we might as well question whether surgeons are aware of the actuation of the instrument. Lastly, since the vast majority of respondents were Dutch, we have to be reticent to extrapolate these findings to Europe as a whole.

Conclusion

This study highlights the clinical importance of well-designed ergonomic laparoscopic instruments. Moreover, the need of haptic feedback in laparoscopic surgery is recognized by surgeons of different disciplines. Both patients and surgeons may well benefit from the implementation of enhanced haptic feedback in laparoscopic instruments.

Acknowledgments The authors acknowledge Otmar Klaas for his contribution to the composition of the questionnaire and the design of handle illustrations.

Contributions of the authors CCJ Alleblas performed the project development, research design, data collection, data analysis, and manuscript writing.

MPH Vleugels performed the project development, research design, data collection, and manuscript writing.

TE Nieboer performed the project development, research design, data collection, and manuscript writing.

Compliance with ethical standards

Funding This study was funded with a grant provided by the European Regional Development Fund.

Informed consent The subjects were informed about the aim of this study. By completing the questionnaire, the participants implicitly declared their agreement with the use of their data for this study.

Appendix

Table 4 Survey questions

Demographics	
What is your age?	N
What is your gender?	S
In which country do you work?	S
In what department do you work?	S
What is your dominant hand?	S
What is your surgical glove size?	N
For how many years are you in practice?	N
For how many years do you perform laparoscopic surgery?	N
How many laparoscopic procedures do you perform per month?	N
Physical symptoms	
Have you ever experienced physical complaints or discomfort that you would attribute to the use of laparoscopic instruments?	S
If applicable, in which parts of the upper extremities have you experienced these physical complaints or discomforts?	M
If applicable, where do you experience discomfort from pressure caused by instruments? (includes the hand map as illustrated in Fig. 2)	M
Handgrip assessment	
In what percentage of laparoscopic procedures do you use these handle types?	N
Which handle type is your favorite for grasping?	S
How do you rate the functionality of each handle type for grasping tasks?	L
How do you rate the comfort of each handle type for grasping tasks?	L
How do you rate the freedom of movement of each handle type for grasping tasks?	L
Which handle type would be your favorite for grasping with an instrument that provides enhanced haptic feedback?	S
User features	
When holding a laparoscopic grasper with rotating function for the instrument tip, what percentage of time do you keep your index finger pointed forward?	N
Do you sometimes "palm" your grip when operating with a scissors handle?	S
If so, in what situations do you do this?	D
Clinical relevance	
If you had a laparoscopic tool with haptic feedback, for what specific scenarios would you consider it useful?	L
- Feeling differences in tissue consistencies	
- Locating a tumor or enlarged lymph node	
- Feeling arterial pulse	
- Feeling how much pressure is being applied	
- Limiting the force on the surgeons' hand	
- Lowering the time to complete surgery	
- Reducing complications	
- Reduction of conversions to open surgery	
- Performing laparoscopy instead of open surgery	

Body parts involved the following: wrists, fingers, thumbs, elbows, and shoulders. Handgrip assessments concerned the evaluation of the following designs: back-hinged scissors handle, front-hinged scissors handle, in-line handle, long-lever pistol grip, and short-lever pistol grip

D descriptive, *L* Likert scale, *M* multiple answers, *N* numeric response, *S* single answer

References

1. Breedveld P, Stassen HG, Meijer DW, Jakimowicz JJ (1999) Manipulation in laparoscopic surgery: overview of impeding effects and supporting aids. J Laparoendosc Adv Surg Tech A 9: 469–480

2. Westebring-van der Putten EP, Goossens RHM, Jakimowicz JJ, Dankelman J (2008) Haptics in minimally invasive surgery—a review. Minim Invasive Ther Allied Technol 17:3–16

3. Ottermo MV, Ovstedal M, Lango T, Stavdahl O, Yavuz Y, Johansen TA, Marvik R (2006) The role of tactile feedback in laparoscopic surgery. Surg Laparosc Endosc Percutan Tech 16:390–400

4. den Boer KT, Herder JL, Sjoerdsma W, Meijer DW, Gouma DJ, Stassen HG (1999) Sensitivity of laparoscopic dissectors—what can you feel? Surg Endosc 13:869–873

5. Bholat OS, Haluck RS, Kutz RH, Gorman PJ, Krummel TM (1999) Defining the role of haptic feedback in minimally invasive surgery. Stud Health Technol Inform 62:62–66

6. Way LW, Stewart L, Gantert W, Liu K, Lee CM, Whang K, Hunter JG (2003) Causes and prevention of laparoscopic bile duct injuries—analysis of 252 cases from a human factors and cognitive psychology perspective. Ann Surg 237:460–469

7. Dekker SW, Hugh TB (2008) Laparoscopic bile duct injury: understanding the psychology and heuristics of the error. ANZ J Surg 78: 1109–1114

8. McKinley SK, Brunt LM, Schwaitzberg SD (2014) Prevention of bile duct injury: the case for incorporating educational theories of expertise. Surg Endosc 28:3385–3391

9. Rodrigues SP, Ter Kuile M, Dankelman J, Jansen FW (2012) Patient safety risk factors for minimally invasive surgery: a validation study. Gynecol Surg 9:265–27

10. Tholey G, Desai JP, Castellanos AE (2005) Force feedback plays a significant role in minimally invasive surgery: results and analysis. Ann Surg 241:102–109

11. Heijnsdijk EA, Dankelman J, Gouma DJ (2002) Effectiveness of grasping and duration of clamping using laparoscopic graspers. Surg Endosc 16:1329–1331

12. Marucci DD, Shakeshaft AJ, Cartmill JA, Cox MR, Adams SG, Martin CJ (2000) Grasper trauma during laparoscopic cholecystectomy. Aust NZ J Surg 70:578–581

13. van der Meijden OA, Schijven MP (2009) The value of haptic feedback in conventional and robot-assisted minimal invasive surgery and virtual reality training: a current review. Surg Endosc 23: 1180–1190

14. Schostek S, Schurr MO, Buess GF (2009) Review on aspects of artificial tactile feedback in laparoscopic surgery. Med Eng Phys 31: 887–898

15. Lucas-Hernandez M, Pagador JB, Perez-Duarte FJ, Castello P, Sanchez-Margallo FM (2014) Ergonomics problems due to the use and design of dissector and needle holder: a survey in minimally invasive surgery. Surg Laparosc Endosc Percutan Tech 24:E170–E177

16. Sari V, Nieboer TE, Vierhout ME, Stegeman DF, Kluivers KB (2010) The operation room as a hostile environment for surgeons: physical complaints during and after laparoscopy. Minim Invasive Ther Allied Technol 19:105–109

17. Van Veelen MA, Meijer DW (1999) Ergonomics and design of laparoscopic instruments: results of a survey among laparoscopic surgeons. J Laparoendosc Adv Surg Tech A 9:481–489

18. Berguer R (1998) Surgical technology and the ergonomics of laparoscopic instruments. Surg Endosc 12:458–462

19. Sutton E, Irvin M, Zeigler C, Lee G, Park A (2014) The ergonomics of women in surgery. Surg Endosc 28:1051–1055

20. Adams DM, Fenton SJ, Schirmer BD, Mahvi DM, Horvath K, Nichol P (2008) One size does not fit all: current disposable laparoscopic devices do not fit the needs of female laparoscopic surgeons. Surg Endosc 22:2310–2313

21. Berguer R, Hreljac A (2004) The relationship between hand size and difficulty using surgical instruments: a survey of 726 laparoscopic surgeons. Surg Endosc 18:508–512

22. Goossens RHM, van Veelen MA (2001) Assessment of ergonomics in laparoscopic surgery. Minim Invasive Ther Allied Technol 10: 175–179

23. Vleugels M, Nieboer B (2015) Real time haptic feedback in endoscopy; the proof of concept. Gynecol Surg 12(Suppl 1):97

24. Santos-Carreras L, Hagen M, Gassert R, Bleuler H (2012) Survey on surgical instrument handle design: ergonomics and acceptance. Surg Innov 19:50–59

25. Jinadu O (2005) A multi-centre survey on the team concept of instrument design in gyn-endoscopy. Minim Invasive Ther Allied Technol 14:345–351

26. Kuijt-Evers LFM (2007) Comfort in using hand tools: theory, design and evaluation. Dissertation, Delft University of Technology

27. Rodrick D, Karwowski W, Marras WS (2012) Work-related upper extremity musculoskeletal disorders. In: Salvendy G (ed) Handbook of human factors and ergonomics. Wiley, New Jersey

28. Buchel D, Marvik R, Hallabrin B, Matern U (2010) Ergonomics of disposable handles for minimally invasive surgery. Surg Endosc 24: 992–1004

29. Tung KD, Shorti RM, Downey EC, Bloswick DS, Merryweather AS (2015) The effect of ergonomic laparoscopic tool handle design on performance and efficiency. Surg Endosc 29:2500–2505

30. Matern U, Kuttler G, Giebmeyer C, Waller P, Faist M (2004) Ergonomic aspects of five different types of laparoscopic instrument handles under dynamic conditions with respect to specific laparoscopic tasks: an electromyographic-based study. Surg Endosc 18:1231–1241

38

A patient-preference cohort study of office versus inpatient uterine polyp treatment for abnormal uterine bleeding

Natalie A. M. Cooper[1] · Lee Middleton[2] · Paul Smith[3,4] · Elaine Denny[5] ·
Lynda Stobert[6] · Jane Daniels[2] · T. Justin Clark[3,7] · on behalf of the OPT trial
collaborative group

Abstract Uterine polyps can cause abnormal bleeding in
women. Conventional practise is to remove them under general
anaesthesia but advances in technology have made it possible
to perform polypectomy in the office setting. We conducted a
patient-preference study to explore women's preferences for
treatment setting and to evaluate the effectiveness and treatment
experience of women undergoing uterine polypectomy. Three
hundred ninety-nine women with abnormal uterine bleeding
who were found to have uterine polyps at diagnostic hysteroscopy were recruited. Office polypectomies were performed in
office hysteroscopy clinics, and inpatient procedures were undertaken in operating theatres. Three hundred twenty-four of
399 (81 %) expressed a preference for office treatment. There
was no difference found between office treatment and inpatient
treatment in terms of alleviating abnormal uterine bleeding as
assessed by patients and in improving disease-specific quality
of life. Acceptability was lower and patient pain scores were
significantly higher in the office group. When offered a choice
of treatment setting for uterine polypectomy, patients have a
preference for office over inpatient treatment. Ambulatory gynaecology services should be available within healthcare systems to meet patient demand.

Keywords Office polypectomy · Abnormal uterine bleeding ·
Patient preference · Ambulatory gynaecology · Uterine polyp

Introduction

Abnormal uterine bleeding affects women of all ages and is
the commonest reason for referral to secondary care [1, 2].
Uterine polyps are commonly found in association with abnormal uterine bleeding in both pre- and postmenopausal
women [3–7] when investigated with ultrasound or office
hysteroscopy. Whilst the risk of occult malignancy within
uterine polyps is low, the available evidence supports the current practise of surgically removing uterine polyps to help
alleviate bleeding symptoms [8, 9] and this has traditionally
been performed under general anaesthesia. However, with advances in endoscopic technology, it is now possible to perform
uterine polypectomy under hysteroscopic guidance in an office setting without the need for hospital admission and anaesthesia [10–12]. Furthermore, treatment can be carried out at
the same time as diagnosis; the "see & treat" approach [13].

Whilst recruiting to a randomised controlled non-inferiority
study which compared office to inpatient polypectomy, we collected data from women who consented to be followed-up, but
had a preference for how they were treated and so could not be
randomised. We designed this parallel observational study

✉ T. Justin Clark
justin.clark@bwhct.nhs.uk

1 Women's Health Research Unit, Queen Mary University of London,
London E1 2AT, UK

2 Birmingham Clinical Trials Unit, University of Birmingham,
Birmingham B15 2TT, UK

3 Birmingham Women's NHS Foundation Trust, Birmingham B15
2TG, UK

4 School of Clinical and Experimental Medicine, University of
Birmingham, Birmingham B15 2TT, UK

5 Centre for Health and Social Care Research, Birmingham City
University, Birmingham B15 3TN, UK

6 School of Allied and Public Health Professions, Birmingham City
University, Birmingham B15 3TN, UK

7 OPT Trial Office, Birmingham Clinical Trials Unit, College of
Medical and Dental Sciences, Robert Aitken Institute for Clinical
Research, University of Birmingham, Edgbaston, Birmingham B15
2TT, UK

because a pilot RCT to aid the final office polyp treatment (OPT) study design (www.birmingham.ac.uk/research/activity/mds/trials/bctu/trials/womens/opt/index.aspx) had suggested that a substantial proportion of women would exert a preference for treatment setting. We therefore wanted to explore women's preferences for treatment setting and to evaluate the effectiveness and treatment experience of women when undergoing uterine polypectomy for alleviating abnormal bleeding according to their preference.

Methods

Population

All women with abnormal uterine bleeding and a uterine polyp diagnosed at office hysteroscopy [13] were eligible to be recruited into the office polyp treatment (OPT) study. Women in equipoise were recruited to the randomised study [14] and those with a preference for treatment were asked to participate in the preference study as we describe here. Abnormal uterine bleeding included heavy menstrual bleeding, intermenstrual bleeding and postmenopausal bleeding. Women were excluded if office polypectomy was considered not feasible, malignancy was suspected or another surgical uterine intervention was needed. All participants provided written informed consent. In clinics which provided a 'see and treat' service, consent was obtained and the patient was registered on the on-line recruitment system prior to the diagnostic hysteroscopy, so that if a uterine polyp was diagnosed and the woman's preference was for office polypectomy, treatment could be performed straight away without an interruption to register the patient into the study.

Procedures

Following the diagnostic hysteroscopy, women who agreed to participate in the preference study had their choice of treatment arranged. Those who chose office polypectomy underwent the procedure immediately following diagnosis in most instances, although some participants had their treatment scheduled within the following 8 weeks. Office polypectomies were performed in the office hysteroscopy clinic and inpatient procedures were performed in operating theatres, under general or regional anaesthesia. Office polyp removal was carried out under direct hysteroscopic vision using miniature mechanical (scissors, biopsy cups and grasping forceps) or electrosurgical instruments (bipolar electrodes), with or without the need for minor degrees of cervical dilatation and local anaesthesia (direct cervical infiltration or paracervical injection). Blind avulsion with small polypectomy forceps was also allowed. Women who chose inpatient polypectomy could have traditional dilatation and curettage or removal under vision using a resectoscope. Clinicians were free to choose the operative technique for polypectomy. Endometrial biopsy and medical therapies were permitted when indicated.

Outcome measures and follow-up

Our main measure of interest was successful treatment, determined by the women's assessment of their bleeding at 6 months using a dichotomous (success/fail) outcome measure. For women with heavy menstrual bleeding, treatment was considered a success if bleeding had reduced to acceptable levels. For women with intermenstrual or postmenopausal bleeding, the definition was cessation of bleeding.

Other patient reported outcome measures were the women's subjective assessment of their bleeding using visual-analogue-scales (0 for no bleeding to 100 heaviest imaginable and 0 for no days bleeding to 100 bleeding every day) and response to the question 'compared to before your treatment, would you say your bleeding is?' on an ordered Likert scale (much better, little better, same, worse). Health-related-quality-of-life was measured using the generic EuroQol EQ-5D-3L [15] and the disease-specific Menorrhagia Multi-Attribute Scale (MMAS) [16]. All clinical data were collected at baseline and then by mail at 6 months post recruitment.

Patient experience was also evaluated; patients were asked to rate their level of pain 1 h after the procedure and on discharge from hospital using visual-analogue-scales (0 no pain to 100 worst imaginable pain). Women undergoing office polypectomy also rated the level of pain during the procedure. Acceptability of the procedure was assessed using Likert scales and structured questions. This was supplemented by a series of semi-structured qualitative telephone interviews in a purposive sample of women (who had consented to be interviewed) 1 week after the procedure. Rates of successful polyp removal and complications were recorded peri-operatively, and postoperative data were collected for adverse events and need further treatment.

Statistical analysis

Analyses were performed including all consenting participants in the group of their preference regardless of whether they received their preference, or indeed any, treatment (i.e. intention–to-treat). Chi-squared and t tests were used to assess if there were any systematic differences between the preference groups in terms of their baseline characteristics. Odds ratios for successful treatment at 6 month were generated using a logistic regression model (odds ratios were favoured over risk ratios as it is more straightforward to generate stable adjusted estimates [17]. Estimates were adjusted for potential confounders that were considered to be the most clinically important by adding the following 12 variables to the model: predominant bleeding complaint at consent (postmenopausal/heavy menstrual/intermenstrual), site of uterine polyp (fundal/non-fundal), type of uterine polyp (glandular/fibrous), number of polyps (1/2/3+), largest polyp size (continuous variable), grade of surgeon (consultant/less experienced), removal technique (blind/hysteroscopic), detachment technique (electrode/mechanical), age (continuous variable), body mass index (continuous variable), parity (0/1/2/3/4+), and centre of recruitment (Birmingham Women's Hospital/Royal Hallamshire Hospital Sheffield/other minor centre). A multiple imputation procedure [18] (assumed data was missing at random) was used in this analysis to impute any missing data items. Variables in the imputation model included the outcome variable of interest together with the parameters listed above; 20 imputed data sets were created using the MCMC method with overall estimates and standard error calculated using Rubin's rules [19]. 95 % confidence intervals were generated along with a p value from the associated two-sided chi-squared test. Other binary outcomes and endpoints measured on a continuous scale (scores from MMAS, EQ-5D and VAS scores) were analysed in a similar fashion to the above (linear regression model adjusting for baseline score for continuous variables). Unadjusted estimates are provided for comparison or where an adjustment was not possible because of low group frequencies. No adjustments were made for operative descriptors. Standard tests were used for other outcome measures: paired t tests for changes from baseline scores within groups and two-sample t tests for continuous data with a normal distribution, Wilcoxon signed rank test for skewed continuous data and chi-squared tests for binary and categorical responses. SAS version 9.2 was used for analyses (PROC MI for the multiple imputation procedure).

Results

Recruitment and qualitative assessment of patients' preference for treatment

Between April 2008 and July 2011, in 30 UK NHS centres, 952 women with abnormal uterine bleeding and a preference for how they wanted to be treated agreed to participate. Three hundred ninety-nine (42 %) women were recruited with the main reason for ineligibility being no polyp present at diagnostic hysteroscopy. Three hundred twenty-four of 399 (81 %) expressed a preference for office treatment (Fig. 1).

Thirteen women underwent qualitative interviews. Women were asked about their treatment preferences, which were mainly down to individual reasons. Most women choosing office treatment wanted it over and done within one hospital visit, and even though for one of these women the procedure could not be completed she still thought it was the right choice. Of the other women, two had a fear of anaesthetics, one had a pre-existing medical condition, one had children to make

arrangements for and one did not want to take time off work. Very few women in the overall preference study chose inpatient treatment and the four interviewed all spoke of a previous bad experience of hysteroscopy or other procedures under local anaesthetic, or embarrassment at being in stirrups, which made them want a general anaesthetic. In both groups of the study, a number of women told of how they had consulted friends and family before attending the clinic, or the nurse in the clinic, in order to make a decision about the procedure, but this had to be weighed up against their personal feelings.

Participants and follow-up

There were no statistically significant differences between groups in the baseline characteristics of the women (Table 1). Overall, for 48 % (192/399) of the women, the initial complaint was postmenopausal bleeding; 25 % (98/399) had heavy menstrual bleeding and the remaining participants had intermenstrual bleeding, 109/399 (27 %). Three hundred two of 324 (93 %) of the office group received their treatment preference compared with 68/75 (91 %) of the inpatient group (Fig. 1). Sixty-three percent of the women allocated to office polypectomy were treated in 'see and treat' clinics. The median time from recruitment to treatment in the office groups and inpatient group were 0 days (IQR = 0, 27) and 31 days (IQR = 7, 55), respectively. Completed primary outcome responses were available from 338/399 (85 %) of participants at 6 months (Fig. 1).

Treatment success

There was no significant difference between treatment success in the office and inpatient polypectomy groups with 82 % in each group reporting successful alleviation of bleeding symptoms at 6 months (231/283 versus 45/55, unadjusted OR = 0.99, 95 % CI = 0.47, 2.09; $p > 0.9$; adjusted OR = 1.12, 95 % CI = 0.47, 2.69; $p = 0.8$).

Operative results

Table 2 details the operative and postoperative results details. Office treatment required less vaginal instrumentation (OR = 0.13, 95 % CI = 0.06, 0.31; $p < 0.001$) and dilatation of the cervix (OR = 0.15, 95 % CI = 0.08, 0.28; $p < 0.001$). Hysteroscopic polypectomy under direct vision was significantly more common (OR = 3.6, 95 % CI = 2.0, 6.4; $p < 0.001$) in the office setting, with electrosurgery being the most popular method of detaching polyps (OR = 2.0, 95 % CI = 1.2, 3.5; $p = 0.02$). Hysteroscopic retrieval of specimens from the uterine cavity was the most common technique in the office setting whereas blind mechanical extraction was preferred in the inpatient group (OR = 5.6, 95 % CI = 3.0, 10.4; $p < 0.001$). The proportion of complete removals was not

Fig. 1 Flow diagram showing enrollment, preference for treatment and follow-up of the study patients

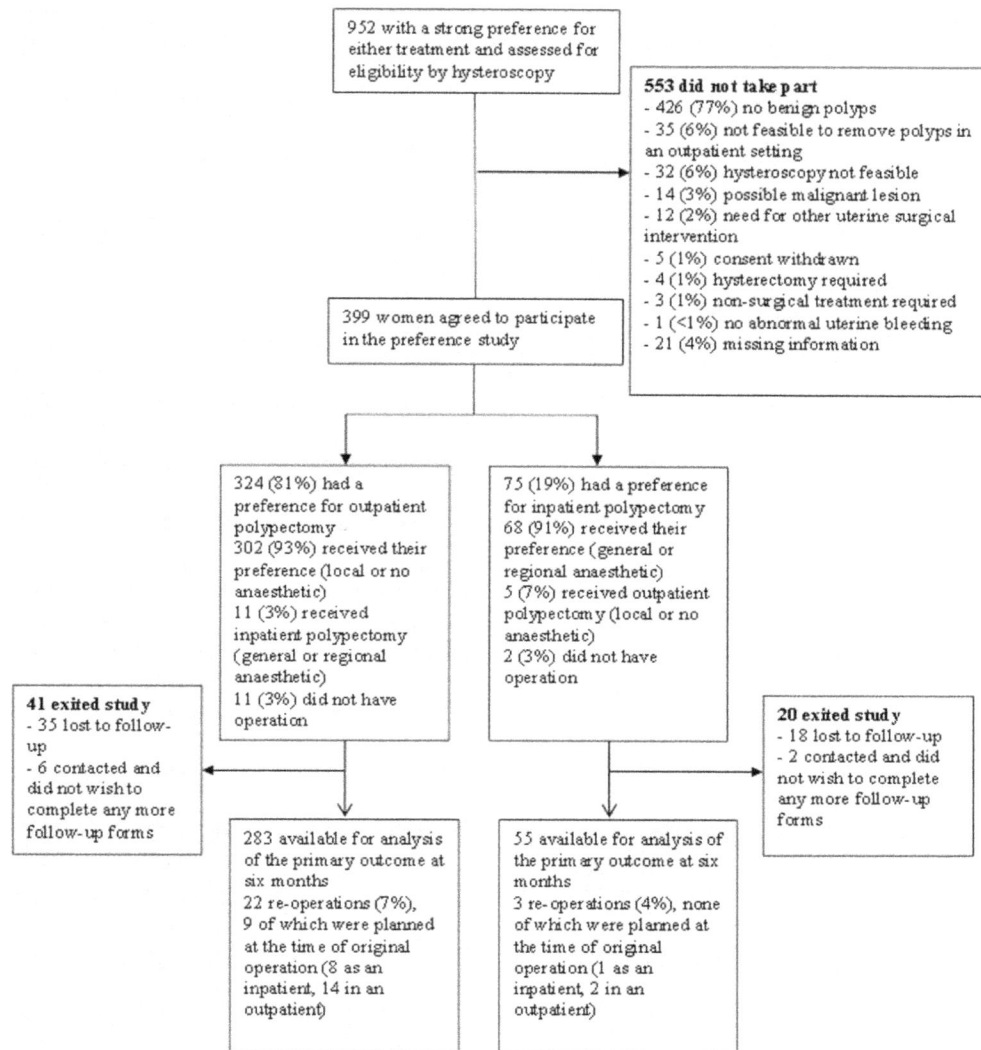

significantly different between groups (282/312 [90 %] versus 68/73 [93 %], unadjusted OR = 1.4, 95 % CI = 0.5, 3.9; $p = 0.5$; adjusted OR = 1.9, 95 % CI = 0.7, 5.6; $p = 0.2$).

Serious adverse events

No serious adverse events occurred in the preference study. The most common perioperative complications in the office group were induced vaso-vagal reactions affecting 6 % of the cohort. Vaso-vagal reactions also occurred postoperatively with a similar percentage in each cohort (5 % of the office group versus 3 % of the inpatient group) (Table 2).

Quality of life and bleeding scores

Condition-specific quality of life and bleeding scores were significantly improved from baseline at 6 months in both groups with no significant differences between them (Table 3). Generic

quality of life scores (Euroqol EQ-5D) were improved from baseline in the office group but not in the inpatient group with no difference between the groups at 6 months. The non-significant increase within the inpatient group may be due to the relatively small number of women in this group.

Procedure acceptability

Mean pain scores were significantly higher in the office polypectomy group compared with the inpatient group at 1-h post procedure and on discharge (Table 3). Two percent (7/299) of women in the office group compared with no women in the inpatient group felt that the procedure they underwent was 'unacceptable'. There was no difference between groups in terms of the number of women who would recommend the procedure to a friend, choose to have the same procedure again or in retrospect would have preferred the alternative treatment. In qualitative interviews, the preference

Table 1 Baseline characteristics of the patients

		Office polypectomy (n = 324)	Inpatient polypectomy (n = 75)	p value
Age (years)	Mean (SD)	53 (11)	51 (12)	p = 0.2
BMI (kg/m²)	Mean (SD)	31 (8)[a]	31 (8)[b]	p = 0.7
Ethnicity	White	263 (91 %)	54 (93 %)	p > 0.9
	Asian	12 (4 %)	2 (3 %)	
	Black	8 (3 %)	1 (2 %)	
	Other	6 (2 %)	1 (2 %)	
	Not given/not known	35	17	
Recruiting centre	BWH[c]	105 (32 %)	24 (32 %)	p = 0.5
	RHH[d]	60 (19 %)	18 (24 %)	
	Others[e]	159 (49 %)	33 (44 %)	
Predominant bleeding complaint at randomisation	Post-menopausal[f]	155 (48 %)	37 (49 %)	p = 0.2
	Heavy menstrual[g]	75 (23 %)	23 (31 %)	
	Intermenstrual[h]	94 (29 %)	15 (20 %)	
Site of uterine polyp	Fundal	118 (36 %)	25 (33 %)	p = 0.6
	Non-fundal	206 (64 %)	50 (67 %)	
Type of uterine polyp	Glandular	229 (71 %)	53 (71 %)	p > 0.9
	Fibrous	95 (29 %)	22 (29 %)	
Number of polyps	1	233 (72 %)	58 (77 %)	p = 0.6
	2	62 (19 %)	11 (15 %)	
	> = 3	29 (9 %)	6 (8 %)	
Parity	0	49 (15 %)	18 (24 %)	p = 0.4
	1	35 (11 %)	6 (8 %)	
	2	121 (37 %)	26 (35 %)	
	3	50 (15 %)	9 (12 %)	
	> = 4	37 (11 %)	8 (11 %)	
	missing	32 (10 %)	8 (11 %)	
Other benign pathology	None	318 (98 %)	74 (99 %)	p = 0.8
	SMF/Adhesion/ Septum	–	–	
	Adhesion/Septum	–	–	
	SMF	5 (2 %)	1 (1 %)	
	Septum	1 (<1 %)	–	

SMF submucosal fibroid

[a] Based on 56 values

[b] Based on 207 values

[c] Birmingham Women's Hospital

[d] Royal Hallamshire Hospital, Sheffield

[e] 28 other centres: median recruitment = 4 (IQR = [2, 9])

[f] 16 (10 %) and 3 (8 %) of these women were currently taking a continuous combined 'no bleed' HRT in the office and inpatient groups, respectively

[g] Includes one post-menopausal woman (1 %) on a sequential HRT (office group)

[h] Includes two post-menopausal women (2 %) on a sequential HRT (office group)

patients reported less pain than the randomised ones, using descriptions such as 'uncomfortable', 'bearable' and 'better than expected'. This group also reported little postoperative pain describing it like 'wind' or 'period pain'. They balanced pain, which they mainly experienced short term, with the convenience of a fast response to their problem.

Additional treatments

There was no difference between groups in the number of women using additional medical treatments for their bleeding, or consulting a healthcare provider during the 6-month follow-up period. Twenty-two women in the office group (7 %)

Table 2 Operative details and complications

	Office polypectomy	Inpatient polypectomy	Mean difference or OR (95 % CI)[b], p value
Largest polyp size, cm (median [IQR], n)[a]	1.1 [0.8–2.0], 286	1.0 [0.8–2.0], 57	0.0 (−0.2, 0.2), p > 0.9
Need for cervical dilation = yes	105/303 (35 %)	52/67 (78 %)	0.15 (0.08, 0.28), p < 0.001
Use of vaginal speculum = yes	152/301 (50 %)	53/60 (88 %)	0.13 (0.06, 0.31), p < 0.001
Use of local anaesthetic = yes	132/313 (42 %)	2/73 (3 %)	25.9 (6.2, 107), p < 0.001
Hysteroscopic removal = yes (vs. blind)	246/299 (82 %)	36/64 (56 %)	3.6 (2.0, 6.4), p < 0.001
Scope diameter (mm)	4.0 [4.0–6.0], 201	5.5 [4.0–6.0], 42	−1.0 (−1.0, −1.0), p < 0.001
Method used to detach	n = 287	n = 65	2.0 (1.2, 3.5)[c], p = 0.02
Electrode	155 (54 %)	24 (37 %)	
Mechanical	102 (36 %)	35 (54 %)	
Combination	30 (10 %)	6 (9 %)	
Method of retrieval	n = 292	n = 62	5.6 (3.0, 10.4)[d], p < 0.001
Hysteroscopic	193 (66 %)	16 (26 %)	
Mechanical	69 (24 %)	43 (69 %)	
Combination	11 (4 %)	–	
None	19 (7 %)	3 (5 %)	
Surgeon grade = consultant	233/305 (76 %)	40/67 (60 %)	2.2 (1.3, 3.8), p = 0.005
Time taken for polypectomy, min (median [IQR], n)	10 [5–15], 290	10 [7–15], 52	−1.5 (3.0, 0.0), p = 0.3
Time in office room/theatre, min (median [IQR], n)	30 [20–35], 285	33 [25–45], 53	−6.0 (−10.0, −2.0), p = 0.003
Removal success	n = 312	n = 73	1.4 (0.5, 3.9)[f], p = 0.5
Complete	282 (90 %)	68 (93 %)	
Partial[e]	22 (7 %)	3 (4 %)	
Failed[e]	8 (3 %)	2 (3 %)	
Operative complications	n = 302	n = 67	
Vaso-vagal episode	17 (6 %)	–	
Patient discomfort	9 (3 %)	–	
Cervical trauma	1 (<1 %)	1 (1 %)	
Uterine perforation	–	–	
Other[g]	1 (<1 %)	–	
Postoperative complications	n = 301	n = 67	
Vaso-vagal episode	14 (5 %)	2 (3 %)	
Vomiting	3 (1 %)	2 (3 %)	
Severe pain	–	2 (3 %)	
Further treatment/procedure given	n = 292	n = 64	
Mirena IUS	42 (14 %)	8 (13 %)	
Tranexamic acid	9 (3 %)	–	
Progestogens	3 (1 %)	–	
Endometrial destruction	2 (1 %)	–	
Local oestrogen cream	2 (1 %)	–	
Mefenamic acid	1 (<1 %)	1 (2 %)	
Contraceptive pill	1 (<1 %)	–	
Missing treatment name	2 (1 %)	1 (2 %)	

Numbers in italics refer to the responses received for that particular question

n = number of responses

[a] Polyp size was estimated hysteroscopically

[b] Mean difference < 0 indicates lower with office, similarly OR < 1 is lower with office. For skewed variables presented with medians, differences in location between groups were calculated using Hodges-Lehmann estimates and Moses' confidence intervals

[c] Odds ratio calculated from 'electrode' versus any other category

[d] Odds ratio calculated from 'hysteroscopic' versus any other category

[e] Nine (3 %) partial or failed patients in the office group and none in the inpatient group were immediately scheduled for reoperation. Six of these were scheduled to be an inpatient. *Partial or failed reasons in the office group* (%'s given of the total number, 312): patient discomfort (9, 3 %), unable to locate blindly (5, 2 %), unable to access under vision (4, 1 %), polyp too large (3, 1 %), failed hysteroscopy (1, <1 %), base cut but unable to remove (1, <1 %), wide base unable to fully resect (1, <1 %), vaso-vagal episode (1, <1 %), difficult access to base of polyp (1, <1 %), missing reason (4, 1 %); *partial or failed reasons in the inpatient group* (%'s given of the total number, 73): unable to access under vision (1, 1 %), unable to locate blindly (1, 1 %), deep sub-mucous fibroid polyp (1, 1 %), too broad base (1, 1 %), missing reason (1, 1 %)

[f] Odds ratio calculated from 'partial' or 'failed' versus complete

[g] Other complications: nausea

Table 3 Results of quality of life assessments, bleeding and pain scores and procedure acceptability

	Office polypectomy Mean (SD, n)	Inpatient polypectomy Mean (SD, n)	Difference (95 % CI)[a], p value	Adjusted difference[h] (95 % CI), p value
MMAS[b]				
Baseline	63 (26, 163)	61 (28, 37)		
6 months	77 (25, 135)[g]	79 (25, 25)[g]	−3 (−12, 7), $p = 0.55$	−4 (−14, 3), $p = 0.18$
EuroQol EQ-5D[c]				
Baseline	0.79 (0.26, 312)	0.72 (0.30, 71)		
6 months	0.82 (0.25, 289)[g]	0.81 (0.30, 56)	0.00 (−0.07, 0.06), $p = 0.88$	0.01 (−0.05, 0.08), $p = 0.64$
EuroQol health thermometer[d]				
Baseline	78 (18, 305)	75 (21, 71)		
6 months	78 (19, 291)	79 (20, 57)	−2 (−7, 3), $p = 0.34$	−1 (−4, 5), $p = 0.81$
Bleeding duration visual analogue scale[e]				
Baseline	39 (26, 74)	38 (26, 23)		
6 months	30 (28, 65)[g]	18 (19, 16)[g]	−13 (−27, 2), $p = 0.09$	−13 (−27, 2), $p = 0.09$
Bleeding amount visual analogue scale[f]				
Baseline	59 (28, 75)	58 (26, 23)		
6 months	32 (28, 68)[g]	26 (27, 16)[g]	−4 (−19, 11), $p = 0.61$	−3 (−20, 14), $p = 0.72$
Operation pain scores				
During procedure[i]	42 (26, 296)	–	–	–
60 min after procedure[i]	27 (24, 247)	20 (24, 60)	−7 (−14, 0), $p = 0.04$	−8 (−11, −4), $p = 0.03$
On discharge[i]	22 (21, 276)	13 (18, 57)	−9 (−15, −3), $p = 0.003$	−9 (−15, −3), $p = 0.002$
	n (%)	n (%)	OR (95 % CI), p value[j]	Adjusted OR[h] (95 % CI), p value
Operation acceptability				
Totally	194 (65 %)	52 (81 %)		
Generally	48 (16 %)	9 (14 %)	0.21 (0.06, 0.69), $p = 0.01$[k]	0.19 (0.05, 0.70), $p = 0.01$[k]
Fairly	50 (17 %)	3 (5%)		
Unacceptable	7 (2 %)	0 (–)		
Exposure embarrassing?				
Extremely	5 (2 %)	2 (3 %)		
Moderately	30 (10 %)	7 (12 %)	1.4 (0.6, 3.0), $p = 0.46$[l]	1.4 (0.6, 3.7), $p = 0.36$[l]
A little	90 (30 %)	8 (13 %)		
No	177 (59 %)	43 (72 %)		
Recommend to a friend?				
Yes/total	282/302 (93 %)	62/64 (97 %)	0.45 (0.10, 2.0), $p = 0.28$	Not possible to compute
Same treatment again?				
Yes/total	283/300 (94 %)	62/63 (98 %)	0.27 (0.04, 2.1), $p = 0.21$	Not possible to compute
Preferred alternative treatment?				
Yes/total	36/299 (12 %)	10/63 (16 %)	1.4 (0.7, 3.0), $p = 0.41$	1.5 (0.7, 3.5), $p = 0.32$

n number of responses

[a] Difference between groups at each time point adjusted for baseline score. Estimates of differences >0 favour office polypectomy, those <0 favour inpatient polypectomy

[b] Menorrhagia Multi-Attribute Scale questionnaire. Scores range from 0 (severely affected) to 100 (not affected). Restricted to those with heavy menstrual and intermenstrual bleeding only

[c] Health-related quality of life questionnaire. Scores range from −0.59 (health state worse than death) to 1.0 (perfect health state)

[d] Health-related quality of life questionnaire. Scores range 0 (worst imaginable health state) to 1.0 (best imaginable health state)

[e] Visual Analogue Scale score. Scores range from 0 (no days of bleeding in the last month) to 100 (bleeding every day in the last month). Restricted to those with heavy menstrual bleeding only

[f] Visual Analogue Scale score. Scores range from 0 (no bleeding in the last month) to 100 (heaviest imaginable bleeding in the last month). Restricted to those with heavy menstrual bleeding only

[g] $p < 0.05$ when compared with baseline score within group (by paired t test)

[h] See statistical methods section for details on adjustments

i Visual Analogue Scale score. Scores range from 0 (no pain at all) to 100 (worst imaginable pain). T test used for analysis

[j] Estimates of OR > 1 favour office polypectomy, those <1 favour inpatient polypectomy

[k] Totally acceptable/generally acceptable vs. fairly acceptable/unacceptable combined categories used to calculate odds ratio

[l] Extremely/moderately vs. a little/no combined categories used to calculate odds ratio

and three in the inpatient group (4 %) had at least one further polyp removal (OR = 1.75, 95 % CI = 0.51, 6.00; p = 0.4). The total number of women undergoing subsequent gynaecological operations other than polyp removal was higher with office polypectomy (27 [8 %] versus 3 [4 %]) but this difference was not statistically significant (OR = 1.86, 95 % CI = 0.55, 6.35; p = 0.3). These operations comprised the following in the office versus inpatient groups, respectively: hysteroscopy, 9 (3 %) versus 2 (3 %); hysterectomy, 9 (3 %) versus 1 (2 %) and endometrial ablation, 3 (1 %) versus 0. The other six operations were in the office group: five cyst removals (2 %) and one ovary removal (<1 %).

Discussion

The results of this study demonstrate that women with abnormal uterine bleeding and uterine polyps, who have a preference for how they are treated, are more likely to choose office polypectomy than an inpatient procedure. At 6 months, we found no differences between office and inpatient treatment in terms of treating abnormal uterine bleeding and over 80 % women reported successful alleviation of symptoms, regardless of initial bleeding complaint. The duration and amount of bleeding were significantly reduced following both office and inpatient treatment, and no differences were identified according to treatment preference. Similarly, a non-differential but significant improvement in disease-specific quality of life was seen following polypectomy, although generic quality of life appeared only marginally improved.

There was no increased risk of partial or failed polypectomy in the office group in the preference study which is contradictory to the results of the randomised OPT study [14] which found that office treatment was more likely to fail. This is likely to be due to unknown confounders and the small sample size in the inpatient group. Overall pain scores were still significantly higher in the office group than in the inpatient group but these differences were small and so their clinical significance is debatable; differences between groups in the amount of postoperative medication may also have affected this to an unknown degree. Only 2 % of office patients felt that the procedure was unacceptable; findings that are consistent with the concomitant RCT. Not all women underwent their preferred treatment. We can hypothesise that women may have changed their mind about which treatment they wanted but we are unable to provide data as the reasons were not recorded.

In the qualitative interviews, women who had a preference for office treatment appeared to report less pain than those who were randomised to the office setting. Although the number of women who were interviewed was small, this may suggest that women who choose to have the office treatment are more motivated to tolerate and complete the procedure,

which may also contribute to the reduced number of failed procedures in the office setting.

The strengths of this study include its size, the multicentre design, a population representative of the UK demographic, the relatively low rates of loss to follow-up and the tailoring of assessment of outcomes to the primary complaint. As this was a preference study, selection bias is an obvious limitation to the interpretation of the results. However, statistical adjustments were made for the obvious confounding factors including type of bleeding, surgical experience, removal method and the site, nature, size and number of uterine polyps.

In comparison to data from the parallel randomised controlled trial [14], the overall level of failed polypectomy in both groups was lower (9 versus 13 %; OR = 0.64, 95 % CI = 0.42 to 0.99; p = 0.05) and treatment success higher (82 versus 76 %; OR = 1.4, 95 % CI = 1.0 to 2.0; p = 0.06). These findings are unlikely to be due to differences in demographics of the two studies as they were largely the same apart from a slightly older population in the preference study (2.4 years, 95 % CI = 0.9 to 3.7). It is more likely to reflect the selection of more favourable, better motivated women and technically 'less challenging' polyps to surgically remove in the office setting by the operating surgeon. However, the effect of counselling by individual surgeons on patient preference for treatment setting or indeed participation in the parallel randomised trial is unclear.

The 4:1 preference for office over inpatient polypectomy resulted in a smaller inpatient cohort and therefore the result estimates are less precise. Additional limitations of our preference study include varying practise between clinicians and a small number of participants failing to get their chosen treatment.

Office polyp treatment appears to be safe, feasible, acceptable and effective for the treatment of abnormal uterine bleeding in women expressing a preference for such treatment. Although this treatment is becoming more widespread, it is not universally available within national healthcare systems. This study demonstrates that when office treatment is available, most women recognise the potential benefits of office treatment and approximately 80 % would choose it over inpatient treatment. In addition, this cohort study and the RCT have both shown that removing uterine polyps appears to alleviate abnormal uterine bleeding, for which data were previously lacking. Thus, there is evidence on both clinical and patient preference grounds, to support prioritising the provision of ambulatory gynaecology services such as office hysteroscopic polypectomy. An important caveat, however, is that women should be informed that office treatment may be associated with more pain and reduced acceptability compared with scheduled inpatient approaches to treatment under general anaesthesia, although they can be reassured that at least eight out of ten women find the procedure to be totally or generally acceptable. Although the preference study did not demonstrate an increased failure rate in the office group, this is likely to be due to confounding factors and the small inpatient group and as the RCT showed that failure was more likely, women should be informed of this, to allow them to make an informed decision about treatment setting. Future research should be directed at evaluating the influence of clinical characteristics and surgical technologies on the feasibility, acceptability and effectiveness of office hysteroscopic polypectomy.

This large, controlled observational study has shown that the majority of women expressing a treatment preference choose to have office treatment of uterine polyps associated with abnormal uterine bleeding. The findings of the study are subject to selection bias; however, they are consistent with the robust data derived from the parallel RCT. The findings, in particular the high levels of patient preference for office treatment, support the conclusions of the RCT that 'ambulatory' gynaecological therapeutic services should be made more widely available within healthcare systems. Currently, some women are being denied a choice of treatment setting and consequently are being subjected to the inconvenience and greater burden of inpatient hospital treatment, which if offered an alternative office treatment option, they could avoid.

Acknowledgments   We thank the many women who participated in the OPT study. We also thank the following people: Richard Grey who provided initial statistical advice; and past and present members of OPT project management team: Laura Gennard, Liz Brettell, Lisa Leighton and Enid Darby (trial management); Tracy Bingham and Susan Sargent (research nurses); Mary Connor and Sian Jones (surgical advisors); Versha Cheed (statistics); Nicholas Hilken (database programmers).

OPT collaborative group   We would like to acknowledge our National Health Service colleagues who supported recruitment for the trial: *Barnsley District General Hospital, South Yorkshire:* K Cannon, KA Farag, K Raychaudhuri, M Reid, A Zahid; *Birmingham Heartlands/ Solihull Hospital, Birmingham:* J Blunn, S Guruswami, S Irani, D Robinson; *Birmingham Women's Hospital, Birmingham:* T Bingham, TJ Clark, NAM Cooper, J Gupta, S Madari, D Mellers, S O'Connor, C O'Hara, M Pathak, V Preece, E Sangha, M Shehmar, P Trinham, A Wilson; *Bishop Aukland General Hospital, County Durham:* J Dent, J Macdonald, P Sengupta; *Blackpool Victoria Hospital, Blackpool:* C Brookes, J Davies; *Bradford Royal Infirmary, Bradford:* M Jackson, S Jones, H Ludkin, S Riddiough; *Castle Hill Hospital, East Yorkshire:* J Allen, T Cathcart, D Cox, S Ford, L Kenny, K Phillips, N Rawal, A Rodgers, J Siddiqui; *Chelsea and Westminster Hospital, London:* A Dine-Atkinson, S Kalkur, G Merriner, J Ben-Nagi, A Raza, R Richardson; *University Hospital of North Staffordshire, Stoke-on Trent:* I Hassan; *City Hospital, Sunderland:* D Edmundson, J Chamberlain, A Barge, P Wake, D Milford, E Walton; *Countess of Chester Hospital, Chester:* S Arnold, M Blake, MJ McCormack, N Naddad, J Hane, S Wood; *Kidderminster Hospital, Worcester:* M Labib, T Martin, S Moss, M Pathak; *Liverpool Women's Hospital, Liverpool:* N Aziz, L Harris, D Pattison; *Manor Hospital, Walsall:* J Pepper; *Musgrove Park Hospital, Taunton:* M Escott, G Fender; *New Cross Hospital, Wolverhampton:* M Saeed; *Newham University Hospital, Plaistow:* A Antoniou, R Chenoy; *Norfolk and Norwich University Hospital, Norwich:* E Morris, M Sule; *Ormskirk and District General Hospital, Southport:* A Cope, S Sharma, T Taylor; *Queen Charlotte's and Chelsea Hospital, London:* N Panay, C Rothan; *Queen's Hospital, Romford:* A Coker; *Royal Blackburn Hospital, Blackburn:* M Abdel-Aty, K Bhatia, S Gardiner, W Myint, M Willett; *Royal Hallamshire Hospital, Sheffield:* V Brown, C Bonner, M Connor, S Stillwell; *Royal Infirmary of Edinburgh, Edinburgh:* A Horne, S Milne, J Rowan; *Sandwell General Hospital, West Midlands:* A Ewies, J Kabukoba; *Shotley Bridge Hospital, County Durham:* J Dent, P Sengupta; *St Mary's Hospital, Manchester:* R Biancardi, K Donnelly, L Dwyer, K Naidoo, I Pinton; *Stafford Hospital, Stafford:* K Chin, T Harrison, J Roger, D Sirdefield, J Stacey; *Royal Oldham Hospital, Oldham:* Z Anjum, N Aziz; *The Royal Victoria Infirmary, Newcastle Upon Tyne:* J Bainbridge, G Cosgrove, A Desai, J Gebbie, D Koleskas, P Ranka, M Roberts; *Whiston Hospital, Merseyside:* C Cunningham, C Nwosu, N Aziz.

Author's contributions   TJC, LM, ED, SJ and JD were involved in designing the study as co-applicants. TJC oversaw the running of the trial and all of the authors contributed to the ongoing management of the trial. NAMC, TJC and the OPT collaborative group recruited patients to the trial. NAMC, TJC, PS, ED, LS and the OPT collaborative group collected data for the trial. LM performed the statistical analysis. ED and LS evaluated the qualitative data. The manuscript was drafted by NAMC and TJC with contributions from LM (statistics) ED (qualitative study). All the authors contributed to the interpretation of the results of the study and revised and reviewed the paper. The Birmingham Clinical Trials Unit did the randomisation and data management and monitoring.

Consent   All persons gave their informed consent prior to their inclusion in the study.

Funding   The study sponsors were the University of Birmingham and Birmingham Women's NHS Foundation Trust, and the study was funded by the National Institute of Health Research (NIHR) Health Technology Assessment Programme (06/404/84). The views and opinions expressed in this article are those of the authors and do not necessarily reflect those of the NIHR Health Technology Assessment Programme, the NIHR, the National Health Service or the English Department of Health.

Role of the funding source   Neither the funder nor sponsor had any role in study design, data collection, interpretation or analysis or in writing the report for publication. The authors had full access to all the data from the study. The authors vouch for the accuracy and completeness of the data and analyses.

Data   The corresponding author affirms that the manuscript is an honest, accurate and transparent account of the study being reported that no important aspects of the study have been omitted and that any discrepancies from the study as planned (and, if relevant, registered) have been explained.

The full dataset is available from the corresponding author. Consent was not obtained but the presented data are anonymised and risk of identification is low.

References

1. Spencer CP, Whitehead MI (1999) Endometrial assessment re-visited. Br J Obstet Gynaecol 106(7):623–632

2. Bradlow J, Coulter A, Brooks P (1992) Patterns of referral. Oxford Health Services Research Unit, Oxford

3. Nagele F, O'Connor H, Davies A, Badawy A, Mohamed H, Magos A (1996) 2500 outpatient diagnostic hysteroscopies. Obstet Gynecol 88(1):87–92

4. Clevenger-Hoeft M, Syrop CH, Stovall DW, Van Voorhis BJ (1999) Sonohysterography in premenopausal women with and without abnormal bleeding. Obstet Gynecol 94(4):516–520

5. van H, CD d, CE J, JB T, FW J (2007) Diagnostic hysteroscopy in abnormal uterine bleeding: a systematic review and meta-analysis. BJOG: Int J Obstet Gynaecol 114(6):664–675

6. Lasmar RB, Dias R, Barrozo PR, Oliveira MA, Coutinho ES, da Rosa DB (2008) Prevalence of hysteroscopic findings and histologic diagnoses in patients with abnormal uterine bleeding. Fertil Steril 89(6):1803–1807

7. Coloma CF, Paya AV, Diago Almela VJ, Costa CS, Valero FV, Lopez-Olmos J (1998) 2,000 out-patient diagnostic hyteroscopies: 8 years of experience [Spanish] dos mil histeroscopias diagnosticas ambulatorias: Experiencia de echo anos. Progresos en Obstetricia y Ginecologia 41(6):347–352

8. Lieng M, Istre O, Qvigstad E (2010) Treatment of endometrial polyps: a systematic review. Acta Obstet Gynecol Scand 89(8): 992–1002

9. Nathani F, Clark TJ (2006) Uterine polypectomy in the management of abnormal uterine bleeding: a systematic review. J Minim Invasive Gynecol 13(4):260–268

10. Marwah V, Bhandari SK (2003) Diagnostic and interventional microhysteroscopy with use of the coaxial bipolar electrode system. Fertil Steril 79(2):413–417

11. Cicinelli E, Tinelli R, Loiudice L, Loiudice I, Francavilla M, Pinto V (2010) Office polypectomy without anesthesia with Alphascope: a randomized controlled study. J Minim Invasive Gynecol 17(6 SUPPL. 1):796–799

12. Clark TJ, Godwin J, Khan KS, Gupta JK (2002) Ambulatory endoscopic treatment of symptomatic benign endometrial polyps. A feasibility study. Gynaecol Endosc 11(2–3):91–97

13. Clark TJ, Gupta JK (2005) Handbook of outpatient hysteroscopy. A complete guide to diagnosis and therapy. First ed. Hodder Education, London

14. Cooper NAM, Clark TJ, Middleton LJ, Diwakar L, Smith P, Denny E, et al. (2015) A randomised trial of outpatient versus inpatient uterine polyp treatment for abnormal uterine bleeding. Br Med J 350:h1398

15. EuroQol Group. EuorQol EQ-5D. http://www.euroqol.org/. 2013. 3–12-2013.

16. Shaw RW, Brickley MR, Evans L, Edwards MJ (1998) Perceptions of women on the impact of menorrhagia on their health using multi-attribute utility assessment. Br J Obstet Gynaecol 105(11):1155–1159

17. Blizzard L, Hosmer DW (2006) Parameter estimation and goodness-of-fit in log-binomial regression. Biom J 48(1):5–22

18. Sterne JA, White IR, Carlin JB, Spratt M, Royston P, Kenward MG, et al. (2009) Multiple imputation for missing data in epidemiological and clinical research: potential and pitfalls. Br Med J 29(338):b2393

19. Rubin DB. Multiple Imputation for Nonresponse in Surveys. http://onlinelibrary.wiley.com/doi/10.1002/9780470316696.fmatter/pdf. 1987. John Wiley and Sons.

Permissions

List of Contributors

Henrik Halvor Springborg and Olav Istre
Department of Minimal Invasive Gynaecology, Aleris Hamlet Hospital, Gyngemose Parkvej 66, 2860 Soeborg, Copenhagen, Denmark

Pietro Gambadauro
Karolinska Institutet, LIME/NASP-C7, 17177 Stockholm, Sweden
Res Medica Sweden, Uppsala, Sweden

Vladimir Carli
Karolinska Institutet, LIME/NASP-C7, 17177 Stockholm, Sweden
WHO Collaborating Centre for Research, Training and Methods Development, and National Centre for Suicide Research and Prevention of Mental Ill-Health, Karolinska Institutet, Stockholm, Sweden

Ramesan Navaratnarajah
St. Bartholomew's and the Royal London Hospital, Bart's Health NHS Trust, Queen Mary University of London, London, UK

Anneleen Reynders and Jan Baekelandt
Department of Obstetrics and Gynaecology, Imelda Hospital, Imeldalaan 9, 2820 Bonheiden, Belgium

Per Istre
Department of Gynecology/Obstetrics, Hvidovre University Hospital, Kettegård Allé 30, 2650 Hvidovre, Denmark

Lars Franch Andersen
Department of Gynecology/Obstetrics, Nordsjællands Hospital Hillerød, Dyrehavevej 29, 3400 Hillerød, Denmark

Henrik Halvor Springborg
Department of Gynecology, Aleris-Hamlet Private Hospital, Gyngemose Parkvej 66, 2860 Søborg, Denmark

Abimbola O. Famuyide
Department of Obstetrics and Gynecology, Mayo Clinic, Rochester, MN, USA

Sherif A. El-Nashar and Sherif A. M. Shazly
Department of Obstetrics and Gynecology, Mayo Clinic, Rochester, MN, USA
Department of Obstetrics and Gynecology, Assiut University, Assiut, Egypt

J. L. Herraiz Roda, J. A. Llueca Abella, C. Catalá Masó, Y. Maazouzi, M. Colecha Morales, A. Serra Rubert, D. Piquer Simó, C. Oliva Martí and E. Calpe Gómez
Department of Obstetrics and Gynecology, General University Hospital of Castellón, Avenida Benicassim, 12004 Castellas, Spain

C. Celle, C. Pomés, G. Durruty, M. Zamboni and M. Cuello
Division of Obstetrics and Gynecology, UC-Christus Health Network, Pontificia Universidad Católica de Chile, Lira 85, 5th floor, Santiago 8330074, Chile

Hosam Abdel-Fattah, Nasser El-Lakkany, Adel Saad Helal, Alaa Mosbah, El-Said Abdel-Hady and Mahmoud Abdel-Shaheed
Department of Obstetrics and Gynecology, Mansoura University, Mansoura, Egypt
Department of Diagnostic Radiology, Mansoura University, Mansoura, Egypt

Carlo De Cicco
Department of Obstetrics and Gynaecology, University Hospital Gasthuisberg, Katholieke Universiteit Leuven, Leuven, Belgium
Department of Gynecology, Campus Bio-Medico University, Rome, Italy

Ron Schonman
Department of Obstetrics and Gynecology, University Hospital Gasthuisberg, Katholieke Universiteit Leuven, Leuven, Belgium
Department of Obstetrics and Gynecology, Tel Aviv University, Tel Aviv, Israel

Philippe R. Koninckx
Department of Obstetrics and Gynecology, University Hospital Gasthuisberg, Katholieke Universiteit Leuven, Leuven, Belgium
Gruppo Italo Belga, Villa del Rosario, Rome, Italy
Vuilenbos 2, 3360 Bierbeek, Belgium

Anastasia Ussia
Gruppo Italo Belga, Villa del Rosario, Rome, Italy

Verguts Jasper
Department of Obstetrics and Gynecology, Jessa Hospital, Stadsomvaart 11, 3500 Hasselt, Belgium
UZ Leuven, Herestraat 49, 3000 Leuven, Belgium

Bosteels Jan
Department of Obstetrics and Gynecology, Imelda Hospital, Bonheiden, Belgium

Corona Roberta
Unit of Reproductive Medicine, Department of Obstetrics and Gynecology, University Hospital Brussels, Brussels, Belgium

Hamerlynck Tjalina and Weyers Steven
Department of Obstetrics and Gynaecology, Ghent University Hospital, Gent, Belgium

Mestdagh Greet
Department of Obstetrics and Gynecology, ZOL, Genk, Belgium

Nisolle Michelle
Department of Obstetrics and Gynecology, University of Liège, Liège, Belgium

Puttemans Patrick
Unit of Reproductive Medicine, Leuven Institute for Fertility and Embryology, Heilig Hart Hospital, Leuven, Belgium

Squifflet Jean-Luc
Department of Obstetrics and Gynecology, Catholique de Louvain, Woluwe-Saint-Lambert, Belgium

Van Herendael Bruno
Department of Obstetrics and Gynecology, ZNA Stuivenberg, Antwerp, Belgium

I. Muller
Faculty of Medical Sciences, University of Groningen, Groningen, The Netherlands

J. van der Palen
Faculty of Behavioral Sciences, University of Twente, Enschede, The Netherlands

D. Massop-Helmink
Department of Obstetrics and Gynaecology, Medisch Spectrum Twente hospital, Enschede, The Netherlands

R. Vos-de Bruin and J. M. Sikkema
Department of Obstetrics and Gynaecology, Ziekenhuisgroep Twente hospital, Zilvermeeuw 1, 7609 PP Almelo/ Hengelo, The Netherlands

Vasileios Minas, Antonios Anagnostopoulos and Nahid Gul
Minimal Access Centre, Department of Obstetrics and Gynaecology, Wirral University Teaching Hospital, Upton, UK

Debjani Mukhopadhyay
The Department of Gynaecology and Obstetrics, Ipswich Hospital NHS Trust, Heath Road, Ipswich, Suffolk IP4 5PD, UK

Thomas E. J. Ind
The Department of Gynaecological Oncology, St. George's Hospital NHS Trust, Blackshaw Road, London SW17 0QT, UK
The Department of Gynaecological Oncology, The Royal Marsden Hospital, Fulham Road, London SW3 6JJ, UK

Nicole M. Donnellan, Suketu Mansuria and Ted Lee
Obstetrics, Gynecology and Reproductive Sciences, University of Pittsburgh, Magee-Womens Hospital of UPMC, 300 Halket Street, Pittsburgh, PA 15213, USA

Nancy Aguwa
School of Medicine, University of Texas Health Science Center at San Antonio, 7703 Floyd Curl Drive, San Antonio, TX 78229, USA

Deirdre Lum
Obstetrics and Gynecology, Stanford University, 900 Blake Wilbur Drive, Palo Alto, CA 94304, USA

Leslie Meyn
Obstetrics, Gynecology and Reproductive Sciences, Magee-Womens Research Institute, 204 Craft Ave, Pittsburgh, PA 15213, USA

Elizabeth A. Pritts and David L. Olive
Wisconsin Fertility Institute, Middleton, WI, USA

David J. Vanness
University of Wisconsin School of Medicine and Public Health, Madison, WI, USA

Jonathan S. Berek
Stanford University School of Medicine, Stanford, CA, USA

William Parker
University of California, Los Angeles, Los Angeles, CA, USA

Ronald Feinberg and Jacqueline Feinberg
Reproductive Associates of Delaware, Newark, DE, USA

Masayuki Endo, Iva Urbankova, Jaromir Vlacil, Andrew Feola and Jan Deprest
Centre for Surgical Technologies, Faculty of Medicine, KU Leuven, Herestraat 49, 3000 Leuven, Belgium

Masayuki Endo, Iva Urbankova, Jaromir Vlacil, Siddarth Sengupta, Thomas Deprest, Andrew Feola and Jan Deprest
Department of Development and Regeneration, Organ Systems Cluster, Faculty of Medicine, KU Leuven, Herestraat 49, 3000 Leuven, Belgium

Masayuki Endo and Jan Deprest
Pelvic Floor Unit, University Hospitals KU Leuven, Leuven, Belgium

Iva Urbankova and Jaromir Vlacil
Institute for Care of Mother and Child, Prague, Czech Republic

Bernd Klosterhalfen
Institute for Pathology, Düren Hospital, Düren, Germany

Anneleen Reynders and Jan Baekelandt
Department of Obstetrics and Gynaecology, Imelda Hospital Bonheiden, Imeldalaan 9, 2820 Bonheiden, Belgium

Zainab Kazmi
University of Manchester School of Medicine, Stopford Building, Oxford Road, Manchester M13 9PT, UK
Women's Health Directorate, Royal Preston Hospital, Sharoe Green Lane North, Preston, Lancashire PR2 9HT, UK

Sujata Gupta
Women's Health Directorate, Royal Preston Hospital, Sharoe Green Lane North, Preston, Lancashire PR2 9HT, UK

Michael Dobson
Department of Radiology, Royal Preston Hospital, Sharoe Green Lane North, Preston, Lancashire PR2 9HT, UK

Grace W. Yeung, Angelos G. Vilos and Hanin Abduljabar
Division of Reproductive Endocrinology and Infertility, Department of Obstetrics and Gynecology, Western University, London, Ontario, Canada
King Abdul Aziz University, Jeddah, Saudi Arabia

Ayman Oraif
Division of Reproductive Endocrinology and Infertility, Department of Obstetrics and Gynecology, Western University, London, Ontario, Canada
King Abdul Aziz University, Jeddah, Saudi Arabia

George A. Vilos
Division of Reproductive Endocrinology and Infertility, Department of Obstetrics and Gynecology, Western University, London, Ontario, Canada

The Fertility Clinic, Room E-3620A, London Health Science Centre, 800 Commissioners Road East, London, ON N6A 4G5, Canada

Basim Abu-Rafea
Dalhousie University, Halifax, Nova Scotia, Canada

P .G Paul, Dimple K. Ahluwalia, Dhivya Narasimhan, Gaurav Chopade, Saurabh Patil, Varsha Rengaraj and Tanuka Das
Centre for Advanced Endoscopy and Infertility, Paul's Hospital, Vattekkattu Road, Kaloor, Kochi, Kerala 682 017, India

Hans Brölmann
Vrije Universiteit Medisch Centrum, Amsterdam, Netherlands

Marlies Bongers
Máxima Medisch Centrum, Veldhoven, Netherlands

José Gerardo Garza-Leal
Universidad Autónoma de Nuevo León, Monterrey, Nuevo Leon, Mexico

Janesh Gupta
Birmingham Women's Hospital, Birmingham, UK

Sebastiaan Veersema
Sint Antonius Ziekenhuis, Nieuwegein, Netherlands

Rik Quartero
Medisch Spectrum Twente, Enschede, Netherlands

David Toub
Gynesonics, Inc., Redwood City, CA 94063, USA
Albert Einstein Medical Center, 5501 Old York Road, Philadelphia, PA 19141, USA

S. Knaepen
Department of Obstetrics and Gynecology, General Hospital Hasselt, Hasselt, Belgium
Rummenweg 57, 3800 Sint-Truiden, Belgium

S. Van Calenbergh
Department of Obstetrics and Gynecology, General Hospital Turnhout, Turnhout, Belgium

J. Mairos and P. Di Martino
Department of Gynecology and Obstetrics, Hospital das Forças Armadas - Pólo de Lisboa, Azinhaga dos Ulmeiros, 1649-020 Lisbon, Portugal

Antoni Llueca, Jose Luis Herraiz, Miguel Rodrigo, Yasmin Mazzouzi, Dolores Piquer, Miriam Guijarro, Arhoa Cañete and Javier Escrig
Multidisciplinary Unit of Abdominal Pelvic Oncology Surgery (MUAPOS), University General Hospital of Castellon, Av Benicasim s/n, 12004 Castellón, Spain

Department of Medicine, University Jaume I, Castellón de la Plana, Spain

L. van den Haak, M. D. Blikkendaal, A. C. M. Luteijn and S. R. C. Driessen
Department of Gynecology, Leiden University Medical Center, 2300 RC Leiden, The Netherlands

F. W. Jansen
Department of Gynecology, Leiden University Medical Center, 2300 RC Leiden, The Netherlands Department BioMechanical Engineering, Delft University of Technology, 2628 CD Delft, The Netherlands

J. P. T. Rhemrev
Department of Obstetrics and Gynecology, Bronovo Hospital The Hague, The Hague, The Netherlands

J. J. van den Dobbelsteen
Department BioMechanical Engineering, Delft University of Technology, 2628 CD Delft, The Netherlands

Attilio Di Spiezio Sardo, Sotirios H. Saravelos, Stephan Gordts, Caterina Exacoustos, Dominique Van Schoubroeck, Carmina Bermejo, Nazar N. Amso, Geeta Nargund, Dirk Timmermann, Apostolos Athanasiadis, Sara Brucker, Carlo De Angelis, Marco Gergolet, Tin Chiu Li, Vasilios Tanos, Basil Tarlatzis, Roy Farquharson, Luca Gianaroli and Rudi Campo
Congenital Uterine Malformations (CONUTA) Common ESHRE/ ESGE Working Group and Invited Experts, Leuven, Belgium

Grigoris F. Grimbizis
Congenital Uterine Malformations (CONUTA) Common ESHRE/ ESGE Working Group and Invited Experts, Leuven, Belgium
1st Department ofObstetrics and Gynecology, Aristotle University of Thessaloniki, Tsimiski 51 Street, 54623 Thessaloniki, Greece

Silvia Baggio, Paola Pomini, Alessandro Zecchin, Simone Garzon, Cecilia Bonin, Anna Festi and Massimo Piergiuseppe Franchi
Department of Obstetrics and Gynaecology, University of Verona, Piazzale L.A. Scuro 10, 37134 Verona, Italy

Lorenza Santi
Department of Endocrinology, University of Verona, Piazzale L.A. Scuro 10, 37134 Verona, Italy

Geertje Callewaert, Ben Van and Jan Deprest
Department of Development and Regeneration, Cluster Organ Systems, Faculty of Medicine, Group Biomedical Sciences, KU Leuven, 3000 Leuven, Belgium

Department of Obstetrics and Gynaecology, University Hospitals Leuven, 3000 Leuven, Belgium

Cleynenbreugel, Frank Van der Aa and Dirk De Ridder
Department of Development and Regeneration, Cluster Organ Systems, Faculty of Medicine, Group Biomedical Sciences, KU Leuven, 3000 Leuven, Belgium
Department of Urology, University Hospitals Leuven, Leuven, Belgium

Susanne Housmans
Department of Obstetrics and Gynaecology, University Hospitals Leuven, 3000 Leuven, Belgium

Jasper Verguts
Department of Obstetrics and Gynaecology, University Hospitals Leuven, 3000 Leuven, Belgium
Department of Obstetrics and Gynaecology, Jessa Hospital, 3500 Hasselt, Belgium

Ignace Vergote
Department of Obstetrics and Gynaecology, University Hospitals Leuven, 3000 Leuven, Belgium
Department of Gynaecologic Oncology, Leuven Cancer Institute, University Hospitals Leuven, KU Leuven, 3000 Leuven, Belgium

Jan Bosteels
Belgian Center for Evidence Based Medicine (CEBAM), Belgian Branch of the Cochrane Collaboration, 3000 Leuven, Belgium

Mohammed Rizk
Obstetrics and Gynecology Department, Ain Shams University, Cairo, Egypt

Haitham Salem
Surgery Department, Cairo University, Cairo, Egypt

Van Peer Sarah and Baekelandt Jan
Department of Obstetrics and Gynaecology, Imelda Hospital Bonheiden, Bonheiden, Belgium

Nataša Kenda Šuster
Department of Obsterics and Gynecology, University of Ljubljana, Šlajmerjeva 3, 1000 Ljubljana, Slovenia

Marco Gergolet
Casa di Cura Sanatorio Triestino, Via Rossetti 62, 34141 Trieste, Italy

Karin Abbink and Dick C. Schoot
Department of Obstetrics and Gynaecology, Catharina Hospital Eindhoven, Michelangelolaan 2, 5623 Eindhoven, The Netherlands

Sameer Sendy
Women's Specialized Hospital, King Fahad Medical City Riyadh, Riyadh, Kingdom of Saudi Arabia

Tawfig H. Gaafar
Maternity Hospital, IVF unit, Sulaiman al Habib Medical Complex, Riyadh, Kingdom of Saudi Arabia

Cheryl T Fitzgerald
Department of Reproductive Medicine, St Mary's Hospital, Manchester Academic Health Science Centre (MAHSC), Central Manchester University Hospital NHS Foundation Trust, Manchester M13 0JH, UK

Oybek Rustamov
Department of Reproductive Medicine, St Mary's Hospital, Manchester Academic Health Science Centre (MAHSC), Central Manchester University Hospital NHS Foundation Trust, Manchester M13 0JH, UK
Present address: Aberdeen Maternity Hospital, University of Aberdeen, Aberdeen AB25 2ZN, UK

Monica Krishnan
Present address: Sheffield Teaching Hospitals, Royal Hallamshire Hospital, Sheffield S10 2JF, UK
Manchester Royal Infirmary, Central Manchester University Hospitals NHS Foundation Trust, Manchester M13 9WL, UK

Stephen A Roberts
Centre for Biostatistics, Institute of Population Health, Manchester Academic Health Science Centre (MAHSC), University of Manchester, Manchester M13 9PL, UK

Carlos Roger Molinas
Neolife Medicina y Cirugía Reproductiva, Avenida Brasilia 760, 1434 Asunción, Paraguay
European Academy of Gynaecological Surgery, Leuven, Belgium

Rudi Campo
European Academy of Gynaecological Surgery, Leuven, Belgium

Arnaud Wattiez
Life Expert Centre, Schipvaartstraat 2 Bus 4, 3000 Leuven, Belgium
European Academy for Gynaecological Surgery, Diestsevest 43/ 0001, 3000 Leuven, Belgium
European Society for Gynaecological Endoscopy, Diestsevest 43/ 0001, 3000 Leuven, Belgium

Rudi Campo
Life Expert Centre, Schipvaartstraat 2 Bus 4, 3000 Leuven, Belgium
European Academy for Gynaecological Surgery, Diestsevest 43/ 0001, 3000 Leuven, Belgium

European Society for Gynaecological Endoscopy, Diestsevest 43/ 0001, 3000 Leuven, Belgium
European Board and College of Obstetrics and Gynaecology, Brussels, Belgium

Marco Puga, Yves Van Belle and Roger Molinas
European Academy for Gynaecological Surgery, Diestsevest 43/ 0001, 3000 Leuven, Belgium

Vasilis Tanos and Peter O'Donovan
European Academy for Gynaecological Surgery, Diestsevest 43/ 0001, 3000 Leuven, Belgium
European Society for Gynaecological Endoscopy, Diestsevest 43/ 0001, 3000 Leuven, Belgium

Diethelm Wallwiener
European Academy for Gynaecological Surgery, Diestsevest 43/ 0001, 3000 Leuven, Belgium
Department of Women's Health, University Hospital Tuebingen, Calwerstraat 7, 72077 Tuebingen, Germany

Ann Lissens
European Academy for Gynaecological Surgery, Diestsevest 43/ 0001, 3000 Leuven, Belgium
Center for Surgical Technologies, Leuven, Belgium
University Hospitals Leuven, Leuven, Belgium

Attilio Di Spiezio Sardo and Grigoris Grimbizis
European Society for Gynaecological Endoscopy, Diestsevest 43/ 0001, 3000 Leuven, Belgium

Sara Brucker
European Society for Gynaecological Endoscopy, Diestsevest 43/ 0001, 3000 Leuven, Belgium
Department of Women's Health, University Hospital Tuebingen, Calwerstraat 7, 72077 Tuebingen, Germany

Jan Deprest
European Society for Gynaecological Endoscopy, Diestsevest 43/ 0001, 3000 Leuven, Belgium
Center for Surgical Technologies, Leuven, Belgium

Rudy Leon De Wilde
European Society for Gynaecological Endoscopy, Diestsevest 43/ 0001, 3000 Leuven, Belgium
Pius-Hospital Oldenburg, Department of Gynecology, Obstetrics and Gynaecological Oncology, Carlvon Ossietzky University, Georgstraße 12, 26121 Oldenburg, Germany

Mahmood Tahir and Chiara Benedetto
European Board and College of Obstetrics and Gynaecology, Brussels, Belgium

Anja Herrmann
Pius-Hospital Oldenburg, Department of Gynecology, Obstetrics and Gynaecological Oncology, Carlvon Ossietzky University, Georgstraße 12, 26121 Oldenburg, Germany

Igno Siebert
African Endoscopic Training Academy, Cape Town, South Africa

Benoit Rabischong
International Centre for Endoscopic Surgery, Clermont-Ferrand, France

Liisu Saavalainen, Oskari Heikinheimo, Aila Tiitinen and Päivi Härkki
Department of Obstetrics and Gynecology, University of Helsinki and Helsinki University Hospital, Sofianlehdonkatu 5, FI-00029 HUS Helsinki, Finland

Chantal C. J. Alleblas andTheodoor E. Nieboer
Department of Obstetrics and Gynecology, Radboud University Medical Center, 6500HB Nijmegen, The Netherlands

Michel P. H. Vleugels
Department of Obstetrics and Gynecology, Riverland Hospital, Tiel, The Netherlands

Natalie A. M. Cooper
Women's Health Research Unit, Queen Mary University of London, London E1 2AT, UK

Lee Middleton and Jane Daniels
Birmingham Clinical Trials Unit, University of Birmingham, Birmingham B15 2TT, UK

Paul Smith
Birmingham Women's NHS Foundation Trust, Birmingham B15 2TG, UK
School of Clinical and Experimental Medicine, University of Birmingham, Birmingham B15 2TT, UK

T. Justin Clark
Birmingham Women's NHS Foundation Trust, Birmingham B15 2TG, UK
OPT Trial Office, Birmingham Clinical Trials Unit, College of Medical and Dental Sciences, Robert Aitken Institute for Clinical Research, University of Birmingham, Edgbaston, Birmingham B15 2TT, UK

Elaine Denny
Centre for Health and Social Care Research, Birmingham City University, Birmingham B15 3TN, UK

Lynda Stobert
School of Allied and Public Health Professions, Birmingham City University, Birmingham B15 3TN, UK

Index